# Handbook of
# Aging and the Social Sciences

## Sixth Edition

Editors
### Robert H. Binstock and Linda K. George

Associate Editors
Stephen J. Cutler, Jon Hendricks, and James H. Schulz

AMSTERDAM • BOSTON • HEIDELBERG • LONDON • NEW YORK • OXFORD
PARIS • SAN DIEGO • SAN FRANCISCO • SINGAPORE • SYDNEY • TOKYO
Academic Press is an imprint of Elsevier

Academic Press is an imprint of Elsevier
30 Corporate Drive, Suite 400, Burlington, MA 01803, USA
525 B Street, Suite 1900, San Diego, California 92101-4495, USA
84 Theobald's Road, London WC1X 8RR, UK

This book is printed on acid-free paper. ⊚

**Library of Congress Cataloging-in-Publication Data**

Handbook of aging and the social sciences / editors Robert H. Binstock and Linda K. George ; associate editors Stephen J. Cutler, Jon Hendricks, and James H. Schulz.– 6th ed.
    p. cm.
  Includes bibliographical references and index.
  ISBN 0-12-088388-0 (alk. paper)
 1. Gerontology. 2. Aging–Social aspects. 3. Life change events in old age. 4. Older people–Care.
I. Title: Aging and the social sciences. II. Binstock, Robert H. III. George, Linda K. IV. Cutler, Stephen J. V. Hendricks, Jon. VI. Schulz, James H.
  HQ1061.H336 2006
  305.26–dc22

                                         2005029192

**British Library Cataloguing-in-Publication Data**
A catalogue record for this book is available from the British Library.

ISBN 13: 978-0-12-088388-2
ISBN 10: 0-12-088388-0

For information on all Elsevier Academic Press publications
visit our Web site at www.books.elsevier.com

Printed in the United States of America
05  06  07  08  09  10  9  8  7  6  5  4  3  2  1

To my cousin, Senator Russ Feingold (D., WI), with the hope that he can
preserve Social Security and Medicare.
—R.H.B.

To my mother, Doretta A. Kaufman, and in memory of my father, Amos D. Kaufman,
with love and gratitude.
—L.K.G.

# Contents

## Part One
## Aging and Time

# Part Two
## Aging and Social Structure

## Part Three
## Social Factors and Social Institutions

## Part Four
## Aging and Society

## 25. Aging and Justice
*Martin Kohli*

# Contributors

Numbers in parentheses indicate the pages on which the authors' chapters begin.

**Duane F. Alwin** (20), Population Research Institute, Pennsylvania State University, University Park, PA 16801

**Jacqueline L. Angel** (94), Lyndon B. Johnson School of Public Affairs, University of Texas, Austin, TX 78713-8925

**Ronald J. Angel** (94), Department of Sociology, University of Texas, Austin, TX 78712

**Robert H. Binstock** (436), School of Medicine, Case Western Reserve University, Cleveland, OH 44106-4945

**Allan Borowski** (360), School of Social Work and Social Policy, La Trobe University, Bundoora (Melbourne), Victoria, Australia 3086

**Don E. Bradley** (76), Department of Sociology, East Carolina University, Greenville, NC 27858-4353

**Stephen J. Cutler** (257), Department of Sociology, University of Vermont, Burlington, VT 05405

**Kenneth F. Ferraro** (238), Department of Sociology, Purdue University, West Lafayette, IN 47907-2059

**Jennifer R. Fishman** (436), Department of Bioethics, Case Western Reserve University, Cleveland, OH 44106

**Linda K. George** (320), Center for the Study of Aging and Human Development, Duke University, Durham, NC 27710

**Carole Haber** (59), Department of History, University of Delaware, Newark, DE 19716

**Melissa Hardy** (201), Gerontology Center, Pennsylvania State University, State College, PA 16801

**Laurie Russell Hatch** (301), Department of Sociology, University of Kentucky, Lexington, KY 40506-0027

**Charles Hatcher** (219), Department of Consumer Science, University of Wisconsin–Madison, Madison, WI 53705

**Jon Hendricks** (301), University Honors College, Oregon State University, Corvallis, OR 97331-2221

**Scott M. Hofer** (20), Department of Human Development and Family Studies, Pennsylvania State University, University Park, PA 16802

**Karen Holden** (219), LaFollette Institute of Public Affairs, University of Wisconsin–Madison, Madison, WI 53706

**Ellen Idler** (277), Institute for Health, Health Care Policy, and Aging Research, Rutgers University, New Brunswick, NJ 08903

**Thomas E. Johnson** (436), Institute for Behavioral Genetics, University of Colorado, Boulder, CO 80303

**Marshall B. Kapp** (419), School of Law, Southern Illinois University, Carbondale, IL 62901-6804

**Martin Kohli** (456), Department of Political and Social Sciences, European University Institute, 50016 San Domenico di Fiesole, Italy

**Neal Krause** (181), School of Public Health, University of Michigan, Ann Arbor, MI 48109-2029

**Kenneth C. Land** (41), Department of Sociology, Duke University, Durham, NC 27708

**Nan Lin** (111), Department of Sociology, Duke University, Durham, NC 27708

**Charles F. Longino, Jr.** (76), Reynolds Gerontology Program, Wake Forest University, Winston-Salem, NC 27109

**Ryan J. McCammon** (20), Survey Research Center, University of Michigan, Ann Arbor, MI 48106-1248

**Phyllis Moen** (127), Department of Sociology, University of Minnesota, Minneapolis, MN 55455

**Marilyn Moon** (380), American Institutes for Research, Silver Spring, MD 20901

**Jennifer L. Moren-Cross** (111), Department of Sociology, Duke University, Durham, NC 27708

**Angela M. O'Rand** (145), Department of Sociology, Duke University, Durham, NC 27708

**James H. Schulz** (360), 557 State Street, Portsmouth, NH 03801

**Richard A. Settersten, Jr.** (3), Department of Sociology, Case Western Reserve University, Cleveland, OH 44106-7124,

**Merril Silverstein** (165), Andrus Gerontology Center, University of Southern California, Los Angeles, CA 90089

**Donna Spencer** (127), Department of Sociology, University of Minnesota, Minneapolis, MN 55455

**Robyn I. Stone** (397), Institute for the Future of Aging Services, American Association of Homes and Services for the Aging, Washington, DC 20009

**Alan Walker** (339), Department of Sociological Studies, University of Sheffield, Sheffield S102TU, United Kingdom

**Yang Yang** (41) Department of Sociology and Center for Demographic Studies, Duke University, Durham, NC 27708-0088

# Foreword

This volume is one of a series of three handbooks of aging: *Handbook of the Biology of Aging, Handbook of the Psychology of Aging,* and *Handbook of Aging and the Social Sciences. The Handbooks of Aging* series, now in its sixth edition, reflects the exponential growth of research and publications in aging research, as well as the growing interest in the subject of aging. Stimulation of research on aging by government and private foundation sponsorship has been a major contributor to the growth of publications. There has also been an increase in the number of university and college courses related to aging. *The Handbooks of Aging* have helped to organize courses and seminars on aging by providing knowledge bases for instruction and for new steps in research.

*The Handbooks* are used by academic researchers, graduate students, and professionals, for access and interpretation of contemporary research literature about aging. They serve both as a reference and as an organizational tool for integrating a wide body of research that is often cross disciplinary. *The Handbooks* not only provide updates about what is known about the many processes of aging, but also offer interpretations of findings by well-informed and experienced scholars in many disciplines. Aging is a complex process of change involving influences of a biological, behavioral, social, and environmental nature.

Understanding aging is one of the major challenges facing science in the 21st century. Interest in research on aging has become a major focus in science and in the many professions that serve aging populations. Growth of interest in research findings about aging and their interpretation has been accelerated with the growth of populations of older persons in developed and developing countries. As more understanding has been gained about genetic factors that contribute to individual prospects for length of life and life-limiting and disabling diseases, researchers have simultaneously become more aware of the environmental factors that modulate the expression of genetic predispositions. These *Handbooks* both reflect and encourage an ecological view of aging, in which aging is seen as a result of diverse forces interacting. These *Handbooks* can help to provide information to guide planning as nations face "age quakes" due to shifts in the size of their populations of young and older persons.

In addition to the rise in research publications about aging, there has been a dramatic change in the availability of scientific literature since the first editions of *The Handbooks of Aging* were published. There are now millions of references available on line. This increases the need for integration of information. *The Handbooks* help to encourage integration of information from across disciplines and methods of gathering data about aging.

With so much new information available, one of the editorial policies has been the selection of new chapter authors and subject matter in each successive edition. This allows *The Handbooks* to present new points of view, to keep current, and to explore new topics in which new research has emerged. The sixth edition is thus virtually wholly new, and is not simply an update of previous editions.

I want to thank the editors of the individual volumes for their cooperation, efforts, and wisdom in planning and reviewing the chapters. Without their intense efforts and experience *The Handbooks* would not be possible. I thank Edward J. Masoro and Steven N. Austad, editors of the *Handbook of the Biology of Aging*; the editors of the *Handbook of Aging and the Social Sciences*, Robert H. Binstock and Linda K. George, and their associate editors, Stephen J. Cutler, Jon Hendricks, and James H. Schulz; and my co-editor of the *Handbook of the Psychology of Aging*, K. Warner Schaie, and the associate editors, Ronald P. Abeles, Margaret Gatz, and Timothy A. Salthouse.

I also want to express my appreciation to Nikki Levy, Publisher at Elsevier, whose experience, long-term interest, and cooperation have facilitated the publication of *The Handbooks* through their many editions.

James E. Birren

# Preface

This sixth edition of the *Handbook of Aging and the Social Sciences* provides extensive reviews and critical evaluations of research on the social aspects of aging. It also makes available major references and identifies high-priority topics for future research.

To achieve these purposes, the *Handbook* presents knowledge about aging through the systematic perspectives of a variety of disciplines and professions: anthropology, bioethics, biology, demography, economics, epidemiology, history, law, medicine, political science, policy analysis, public administration, social psychology, social work, and sociology. Building on five previous editions (1976, 1985, 1990, 1996, and 2001), this edition reflects the tremendous growth of ideas, information, and research literature on the social aspects of aging that has taken place during the last five years.

The *Handbook* is intended for use by researchers, professional practitioners, and students in the field of aging. It is also expected to serve as a basic reference tool for scholars, professionals, and others who are not presently engaged in research and practice directly focused on aging and the aged.

When the first edition of this *Handbook* was being prepared by Bob Binstock and Ethel Shanas in the early 1970s, only a small number of social scientists were equipped to address any specific topic in a first-rate fashion. More than a quarter of a century later, the field has burgeoned in such quality and quantity that a great many scholars would be outstanding contributors for each of the various subjects chosen for this volume.

Accordingly, this sixth edition was planned and implemented so as to enlist predominantly new contributors from among the rich variety of distinguished scholars and path-breaking perspectives now constituting the field. Of the 37 authors and coauthors in this edition, 24 are contributing to the *Handbook* for the first time. One author has contributed to all 6 editions; one is contributing for the fifth time; 3 are contributing for the fourth time; 4 are contributing for the third time; and 4 are contributing for a second time.

In several respects the contents of this sixth edition are also substantially different from those of its predecessors. Seventeen chapters are on subjects that were not in the fifth edition. Seven topics that were maintained from the previous edition have been addressed by different authors who bring their own perspectives to bear on the subject matter. The other chapter has been substantially revised and brought up to date by its author.

The 17 chapters in this volume that address new topics include the following: "Aging and the Life Course"; "Modeling the Effects of Time: Integrating Demographic and Developmental Perspectives"; "Morbidity, Disability, and Mortality; Internal and International Migration"; "Social Networks and Health"; "Converging Divergences in Age, Gender, Health, and Well-Being: Strategic Selection in the Third Age"; "Intergenerational Family Transfers in Social Context"; "Social Relationships in Late Life"; "Health and Aging"; "Technological Change and Aging"; "Religion and Aging"; "Lifestyle and Aging"; "Perceived Quality of Life"; "Economic Security in Retirement: Reshaping the Public-Private Pension Mix"; "Aging and the Law"; "Anti-Aging Medicine and Science: Social Implications"; and "Aging and Justice."

The continuing topics dealt with by new authors have been treated from rather different viewpoints than in previous editions. The chapter on aging and politics, for example, emphasizes an international perspective, including attention to multinational organizations such as the World Bank and the European Community, in contrast to previous chapters that focused primarily on the United States. Another example is the chapter on diversity and aging, which pays far more attention to issues related to immigration than previous *Handbook* treatments of this subject area.

As implied by this design, to have continuing topics addressed from new but complementary perspectives, the editors and associate editors regard the earlier editions of the *Handbook* as part of the active literature in the field. The chapters in them remain important reference sources for topics and perspectives not

represented in this sixth edition. Indeed, because of the ongoing life of those earlier chapters, it was feasible to introduce new dimensions within the limited space available in the present volume. Some of the present chapter authors, in fact, build explicitly and actively on the work of their predecessors in the earlier editions. By the same token, it seemed reasonable not to allocate space in this volume to updating certain subjects that were treated in excellent chapters published in the fifth edition only five years ago.

The 25 chapters of this sixth edition are organized in four sections: Part I, Aging and Time; Part II, Aging and Social Structure; Part III, Social Factors and Social Institutions; and Part IV, Aging and Society. Each chapter was conceived and written specifically for this volume. The book includes a thorough subject matter index and a comprehensive bibliography on the social aspects of aging. The research literature cited and referenced in each chapter is also indexed by author at the end of the volume.

The contributors to this sixth edition successfully met a number of challenges. They organized their chapters in terms of analytical constructs that enabled them to sift through a great deal of literature bearing on their topics. They provided historical perspectives on these subjects, drawing on classic and contemporary references in the field, and constructed their presentations so as to ensure that the usefulness of the volume would not be limited by specific time referents. Most impressively, they were able to present their knowledge and viewpoints succinctly and to relate their treatments to those of their fellow authors.

In developing the subject matter for this volume and in the selection of contributors, the editors were assisted by three associate editors: Stephen J. Cutler, Jon Hendricks, and James H. Schulz. They also helped the editors substantially in the process of editorial review in which critical comments and suggestions were forwarded to the authors for their consideration in undertaking revised drafts. In addition, Megan M. Johnson assisted us in reviewing the formatting and accuracy of citations and references.

Steve Cutler and Joe Hendricks joined our editorial team for the first time in this edition and were tremendous assets. Jim Schulz has been an associate editor for five editions of the *Handbook* and has authored five different chapters starting with the first edition; we take this opportunity to express our great appreciation and admiration for his outstanding contributions over a 30-year journey with the *Handbook*.

The success of this volume is due primarily to the seriousness with which the chapter authors accepted their assignments and to the good will with which they responded to editorial criticism and suggestions. To these colleagues, the editors and associate editors would like to express their special appreciation.

Finally, we report sadly that Ethel Shanas, co-editor of the first and second editions of the *Handbook*, died not long ago. Ethel was a pioneering leader in social scientific studies of aging. During the height of her professional career, she was internationally recognized as a giant in the field of scholarship on the social aspects of aging. A former president of the Gerontological Society of America, she was a superb colleague and excellent editor. Her retirement in the 1980s was a great loss to the field of gerontology.

Robert H. Binstock
Linda K. George

# About the Editors

## Robert H. Binstock

is Professor of Aging, Health, and Society at Case Western Reserve University. A former president and fellow of the Gerontological Society of America (1976), and Chair of the Gerontological Health Section of the American Public Health Association (1996–1997), he has served as director of a White House Task Force on Older Americans for President Lyndon B. Johnson, and as chairman and member of a number of advisory panels to the United States government, state and local governments, and foundations. Professor Binstock is the author of more than 250 articles and book chapters, most of them dealing with politics and policies related to aging. His 24 authored and co-edited books include *The Fountain of Youth: Cultural, Scientific, and Ethical Perspectives on a Biomedical Goal* (2004); *The Lost Art of Caring: A Challenge to Health Professionals, Families, Communities, and Societies* (2001); and six editions of the *Handbook of Aging and the Social Sciences*. Among the honors he has received for contributions to gerontology and the well-being of older persons are the Kent and Brookdale awards from the Gerontological Society of America; the Lifetime Achievement and Key awards from the Gerontological Health Section of the American Public Health Association; the American Society on Aging Award; and the Arthur S. Flemming Award from the National Association of State Units on Aging.

## Linda K. George

is Professor of Sociology at Duke University, where she also serves as Associate Director of the Duke University Center for the Study of Aging and Human Development. She is a fellow and past president of the Gerontological Society of America. She is former chair of the Aging and Life Course Section of the American Sociological Association. She is former editor of the *Journal of Gerontology, Social Sciences Section*. She currently serves on the editorial boards of the *Journal of Gerontology: Social Sciences* and the *Journal of Aging and Health*. Professor George is the author or editor of seven books and author of more than 200 journal articles and book chapters. She co-edited the third, fourth, and fifth editions of the *Handbook of Aging and the Social Sciences*. Her major research interests include social factors and illness, stress and coping, and the aging self. Among the honors Professor George has received are Phi Beta Kappa, the Duke University Trinity College Distinguished Teaching Award, the W. Fred Cottrell Award for Outstanding Achievement in the Field of Aging, the Mentorship Award from the Behavioral and Social Sciences Section of the Gerontological Society of America, the Kleemeier Award from the Gerontological Society of America, the Dean's Mentoring Award from Duke University, and the Matilda White Riley Award from the American Sociological Association.

## Stephen J. Cutler

is Professor of Sociology and the Bishop Robert F. Joyce Distinguished University Professor of Gerontology at the University of Vermont. He is a fellow and past president of the Gerontological Society of America, a past chair of GSA's Behavioral and Social Sciences Section, and a past chair of the Aging and Life Course Section of the American Sociological Association. Professor Cutler is also a fellow of the Association for Gerontology in Higher Education and has served as an elected and an appointed member of AGHE's Executive Committee. He is a former editor of the *Journal of Gerontology: Social Sciences* and is on the editorial boards of *Research on Aging*, the *Journal of Applied Gerontology*, the *International Journal of Aging and Human Development*, and the *American Journal of Alzheimer's Disease*. He received the Clark Tibbitts Award from the Association for Gerontology in Higher Education, has been designated as a University Scholar by the University of Vermont, was a Petersen Visiting Scholar at Oregon State University, and has taught and conducted research in Romania as a Senior Fulbright Scholar. His research and

publications have been in the areas of caregiving, transportation, household composition, social and political attitude change, voluntary association participation, social aspects of cognitive change, and ethics.

## Jon (Joe) Hendricks

is Dean, University Honors College, and Professor of Sociology at Oregon State University. He is a past president of the Association for Gerontology in Higher Education and has served as Behavioral and Social Sciences section chair of GSA and as chair of the Aging and the Life Course Section of the American Sociological Association. Hendricks is widely published in social gerontology and has edited two book series for Little, Brown and for Baywood. Hendricks assists editorial boards for *Journal of Gerontology: Social Sciences*; *The Gerontologist*; *Journal of Aging Studies*; *Ageing International*; *International Journal of Aging & Human Development* and is co-editor-in-chief, *Hallym International Journal of Aging*. He is a Fellow in GSA and AGHE and received the latter's 2004 Clark Tibbitts Award.

## James H. Schulz

is Professor Emeritus, Brandeis University. He is an economist (Ph.D., Yale, 1966) specializing in the economics of aging, pension and retirement policy, and international aging issues. A former president of the Gerontological Society of America, he received the Society's 1983 Kleemeier Award for outstanding research in aging; the 1998 Clark Tibbitts Award for contributions to the field of gerontology; and a 1999 Testimonial Award from the United Nations Secretary General for his international aging research and other activities related to the "International Year of Older Persons." His books include *Providing Adequate Retirement Income*;

*The World Ageing Situation, 1991; Economics of Population Aging; When Life-Time Employment Ends: Older Worker Programs in Japan;* and *Social Security in the Twenty-first Century.* His most recent research is on social security privatization issues and includes *Older Women and Private Pensions in the United Kingdom.* His best-known book is *The Economics of Aging* (which has been translated into Japanese and Chinese and is currently available in its 7th edition).

## Part One

# Aging and Time

# One

# Aging and the Life Course

Richard A. Settersten, Jr.

The maturation of the life-course perspective is one of the most significant social science developments of the last quarter century. This chapter builds a case for why gerontology needs the life-course perspective and how life-course principles, methods, and data will continue to change the face of research on aging. The first section outlines the potentials of life-course ideas for gerontology. As attention to the life course increases, however, gerontologists will need to clarify how old age is distinct from periods before it; the second section considers this issue. The third section briefly highlights some empirical evidence on connections between old age and earlier periods of life and some of the theoretical and methodological complexities of making such connections. As life-course studies grow, one begins to wonder whether age-based fields, including gerontology, will lose some of their significance or even disappear; the fourth section concludes with a few reflections on this provocative question. The chapter concludes with a few additional thoughts on how life-course ideas might be infused into gerontology to both broaden and deepen our view and knowledge base.

This chapter builds on the foundation laid in four chapters from earlier editions of this handbook. The first two chapters (Neugarten & Hagestad, 1976; Hagestad & Neugarten, 1985) focused on the social meanings and uses of age, and paid special attention to systems of age structuring, particularly age norms for life-course transitions (for a recent review of this topic, see Settersten, 2003a). The latter two chapters (Hagestad, 1990; Hagestad & Dannefer, 2001) focused on variability in transition patterns and the importance of social perspectives in countering trends toward "microfication" in gerontology. The current chapter, like the prior one, emphasizes the need to reclaim the *social* in "social gerontology." The task of more completely infusing life-course ideas into gerontology is central to that mission.

## I. Why Gerontology Needs the Life Course

It was not until the latter half of the twentieth century that the field of human development turned its attention more seriously to adulthood and aging,

*Handbook of Aging and the Social Sciences, Sixth Edition*

prompted in part by early longitudinal studies that demanded new theories and methods for understanding development in lifelong terms (Elder & Johnson, 2003; Settersten, 2003b). The principles and concepts related to children and adolescents, which had been the targets of inquiry through the first half of the twentieth century, could not simply be extended to adults. New and difficult questions were raised about continuity and change in adult lives over time, the social settings that structure movement through adulthood, and connections between lives, time, and place. These remain the most important challenges for understanding adult development and aging in the twenty-first century. The growing recognition of these challenges is reflected in recent surges in references to the "life span" and "life course," driven by advances in the respective disciplines of psychology and sociology (e.g., in psychology, see Baltes, Lindenberger, & Staudinger, 1998; in sociology, see Mortimer & Shanahan, 2003; for an integrated view, see Settersten, 2003b).

Understanding the life course is about describing individual and collective experiences and statuses over long stretches of time and explaining the short- and long-range causes and consequences of these patterns. It is also about addressing a range of social, historical, and cultural forces that determine the structure and content of life experiences and pathways. And just as the life-course perspective takes a dynamic view of individuals and groups, it takes a dynamic view of environments, probing when and how environments change and probing reciprocal connections between changing individuals and changing environments. For all of these reasons, there is a natural, mutual attraction between scholarship on the life course and scholarship on aging.

A central premise of this chapter is that greater attention to the life course will continue to transform and even revolutionize theories, questions, methods, and data in gerontology. These include the need to describe and explain:

- Aging along multiple dimensions (e.g., physical, cognitive, psychological) and in multiple social spheres (e.g., family, work, education, leisure).
- Aging in multiple directions (e.g., dynamics related to both decline *and* growth).
- Aging as a joint set of interdependent trajectories (e.g., interactions among dimensions and spheres over time).
- How experiences in old age are shaped by those in earlier periods. This includes examining connections both near and far away in time, as well as the processes and mechanisms that drive these connections. It also includes examining the timing, sequencing, spacing, density, and duration of experiences up to and through old age.
- How old age involves distinct and important developmental experiences relative to earlier periods.
- How aging-related experiences are shaped by specific characteristics of and processes in a wide range of interconnected, and even nested, social settings. These include proximal settings of everyday life (such as families, peer and friendship groups, schools, neighborhoods, work organizations, or health care institutions), distal settings (such as the state and its policies, historical events and changes, demographic parameters, the economy or culture), and connections among them. Distal settings are not only important in their own right but also in how they shape the proximal settings beneath them.
- Differentiation in aging-related experiences across cohort, sex, race, and social class groups, generations within families, and nations.

The importance of these and other propositions of life-course research is illustrated throughout the chapter. Although the term *life course* is associated with the discipline of sociology, this chapter does not take life-course scholarship to be the exclusive terrain of sociology. Instead, it takes the view that understanding the life course, as it was just described, requires the active integration of the human sciences and rests especially on a stronger partnership between life-course sociology and life-span psychology (see Settersten, 2003b, 2005a). I now briefly consider how tending to the life course might strengthen research on aging in the areas of work and retirement, leisure, family, and health and illness.

## A. Work and Retirement

Research on work and retirement in late life has often been at least partially conducted in ways consistent with a life-course perspective, especially in pointing to the roles of work environments and policies, prior work histories, and the needs and resources of family members in determining work and retirement experiences. Furthering a life-course perspective on this topic requires more careful attention to the institutional level of analysis, the individual life course, and the relationship between them (for illustrations, see Henretta, 2003). At the institutional level, for example, there is much to learn about how employment institutions organize the life course. This is especially important because there is great variability in the characteristics of work organizations. These organizations must also be understood in conjunction with other social forces that allocate education, work, and leisure experiences to the early, middle, and final decades of life, thereby leaving these activities and spheres as largely "age segregated" rather than "age integrated" (Riley, Kahn, & Foner, 1994; Uhlenberg & Riley, 2000). Important shifts in the boundaries

between the three "boxes" of education, work, and leisure have occurred in recent decades—extensions in education at the front end, earlier retirement and increased longevity at the back end, and a shorter period of gainful employment in the middle. Yet the "3-box" structure largely remains intact, salient in both individual and cultural thought (Settersten, 2003b) and embedded in the policies and programs of the state, especially in the United States (for illustrations, see Settersten, 2003c).

There is growing evidence, however, that the education-work-leisure lock-step is beginning to dissolve, and for a wide variety of reasons related to both choice and circumstance. More significant shifts are apparent in the first two boxes, as education and work are now more often pursued concurrently (Settersten, Furstenberg, & Rumbaut, 2005). Modernization and rapid technological change have also made it necessary for adults to periodically update their skills and knowledge if they are to compete in contemporary markets, especially as "lifetime" models of work erode and stable work becomes uncertain or "contingent" (see also Heinz, 2003; Pallas, 2003). In the third box, a wider array of patterns into retirement are now common, though most people nonetheless desire and strive for a fairly long period of retirement (O'Rand & Henretta, 1999).

These changes have the net result of producing a more flexible life course, but they also bring more fragmentation and risk because the experimental nature of individualized pathways makes them more likely to break down (Beck, 2000; O'Rand, 2003; Settersten, 2003c, 2005b). When individuals choose or find themselves on pathways that are not widely shared by others or reinforced in institutions or policies, they may lose important sources of informal and formal support. These vulnerabilities may be especially apparent for members of cohorts who are now navigating the transition to adulthood (see Settersten, Furstenberg, & Rumbaut, 2005) and retirement (see Hardy, this volume) in brand new ways.

There is much to learn about how and how much individual lives are rooted in the institutional life course—how "loosely" or "tightly" coupled they are, and the causes and consequences of adherence to or departure from institutional norms (for illustrations, see Henretta, 2003). This is particularly important in the case of employment in that individuals spend a large portion of their lives at work and, increasingly, in different work environments because they more often change positions or organizations. Yet the life course is derived only partly from employment activities and institutions, and we must understand the full range of individual factors, especially those related to family and health, that combine with institutional factors to determine work and retirement experiences in late life.

## B. Leisure

In the second half of the twentieth century, the emphasis on full-time continuous work in the middle box of life, coupled with new versions of childhood that occurred even earlier in the century as a result of compulsory schooling and the regulation of child labor, meant that most leisure was relegated to the beginning and end of life. In the years ahead, new opportunities for leisure may result from changing patterns of education, work, family, and health—such as extended schooling, delayed parenting and reduced fertility, later entry into full-time work and less stable or continuous employment, earlier or more gradual retirement, longer lives, and better health. These and other patterns suggest that in the future, and again because of factors related to both social forces and individual choices, leisure will not only assume a bigger place in the lives of old people but may also be more evenly distributed across life (for other illustrations, see Hendricks & Cutler, 2003). Leisure is also likely to become a clearer and more significant source of identity in determining the choices individuals make and the actions individuals take to define themselves and anchor their relationships (Hendricks & Cutler, 2003).

Life-course studies are especially well poised to analyze individual- and societal-level dynamics in the allocation, forms, and meanings of leisure—or their relative absence in some societies or social strata therein. These dynamics will become increasingly important as large cohorts now on the threshold of old age move through their later years in ways that are different from their predecessors, and as younger cohorts now moving into and through adulthood face life circumstances and prospects very different from cohorts past (see also Cutler, this volume; Hendricks & Hatch, this volume).

## C. Family

Families are front and center in a life-course perspective because they are the primary setting in which individuals of many ages are assembled together and have relationships that span many decades. The life chances and options of individuals are intimately tied to family members (e.g., educational and occupational attainment, marital and fertility patterns, and health outcomes are all strongly conditioned by family background and resources) and the experiences of particular family members or generations may have ripple effects throughout the extended family matrix (e.g., economic hardship or prosperity in one generation potentially may bring both immediate and long-ranging effects on a wide array of outcomes for generations above or below it; teenage pregnancy in one generation prompts early entry into grandparenthood in the generation above and likely changes the constellation of roles and responsibilities for everyone involved).

A life-course perspective on families emphasizes the need to capture the interdependence of lives across three levels: the interdependence of cohorts in societies, of generations in the family (members of which also belong to different cohorts), and of individual life paths in connection to these and other social relationships (Hagestad, 2003). At the societal level, intergenerational models are critical to understanding aging because of political debates and public dialogue in many nations about both intergenerational equity and intragenerational justice (Esping-Andersen, 2002; Myles, 2002; see also Walker, this volume; Kohli, this volume). At the family level, intergenerational models are naturally relevant to understanding aging because families and family-like relationships influence the course of aging by fulfilling (or failing to fulfill) important human needs and support, just as the course of aging also affects the vitality of these relationships (Elder & Johnson, 2003; see also Chapters 10 and 11).

A life-course perspective on families also emphasizes three types of temporal location: individual, family, and historical time (for illustrations, see Hagestad, 2003). Individual time is roughly expressed through chronological age, which serves as a gauge for social roles and expectations, rights, and responsibilities. These are also conditioned by family time, which is roughly expressed through the generational position of an individual in the extended family matrix, and which also changes as older generations die and new ones are born.

Attention to historical time is a particularly important contribution of a life-course perspective. Members of different generations in the family come from different cohorts, which have been exposed to different economic, political, and social conditions, and which have different attitudes, values, and behaviors. The family is the immediate context in which "generation gaps" are personally felt and

played out, as well as the intermediate context through which the effects of macro-level phenomena on individuals are mediated or moderated, a theme to which we later return. Historical shifts in demographic parameters (especially fertility, mortality, and morbidity) have also altered the very structure and experience of family life, bringing both new problems and possibilities for family relationships (for further discussion, see Settersten, 2002).

## D. Health and Illness

There are strong natural links between the life-course perspective and the study of health and illness, for which the strongest body of empirical evidence exists on the connections between earlier and later experiences and statuses. Health and illness are not only states but also *processes* that grow and have consequences over time (George, 2003a). This has long been recognized by scholarship on social factors and illness, especially that which explores the impact of social and behavioral processes *on* health and the social and behavioral consequences *of* illness (for illustrations, see Ferraro, this volume; George, 2003a).

A marriage between the stress paradigm and the life-course perspective offers a particularly important avenue for studying social factors and illness. Drawing on research related to physical disability, functional impairments, and mental health, George (2003a) offers many good illustrations of three key strategies. First, it is possible to analyze trajectories as pathways of vulnerability and resistance using (1) specific antecedents to predict health trajectories as outcomes, (2) risk trajectories to predict specific health outcomes, or (3) risk trajectories to predict health trajectories. For each of these approaches, both aggregated and disaggregated strategies can be used, with the former producing trajectories that best describe long-term patterns of stability and change for a sample as a whole and the latter producing distinctive patterns within a sample. Second, it is possible to trace long-term pathways using nontrajectory approaches such as time series and path analyses. Third, it is possible to address pervasive problems of social selection (that is, relationships between social risk factors and health may not be caused by the risk factors themselves, such as socioeconomic status, exposure to stress, or social support, but instead by the things that determine these factors) by taking these to be life-course processes to be explicitly modeled in their own right rather than statistically controlled. This strategy thereby transforms how we approach one of the most challenging problems at the heart of the field.

In prompting movement in these directions, the life-course perspective reinforces and extends the existing emphasis on process in research on health and aging by suggesting that even longer views will provide valuable information on the precursors and consequences of health and illness experiences in late life. It especially points to the need to gather and analyze data on long-term patterns of social factors and illness, differentials in vulnerability and resistance to illness, and variability in illness outcomes. This knowledge is vital to ensuring the well-being of elders, their families, and societies through more effective policies and practices.

## II. Clarifying the Distinctiveness of Old Age

As noted earlier, a central life-course proposition concerns variability, themes of which are now pervasive throughout gerontology. Research on aging routinely references the notion that the degree of variability among old people is not only great but is often greater than that which exists in other age groups. The important new consciousness of variability has been promoted especially by theories of cumu-

lative advantage and disadvantage over the life course (e.g., Dannefer, 2003a), though the field is in need of comprehensive empirical treatments of variability, its sources, and its consequences.

Gerontologists now assume that there is so much variability among old people, however, that only rarely do we consider the things that old people may have in common. This trend, coupled with more attention to the life course as a whole, makes it increasingly important *and* difficult to clarify how old age is distinct from periods before it. When we lose sight of commonness, we lose sight of the things that make our subject matter distinct. To what extent are the challenges of old age simply those of earlier periods that are prolonged or revisited? To what extent does old age pose unique developmental challenges and opportunities? What are the markers that define entry into old age and movement through the "young-old," "old-old," and "oldest-old" periods so commonly cited in research on aging? To what degree do such phases actually exist?

This is not to say that gerontologists should return to rigid or all-encompassing "stage" theories of psychological development (e.g., Erikson, 1980) or to narrow social theories of aging that make assumptions that do not reflect the realities of most old people or the contemporary world (e.g., Cumming & Henry, 1961). Indeed, few developmental scientists today value theories or models that are proposed as fixed and universal, or that ignore the ways in which lives are self-regulated. It is instead to say that we must be as open to things that are shared by old people, experiences that may persist across time and context, as we are to the things that make old people different and may vary across time and context. Early scholarship on aging focused on commonness to the exclusion of difference; current scholarship focuses on difference to the exclusion of commonness. When things that old people share—and potentially unite them—are neglected, the political activities and policy agendas that serve their interests and needs are also risked.

Gerontology would therefore benefit from systematic attention to both difference and commonness among "old people," however they might be defined. These tensions are healthy and need not be reconciled as much as actively seized in an effort to foster innovative scholarship on aging. Our dual task must be (1) to identify core features of human growth and maturation, as well as fundamental needs that must be met, in old age; and (2) to elaborate the differential expression of these needs and how they are or might be better met in a range of particular contexts.

In considering what makes old people different from other adults, and old age different from the rest of adulthood, several possibilities can be gleaned from the literature (for further discussion, see Settersten, 2005c). These include normative losses in physical and cognitive capacities and the increased likelihood of failing health or chronic health conditions; the centrality of health concerns in self-definitions; a shorter time horizon and more pressing need to come to terms with one's mortality; a growing emphasis on achieving integrity and searching for meaning in life; bereavement associated with the death of parents, spouses, and friends; more restricted but intense social relationships and networks; being perceived or treated by others in ageist ways; and greater acceptance of things that cannot be controlled *in* life, coupled with greater fear of losing control *over* one's life.

This latter point, on letting go of things that cannot be controlled but being frightened by the possibility of losing control, seems especially important. Much scholarship in gerontology in the last few decades has been characterized by models of *agency without structure* (Settersten, 1999), which emphasize the significance of individual decisions and actions in determining life outcomes. A wide range of concepts—such as "self-efficacy,"

"self-determination," "locus of control," "proactivity," "effort," "mindfulness," "resourcefulness," "mastery," and "autonomy"—is often used to index agency. This trend has especially been promoted by popular models of "successful" aging (e.g., Baltes & Baltes, 1990; Kahana & Kahana, 2003; Rowe & Kahn, 1998; Vaillant & Mukamal, 2001). What is needed is a more balanced treatment of agency and structure, especially models of *agency within structure* (Settersten, 1999), which explicitly seek to understand how individuals set goals, take actions, and create meanings within the parameters imposed by social settings, and even how individuals may change those parameters through their own actions (see also Hendricks & Hatch, this volume). These models are key to advancing knowledge about human development in all life periods, though issues related to control, autonomy, and independence are especially important during the first and last few decades of life (for illustrations, see Settersten, 2005c).

One critical difference between late life and earlier periods is that levels and types of human agency in late life are more heavily conditioned by losses in physical, cognitive, psychological, and social capacities and by increased dependence on others. For these reasons, and because time is more limited, opportunities for action—and those actions taken—may be especially meaningful in old age. While life is characterized by gains as well as losses, gains in old age surely pale in comparison to those made early in life, just as losses early in life surely pale in comparison to those experienced in old age. By advanced old age, the balance between gains and losses becomes less positive, if not negative. As the life span approaches its maximum biological limits, the "plasticity" of human potential decreases and the optimization of development becomes increasingly difficult (Baltes et al., 1998).

## III. Exploring Connections Between Old Age and Prior Life Periods

Given the lifelong nature of human development, old age cannot be adequately understood in isolation from other periods. More than any other period, old age must be understood in relation to a long past, making the life course a sort of "endogenous causal system," to use Mayer and Tuma's (1990) phrase, in understanding the present. Present experiences, too, must be understood in relation to an anticipated, but more limited, future. The goal of understanding lives over many decades makes demanding requests of theories, methods, and data. The longer a life is studied, the more difficult it becomes to trace connections, and the possible connections seem endless and often tenuous.

This process is especially difficult because there is little time-based theory to guide the selection of data points and variables. Significant theoretical advances, whether through the development of new theories or the revision of existing ones, are necessary to help determine *which* variables are important, *when* they are important, *how* they might be arrayed in sequence, and *what* processes and mechanisms drive them. It is also made difficult because variables may be multiply confounded not only at single time points but also across multiple points. Temporal connections therefore become major "leaps of faith," especially when the intervals between data points are wide and when experiences from long ago are included. Future theoretical advances can be made only to the extent that measures and observations can be meaningfully linked over time.

Theoretical limitations aside, few longitudinal studies are long enough to explore connections between old age and earlier life periods. Such connections cannot really be considered in most of the data sets commonly used in gerontology. Most "longitudinal" studies of aging begin with individuals who are already in late life (or midlife, at best), extend over just a few years (few span as many as 10 years), and contain little to no information on the developmental histories of individuals, the social settings in which they have existed, or historical or other macro-level conditions to which they have been exposed. There is a particular need to collect data on the economic, political, and historical contexts that affect aging, for longitudinal data on individuals can be fully understood only if they are explicitly considered against these contexts, as well as against *changes* in these contexts. Even most sociological data sets (e.g., life history studies, economic panels) come up short in this regard, containing much information on the social and economic roles and statuses of individuals but little on contexts beyond the household or family (see also Diewald, 2001). Most important, there is great need for gerontologists to more often couple physical, psychological, and contextual data (for illustrations, see Settersten, 2005a). Such mergers are necessary if we are to understand aging as the interplay among species, social, and individual influences.

Despite these problems, there are creative and less demanding methodological strategies that can be used to gather and analyze data, even retrospectively, in ways that are consistent with a life-course perspective (see Alwin, Hofer, & McCammon, this volume; and Giele & Elder, 1998; Settersten, 1999). Particularly important are life-history calendars, which allow investigators to reconstruct residential, educational, employment, marriage, and parenting histories with relative ease and accuracy. Life-history calendars can be used flexibly in single-point studies or to fill in intervals between data points in prospective studies. Excellent illustrations of life-history calendars can be found in the Berlin

Aging Study (BASE) and the German Life History Study (GLHS) (e.g., Baltes & Mayer, 1999; Mayer & Brueckner, 1998). In the GLHS, for example, complete event histories (from birth to the present) were collected in a variety of life domains, beginning with the residential history because it provides a good anchor for the recollection of information on other domains. In the case of residential history, data were gathered on every residential location, including the month and year of arrival and departure, the size and type of residence, geographic location, and household composition. Data were then gathered on marriage and family, education and training, primary and secondary employment, and military service and were reviewed for any unaccounted periods. This strategy results in rich, time-continuous data on statuses in multiple life domains, which are simultaneously mapped onto a single frame.

Data sets that have permitted the analysis of connections between old age and earlier life periods have yielded powerful findings. These include a handful of long-standing prospective studies started in the early to middle parts of the last century (e.g., the Berkeley Guidance, Berkeley Growth, and Oakland Growth Studies; Longitudinal Study of Generations; Scottish Mental Survey; Terman Study of the Gifted; Whitehall Study) and many shorter-term longitudinal projects begun later (e.g., the Seattle Longitudinal Study; Normative Aging Study; Framingham Study; the Berlin Aging Study; German Life History Study), most of which include retrospective components (see also Phelps, Furstenberg, & Colby, 2002).

Many of these early studies, however, were not initially conceived as general studies of human development, or even longitudinal studies, but were first launched to examine restricted topics or samples and then later broadened in coverage or design. This constrains the range of analyses that can be conducted, as well

as the degree to which findings can be generalized. The advantages that come with being able to address temporal connections also come with disadvantages related to selectivity, especially attrition (resulting from the difficulties of tracking and maintaining relationships with individuals over time) and selective mortality (that is, there are important differences between individuals who manage to survive to old age, especially advanced old age, and those who do not; in examining survivors, many of the processes that underlie the phenomena of interest cannot be observed). Of course, problems associated with selective mortality plague most research on late life, not just that which explicitly seeks to examine connections between old age and prior periods. This is particularly true of health-related research.

Some of the research that has examined connections between late life and earlier periods has focused on charting stability and change, from as early as childhood, in single domains over time, especially dimensions of abilities (e.g., Deary, Whalley, Lemmon, Crawford, & Starr, 2000; McArdle, Hamagami, Meredith, & Bradway, 2000) and personality (e.g., Helson, Jones, & Kwan, 2002; Jones & Meredith, 2000; Roberts & DelVecchio, 2000). From a life-course perspective, however, the most interesting questions are found in connecting different domains and linking resulting patterns to social factors and forces. This approach is at least implicit in research that associates statuses in a variety of social domains early in life with abilities, psychological health, and/or physical health and mortality late in life (e.g., Aldwin, Spiro, Levenson, & Cupertino, 2001; Bosworth, Schaie, Willis, & Siegler, 1999; Breeze et al., 2001; Crosnoe & Elder, 2004; Danner, Snowdon, & Friesen, 2001; Holahan & Suzuki, 2004; Luo & Waite, 2005; Starr, Deary, Lemmon, & Whalley, 2000). Just a few illustrations are offered next to demonstrate the explanatory power and potential of this perspective.

Using prospective data from the Terman Study of the Gifted, begun in 1922, Crosnoe and Elder (2004) found that four holistic profiles of aging ("less adjusted," "career-focused but socially disengaged," "family focused," and "well-rounded"—all of which are based on late-life satisfaction, vitality, family engagement, occupational success, and civic involvement) we associated with three family experiences in childhood or adolescence (socioeconomic status, parental divorce, and parent-child attachment). This study is noteworthy because it attempts to link these distal experiences through "mediational pathways," in which early family experiences predict later adult experiences (e.g., educational attainment, long-term intact marriage, persistent alcoholism) and other current circumstances (e.g., retirement status, income level, physical health, emotional health, and marital status), which in turn predict the aging profiles; and through "supplemental pathways," in which the effects of early family experiences on aging profiles are not filtered through adult experiences and other current circumstances.

The best illustrations of life-course research, elements of which can be extended to studies of aging, relate to probing more fully the intersections between individuals, family environments, and social change. As noted earlier, the life-course perspective places families center stage in research, and intergenerational models are natural to this perspective. For example, how do members of different family generations, who belong to different cohorts, experience and bridge potential chasms in attitudes, values, and behaviors? An innovative model for addressing this question can be found in recent analyses of the Longitudinal Study of Generations (LSOG), which take a fresh look at age-

old concerns about gaps in achievement and value orientations across family generations (Bengtson, Biblarz, & Roberts, 2002). These investigators capitalize on the unique design and data of the LSOG in an attempt to dispel several "myths" about contemporary youth and their families, including the notion that the achievement and value orientations of young people have declined since the social upheaval of the 1960s. As such, this is a good example of work that attempts to connect larger periods of social change to family dynamics and, in turn, connect family dynamics to individual outcomes.

There are also excellent models for exploring the effects of specific historical events on the social and psychological outcomes of individuals. The research of Elder and colleagues, which has focused on two large-scale events—the Great Depression and World War II—has been especially important in this regard (for an overview, see Elder & Johnson, 2003). The model at the foundation of the classic *Children of the Great Depression* (Elder, 1974/1999), for example, can be extended to research in gerontology to better link social change, life experiences, and aging. Elder examined how the economic deprivation caused by the Depression changed household economies, altered family relations, and created other significant strains, which, in turn, had serious but differential effects on the development of children depending on how old they were at the time of the deprivation, the severity of family deprivation, and other factors. Models such as this are important ventures because they trace how distal phenomena, such as historical conditions, have direct and indirect effects on individuals and cohorts, and they illustrate the strength of personal and familial characteristics and resources in mediating or moderating those effects. The mix of both negative and positive outcomes also serves as a reminder that even very difficult circumstances, such as those stemming from economic hardship or wartime military service, may prompt and even demand innovation, resilience, and psychological growth (see also Spiro, Schnurr, & Aldwin, 1997).

These connections nicely illustrate an important caveat in understanding all contemporary knowledge of aging: it is based on cohorts born in the first few decades of the twentieth century, and these cohorts have experienced dramatic historical events and rapid social change in their lifetimes. There is a great need for gerontologists to assess the ways in which the conditions of the last century may lurk beneath current knowledge of aging and limit the degree to which it can be generalized to future cohorts whose lives have been or will be radically different from those of prior cohorts.

## IV. The End of Gerontology?

Most gerontologists are interested in *aging* as a lifelong process but generally study *old age* as a discrete period, paying little to no attention to earlier experiences or statuses. Even inquiry into "old age" proper, at least as it is traditionally defined in many Western nations through eligibility for old age programs and entitlements or retirement from work (e.g., Phillipson, 1998), potentially spans three or more decades and requires a dynamic view. For these reasons, Neugarten (1996) once argued that gerontology would eventually disappear as a field in part because age-based specialties belittle the idea of lifelong development. She also suggested that gerontology would disappear as age-related entitlements are called into question and as service providers recognize that it is difficult to design and provide services for clients based solely on age.

Consistent with Neugarten's prediction, references to the "life span" and especially "life course" in research on aging have risen significantly in the last decade. Still, more attention to the life course will not likely bring the *end* of gerontology—though it will transform the field as we know it, and there is strong evidence that such transformations are under way. Too exclusive a focus on old age, or any particular life period for that matter, loses what is best in life-course research: a dynamic and process-based approach to understanding trajectories and transitions for individuals and cohorts as they grow up and older. This requires the development of new theories and methods, as well as further commitments to gathering and analyzing longitudinal and archival data. It also requires scientists to monitor advances in knowledge on all life periods, sift through mounting evidence, and make connections and build theories that transcend age- and discipline-based divisions.

This is clearly a tall order. But highly skilled and broadly trained gerontologists will be well suited for these tasks because gerontologists, more than other developmental scientists, must naturally account for a long past in understanding old age. This is not to say, of course, that temporal matters are unimportant in understanding childhood or other earlier periods. Indeed, concerns about the long-ranging effects of early experiences underlie much scholarship on child development and many child policies. It is instead to say that temporal matters cannot justifiably be ignored in gerontology, for even if the primary focus of our subject matter concerns experiences in the last few decades of life, there are six to nine (or more) decades of lived experiences that precede and profoundly shape it. It is important to note, though, that if gerontologists are to take the lead on these tasks, a major paradigm shift will be required; that is, we will need to transcend the very thing that now defines our field: age.

Many aspects of the social organization of science, however, reinforce rather than dissolve age- and discipline-based boundaries, including the structure of academic institutions, criteria for tenure and promotion, the scope of professional societies, the emphases of publication venues, and the priorities of funding agencies. In addition, age-based specializations such as gerontology will always exist because there *are* important and unique matters to be understood in different life periods, as discussed earlier.

Gerontology should also continue to thrive for other reasons. These include the need to reveal the nature, sources, and consequences of variability among old people, which is important for developing social programs and policies; the explosive growth in the numbers and proportion of old people in the population, which will prompt major social changes; and the fact that retirement and health care policies are significant and controversial issues in most nations (Hendricks & Cutler, 2002). These concerns will only be heightened amidst the growing anti-aging movement and an increasingly "prolonged" old age in "long-lived" societies (for illustrations, see Post & Binstock, 2004).

Professional organizations focused on particular age groups, such as the Gerontological Society of America or the Society for Research on Child Development, will also continue to attract scholars and practitioners who work on those periods and value interdisciplinary exchange and collaboration. These organizations were especially important when disciplinary organizations did not have critical masses interested in development during specific life periods. Since then, many disciplinary organizations have built flourishing sections devoted to particular periods, such as the American Sociological Association's recently renamed section on Aging *and the Life Course* and the

American Psychological Association's division on Adult Development and Aging. These groups offer important opportunities to foster disciplinary networks and strengthen disciplinary treatments of aging. But these alternatives have also somewhat competed with interdisciplinary organizations rather than supplemented them, which should be worrisome to gerontologists and others committed to interdisciplinary inquiry.

At the same time, there are indications that gerontology has vitality as an interdisciplinary field. Its vitality can be seen in the proliferation of interdisciplinary journals and sessions at professional meetings; the stability and popularity of both undergraduate and graduate interdisciplinary programs; the increased investments of faculty in training the next generation in broader ways; and new funding opportunities, especially predoctoral and postdoctoral training programs and research program projects (see also Bass & Ferraro, 2000; Clair & Allman, 2000).

The wide array of age-based organizations, programs, and activities suggests that age-based divisions remain firmly entrenched in the organization of developmental science. Nonetheless, age-specific inquiry inevitably loses some significance—or at least must become more modest—as it confronts the whole of life in all its richness and complexity. But rather than assume that increased attention to the life course might mean the end of gerontology, it might instead be taken as a symbol of the maturity of our field and its promising future (see also Hendricks & Cutler, 2002).

## V. Conclusion

Research on aging has much to gain by more comprehensively adopting life-course ideas—despite, or rather, precisely because of—the many theoretical and methodological complexities that time and place bring to our work, and the advances that may lie in their wake. This seems especially important in light of the changing and often declining mix of personal capacities and social resources in the final decades of life. The better gerontology can address developmental influences at multiple levels of analysis and understand these interactions over time, the better our science will be. Progress in these directions requires, and will flourish with, cross-disciplinary exchange and collaboration, especially among biological sciences, the behavioral and social sciences, clinical medicine, and policy studies.

Two clear traditions exist in life-course research (George, 2003b). One tradition takes the life course itself to be the primary target of inquiry—for example, in describing the structure and content of the life course, how it has changed over time or varies across place, or how it is reinforced or altered by the policies of the state or by historical events. The other tradition views the life course as a framework of common elements meant to guide research. From the vantage point of this second tradition, the life course is not a separate research topic as much as it is a set of principles and concepts (and, by extension, a set of methods) for understanding the many domains and dimensions of human life and functioning. As such, it is probably most effectively used in conjunction with other social and behavioral paradigms.

While both traditions bring important insights, it is the second tradition that offers greater promises for the field of gerontology. Research on circumscribed topics on aging will be greatly enriched through the infusion of life-course approaches, as outlined in the first section. An excellent example of the success of this strategy can also be found in the field of criminology, which has been transformed by the application of life-course ideas (e.g., Laub & Sampson, 2003). These ideas have enlarged the view implicit in traditional approaches, which have emphasized or assumed stability in offending and individual traits, by demanding empirical examination of long-term trajectories and promoting the possibilities of desistance from crime and malleability of character (Laub & Sampson, 2003). The life-course perspective has matured over several decades, but its potentials have yet to be fully realized. And although this perspective *grew out of* scholarship on aging, more complete *applications* of life-course models in substantive areas of aging have only just begun. To move forward, gerontologists must actively generate substantive theory, ask questions, collect data, and choose methods with the life course in mind.

It is important to note, however, that there is not, and will never likely be, an all-encompassing "theory" of the life course (see also George, 2003b; Settersten, 2003b). Nor can all elements of a life-course perspective be managed well in single studies. Any research agenda that embraces temporal, individual, and sociocultural phenomena becomes quickly complicated, which is precisely what makes the life course one of the greatest challenges to handle scientifically (Fry, 2003). Individual scientists must inevitably direct their work toward specific aspects of the framework or incorporate limited parts of it. The life-course perspective, like other meta-theoretical frameworks, is a broad heuristic device for coordinating research, facilitating communication, interpreting research, and integrating the growing knowledge base.

One of the most important consequences of infusing life-course ideas more fully into gerontology is that the *social* in "social gerontology" will be expanded. That is, gerontologists can compensate for the still heavy emphasis on biological and psychological factors by strengthening the treatment of sociocultural forces and by making more apparent the social complexities and ambiguities of old age and aging in contemporary societies. This task is very important in light of the dramatic social change of recent decades, and as traditional social institutions and scripts for life change and even crumble before us. Also, in more often looking beyond our own time and place, we will realize how irrelevant Western descriptions and explanations of life-course and aging patterns are in much of the world (Dannefer, 2003b). We will also achieve new awareness of the interdependence of lives across the globe and the ways in which the actions of individuals, groups, and nations intimately determine the life chances and welfare of others in faraway places and in unknown or unintended ways.

Another important consequence of adopting life-course ideas is that gerontology will not only pursue immediate answers to current problems by focusing on individuals who are already old, but we will also become more focused on predicting the future needs of those who are not yet old—what Cain (2003) called "ameliorative" versus "anticipatory" gerontology, respectively. Understanding the life course is central to producing a more anticipatory gerontology, especially within emphasizing cohort and generational phenomena, dynamic social systems, and earlier antecedents of late-life experiences. As Cain (2003) also noted, a more anticipatory gerontology will enrich the field by fostering the perspective of jurisprudence, not just politics, in confronting issues of equitability within and across age groups. These prospects will not only foster more effective social planning and policy making but will bring important opportunities *and* obligations to build greater compassion and concern for people of all ages and for all of the world's people.

## References

Aldwin, C. M., Spiro, A., III, Levenson, M. R., & Cupertino, A. P. (2001). Longitudinal findings from the Normative Aging Study: III. Personality, individual health trajectories, and mortality. *Psychology and Aging, 16*, 450–465.

Baltes, P. B., & Baltes, M. M. (Eds.). (1990). *Successful aging: Perspectives from the behavioral sciences.* New York: Cambridge University Press.

Baltes, P. B., Lindenberger, U., & Staudinger, U. M. (1998). Life-span theory in developmental psychology. In R. M. Lerner (Ed.), *Handbook of child psychology: Vol. 1. Theoretical models of human development* (pp. 1029–1143). New York: Wiley.

Baltes, P. B., & Mayer, K. U. (Eds.). (1999). *The Berlin Aging Study: Aging from 70 to 100.* Cambridge, UK: Cambridge University Press.

Bass, S. A., & Ferraro, K. F. (2000). Gerontology education in transition: Considering disciplinary and paradigmatic evolution. *Gerontologist, 40*, 97–106.

Beck, U. (2000). Living your own life in a runaway world: Individualisation, globalisation, and politics. In W. Hutton & A. Giddens (Eds.), *Global capitalism* (pp. 164–174). New York: The New Press.

Bengtson, V. L., Biblarz, T. J., & Roberts, R. E. L. (2002). *How families still matter: A longitudinal study of youth in two generations.* Cambridge, UK: Cambridge University Press.

Bosworth, H. B., Schaie, K. W., Willis, S. L., & Siegler, I. C. (1999). Age and distance to death in the Seattle Longitudinal Study. *Research on Aging, 21*, 723–738.

Breeze, E., Fletcher, A. E., Leon, D. A., Marmot, M. G., Clarke, R. J., & Shipley, M. J. (2001). Do socioeconomic disadvantages persist into old age? Self-reported morbidity in a 29-year follow-up of the Whitehall Study. *American Journal of Public Health, 91*, 277–283.

Cain, L. (2003). Age-related phenomena: The interplay of the ameliorative and the scientific. In R. A. Settersten, Jr. (Ed.), *Invitation to the life course: Toward new understandings of later life* (pp. 295–325). Amityville, NY: Baywood Publishing.

Clair, J. M., & Allman, R. M. (Eds.). (2000). *The gerontological prism: Developing interdisciplinary bridges.* Amityville, NY: Baywood Publishing Company.

Crosnoe, R., & Elder, G. H., Jr. (2004). From childhood to the later years: Pathways of human development. *Research on Aging, 26*(6), 623–654.

Cumming, E., & Henry, W. (1961). *Growing old: The process of disengagement.* New York: Basic Books.

Dannefer, D. (2003a). Cumulative advantage/disadvantage and the life course: Cross-fertilizing age and social science theory. *Journal of Gerontology: Social Sciences, 58B,* S327–337.

Dannefer, D. (2003b). Whose life course is it, anyway? Diversity and "linked lives" in global perspective. In R. A. Settersten, Jr. (Ed.), *Invitation to the life course: Toward new understandings of later life* (pp. 259–268). Amityville, NY: Baywood Publishing.

Danner, D. D., Snowdon, D. A., & Friesen, W. V. (2001). Positive emotions in early life and longevity: Findings from the Nun Study. *Journal of Personality and Social Psychology, 80,* 804–813.

Deary, I. J., Whalley, L. J., Lemmon, H., Crawford, J. R., & Starr, J. M. (2000). Stability of individual differences in mental ability from childhood to old age: Follow-up of the 1932 Scottish Mental Survey. *Intelligence, 28,* 49–55.

Diewald, M. (2001). Unitary social science for causal understanding: Experiences and prospects of life course research. *Canadian Studies in Population, 28*(2), 219–248.

Elder, G. H., Jr. (1999). *Children of the Great Depression: Social change in life experience* (25th anniversary ed.). Boulder, CO: Westview Press. (Original work published 1974.)

Elder, G. H., Jr., & Johnson, M. K. (2003). The life course and aging: Challenges, lessons, and new directions. In R. A. Settersten, Jr. (Ed.), *Invitation to the life course: Toward new understandings of later life* (pp. 49–81). Amityville, NY: Baywood Publishing.

Erikson, E. (1980). *Identity and the life cycle.* New York: W. W. Norton Press.

Esping-Andersen, G. (2002). Towards the good society, once again? In G. Esping-Andersen (with D. Gallie, A. Hemerijck, and J. Myles), *Why we need a new welfare state* (pp. 1–25). Oxford: Oxford University Press.

Fry, C. (2003). The life course as a cultural construct. In R. A. Settersten, Jr. (Ed.), *Invitation to the life course: Toward new understandings of later life* (pp. 269–294). Amityville, NY: Baywood Publishing.

George, L. K. (2003a). What life-course perspectives offer the study of aging and health. In R. A. Settersten, Jr. (Ed.), *Invitation to the life course: Toward new understandings of later life* (pp. 161–190). Amityville, NY: Baywood Publishing.

George, L. K. (2003b). Life course research: Achievements and potential. In J. Mortimer & M. Shanahan (Eds.), *Handbook of the life course* (pp. 671–680). New York: Kluwer Academic/Plenum Publishers.

Giele, J., & Elder, G. H., Jr. (Eds.). (1998). *Methods of life-course research: Qualitative and quantitative approaches.* Newbury Park, CA: Sage Publications.

Hagestad, G. O. (1990). Social perspectives on the life course. In R. Binstock & L. George (Eds.), *Handbook of aging and the social sciences* (3rd ed., pp. 151–168). New York: Academic Press.

Hagestad, G. O. (2003). Interdependent lives and relationships in changing times: A life-course view of families and aging. In R. A. Settersten, Jr. (Ed.), *Invitation to the life course: Toward new understandings of later life* (pp. 135–160). Amityville, NY: Baywood Publishing.

Hagestad, G. O., & Dannefer, D. (2001). Concepts and theories of aging: Beyond microfication in social science approaches. In R. Binstock & L. George (Eds.), *Handbook of aging and the social sciences* (5th ed., pp. 3–21). San Diego, CA: Academic Press.

Hagestad, G. O., & Neugarten, B. L. (1985). Age and the life course. In E. Shanas & R. Binstock (Eds.), *Handbook of aging and the social sciences* (2nd ed., pp. 36–61). New York: Van Nostrand Reinhold Company.

Heinz, W. R. (2003). From work trajectories to negotiated careers: The contingent work life course. In J. Mortimer & M. Shanahan (Eds.), *Handbook of the life course* (pp.

185–204). New York: Kluwer Academic/ Plenum Publishers.

Helson, R., Jones, C., & Kwan, V. S. Y. (2002). Personality change over 40 years of adulthood: Hierarchical linear modeling analyses of two longitudinal samples. *Journal of Personality and Social Psychology, 83,* 752–766.

Hendricks, J., & Cutler, S. J. (2002). The future of gerontology and geriatrics. *Contemporary Gerontology, 9,* 7–10.

Hendricks, J., & Cutler, S. J. (2003). Leisure in life-course perspective. In R. A. Settersten, Jr. (Ed.), *Invitation to the life course: Toward new understandings of later life* (pp. 107–134). Amityville, NY: Baywood Publishing.

Henretta, J. C. (2003). The life-course perspective on work and retirement. In R. A. Settersten, Jr. (Ed.), *Invitation to the life course: Toward new understandings of later life* (pp. 85–106). Amityville, NY: Baywood Publishing.

Holahan, C. K., & Suzuki, R. (2004). Adulthood predicators of health promoting behavior in later aging. *International Journal of Aging and Human Development, 58,* 289–313.

Jones, C. J., & Meredith, W. (2000). Developmental paths of psychological health from early adolescence to later adulthood. *Psychology and Aging, 15,* 351–360.

Kahana, E., & Kahana, B. (2003). Contextualizing successful aging: New directions in an age-old search. In R. A. Settersten, Jr. (Ed.), *Invitation to the life course: Toward new understandings of later life* (pp. 225–255). Amityville, NY: Baywood Publishing.

Laub, J., & Sampson, R. (2003). *Shared beginnings, divergent lives: Delinquent boys to age 70.* Cambridge, MA: Harvard University Press.

Luo, Y., & Waite, L. (2005). The impact of childhood and adult SES on physical, mental, and cognitive well-being in later life. *Journal of Gerontology: Social Sciences, 60B,* S93–S101.

Mayer, K. U., & Bruekner, E. (1998). Collecting life history data: Experiences from the German Life History Study. In J. Giele & G. H. Elder, Jr. (Eds.), *Methods of life course research: Qualitative and quantitative approaches* (pp. 152–181). Thousand Oaks, CA: Sage Publications.

Mayer, K. U., & Tuma, N. B. (1990). Life course research and event history analysis: An overview. In K. U. Mayer & N. B. Tuma (Eds.), *Event history analysis in life course research* (pp. 3–20). Madison, WI: University of Wisconsin Press.

McArdle, J. J., Hamagami, F., Meredith, W., & Bradway, K. P. (2000). Modeling the dynamic hypotheses of Gf-Gc theory using longitudinal life-span data. *Learning and Individual Differences, 12,* 53–79.

Mortimer, J., & Shanahan, M. (Eds.). (2003). *Handbook of the life course.* New York: Kluwer Academic/Plenum Publishers.

Myles, J. (2002). A new social contract for the elderly? In G. Esping-Andersen (with D. Gallie, A. Hemerijck, and J. Myles), *Why we need a new welfare state* (pp. 130–174). Oxford: Oxford University Press.

Neugarten, B. L. (1996). The end of gerontology? In D. Neugarten (Ed.), *The meanings of age: Selected papers of Bernice L. Neugarten* (pp. 402–403). Chicago: University of Chicago Press.

Neugarten, B. L., & Hagestad, G. O. (1976). Age and the life course. In R. Binstock & E. Shanas (Eds.), *Handbook of aging and the social sciences* (pp. 35–55). New York: Van Nostrand Reinhold Company.

O'Rand, A. M. (2003). The future of the life course: Late modernity and life course risks. In J. Mortimer & M. Shanahan (Eds.), *Handbook of the life course* (pp. 693–702). New York: Kluwer Academic/Plenum Publishers.

O'Rand, A. M., & Henretta, J. C. (1999). *Age and equality: Diverse pathways through later life.* Boulder, CO: Westview Press.

Pallas, A. M. (2003). Educational transitions, trajectories, and pathways. In J. Mortimer & M. Shanahan (Eds.), *Handbook of the life course* (pp. 164–184). New York: Kluwer Academic/Plenum Publishers.

Phelps, E., Furstenberg, F. F., Jr., & Colby, A. (Eds.). (2002). *Looking at lives: American longitudinal studies of the 20th century.* New York: Russell Sage.

Philipson, C. (1998). *Reconstructing old age: New agendas in social theory and practice.* London: Sage Publications.

Post, S.G., & Binstock, R.H. (Eds.). (2004). *The fountain of youth: Cultural, scientific, and* ethical perspectives on a biomedical goal. New York: Oxford University Press.

Riley, M. W., Kahn, R. L., & Foner, A. (Eds.). (1994). *Age and structural lag: Society's failure to provide meaningful opportunities in work, family, and leisure.* New York: John Wiley & Sons.

Roberts, B., & DelVecchio, W. (2000). The rank-order consistency of personality traits from childhood to old age: A quantitative review of longitudinal studies. *Psychological Bulletin, 126,* 3–25.

Rowe, J., & Kahn, R. (1998). *Successful aging.* New York: Pantheon.

Settersten, R. A., Jr. (1999). *Lives in time and place: The problems and promises of developmental science.* Amityville, NY: Baywood Publishing.

Settersten, R. A., Jr. (2002). Socialization and the life course: New frontiers in theory and research. In R. A. Settersten, Jr. & T. Owens (Eds.), *New frontiers in socialization* (pp. 13–40). London: Elsevier.

Settersten, R. A., Jr. (2003a). Age structuring and the rhythm of the life course. In J. Mortimer & M. Shanahan (Eds.), *Handbook of the life course* (pp. 81–98). New York: Kluwer Academic/Plenum Publishers.

Settersten, R. A., Jr. (2003b). Propositions and controversies in life-course scholarship. In R. A. Settersten, Jr. (Ed.), *Invitation to the life course: Toward new understandings of later life* (pp. 15–48). Amityville, NY: Baywood Publishing.

Settersten, R. A., Jr. (2003c). Rethinking social policy: Lessons of a life-course perspective. In R. A. Settersten, Jr. (Ed.), *Invitation to the life course: Toward new understandings of later life* (pp. 191–222). Amityville, NY: Baywood Publishing.

Settersten, R. A., Jr. (2005a). Toward a stronger partnership between life-course sociology and life-span psychology. *Research in Human Development, 2,* 25–41.

Settersten, R. A., Jr. (2005b). Social policy and the transition to adulthood: Toward stronger institutions and individual capacities. In R. A. Settersten, Jr., F. F. Furstenberg, Jr., & R. G. Rumbaut (Eds.), *On the frontier of adulthood: Theory, research, and public policy* (pp. 534–560). Chicago: University of Chicago Press.

Settersten, R. A., Jr. (2005c). Linking the two ends of life: What gerontology can learn from childhood studies. *Journal of Gerontology: Social Sciences, 60B,* S173–S180.

Settersten, R. A., Jr., Furstenberg, F. F., Jr., & Rumbaut, R. G. (Eds.). (2005). *On the frontier of adulthood: Theory, research, and public policy.* Chicago: University of Chicago Press.

Spiro, A., Schnurr, P., & Aldwin, C.M. (1997). A life-span perspective on the effects of military service. *Journal of Geriatric Psychiatry, 30,* 91–128.

Starr, J. M., Deary, I., Lemmon, H., & Whalley, L. (2000). Mental ability age 11 years and health status age 77 years. *Age and Ageing, 29,* 523–528.

Uhlenberg, P., & Riley, M. W. (Eds.). (2000). Essays on age integration. *The Gerontologist, 40,* 261–307.

Vaillant, G. E., & Mukamal, K. (2001). Successful aging. *American Journal of Psychiatry, 158,* 839–847.

# Two

# Modeling the Effects of Time
## Integrating Demographic and Developmental Perspectives

Duane F. Alwin, Scott M. Hofer, and Ryan J. McCammon

There is an emerging consensus that longitudinal measurements of the same persons have a number of desirable features for the study of aging. Indeed, some of the most important quantitative developments in recent decades are the advances that have been made in the modeling of longitudinal trajectories, allowing researchers to study processes occurring in time (e.g., McArdle & Nesselroade, 2003; Schaie & Hofer, 2001). While investigators interested in aging and human development are increasingly turning to large-scale, multi-wave longitudinal studies to investigate processes of *intra-individual* (i.e., within-person) *change* and their causes, the application of these methods is neither straightforward nor unproblematic. For example, many of the problems identified in the use of repeated cross-sectional designs, particularly the problem of the confounding of the effects of aging with cohort and period effects, are also problematic in panel (or repeated measures) designs.

There are a number of additional problems, from nonresponse (and/or attrition) to retest effects. In this chapter, we focus on some of the problems involved in *the analysis of within-person change* using panel survey designs. The chapter focuses on this topic, in part because the tools for "growth modeling" have become very popular and widely available, but also because several conceptual and methodological issues must be addressed to make effective use of these techniques.

## I. Conceptions of Time

In this chapter we focus attention on several aspects of time and the way in which processes of within-person change can be modeled using repeated measures in longitudinal designs. We emphasize the utility of different conceptualizations of time and the way in which different time structures permit alternate accounts of individual change. The metric of time is arbitrary,

*Handbook of Aging and the Social Sciences, Sixth Edition*

but it is typically marked in a *celestial* metric (i.e., days, months, or years). The particular choice of a metric of time is driven by (1) substantive considerations and (2) the available data. In addition, time is measured from a substantively defined zero point—an *event* that gives time meaning. Although the science of aging aspires to measure "biological age" (see Kirkwood, 1999), the most common metric for assessing "age" is simply years from birth, or chronological age, or some linear transformation of it (e.g., time since baseline of the study). Other valuable time metrics designate the origins of time with respect to significant *events*, such as widowhood (e.g., time since the death of spouse), death (e.g., time to death), or diagnosis of a chronic illness or condition (e.g., time to dementia).

## A. Historical Time

Perhaps the most basic distinction to be made is that between *historical time* and *biographical time* (Alwin, 1995; Hareven, 1982) (Table 2.1). Historical time is measured in years, decades, centuries, and so

on, and these broad spans of time, reflecting historical periods, eras, epochs and the like, capture the effects of macro-level changes that affect individuals' private and collective lives. Two important sources of influence on human lives assessed in terms of historical time are "period" and "cohort" effects. Such effects refer to the sources of individual change and/or stability that come about through people's responses to historical events and processes. When an entire population of interest, an entire society, is affected by historical events, such as a war, an economic depression, or a social movement, the widespread changes occurring are conceptualized as *period effects*. Such influences are captured in research investigations by including variables tied to *occasions of measurement*, although the potential effects of time of measurement are often ignored (but see Rodgers, Ofstedal, & Herzog, 2003).

When events occurring in historical time affect only distinctive (or unique) subpopulations, concepts other than period effects are used. One such type of effect refers to the potential for historical

---

**Table 2.1**
Conceptions of Time with Examples

A. *Historical Time* (key concepts: periods, eras, epochs)

B. *Biographical Time* (key concepts: life cycle and aging)
1. Life stage/phase (e.g., childhood, adolescence, early adulthood, midlife, retirement age)
2. Life course events (e.g., transition to first marriage, transition to first parity, transition from school to work, transition to retirement)
3. Chronological age
4. Age-related timing of events (e.g., age at first marriage, age at first parity, age at first divorce, age at retirement, etc.)
5. Event-based time structures (e.g., time to death, time to dementia, time since death of one's spouse, time to retirement, time since retirement, etc.)

C. *Intersection of Historical and Biographical Time* (key concept: cohorts)
1. Birth cohort membership (e.g., being born at a particular time in a cohort with particular characteristics)
2. Other types of cohort membership (e.g., marriage cohorts, retirement cohorts)

events to affect only one segment of the age distribution (e.g., the young), and we use the term *cohort effects* to refer to stable differences among birth cohorts as a result of the historical circumstances of their development (Ryder, 1965). The definition of cohort effects in this way, as the effect of historical events on one segment of the age distribution, is not in theory limited to the young, but this is the way the concept tends to be applied.

## B. Biographical Time

The dimension of time concerned with the lives of individuals, usually conceptualized in terms of the biological, psychological, and social processes (and their interaction) that shape the life cycle and aging of individuals, is referred to as *biographical time* (see Table 2.1). We use the term *biographical time* rather than simply *age* to draw attention to the fact that a concern with human development considers the life cycle and other events, transitions, and trajectories of roles that fill persons' lives. A number of different conceptions of time are useful as a way of thinking about individual development and change. The most common are *age* and *life cycle*, one continuous and one discrete, both of which measure time from birth.

The uniqueness of individual biographies and the diversity of life patterns stimulated the life course approach to human development within the social and behavioral sciences. The primary concerns are with the social pathways, that is, the sequences of roles and experiences followed by individuals over particular phases of their lives, defined by events and transitions within particular life domains (e.g., Elder, Johnson, & Crosnoe, 2003; Ferraro, 2001; Macmillan & Eliason, 2003; Rindfuss, 1991). Although the life course perspective, and its focus on events, transitions, and social pathways, is valuable, we should

also emphasize the importance of the *life-span developmental* perspective, which conceptualizes human development as multidimensional and multidirectional processes of growth involving both gains and losses (Baltes, 1987; Baltes, Staudinger, & Lindenberger, 1999). From this perspective, development is embedded in multi-layered social and cultural contexts and is conceived of as a dynamic process involving the interaction of the developing organism with the social and physical environment (Alwin, Cohen, & Newcomb, 1991; Bronfenbrenner, 1979).

Human development and aging are lifelong processes, and a complete understanding of processes occurring in biographical time requires a multiplicity of concepts. It is important for present purposes that we distinguish among all of these concepts—the *life span, life cycle*, and the *life course*—in modeling the effects of time. From a demographic point of view, the *life span*, the length of life for an individual organism (see Carey, 2003), draws attention to the biological limits on development. It also signals the temporal scope of inquiry, and a life-span developmental perspective focuses therefore on the effects of events and processes occurring throughout the entire life span. And as noted previously, the life-span developmental perspective emphasizes how the age-graded ontogeny of human development interacts with the social environment. Historically, *life cycle* refers to "maturational and generational processes driven by mechanisms of reproduction in natural populations" (O'Rand & Krecker, 1990, p. 242). It refers to a fixed sequence of irreversible stages, tied specifically to sexual reproduction. The irreducible properties of the life cycle, therefore, are successive forms (stages), irreversible development (maturation), and the reproduction of form (generation). These elements of the life cycle define the biological bases of changes over time (Hogan, 2000). By contrast, the *life course* refers to the structure, sequence, and dynamics of events, and their trajectories (social pathways) that take place across life-cycle stages or phases of the life span. The concept of life course is often misunderstood in that it is often used as a synonym for life cycle or life span, but it refers to something quite different (Settersten, 2003). Each phase of the life span has a set of potential life course patterns. These include, for example, role transitions such as entering and leaving school, acquiring a full-time job, and the first marriage, or in old age transition into retirement, or into a long-term care facility.

## C. The Intersection of Historical and Biographical Time

Demographers and others have frequently considered *the intersection of historical and biographical time* (i.e., being born at a particular time) as a set of factors that have important consequences for human development. A *cohort*, in general, is a group of people who experience an event during the same interval of time. For example, people marrying in a given year are called a *marriage cohort*, people who enter college in a given year are referred to as an *entering cohort*, and those who graduate in the same year are called a *graduating cohort*. Similarly, persons born in the same year are members of a *birth cohort*, and this is how the term is used in demographic studies of aging. Defined in this way, knowing a person's *cohort* membership may be thought to index the unique historical period in which a group's common experiences are embedded, but as we have argued elsewhere, this does not necessarily make a cohort (or a set of cohorts) a generation (Alwin & McCammon, 2003).

## II. Population Concepts

The concept of a "population" is important for three reasons. First, issues related to population composition and related processes urge the clear specification of the population of interest in demographic studies of aging and human development (Siegel & Swanson, 2004). Second, statistical concerns with inference and generalization emphasize the standard of external validity as a criterion against which to evaluate the quality of statistical inferences, and specification of the relevant population for these inferences and the systematic sampling from that population provide a means to meet that standard (Kish, 1987). Third, substantive questions are almost always linked to a specific population, and the clear definition of the population of interest brings the requirements of research design into sharper relief. The concept of cohort as used here, that is, a birth cohort, refers to a central component of population composition. Although many studies wish to generalize about the effects of historical events on cohort experiences, this may be futile without data from representative samples of those cohorts for the period studied.

In the general case, we think of populations as being defined by an event or the aggregation of events (e.g., birth, widowhood, retirement, or death). Depending on the substantive question at hand, researchers using longitudinal data may wish to generalize to one of a number of different populations (Nesselroade, 1988). First, there are several natural groups of interest to aging researchers (e.g., nursing home residents, Medicare recipients, or retired persons). Second, the concept of birth cohort is critical for studying population composition. In this case birth is an event that defines the subpopulation of interest, and typically the division of the population into groups defined by cohort membership is the focus of the analysis (e.g., Alwin & McCammon, 2001). Third, survivorship (for example, surviving members of birth cohorts) is often a possible basis of inference. Here issues of mortality selection are made explicit in defining the population. Fourth, mortality or death can be considered as a population-defining event; longitudinal data before death permit the study of processes linked to "time to death." We discuss other possible event-based uses of time next.

In some circumstances, it may be desirable to generalize to baseline respondents, who, in the case of a total population survey, are themselves a subset of the universe of people ever born. Even in the most inclusive population surveys, the initial sample is frequently bound by geography and is always limited to those individuals alive at the time of sampling. When sampling with age restrictions, the universe of eligible respondents, and thus the reference population, is limited to only those members of the birth cohorts sampled that have survived to the age of study eligibility. Despite this potential censoring, the population of "baseline survivors" is potentially quite different from another possible population of interest to researchers, namely, "endpoint survivors." By this, we typically mean the population of sampling units alive and study-eligible at baseline and alive and study-eligible at some later occasion of measurement. If one is interested in aging and is willing to put aside the possibility of period and/or cohort differences, this form of survivorship can be thought of as merely referring to those individuals who attained a given chronological age. For example, in the context of modeling longitudinal trajectories of cognitive aging from age 80 to 89, it is not necessary for all respondents to be age 80 at baseline. Rather, if one wishes to generalize to individuals who live to be at least 89, the important factor is that the respondents

reach age 89 sometime between $wave_1$ and $wave_n$, inclusively.

## III. Analysis Issues

Several statistical issues arise in the analysis of longitudinal data that must be briefly mentioned, although we cannot treat these in any detail: (a) population sampling, (b) sample design effects, (c) statistical power, (d) measurement issues, and (e) handling nonresponse and/or attrition.

### A. Population Sampling

In some areas of social and behavioral science, population sampling may not be critical because the processes involved are so basic that any set of individuals available for study will suffice. This is seldom the case, however, and in order to generalize to a given population of interest, probability sampling of that population is assumed and required. There is no known way to demonstrate the external validity of research results (i.e., being able to generalize beyond a particular study) without meeting some basic requirements of sampling, and apart from some method of probability sampling, one cannot know how generalizable the results are. Fortunately, there are increasing numbers of age-heterogeneous longitudinal data sets that are true "samples" in the sense that they rely on state-of-the art methods of statistical sampling of well-defined populations. Therefore the selection of cases is governed by a replicable process such that their presence in the sample has a known probability.

### B. Sample Design Effects

Data from population-based longitudinal sample are typically based on complex multistage household samples that involve some geographical clustering within primary sampling units. In this sampling design, respondents within clusters are more homogenous than they would be if simple random sampling were possible. As a result, standard errors that do not adjust for sample design effects are often too small and may lead to incorrect inferences. A design effect (Deff) is defined as the ratio of the estimate of sampling variance obtained by taking the complex nature of the sampling design into account to the sampling variance estimate computed using formulae based on a simple random sample (Kish, 1965). Design effects vary depending on the variables under consideration. Generally, statisticians advise that analysts take design effects into account (e.g., Johnson & Elliot, 1998; Korn and Graubard, 1991). Increasingly, general statistical software packages (e.g., STATA) and more specialized packages for structural equation modeling (SEM) and hierarchical modeling (e.g., Mplus and HLM) include the capability of obtaining correct standard errors, given access to case-level stratum and primary sampling unit identifiers. As the ease of implementation of methods that account for complex sample designs continues to increase, it is likely that their use will become more widespread.

In addition to the cost efficiencies introduced by multistage cluster samples, to better represent certain minority populations, disproportionate sampling rates are often used that result in over-samples of certain groups. The impact of over-sampling on results should always be considered; however, there is less consensus on how to handle sample post-stratification weights that adjust for unequal selection probabilities and differential nonresponse. One common argument is that if the variables linked to disproportionate rates of sampling and differential rates of response (e.g., race and/or gender) are in the statistical model, adjusting for their effects is not informative (e.g., Korn & Graubard, 1991). When weights are used, estimates

may be less efficient than their unweighted counterparts, and standard errors may be biased in unpredictable ways (Winship & Radbill, 1994). Again, with some notable exceptions (e.g., AMOS) SEM packages available for growth curve analyses now permit the use of post-stratification weights, and one must carefully consider their use in light of the population of interest and the model specified.

## C. Statistical Power

Although researchers have long wanted to set low probabilities of making Type I errors—the probability of rejecting the null hypothesis when it is true—they have historically not given equal consideration to Type II errors—the likelihood of failing to reject the null hypothesis when there is in fact a real effect. A test has *statistical power* when it leads the researcher to correctly reject the null hypothesis (Murphy & Myors, 2004). Although analysts of large data sets are typically comfortable with the adequacy of their sample sizes for the hypotheses of interest, in some cases statistical power can be an issue. Ferraro and Wilmoth (2000) illustrated the importance of statistical power when examining effects of health conditions that are rare and/or when there are small effect sizes relative to the dependent variable. When rare outcomes are of interest, researchers may wish to pool data across major studies.

Most of the available research on statistical power has been developed within the framework of ANOVA and OLS regression models; although less attention has been devoted to statistical power analysis in SEM growth modeling of the type discussed here, this is clearly an important consideration (Muthén & Muthén, 2002). In cross-sectional data, power is a function of sample size in the groups being compared. In the longitudinal case, power to detect group differences can also be improved through increasing the number of occasions of data collection (Muthén & Curran, 1997).

## D. Measurement Issues

For several years, researchers have been aware of the need to compensate for the poor quality of measurement that is often encountered in social and behavioral science. There are at least three methods of tackling the problem of weak measurement: (a) the use of composite scores, (b) incorporating measurement error properties directly into analyses, and (c) the specification and estimation of multiple indicator models within a SEM framework. The presence of multiple indicators assists in the identification of the parameters of the model, although the use of multiple indicators raises issues of scaling of factors and factorial invariance.

Issues of factorial invariance can be traced to the early origins of factor analytical conceptions of measurement structures wherein concern was registered about the importance of establishing *invariant* relationships among variables. There is a hierarchy of factorial invariance constraints (Meredith, 1993; Meredith & Horn, 2001) that build on one another (each type assumes the existence of the prior form): (1) *Configural Invariance*: same pattern of factor loadings across groups; (2) *Weak or Metric Invariance*: factor pattern coefficients are equal across groups (identification of factor obtained by either a fixed loading or fixed factor variance); (3) *Strong Factorial Invariance*: manifest intercepts are equal across groups (with the factor mean in one group constrained for identification); (4) *Strict Factorial Invariance*: unique variances are equal across groups. Although it is desirable to have *strong* or *strict* factorial invariance in substantive situations (e.g., because mean level and group mean differences are often of interest), the minimal form for covariance analysis is *weak or metric* invariance (Horn & McArdle, 1992; Widaman & Reise, 1997). Weak or metric invariance is essential for making comparisons of factor-level constructs across groups and time. These issues are highly relevant to investigations using multiple measures and/or multiple indicators of theoretical constructs in a SEM framework.

## E. Handling Nonresponse

In longitudinal research there is often substantial nonresponse and/or attrition across different waves of the study, and given the potential for bias, analysts must take such matters seriously. Here we focus on *unit nonresponse*—that is, the presence or absence of a case in a particular wave of the survey—rather than on *item nonresponse*. Item nonresponse is a separate issue from cross-wave nonresponse, although from a practical point of view they are often treated in the same way. In some instances, respondents may be absent from one wave of the study but return for later waves. In other cases, because of death or other forms of permanent nonresponse, there can be substantial attrition from one wave to the next. Fortunately, advances in data-analytical methods for longitudinal data (e.g., structural equation models, multilevel models, and mixture regression models) make it possible to analyze longitudinal data structures without having a complete set of observations on each individual across all waves of the study (e.g., Allison, 2001; Arbuckle, 2000; Bryk & Raudenbush, 1992; Diggle, Liang, & Zeger, 1994; McArdle & Bell, 2000; McArdle & Hamagami, 1992; Muthén & Muthén, 2004; Wothke, 2000). However, the nonresponse in most longitudinal studies is relatively complex, resulting from a combination of factors, including mortality, other forms of attrition, and wave nonresponse. Thus, dealing with nonresponse is not always straightforward.

Nonresponse may not be problematic in some instances because it can be assumed that cases are lost at random. This is seldom the case, however, and it is widely accepted that nonresponse in longitudinal research produces potentially biased results. Nonetheless, some analysts will wish to analyze complete cases only, sometimes referred to as "listwise" deletion of cases. This is one possible strategy, but using it assumes that the nonrespondents are "missing completely at random" (MCAR); that is, for the variables analyzed, nonresponse is completely independent of either the true values of the variables of interest or any other variable (Little & Rubin, 1987, pp. 14–17). In some cases, the analyst has no choice when, for example, the longitudinal data archived for public use contain only those cases with complete data across waves. If the strategy of complete cases is used, the MCAR assumption should be tested to the extent possible. One useful approach (Allison,1987) treats each unique pattern of "incomplete" data resulting from differences in the timing of "attrition" as a separate group in a multiple-group SEM model, where variables from absent waves are treated as "unobserved" latent variables. This approach takes advantage of the flexibility of modern SEM software that allows data to be missing "by design" (Wothke, 2000, p. 239). To implement Allison's (1987) approach, a multiple-group model is estimated where the model parameters are assumed equal across groups (see McArdle & Hamagami, 1992, for an application using growth models). If the constrained model fits the data, the nonresponse is MCAR (Allison, 1987, p. 88), and the listwise-present parameter estimates will be unbiased. On the other hand, the deviation from perfect fit reflects the failure of the model parameters to reproduce the means and covariance structure across groups. This suggests the model parameters are differ-

ent in groups defined by differing patterns of complete data and a violation of the MCAR assumption.

There are typically better solutions to nonresponse than the "listwise" approach, especially given the inefficiency and likely bias involved. State-of-the-art solutions to nonresponse typically make the weaker assumption that cases are "missing at random" (MAR) (Little & Rubin, 1987, pp. 14–17); that is, the nonresponse is completely independent of the true values of the variable of interest after controlling for the other variables in the model. We will not consider these approaches here. Suffice it to say that assumptions of *randomness* of nonresponse in longitudinal research may be problematic in practice and one of a variety of solutions is advisable, including (a) direct estimation using full-information maximum-likelihood, or (b) multiple imputation (Schafer, 1997; Schafer & Graham, 2002).

It is important, however, to distinguish between types of nonresponse in devising strategies for dealing with the absence of data. It may be useful, at a minimum, to distinguish between two types of nonresponse at any given wave: (a) nonrespondents known to be dead, and (2) nonrespondents not known to be dead. Differential rates of nonresponse from mortality and other sources could be due to (among other things) health, disability, cognitive and sensory function, socioeconomic factors, and age itself. If the topic of the study is health, it is unlikely that mortality will be all that similar to other forms of nonresponse. Once the nature of the nonresponse problems has been identified, it is advisable to implement a set of strategies for dealing with the various types. Rather than simply treating cases of mortality as MAR, which they likely are not, two alternative strategies may make sense, depending on the substantive issues at hand. First, one may keep deceased respondents in the analysis, but include a dummy variable reflecting "mortality status" (but see Allison, 2001, pp. 9–11), or age at death can be included in the models to permit conditional population inferences (see later). An alternative method is to include "age at death" or "months until death" at baseline as a predictor in the model. This is not a problem for studies with complete follow-up (nonmissing age at death). For ongoing studies or studies *without mortality surveillance*, however, two-stage multiple imputation (Harel, Hofer, & Schafer, 2003), or full information, maximum likelihood methods (e.g., Johansson et al., 2004) may be used for estimation when members of the sample have not yet experienced mortality.

## IV. Modeling the Effects of Time

Contemporary methods of growth curve analysis are rooted in the historical concerns of educational and psychological researchers with the measurement and analysis of change (Harris, 1963). Early fixed-effects ANOVA models were formulated for repeated measures designs involving two or more groups of subjects in which each subject had measurements on two or more occasions (Lindquist, 1953). These early statistical models focused explicitly on *within-person change*, although notions of individual differences in growth or development were fairly primitive in these early statistical treatments. Early methodological contributions concentrated primarily on the problems and limitations of "difference scores" for assessing change (Cronbach & Furby, 1970; Lord, 1963). More recently, modern statistical models for the analysis of growth (and decline) were stimulated in part by early applications of growth curve analysis to the measurement of change (Rogosa, Brandt, & Zimowski, 1982). Somewhat parallel developments occurred with respect to

the analysis of change using causal models of change in panel data (Jöreskog, 1979). This separate regression-based tradition for the analysis of change grew out of causal modeling and structural equation developments in sociology and econometrics (Alwin, 1988). Major shortcomings of this approach for analyzing change, however, are that it focused primarily on inter-individual differences rather than intra-individual change and had no readily available way to incorporate trends in means and individual-level trajectories of change.

In recent years, pioneering work has brought these two traditions together into models of individual growth that can be conceptualized within the general framework offered SEM or covariance structure analysis (e.g., McArdle & Bell, 2000; McArdle & Hamagami, 2001; Meredith & Tisak, 1990; Willett & Sayer, 1994). This approach is referred to as *latent growth curve* (LGC) analysis because the variables representing individual-level intercepts and slopes are incorporated as latent common factors. Given this formulation, LGC models can be embedded in the general SEM approach, and thus have a natural kinship to confirmatory factor models and models for factorial invariance (Alwin, 1988).

Growth models are well suited to the study of aging because they focus on continuous processes of change and can allow for measurement errors in the variables assessed over time. Designs that repeatedly measure the same persons over time are uniquely suited to the analysis and investigation of these issues (Baltes, Cornelius, & Nesselroade, 1979; Baltes & Nesselroade, 1979). Here we discuss several issues (identified by the subheadings in this section) that focus on fundamental strategies of modeling *within-person change relative to events occurring in time*, events that give meaning to individual differences in patterns of change. Because of space limitations, we have been selective in our coverage, leaving out some areas of potential interest (e.g., growth mixture modeling), and we have not been able to consider any single area in great depth. It is hoped that our discussion of these matters will orient the reader to the relevant issues and point to other literature that can encourage a deeper appreciation than we can provide.

## A. Occasion-Based Strategies

There are several alternate ways to construct individual latent growth models (e.g., McArdle & Bell, 2000; Meredith & Tisak, 1990; Willett & Sayer, 1994). In this chapter we conceptualize the models in a SEM framework, but there is an equally common approach in the multilevel regression analysis tradition. For example, such models can also be viewed as a special application of multilevel models in which occasions of measurement are nested within persons, where the level-1 model is used to specify the population function of change (i.e., time in study, chronological age, time to event; e.g., Bryk & Raudenbush, 1992; Hox, 2002). The LGC model is statistically equivalent to a random coefficients model for change over time when time values are discrete across occasions. Because the multilevel modeling approach includes time as a variable in the regression model rather than as a basis parameter (Figure 2.1), it permits a more flexible specification of time in that its values can be different for each individual at each occasion of measurement.

All growth models begin with the specification of a within-person (i.e., intra-individual) model for change over the period of measurement; these are often referred to as time-based or occasion-based models, though for individuals measured longitudinally, there is a perfect correlation between time of measurement and age. When these models are aggregated across individuals, the latent factor means repre-

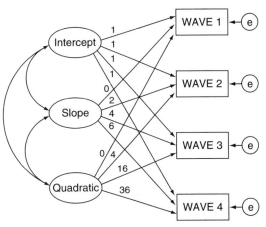

**Figure 2.1**  Causal diagram for occasion-based latent growth model using structural equation methods (Zimprich, Hofer, & Aartsen, 2004)

sent the average trajectory, whereas the factor variances reflect the person-to-person variability of the individual-level curves. Capitalizing on the heterogeneity of birth cohorts that may exist in a data set, separate occasion-based models can be specified for each cohort, and with the appropriate between-person model constraints, the cohort-specific models can then be combined to relatively quickly construct age trajectories that represent the processes of aging across an age range equal to the span of measurement (in years) plus the number of the birth cohorts in the sample. Models such as these, in which within- and between-person models are combined, are referred to as age-based or convergence models.

The causal diagram in Figure 2.1 presents an illustration of a generic occasion-based growth curve model for four waves of data. Although we do not present the mathematical formula here, this is a model for latent intra-individual change in a given variable that is derived from the specification of two models: (a) a measurement model and (b) a model for intra-individual change, where the measurement model for the pth person for a given observed variable y measured at time t is assumed to follow the assumptions of classical measurement theory, and the intra-individual change model is stated for a single true score measured over time (Willett & Sayer, 1994). Note that this model can be readily generalized to the situation where multiple congeneric true scores thought to measure a "factor" may be assessed. In such a case the change process would be modeled for the factor relating the true scores of separate indicators rather than for true scores themselves.

The intra-individual growth model is sometimes called a *level-1* model. Once this model is formulated and estimated, one can examine a *level-2* model for explaining inter-individual differences in levels (intercepts) and rates of change (slopes) in the *level-1* model (Willett & Sayer, 1994, pp. 363–364). Although not represented in Figure 2.1, one of the purposes of the level-2 model is to include covariates to account for variation in the intercepts and slopes. These are often referred to as random coefficients models, as the groups (individuals) are conceptualized as, and in many cases are, a sample from a larger population. Of particular interest is the inclusion of covariates that represent some function of time to account for levels (intercepts) and the rates of change of the dependent variable of interest.

The growth model for *within-person change* in the generic case (Figure 2.1) expresses change as a function of time, where an individual's score at a given point in time is a function of an intercept (or level) parameter, a linear slope parameter, a quadratic slope parameter reflecting some form of curvature, and a disturbance term. The arrows connecting the latent variables and the observed variables are called *latent basis parameters* or *factor loadings*, which are fixed to reflect the nature of the growth function. The particular form of the model is then fit to the data and the model is assessed using standard strategies for evaluating goodness of fit. For example, if change is theorized to be a simple linear function of time, the quadratic latent variable would be omitted and the latent basis parameters for the slope factor would be fixed, for example, at "years since initial testing" (where t = 0, 1, 2, 3 in waves separated by one-year intervals, or some linear transformation of these values). Or, the time-basis parameters might be fixed to represent some form of curvature (e.g., in a quadratic form). One does not *generally* assume that individual change is a linear function of time, and therefore one should use these coefficients to formulate various hypotheses to be tested against the data, or as group-level parameters to be estimated (see McArdle & Bell, 2000, pp. 81–82).

## B. Age-Based or Convergence Models

As mentioned previously, it is possible to aggregate models of intra-individual change across individuals from different birth cohorts, combining observed within-person change and between-person differences, to construct trajectories for a broad range of ages that follow the same overall age function. Such approaches are referred to by a variety of names, including convergence models (McArdle, Anderson, & Aber, 1987; McArdle & Bell, 2000; McArdle & Hamagami, 2001), accelerated longitudinal designs (Bell, 1953, 1954; Miyazaki and Raudenbush, 2000; Raudenbush & Chan, 1992), cohort sequential designs (Baltes & Nesselroade, 1979; Muthén & Muthén, 2000, 2002), or simply age-based modeling. We like the *convergence* terminology for these models, but we also find it somewhat more accurate to refer to these as age-based models because this is how time is modeled in the basis parameters.

A strict age-based model specifies complete convergence between the within-person and between-person models, and therefore it specifies the same functional form in both parts of the model. If one hypothesizes the overall age trajectory to be curvilinear, it *generally* makes little sense to specify a linear trend in the within-person model, though if the period of measurement is short, this may, in practice, make little difference. Note that in the occasion-based models discussed above, the age-specific factor means were unconstrained—their values were determined entirely by the effects of age and age$^2$ estimated in the data. The between-person effects of age are therefore modeled by changing the slope and intercept for each age according to a set of regression coefficients. In a *convergence* model, the function of age is directly in the growth model, rather than including age and age$^2$ as covariates. In the "age-based" convergence model, there is a fixed intercept and slope, but the basis parameters vary across birth cohorts. The *convergence* model requires the age-specific factor means to have the same intercept and slope (and quadratic) means across groups defined by birth cohorts (e.g., the cohort differences and within-person change estimates should "converge" to the same value). The model can be specified as a multiple-group model in which there is a different group for each baseline age group (i.e., birth cohort), and the basis parameters in each group model growth as a function of age rather than time since first measurement. Imagine a separate version of Figure 2.1 for each birth cohort, such that within groups there is age-homogeny at each occasion of measurement. Note that although it is possible to fit the age-based model as a single-group model with some data missing by design, there are a variety of hypotheses regarding the nature of age and cohort differences that are best addressed in a multiple-group framework.

In the occasion-based approach, specific nonlinearities in the age function can be modeled by the inclusion of predictors constructed to fit the needs of theory. For example, instead of using age-squared as a predictor, one could construct a predictor variable that was zero for all cases up to some age, and then increased as a linear function. Age-specific residuals can be modeled in the same way. In the age-based models, such things would be modeled through the inclusion of additional latent factors for the relevant cohort groups. The point is that many of the same hypotheses can be tested in either model.

## C. Testing for Cohort Effects

The demographic literature concerned with cohort effects has focused primarily on differences between cohorts in levels (or intercepts) of variables (Siegel & Swanson, 2004). By contrast, in the developmental literature, cohort variation has been phrased in terms of the existence (or lack thereof) of "simple age-graded nomothetic and universal patterns of behavioral development" (Baltes et al., 1979, p. 86). Both of these issues may be investigated using growth models by examining the differences between two sets of models, one that posits *intra-individual change* across all cohorts follows the same overall age-based trajectory (i.e., the convergence model) (Bell, 1953, 1954; McArdle & Bell, 2000) and one that posits differences in intercepts and slopes across cohorts. Building on modeling strategies used by Miyazaki and Raudenbush (2000), McArdle, Anderson, and Aber (1987), and Muthén and Muthén (2000), a comparison between age-based and occasion-based LGC models can be constructed in a way that tests for cohort differences in slopes and intercepts. This comparison can be implemented using the multiple-group model described previously, where the groups are defined by birth year.

## D. Event-Centered Time Structures

Given an event of substantive interest, it may be useful to describe processes of change that precede or follow the event, regardless of the age of the individual. These event-centered strategies permit a potentially more nuanced version of within-person change than that captured by relying on *time in study* or *age*. For example, one might define widowhood as an event, studying patterns of depression or other measures of psychological well-being as a function of time since the event. A number of process-based time structures and event-centered approaches provide exemplars of the fruitfulness of the approach (e.g., time to death, time to dementia diagnosis). For example, Sliwinski, Hofer, and Hall (2003) used alternative time specifications in mixed models to show how memory loss in aging adults may be due to the progression of preclinical dementia and other nonnormative aging processes that are not captured by chronological age, and how the interpretation of fixed and random effects changes under alternative specifications of time.

As discussed earlier, models based on *time in study* include covariates such as chronological age and other covariates to account for the heterogeneity in individual differences in level and change. Age-based models, as described previously, model age-differences and age-changes as average or fixed effects and often include other covariates as well. Alternatively, event-centered time structures can be used to account for heterogeneity in initial status and rate of change in terms of common patterns of change that occur before or after a discrete time-based structure or event. In the results of Sliwinski et al. (2003), representing cognitive loss as a function of disease progression (indexed by time to diagnosis) provided a much better fit to the data than did representing cognitive change as a function of chronological age. These types of alternative time specifications will lead to different interpretations of the same data. In non-informative time metrics (e.g., time in

study), the heterogeneity of initial status and change (random effects) is accounted for by covariates, whereas in models with informative time metrics, the heterogeneity is accounted for by the alignment of individual change with the time structure and fixed effects specified in the model.

### E. Examining Retest Effects

Retest or practice effects have been reported in a number of longitudinal studies on aging (e.g., Ferrer, Salthouse, Stewart, & Schwartz, 2004; Hultsch, Hertzog, Dixon, & Small, 1998). In longitudinal studies on aging, within-individual change may be attenuated by the observed gains produced by repeated testing (e.g., Schaie, 1996; Willis & Schaie, 1994). For example, Hofland, Willis, and Baltes (1981) found improvements over eight occasions spaced at half-week intervals in adults 60 to 80 years old on several measures of reasoning ability. Complicating matters is the potential for improvement to occur differentially in individuals differing in age, ability, and health (e.g., Rabbitt, 1993; Rabbitt, Diggle, Smith, Holland, & McInnes, 2001). Such retest effects may be due to any number of overlapping influences, including warm-up effects and initial anxiety. Short-term gains from repeated testing, related to test-specific learning of content and strategies for improving performance, can be of direct interest. For example, Zimprich, Hofer, and Aartsen (2004) found that short-term practice gains in processing speed were positively associated with long-term (6-year) changes in processing speed in elders.

Although design-based strategies for controlling retesting effects have been used (McArdle & Woodcock, 1997), recent innovations in estimating practice effects are based on a specification of the piecewise linear growth curve model. There are now several proposed procedures to directly model retest effects (e.g., Ferrer et al., 2004; McArdle, Ferrer-Caja, Hamagami, & Woodcock, 2002; Rabbitt et al., 2001). These procedures require age-based modeling (as described previously) and make use of between-person age differences to correct within-person changes. This approach requires study designs where age is heterogeneous and not highly related to time-in-study in order to estimate separate parameters related to exposure to test (i.e., number of repeated occasions or time in study) and age-based trajectories.

## F. Dual Change Score Models

The analysis of change using growth models is often contrasted with traditional multi-wave panel analysis (autoregressive or quasi-Markov simplex models; see Jöreskog, 1970). Growth models are sometimes presented as if they provide an alternative to the autoregressive approaches. Although we do not cover autoregressive models in this chapter, we believe they assess a complementary set of issues—the stability of individual differences—and both are valuable in the study of human development and aging (see Curran & Bollen, 2001, and McArdle & Hamagami, 2001, for contrasting views).

McArdle and Nesselroade (1994, pp. 234–236) proposed a model that included two components of individual change, constant change over time, and proportional (autoregressive) change across occasions. The constant change component is typically emphasized in linear growth curve models, whereas the proportional change model is associated with the "stability" coefficient in autoregressive models of change. The two components of individual change have been parameterized within the dual change score model (McArdle & Hamagami, 2001). Curran and Bollen (2001) proposed a different model in which they include both autoregressive change and linear growth over time. In more general terms, Rovine and Molenaar (2005) showed that linear growth curve models are a special case of the general autoregressive model with structured means. This illustrates that new methods for modeling change are continually being developed, and aging researchers should watch these developments carefully.

## G. Multivariate Models

We have proposed a framework for the consideration of time that draws attention not only to developmental perspectives, but also to historical and life course conceptions of time. The study of social and behavioral processes in time often requires a multivariate perspective. The level-1 models discussed in the previous sections are, in a sense, univariate models and represent the basic building blocks for developing theories and/or models of aging. While the time structure incorporated in the model may inform a particular hypothesis, thus obviating the utility of statistical controls, it is often useful to incorporate additional covariates to account for individual heterogeneity in the latent trajectories. The most obvious way to create multivariate models of growth is to simply include the covariates in the model. This can be done in three different ways used alone or in combination: (1) variables can be controlled by selection—for example, by sex of respondent; (2) variables can be included as predictors of the latent intercept and slope factors; and (3) variables may be included as direct predictors of the observed variables. The most appropriate approach depends on the substantive objectives of the investigator.

The manner of inclusion of covariates and their interpretation is contingent on the time structure specified in the latent curve model. For instance, when a fixed covariate, such as educational attainment, is thought to have a linear effect on the observed dependent variables, this can be modeled in one of two equivalent ways. Either the covariate can be allowed to predict the observed variable at each occasion of measurement, with the regression weights constrained equal, or the covariate can simply be allowed to predict the latent intercept. If the effect of the covariate was thought to vary as a function of some time structure, then the method of entry depends on the time structure built into the latent curve model. If educational attainment is entered in an occasion-based model as a predictor of the latent intercept and slope(s), it implies that the effect of education on the observed variables differs as a function of time in study, a hypothesis that, although possible, is likely not what is intended by the researcher. Rather, if the effect of the covariate on the observed dependent variable is thought to vary as a function of age, then in an occasion-based model, one approach would be to construct an interaction term between age and the variable in question. Alternatively, if age is built into the time structure of the model (i.e., an age-based model), then this interaction is implied, not by an interaction term, but by allowing the covariate to predict the latent slope.

If instead of being constant over time (fixed), the value of the covariate differs over the occasions of measurement (time-varying), as in the case of a variable such as visual acuity or self-reported health, then the covariate is included in the latent curve model in one of two ways. First, the covariate at each occasion of measurement can simply be allowed to predict the observed dependent variable at the same occasion (or at the subsequent occasion, depending on the hypothesized or observed lag). Alternatively, the time-varying covariate can be modeled according its own latent curve trajectory, the parameters of which then also become available as predictors of either

the dependent latent factors or dependent observed variables. Multivariate change can be assessed in terms of correlated slopes, as well as correlations among time-specific residuals (within-person correlation or coupling). The bivariate dual change score model (McArdle, 2001; McArdle & Hamagami, 2001; McArdle, Hamagami, Meredith, & Bradway, 2000) permits an alternative specification of change involving both correlated slopes and evaluation of lead-lag associations among detrended difference scores. Such approaches offer a wealth of possibilities to the modeler; however, we urge careful consultation of theory in the specification and interpretation of such models, including the temporal sampling of predictors and outcomes (e.g., Martin & Hofer, 2004).

## V. Conclusions

In this chapter we argued that studies of human development and aging can benefit from the phrasing of hypotheses within the framework of studies of *within-person* change. We focused on five central issues that are uniquely suited to longitudinal analysis using growth curve models: (1) specifying individual trajectories of within-person change, (2) modeling individual differences in trajectories of within-person change, (3) specifying the determinants and/or predictors of individual differences in patterns of change (e.g., age), (4) testing for cohort differences in patterns of within-person change, and (5) modeling the effects of events and transitions on processes of change (Baltes & Nesselroade, 1979; Baltes, Cornelius & Nesselroade, 1979).

We conclude that when combined with sampling designs that are adequate for the generalization of findings to populations of interest, along with strategies for handling cross-wave panel nonresponse, new longitudinal investigations can take advantage of the significant improvements that have been made in studying *change within individuals as they age*, and that a variety of conceptions of time, including components that represent events in both historical and biographical time, can be used creatively to provide theoretically informed interpretations of individual change.

## Acknowledgments

Supported by research grant (AG-20099-03) for the project "Latent Growth Models of Cognitive Aging" from the National Institute on Aging (D.F. Alwin and W.L. Rodgers, Principal Investigators).

## References

Allison, P. D. (1987). Estimation of linear models with incomplete data. In C. Clogg (Ed.), *Sociological methodology 1987* (pp. 71–103). Washington DC: American Sociological Association.

Allison, P. D. (2001). *Missing data*. Sage University Papers Series on Quantitative Applications in the Social Sciences, 7–136. Thousand Oaks, CA: Sage.

Alwin, D. F. (1988). Structural equation models in research on human development and aging. In K. W. Schaie, R. T. Campbell, W. Meredith, & S. Rawlings (Eds.), *Methodological issues in aging research* (pp. 71–170). New York: Springer.

Alwin, D. F. (1995). Taking time seriously: Studying social change, social structure and human lives. In P. Moen, G. H. Elder, Jr., & K. Lüscher (Eds.), *Examining lives in context: Perspectives on the ecology of human development* (pp. 211–262). Washington, DC: American Psychological Association.

Alwin, D. F., Cohen, R. L., & Newcomb, T. M. (1991). *Political attitudes over the life span: The Bennington women after fifty years.* Madison: University of Wisconsin Press.

Alwin, D. F., & McCammon, R. J. (2001). Aging, cohorts and verbal ability. *Journal of Gerontology: Social Sciences, 56B*, S1–S11.

Alwin, D. F., & McCammon, R. J. (2003). Generations, cohorts, and social change. In J. Mortimer & M. Shanahan (Eds.), *Handbook of the life course* (pp. 23–49). New York: Plenum Publishing.

Arbuckle, J. L. (2000). Customizing longitudinal and multiple-group structural modeling procedures. In T. Little, K. Schnabel, & J. Baumert (Eds.), *Modeling longitudinal and multilevel data: Practical issues, applied approaches and specific examples* (pp. 241–248). Mahwah, NJ: Lawrence Erlbaum Associates, Publishers.

Baltes, P. B. (1987). Theoretical propositions of life-span developmental psychology: On the dynamics between growth and decline. *Developmental Psychology, 23*, 611–626.

Baltes, P. B., Cornelius, S. W., & Nesselroade, J. R. (1979). Cohort effects in developmental psychology. In J. R. Nesselroade & P. B. Baltes (Eds.), *Longitudinal research in the study of behavior and development* (pp. 61–87). New York: Academic Press.

Baltes, P. B., & Nesselroade, J. R. (1979). History and rationale of longitudinal research. In J. R. Nesselroade & P. B. Baltes (Eds.), *Longitudinal research in the study of behavior and development* (pp. 1–39). New York: Academic Press.

Baltes, P. B., Staudinger, U.M., & Lindenberger, U. (1999). Lifespan psychology: Theory and application to intellectual functioning. *Annual Review of Psychology, 50*, 471–507.

Bell, R. Q. (1953). Convergence: An accelerated longitudinal approach. *Child Development, 27*, 45–74.

Bell, R. Q. (1954). An experimental test of the accelerated longitudinal approach. *Child Development, 25*, 281–286.

Bronfenbrenner, U. (1979). *The ecology of human development*. Cambridge, MA: Harvard University Press.

Bryk, A. S., & Raudenbush, S. W. (1992). *Hierarchical linear models: Applications and data analysis methods*. Newbury Park, CA: Sage Publications.

Carey, J. R. (2003). Life span: A conceptual overview. *Population and Development Review, 29* (Supplement), 1–18.

Cronbach, L. J., & Furby, L. (1970). How should we measure "change"—or should we? *Psychological Bulletin, 74*, 8–80.

Curran, P. J., & Bollen, K. A. (2001). The best of both worlds: Combining autoregressive and latent curve models. In L. Collins, & A. Sayer (Eds.), *New methods for the analy-*

sis of change (pp. 105–135). Washington, DC: American Psychological Association.

Diggle, P. J., Liang, K. Y., & Zeger, S. L. (1994). Analysis of longitudinal data. New York: Oxford University Press.

Elder, G. H., Jr., Johnson, M. K., & Crosnoe, R. (2003). The emergence and development of life course theory. In J. Mortimer & M. Shanahan (Eds.), Handbook of the life course (pp. 3–19). New York: Plenum Publishing.

Ferraro, K. F. (2001). Aging and role transitions. In R. Binstock & L. George (Eds.), Handbook of aging and the social sciences (5th ed., pp. 313–330). New York: Academic Press.

Ferraro, K. F., & Wilmoth, J. M. (2000). Measuring morbidity: Disease counts, binary variables, and statistical power. Journal of Gerontology: Social Sciences, 55B, S173–S189.

Ferrer, E., Salthouse, T. A., Stewart, W. F., & Schwartz, B. S. (2004). Modeling age and retest processes in longitudinal studies of cognitive abilities. Psychology and Aging, 19, 243–259.

Harel, O., Hofer, S. M., & Schafer, J. L. (2003). Analysis of longitudinal data with missing values of two qualitatively different types. Paper presented at the annual meeting of the International Biometric Society (Eastern North American Region), Tampa, FL, March.

Hareven, T. K. (1982). Family time and industrial time. Cambridge, UK: Cambridge University Press.

Harris, C. W. (Ed.). (1963). Problems in measuring change. Madison: The University of Wisconsin Press.

Hofland, B. F., Willis, S. L., & Baltes, P. B. (1981). Fluid intelligence performance in the elderly: Intraindividual variability and conditions of assessment. Journal of Educational Psychology, 73, 573–586.

Hogan, D. P. (2000). Life cycle. In E. Borgatta and R. Montgomery (Eds.), Encyclopedia of sociology (2nd ed., pp. 1623–1627). New York: Macmillan.

Horn, J. L., & McArdle, J. J. (1992). A practical and theoretical guide to measurement invariance in aging research. Experimental Aging Research, 18, 117–144.

Hox, J. J. (2002). Multilevel analysis: Techniques and applications. Mahwah, NJ: Erlbaum.

Hultsch, D. F., Hertzog, C., Dixon, R. A., & Small, B. J. (1998). Memory changes in the aged. New York: Cambridge University Press.

Johansson, B., Hofer, S. M., Allaire, J. C., Maldonado-Molina, M., Piccinin, A. M., Berg, S., Pedersen, N., & McClearn, G. E. (2004). Change in memory and cognitive functioning in the oldest-old: The effects of proximity to death in genetically related individuals over a six-year period. Psychology and Aging, 19, 145–156.

Johnson, D. R., & Elliott, L. A. (1998). Sampling design effects: Do they affect the analyses of data from the National Survey of Families and Households? Journal of Marriage and the Family, 60, 993–1001.

Jöreskog, K. G. (1970). Estimating and testing of simplex models. British Journal of Mathematical and Statistical Psychology, 23, 121–145.

Jöreskog, K. G. (1979). Statistical estimation of structural models in longitudinal developmental investigations. In J. R. Nesselroade & P. B. Baltes (Eds.), Longitudinal research in the study of behavior and development (pp. 303–374). New York: Academic Press.

Kirkwood, T. (1999). Time of our lives: The science of human aging. New York: Oxford.

Kish, L. (1965). Survey sampling. New York: Wiley.

Kish, L. (1987). Statistical design for research. New York: Wiley.

Korn, E., & Graubard, B. (1991). Epidemiological studies utilizing surveys: Accounting for sample design. American Journal of Public Health, 81, 1166–1173.

Lindquist, E. F. (1953). Design and analysis of experiments in psychology and education. Boston: Houghton Mifflin.

Little, R. J., & Rubin, D. B. (1987). Statistical analysis with missing data. New York: Wiley.

Lord, F. M. (1963). Elementary models for measuring change. In C. Harris (Ed.), Problems in measuring change (pp. 21–38). Madison WI: University of Wisconsin Press.

Macmillan, R., & Eliason, S. R. (2003). Characterizing the life course as role configurations and pathways: A latent structure approach. In J. Mortimer & M. Shanahan (Eds.), Handbook of the life course (pp. 529–554). New York: Plenum Publishing.

Martin, M., & Hofer, S. M. (2004). Intraindividual variability, change, and aging: Conceptual and analytical issues. Gerontology, 50, 7–11.

McArdle, J. J. (2001). A latent difference score approach to longitudinal dynamic structural analyses. In R. Cudeck, S. du Toit, & D.

Sörbom (Eds.), *Structural equation modeling: Present and future* (pp. 342–380). Lincolnwood, IL: Scientific Software International.

McArdle, J. J., Anderson, E., & Aber, M. (1987). Convergence hypotheses modeled and tested with linear structural equations. In *Proceedings of the 1987 Public Health Conference on Records and Statistics* (pp. 351–357). Hyattsville, MD: National Center for Health Statistics.

McArdle, J. J., & Bell, R. Q. (2000). An introduction to latent growth models for developmental data analysis. In T. Little, K. Schnabel, & J. Baumert (Eds.), *Modeling longitudinal and multilevel data: Practical issues, applied approaches and specific examples* (pp. 69–107). Mahwah, NJ: Lawrence Erlbaum.

McArdle, J. J., Ferrer-Caja, E., Hamagami, F., & Woodcock, R. W. (2002). Comparative longitudinal structural analyses of the growth and decline of multiple intellectual abilities over the life span. *Developmental Psychology, 38*, 115–142.

McArdle, J. J., & Hamagami, F. (1992). Modeling incomplete longitudinal and cross-sectional data using latent growth structural models. *Experimental Aging Research, 18*, 145–166.

McArdle, J. J., & Hamagami, F. (2001). Latent difference score structural models for linear dynamic analyses with incomplete longitudinal data. In L. Collins & A. Sayer (Eds.), *New methods for the analysis of change* (pp. 137–175). Washington DC: American Psychological Association.

McArdle, J. J., Hamagami, F., Meredith, W., & Bradway, K. P. (2000). Modeling the dynamic hypotheses of Gf-Gc theory using longitudinal life-span data. *Learning and Individual Differences, 12*, 53–79.

McArdle, J.J., & Nesselroade, J.R. (1994). Using multivariate data to structure developmental change. In S. Cohen & H. Reese (Eds.), *Life-span developmental psychology*. Hillsdale NJ: Lawrence Erlbaum.

McArdle, J. J., & Nesselroade, J. R. (2003). Growth curve analysis in contemporary psychological research. In J. Schinka & W. Velicer (Eds.), *Handbook of psychology: Research methods in psychology* (vol. 2, pp. 447–480). New York: John Wiley & Sons, Inc.

McArdle, J. J., & Woodcock, R. W. (1997). Expanding test-retest designs to include developmental time-lag components. *Psychological Methods, 2*, 403–435.

Meredith, W. (1993). Measurement invariance, factor analysis and factorial invariance. *Psychometrika, 58*, 525–543.

Meredith, W., & Horn, J.L. (2001). The role of factorial invariance in modeling growth and change. In L. Collins & A. Sayer (Eds.), *New methods for the analysis of change* (pp. 204–240). Washington, DC: American Psychological Association.

Meredith, W., & Tisak, J. (1990). Latent curve analysis. *Psychometrika, 55*, 107–122.

Miyazaki, Y., & Raudenbush, S. W. (2000). Tests for linkage of multiple cohorts in an accelerated longitudinal design. *Psychological Methods, 5*, 44–63.

Murphy, K. R., & Myors, B. (2004). *Statistical power analysis: A simple and general model for traditional and modern hypothesis tests* (2nd ed.). Mahwah, NJ: Lawrence Erlbaum Associates.

Muthén, B. O., & Curran, P. J. (1997). General longitudinal modeling of individual differences in experimental designs: A latent variable framework for analysis and power estimation. *Psychological Methods, 2*, 371–402.

Muthén, B. O., & Muthén, L. K. (2000). The development of heavy drinking and alcohol-related problems from ages 18 to 37 in a U.S. national sample. *Journal of Studies on Alcohol, 6*, 290–300.

Muthén, L. K., & Muthén, B. O. (2002). How to use a Monte Carlo study to decide on sample size and determine power. *Structural Equation Modeling, 4*, 599–620.

Muthén, L. K., & Muthén, B. O. (2004). *Mplus: The comprehensive modeling program for applied researchers. User's guide*. Version 3.1. Los Angeles, CA.

Nesselroade, J. R. (1988). Sampling and generalizability: Adult development and aging research issues examined within the general methodological framework of selection. In K. W. Schaie, R. T. Campbell, W. Meredith, & S. Rawlings (Eds.), *Methodological issues in aging research* (pp. 13–42). New York: Springer Publishing Company.

O'Rand, A. M., & Krecker, M. L. (1990). Concepts of the life cycle: Their history, meanings, and uses in the social sciences. In

W. Scott & J. Blake (Eds.), *Annual Review of Sociology* (vol. 16, pp. 241–262). Palo Alto CA: Annual Reviews Inc.

Rabbitt, P. (1993). Does it all go together when it goes? The Nineteenth Bartlett Memorial Lecture. *Quarterly Journal of Experimental Psychology: Human Experimental Psychology, 46A,* 385–434.

Rabbitt, P., Diggle, P., Smith, D., Holland, F., & McInnes, L. M. (2001). Identifying and separating the effects of practice and of cognitive ageing during a large longitudinal study of elderly community residents. *Neuropsychologia, 39,* 532–543.

Raudenbush, S. W., & Chan, W.-S. (1992). Growth curve analysis in accelerated longitudinal designs. *Journal of Research in Crime and Delinquency, 29,* 387–411.

Rindfuss, R. R. (1991). The young adult years: Diversity, structural change, and fertility. *Demography, 28,* 493–512.

Rodgers, W. L., Ofstedal, M. B., & Herzog, A. R. (2003). Trends in scores on tests of cognitive ability in the elderly U.S. population, 1993–2000. *Journal of Gerontology: Social Sciences, 58B,* S338–S346.

Rogosa, D. R., Brandt, D., & Zimowski, M. (1982). A growth curve approach to the measurement of change. *Psychological Bulletin, 90,* 726–748.

Rovine, M. J., & Molenaar, P. C. M. (2005). Relating factor models for longitudinal data to quasi-simplex and NARMA models. *Multivariate Behavioral Research, 40,* 83–114.

Ryder, N. B. (1965). The cohort as a concept in the study of social change. *American Sociological Review, 30,* 843–861.

Schafer, J. L. (1997). *Analysis of incomplete multivariate data.* New York: Chapman and Hall.

Schafer, J. L., & Graham, J. W. (2002). Missing data: Our view of the state of the art. *Psychological Methods, 7,* 147–177.

Schaie, K. W. (1996). *Intellectual development in adulthood: The Seattle longitudinal study.* Cambridge UK: Cambridge University Press.

Schaie, K. W., & Hofer, S. M. (2001). Longitudinal studies in aging research. In J. E. Birren & K. W. Schaie (Eds.), *Handbook*

of the psychology of aging (5th ed., pp. 53–77). San Diego: Academic Press.

Settersten, R. A., Jr. (2003). Propositions and controversies in life-course scholarship. In R. A. Settersten, Jr. (Ed.), *Invitation to the life course: Toward new understandings of later life* (pp. 15–45). Amityville NY: Baywood Publishing Co. Inc.

Siegel, J. S., & Swanson, D. A. (2004). *The methods and materials of demography* (2nd ed.). New York: Elsevier Academic Press.

Sliwinski, M. J., Hofer, S. M., & Hall, C. (2003). Correlated and coupled cognitive change in older adults with and without clinical dementia. *Psychology and Aging, 18,* 672–683.

Widaman, K., & Reise, S. P. (1997). Exploring the measurement invariance of psychological instruments: Applications in the substance use domain. In K. Bryant, M. Windle, & S. West (Eds.), *The science of prevention: methodological advances from alcohol and substance abuse research* (pp. 281–324). Washington, DC: American Psychological Association.

Willett, J. B., & Sayer, A. G. (1994). Using covariance structure analysis to detect correlates and predictors of individual change over time. *Psychological Bulletin, 116,* 363–381.

Willis, S. L., & Schaie, K. W. (1994). Cognitive training in the normal elderly. In F. Forette, Y. Christen, & F. Boller (Eds.), *Plasticité cérébrale et stimulation cognitive* (pp. 91–113). Paris: Fondation Nationale de Gérontologie.

Winship, C., & Radbill, L. (1994). Sampling weights and regression analysis. *Sociological Methods and Research, 23,* 230–257.

Wothke, W. (2000). Longitudinal and multigroup modeling with missing data. In T. Little, K. Schnabel, & J. Baumert (Eds.), *Modeling longitudinal and multilevel data: Practical issues, applied approaches and specific examples* (pp. 219–240). Mahwah, NJ: Lawrence Erlbaum Associates, Publishers.

Zimprich, D., Hofer, S. M., & Aartsen, M. J. (2004). Short-term versus long-term longitudinal changes in processing speed. *Gerontology, 50,* 17–21.

## Part Two

# Aging and Social Structure

# Three

# Morbidity, Disability, and Mortality

Kenneth C. Land and Yang Yang

Levels of, and trends in, morbidity, disability, and mortality often are interpreted as indicators of population health and are used to study how health is impacted by demographic and social structures and changes therein (Pol & Thomas, 1992). *Morbidity* refers to the extent and type of illness, disease, or sickness in a society, both physical and mental. Because it often is difficult to obtain measures of incidence or prevalence of sickness for representative samples of a large population, analysts often focus on measures of *disability*, which is defined in terms of restrictions in schooling, work, or normal activities of daily living. For reasons that will become evident later in this chapter, measures of disability actually function quite well as indicators of illness in older populations and thus are good measures of morbidity. *Mortality* refers to the rate of the event of death characterizing a population.

The morbidity, disability, and mortality of populations have been a focus of study in demography, social epidemiology, and medical sociology. Each of these disciplines brings to bear on these subjects a characteristic set of theories, modes of analysis, and explanatory variables.

*Demographers* are concerned with distributions of vital rates in populations, sources of variations in these rates or population dynamics, demographic consequences of changes in the age-sex structures of populations over time, and forecasting. They tend to emphasize population-level models of survival across the entire life course (or a substantial segment thereof) such as the life table and thus emphasize age as the key explanatory variable (Preston, Heuveline, & Guillot, 2001). When they study sample rather than complete population data, demographers often use sample-based models of survival analysis such as hazard regression models. *Social epidemiologists* are concerned with social variations in diseases and measures of prevalence and incidence rates of age-specific morbidity. They are more likely to focus on a shorter time interval and a fixed event, such as whether individuals have or do not have a particular disease or health condition or do or do not respond to a treatment. Thus, the prototypical analytical model is either a logistic regression model or, like demographers, a hazard regression model (Rockett, 1999).

The basic demographic variables of age, sex, and race/ethnicity are of central

*Handbook of Aging and the Social Sciences, Sixth Edition*

interest to demographic studies. In addition, many demographic and social epidemiologic studies introduce various measures of social statuses (e.g., socioeconomic status, marriage and family relations) and behavioral and health factors (e.g., exercise patterns, religious participation, cigarette smoking, dietary practices and food consumption, mental and addictive disorders) that may impact morbidity, disability, and mortality outcomes.

*Medical sociologists* adopt a structural approach to sociological research on illness and health. The major goal is to explain how health is affected by systems of social stratification and inequality. This approach has used the stress process model (Holmes & Rahe, 1967; Pearlin, Lieberman, Menaghan, & Mullan, 1981) as the connection between social structure and health outcomes: High levels of illness and disease among some segments of society can be attributed to their extreme exposure to social stressors or limited access to ameliorative psychosocial resources to cope with stress. Medical sociologists emphasize the interplay of a complex array of social and psychological processes, such as the social origins of stress and psychosocial coping resources that affect disease, disability, and mortality outcomes, often measured in the form of scaled or continuous variables that measure health or mental health. Accordingly, conventional regression models and their extension to structural equation (simultaneous-equation) models that can represent the interconnectedness of multiple explanatory variables tend to be a major tool in medical sociology. Variables that have been commonly studied include life events, acute and chronic stressors, indicators of social class and socioeconomic status such as education, income, and occupation, social support, personal coping resources such as self-esteem and sense of control, and lifestyle and behavioral factors such

as drinking and smoking, to name but a few.

This chapter surveys some of the key theories, models, and findings regarding human morbidity, disability, and mortality, with a focus on aging and the health of older people. It commences with a review of epidemiological transition theory and a description of recent trends in overall adult mortality and mortality by cause-of-death over the past four decades in the United States. The focus then shifts to models and findings from medical demography, the subject of which is dynamics of morbidity, disability, and mortality in the context of adulthood and aging. This is followed by a section—which draws on the research literatures of social demography, social epidemiology, and medical sociology—on findings concerning the diversity of morbidity, disability, and mortality outcomes by demographic, social, and behavioral characteristics (i.e., of the health effects of demographic and social structures and changes therein). The chapter ends with a brief statement of conclusions and important directions for future research.

# I. Epidemiologic Transition Theory and Recent Trends in Adult Mortality

The twentieth century was a period of large increases in life expectancy in the United States. Life expectancy for all races and both sexes combined increased from 47.3 years in 1900 to 77.2 years in 2001 (National Center for Health Statistics, 2004). This is a gain of nearly 30 years, or, in relative terms, a remarkable increase of 62.6%. The rapid increase in life expectancy was accompanied by a substitution of degenerative causes of death such as heart disease and cancer for deaths that previously were caused by infectious and parasitic diseases.

This shift in mortality-related disease patterns is termed the *epidemiologic transition*. Epidemiologic transition theory was given its original statement by Omran (1971). According to the theory, as nations modernized in the twentieth century, they improved their social, economic, and health conditions. Part of the modernization process is the replacement of life conditions that previously were conducive to the spread of infectious and parasitic diseases by more sanitary conditions, improved medical technology, and better lifestyles. This reduces the population risk of dying from infectious diseases. Those saved from dying from such diseases survive into middle and older ages where they face the elevated risk of dying from degenerative diseases. Because degenerative diseases tend to kill at much older ages than infectious diseases, this transition in causes of death is characterized generally by a redistribution of deaths from younger to older ages.

Omran's original statement of epidemiologic transition theory focused on population-level consequences of the modernization of societies and identified *three stages of epidemiologic transition*: the *age of pestilence and famine*, the *age of receding pandemics*, and the *age of degenerative and man-made diseases*. More recent reformulations of the theory stress the fundamental importance of proximate determinants of disease and mortality outcomes such as cigarette smoking, dietary patterns, exercise, and sexual behavior for understanding health and survival (Olshansky, Carnes, Rogers, & Smith, 1997). Two reformulations have articulated a fourth stage of epidemiological transition (Olshansky & Ault, 1986; Rogers & Hackenberg, 1987).

To contextualize these reformulations, note that at the time of Omran's original statement of epidemiological transition theory, the United States had experienced relatively stable mortality rates for the decade from 1958 to 1968. Beginning in the late 1960s, however, the United States and other developed nations began to experience unexpectedly rapid declines in mortality rates for the major degenerative diseases. Olshansky and Ault (1986) identified several factors, including a pronounced shift in the age structure toward older ages, advances in medical technology and public health measures that favored the old over the young, federal health care programs that favored elderly adults and the poor, and reductions in risk factors on a population scale, that are responsible for this new era in human epidemiological history.

Olshansky and Ault (1986) argued that the timing and magnitude of this mortality transition is significant and distinct enough from the previous three stages to qualify as a *fourth stage of epidemiologic transition*, which they termed the *age of delayed degenerative diseases*. This fourth stage is characterized, firstly, by rapidly declining age-specific death rates that are concentrated mostly in advanced ages and that occur at nearly the same pace for males and females. Second, the age pattern of mortality by cause remains largely the same as in the third stage, but the age distribution of deaths from degenerative causes shifts progressively toward older ages. Third, relatively rapid improvements in survival across the life course and life expectancy are concentrated among the population at advanced ages. The result is that the expectation of life at birth in the United States has risen rapidly in recent years to the upper end of the seventh decade of life, and, among some populations in the developed world, to more than eight decades.

In brief, in the fourth stage of epidemiologic transition posited by Olshansky and Ault (1986), the major degenerative causes of death that prevailed during the third stage continue to be the major killers, but the risk of dying from these diseases is redistributed to older ages.

Olshansky and Ault (1986) examined trends in life expectancy, survival curves, and the percentage distributions by age of deaths from all causes and from three degenerative causes of death—ischemic heart disease, cerebrovascular disease, and malignant neoplasms—for the years 1960, 1970, and 1980 and found evidence in support of the postulated fourth stage.

Have the trends implied by the fourth stage of the epidemiologic transition con-tinued in the two decades since 1980? Consider a key characteristic of this phase, namely, shifts in the age distribu-tion of death toward older ages. A consis-tent pattern of redistribution of deaths from younger to older ages means that deaths that previously had occurred in younger ages were delayed, and, as a result, there should be a larger proportion of deaths in advanced ages in more recent decades. Figure 3.1 exhibits the percent-age distributions of deaths at ages 40 and

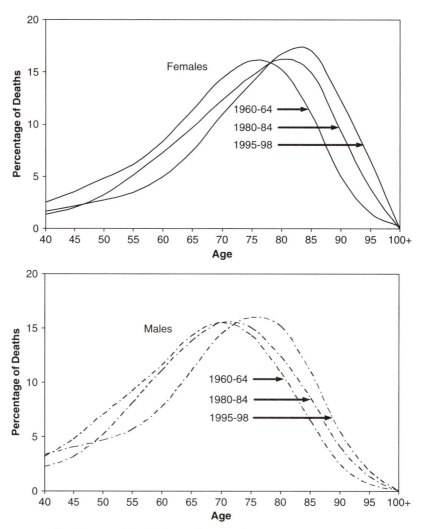

**Figure 3.1** Percentage distribution of deaths from all causes for the U.S. population at ages 40 and above by sex: 1960–1998.

over from all causes combined for three historical periods across the late twentieth century: 1960–1964, 1980–1984, and 1995–1998.

It can be seen from Figure 3.1 that the distributions of deaths have progressively shifted toward older ages for both sex groups from the 1960s to the late 1990s. The overall distributions of female deaths are more skewed to the right than those of male deaths. The peak ages at death are also older for females in all periods, and the difference is the largest in the most recent years: 80 to 90 for females, compared to 72 to 82 for males. Similar patterns are evident in the percentage distributions by age of four leading causes of death—heart disease, stroke, lung cancer, and female breast cancer—but are not presented because of space limitations. In brief, the fundamental conclusion from Figure 3.1 and related cause-specific analyses is that, in the last two decades of the twentieth century, just as in the previous two decades, the percentage distributions of deaths from all causes and from heart disease, stroke, lung cancer, and breast cancer continued to shift toward older ages at death. This is consistent with predictions from the fourth stage of the epidemiologic transition.

## II. The Dynamics of Morbidity, Disability, and Mortality

To further describe how morbidity, disability, and mortality interact, we next review some key findings from studies in medical demography. *Medical demography* is a branch of demography that studies the interactions of chronic disease, disability, and mortality in mature and aging populations (Manton & Stallard, 1994). Many of the key analyses of disease/disability/mortality dynamics have centered around the development and application of the *random-walk model of human mortality and aging* (the "random

walk" name derives from the branch of probability theory on which the model is based) initially proposed by Woodbury and Manton (1977, 1983; see also Manton & Stallard, 1992; Manton, Stallard, & Singer, 1994; Manton, Stallard, Woodbury, & Dowd, 1994). This model is ideally suited to the study of the evolution of morbidity and mortality dynamics over time in a longitudinal cohort design in which some of the explanatory variables/covariates/risk factors may change over time as a consequence of aging and/or mortality selection.

The random-walk model has two basic equations, or sets of equations, for describing the evolution of the health, disability, and survival dynamics of a cohort (or a sample thereof) followed longitudinally over time as a panel with periodic waves of measurements. First, there is a set of autoregressive or recursive *state-space equations* that describe changes over time (age) in state variables. The state variables could be measures of risk factors or factors that affect the mortality risk of individuals. Examples are measures of physiological functioning, such as blood pressure and cholesterol, that are taken periodically on a longitudinal panel. Alternatively, the state variables could be measures of various forms of disability such as ability to feed or dress oneself. For a vector of $J$ state variables measured at time $t$ on individual $i = 1, ..., I, x_{it}$, a simple version of the recursive state-space equations might be:

$$x_{it+1} = \alpha_0 + \alpha_1 x_{it} + \alpha_2 Age_{it} + \alpha_3 z_i + \alpha_4 y_{it} + \varepsilon_{it} \tag{1}$$

where the $a_i$'s are parameters or vectors of parameters to be estimated, $x_{it}$ denotes the vector of state variables measured at the previous time period $t$, $Age_{it}$ is individual $i$'s age at time $t$, $z_i$ is a vector of fixed covariates for individual $i$, $y_{it}$ is a vector of time-varying exogenous covariates for individual $i$, and $\varepsilon_{it}$ is a stochastic shock or error term for individual $i$ at time $t$. A more complex and sophisticated representation of the state-space equations of the random-walk model that incorporates interactions and other contingencies can be found, for example, in Manton and Stallard (1994). However, Eq. (1) captures the essential recursive features of the state-space equations, the purpose of which is to track changes over time in the physiological or disability functioning of members of a longitudinal panel over time.

The second process in the random-walk model is termed a *quadratic survival function*, which can be written:

$$\mu\left(x_{it}, Age_{it}\right) = \left[\mu_0 + x_{it}^T \beta + \frac{1}{2} x_{it}^T B x_{it}\right] e^{\theta Age_{it}}. \tag{2}$$

Equation (2) is a multidimensional generalization of the conventional Gompertz or exponential hazard or force of mortality function often used to model the growth of the risk of mortality in the adult ages. As in conventional Gompertz hazard models, the exponential term in Eq. (2) has a parameter, $\theta$, which estimates the rate of increase in the mortality risk for individual $i$ at time $t$, net of the effects of measured state-space variables contained in the $x_{it}$ vector. Thus, $\theta$ represents the effects of unobserved age-related variables on mortality. In addition, however, the scale parameter $\mu_0$ of the conventional Gompertz model is generalized to include linear and quadratic effects of the vector $x_{it}$ of state variables measured for individual $i$ at time $t$. The linear effects of the state variables are measured by coefficients in the $\beta$ vector corresponding to the $x_{it}$ vector, and the quadratic effects are measured by coefficients in the $B$ matrix corresponding to the quadratic form $x_{it}^T B x_{it}$. In brief, the hazard function in Eq. (2) is dependent on time-varying covariates.

As shown, for example, by Manton and Stallard (1994), the quadratic survival function implies that, for each age and

each state-space variable, there is an optimal point or value at which mortality is minimized. As the values of individual $i$ on a state-space variable deviate from a region near the minimal-mortality point on a state variable, her/his risk of mortality increases. Manton and Stallard noted that this functional specification describes the relation of mortality to many risk factors that have been found in empirical studies.

In sum, the random-walk model embodies the interaction of a quadratic hazard function of mortality and linear dynamics among a set of state variables. It has been widely applied empirically. Some findings can be summarized here.

Given that the parameter $\theta$ represents the age-dependence of human mortality that is due to unobserved factors associated with age, Manton and Stallard (1994) studied the reduction in the value of $\theta$ that could be produced from the analysis of two sets of data. First, using data from the 34-year follow-up of the famous Framingham Heart Study, Manton and Stallard (1994) estimated $\theta = 0.0939$ in a random-walk model for males with no controls for state variables (risk factors) and 0.1002 for females. In other words, without controls for risk factors, the gross mortality risk is estimated to grow at about 9.4% per year of age for males and 10.02 for females. This rate of growth implies a doubling of mortality risk in about 7.45 years. Adding controls for 10 risk factors that have been measured on a biennial basis in the Framingham Study (pulse pressure, diastolic blood pressure, body mass index, cholesterol, blood sugar, hematocrit, vital capacity, cigarette consumption, left ventricular capacity, and ventricular rate), Manton and Stallard estimated $\theta = 0.0805$ for males and 0.0812 for females. Thus, controls for the biological and lifestyle risk factors and their linear dynamics across the state space reduce the age-dependence of mortality by 14% for males and by 19% for females. In terms of chi-squared measures of variance explained, Manton and Stallard further found that the inclusion of the risk factors explain about 70% of the chi-squared explained by the age dependence of mortality.

Manton and Stallard (1994) conducted a similar analysis of data from the 1982, 1984, and 1989 waves of the National Long-Term Care Surveys (NLTCS), which are surveys of the age 65 and over population of the United States in which sampled-in respondents are followed longitudinally until they die. Using mortality data for 1982–1991, Manton and Stallard estimated $\theta = 0.0815$ in a random-walk model for males with no controls for state variables and 0.0910 for females. Then, after controlling for seven indices of physical mobility and functioning (based on 27 functional and physical performance items in the NLTCS) as state variables in the random-walk model, $\theta = 0.0401$ for males and 0.0364 for females. In other words, conditioning $\theta$ on functional status reduces the mortality increase with age to 3.6% to 4.0% per year. This is a reduction in the age-dependence of mortality risk of 51% for males and 60% for females. Manton and Stallard reported that controlling for income and education produces an even further reduction of $\theta$ to 2.6% per year of age, which, for a base $\theta$ of 10% per year of age is about a 74% reduction in the age-dependence of mortality. Also, a $\theta$ of 2.6% corresponds to a doubling of mortality risk in about 27 years. In terms of a reduction in the chi-squared index of variation accounted for by age, physical functioning/disability accounts for 79% and 87% (for males and females, respectively) of the chi-squared explained by age. Thus, controlling for measures of physical functioning described the age dependence of death better than controlling for conventional physiological risk factors. These findings are quite remarkable and are consistent with increased disability/

decreased physical activity being a major risk factor in the age 65 and over population. An implication is that diseases associated with decreased physical activity should be prevalent among the elderly, and, indeed, Gross, Quinan, Rodstein, LaMontagne, Kaslow et al. (1988) found that 56% of deaths in a population whose mean age was 84.5 years were due to pulmonary embolism, congestive heart failure, or pneumonia.

These findings regarding the interaction of disease, disability, and mortality imply that individuals can substantially reduce their mortality risk by the use of lifestyle and health care practices that help them to maintain values on physiological variables that are at or near the optimal values for their age and sex groups and/or maintaining physical activity and functioning. Analyses using the random-walk model have been extended by Manton, Stallard, and Corder (1997) and Manton and Land (2000) to the study of *active life expectancy* (ALE), defined as years of remaining life free of disability in activities of daily living (ADLs), instrumental activities of daily living (IADLs), or physical performance limitations (e.g., Nagi, 1976). ADLs are personal maintenance tasks performed daily, such as eating, getting in and out of bed, bathing, dressing, toileting, and getting around indoors (Katz & Akpom, 1976). IADLs refer to household maintenance tasks associated with independent living such as cooking, doing the laundry, grocery shopping, traveling, and managing money (Lawton & Brody, 1969).

Manton and Land (2000) used data from the 1982, 1984, 1989, and 1994 NLTCS and mortality data for 1982 to 1996 together with the random-walk model to study active life expectancy. In this application, following Manton and Stallard (1994), they used seven indices of physical mobility and functioning (based on 27 functional and physical performance items in the NLTCS) as state variables in the random-walk model. A number of findings were reported. For instance, at age 65, females have a total life expectancy (TLE) of 22.2 years with 15.7 years of ALE; by age 85, the corresponding numbers are 9.3 years of TLE of which only 3.1 years are active. For males, the corresponding estimates at age 65 are 15.7 years of TLE and 13.7 years ALE; at age 85, the numbers for males are 6.4 years TLE and 4.2 years of ALE. The analyses also showed an ALE crossover for males and females. Females have longer TLE and longer ALE at age 65, but, by age 80, although females continue to have a longer TLE than males, their ALE has become 0.54 year shorter. By age 85, males have a full year more of ALE than females, and the male advantage continues to the end of life.

## III. Demographic, Social, and Behavioral Differentials in Morbidity, Disability, and Mortality

We next review the heterogeneity of morbidity, disability, and mortality outcomes among members of human populations. Again, for purposes of illustration, we concentrate on findings from studies of the United States. We approach this topic from the problem of how variations or differentials in morbidity, disability, and mortality among two demographic characteristics, sex and race/ethnicity, and one key measure of position in the social structure, socioeconomic status (SES), can be explained. Findings from medical demography, just reviewed, show that the age-dependence of mortality can be substantially reduced or explained by taking into account several measures of biological functioning. And it can be reduced even more by taking into account several measures of functional limitations/disability. Thinking of these explanatory factors in terms of proximity to mortality, and

using their relative explanatory powers in longitudinal panel studies such as those reviewed above as a benchmark of "closeness" to the death event, this implies that measures of functional limitations/disabilities are closest to mortality, even closer than physiological measurements. In a general framework depicting factors related to adult mortality (Rogers, Hummer, & Krueger, 2005), however, both functional limitations and physiological measures are considered "proximate" factors in the sense that they are close to the death event. In addition, however, both levels of functional limitations/ disabilities and physiological functioning vary dramatically by other more "distal" demographic characteristics such as sex and race/ethnicity and by measures of socioeconomic status. These factors depict the social-structural contexts within which health is protected or put at risk.

### A. Sex

Consider first the differentials in older age morbidity and disability between males and females. The gender gap in disability prevalence in relation to life expectancy and disability incidence has been a source of controversy. As indicated previously, females have longer TLE and ALE in absolute years, although they do not usually enjoy the advantages proportionally (Crimmins, Saito, & Ingegneri, 1997). This is to say that, because of their lower mortality, duration of disability is longer in women, and this leads to higher prevalence of disability in women at old age. One explanation attributes this difference to higher incidence of disability in old females (Leveille, Penninx, Melzer, Izmirlian, & Guralnik, 2000). The multistate life table approach, however, shows that longer female life expectancy, rather than incidence, contributes to the shorter ALE or smaller increases in ALE for females (Manton, 1988; Manton, Corder, & Stallard, 1993).

Consistent sex differences also have been found with regard to mortality. Both sexes enjoyed substantial improvements in life expectancy at birth across the twentieth century in the United States, with females increasing from 48.3 years in 1900 to 79.8 years in 2001 and males increasing from 46.3 years to 74.4 years in the same years. The sex differential in life expectancy, which was two years longer for females in 1900, decreased to a low point of 1 year in 1920. Then the advantage for females increased to its largest value of 7.8 years in 1975, stayed relatively constant around that level through the 1970s, and then began a narrowing to 5.4 years in 2001 (National Center for Health Statistics, 2004; Rogers et al., 2005).

What accounts for the differences in mortality by sex? Biological factors are important, including hormonal differences and childbearing among women, which have been shown to reduce risks of heart disease and cancer (Carey, 1997; Waldron, 1983). Biology may account for the fact that the trends just cited reached a low point in the sex differential of mortality of only one year in 1920, and it may imply that the female advantage in mortality may never be totally reduced.

But the large increase of the sex differential in mortality into the last quarter of the twentieth century is more closely related to socioeconomic, lifestyle, and behavioral factors. For instance, in an analysis of mortality risks for the period 1990–1995, Rogers, Hummer, and Nam (2000) found that controlling for social and economic factors (employment status, income, education, and marital status) *increased* the sex mortality gap because, compared to males, females are more likely to be disadvantaged by earning less money from paid employment, obtaining lower levels of education (at least in the older cohorts), working at lower quality jobs, and living more years unmarried. On the other hand, the intro-

duction of controls for lifestyle/behavioral factors such as cigarette smoking, excessive drinking of alcohol, drug use, and being overweight tends to close the sex gap in adult mortality. In fact, they estimated that cigarette smoking alone accounts for about 25% of the overall sex mortality difference and a much larger percentage of sex differences in mortality resulting from cancer and respiratory disease, because males are more likely than females to smoke, drink excessively, use drugs, and be overweight. These lifestyle/behavioral factors produce increased mortality risks, especially because of accidents, homicide, cancer, circulatory disease, and respiratory diseases. Taking into account the complete set of social, economic, and behavioral factors, however, left the overall odds ratio of mortality basically unchanged. That is, the social/economic factors, which tended to favor men with respect to mortality risk in the last decade of the twentieth century, were counterbalanced by the lifestyle/behavioral factor, which tended to favor females.

One implication of these findings is that trends in the sex differential in mortality across the last century may be indicative of changes between males and females in social, economic, and lifestyle/behavioral factors. That is, as social, economic, and lifestyle/behavioral differences between males and females narrow, it would follow that the sex gap in mortality would decrease. In a partial, but significant, corroboration of this inference, Pampel (2002) demonstrated that increased rates of cigarette smoking among U.S. females from the 1960s through the 1980s fully accounts for the recent narrowing of the sex gap in mortality.

## B. Race/Ethnicity

Racial differences in health in the United States have been widely documented in medical and social research. It is now well established that African Americans fare worse than their Caucasian counterparts in a wide range of health conditions (Clark & Maddox, 1992; Hummer, 1996), are at higher risk for degenerative diseases such as diabetes, cardiovascular disease, stroke, and cancers, have much poorer physical functioning (Clark & Maddox, 1992; Ferraro, Farmer, & Wybraniec, 1997; Kelley-Moore & Ferraro, 2004; Schoenbaum & Waidmann, 1997), and have higher mortality rates (Rogers et al., 2005).

Recent research on racial differences in disability focuses on the dynamics of the disablement process. Although there is evidence of racial differences in disability levels (Clark & Maddox, 1992; Ferraro, et al., 1997; Schoenbaum & Waidmann, 1997), the findings are inconsistent with regard to how the racial inequality in disability changes over time in later life (Kelley-Moore & Ferraro, 2004). Some studies show that the racial gap in disability grows over the life course (Clark, 1997; Liao, McGee, Cao, & Cooper, 1999), but others suggest the reverse: the gap decreases and converges for the oldest old (Guralnik, Land, Blazer, Fillenbaum, & Branch, 1993; Mendes de Leon, Beckett, Fillenbaum, Brock, Branch, & Evans, 1997). Furthermore, additional evidence indicates a "disability crossover" around the age of 80, where surviving African-American elderly have fewer disabilities than Caucasians (Clark, 1996; Guralnik et al., 1993; Johnson, 2000). In a recent attempt to resolve the issue, Kelley-Moore & Ferraro (2004) identified both conceptual and methodological sources of the inconsistency. They examined African-American/Caucasian differences in disability trajectories over six years and found support for the "persistent inequality" hypothesis, indicating that African-American elderly have higher morbidity and disability earlier on, and the gap between African-American and Caucasian older adults stays stable throughout late life.

As mentioned previously, morbidity is the key antecedent of disability, and therefore changes in chronic health conditions such as heart attack, hip fracture, stroke, and diabetes are closely related to decrements in physical functioning (Verbrugge & Jette, 1994; Guralnik et al., 1993). African Americans have higher rates of morbidity incidence than Caucasians and therefore are more susceptible to developing disability in late life.

Racial differences in disability among the elderly have also been attributed to differences in SES. African Americans typically experience socioeconomic disadvantages from birth to late life. Research finds that the disability gap is greatly reduced, if not disappears, after controlling for differences in education and income (Guralnik et al., 1993; Liao et al., 1999; Schoenbaum & Waidmann, 1997), wealth in the form of home ownership, and occupational history (Kelley-Moore & Ferraro, 2004).

Differentials in mortality among the major race and ethnic groups at the end of the twentieth century were as follows. Caucasians had a life expectancy at birth of 77.7 years in 2001; African Americans had a considerably lower life expectancy of 72.2 years (National Center for Health Statistics, 2004). The life expectancy of Hispanics was similar to that of Caucasians, with that of Native Americans falling between the Caucasian and African-American life expectancy (Rogers et al., 2005). Asian Americans had the highest life expectancy of all, estimated at 82.1 years in 1992 for Japanese Americans, 81.7 for Chinese Americans, and 80.6 for Filipino Americans (Hoyert & Kung, 1997). These estimates are subject to errors, especially for non-Caucasian populations, as a result of age-misreporting in the numerators of death rates and under-coverage in the denominators. A study of these data problems by

Rosenberg and colleagues (1999) and a subsequent adjustment of the race/ethnic mortality rates showed that Asian and Pacific Islander death rates remained the lowest, followed by death rates for Hispanics, Native Americans, and non-Hispanic blacks.

These differentials in death rates and life expectancy are not static, however. For instance, the African-American/Caucasian gap in life expectancy at birth was estimated to be 15.8 years in 1900–2002, 6.9 in 1989–1991, and 5.9 in 1999 (Anderson & DeTurk, 2002). Except for chronic obstructive pulmonary disease, African Americans continue to experience higher risks from most causes of death.

What accounts for the race/ethnic differentials in life expectancy? Rogers (1992) found that differences in age, sex, marital status, family size, and income accounted for almost all of the African-American/Caucasian gap. Oliver and Shapiro (1995) found that, compared to Caucasians, African Americans are less likely to be employed, married, or wealthy and are more likely to live in poverty. Research has shown that all of these factors influence the adult mortality gap between the two populations (Bond Huie, Hummer, & Rogers, 2002; Rogers, 1992). Access to health care also has an influence. Sickles and Taubman (1997) found that the African-American/Caucasian gap in life expectancy at birth narrowed from 7.5 to 5.4 years during the period 1965–1975 when Medicare and Medicaid were introduced.

Blacks do not experience higher mortality than Caucasians in all the adult years. Researchers consistently find a African-American/Caucasian "mortality crossover" among the oldest old (Nam, 1995). That is, around ages 85 to 90, blacks begin to experience lower age-specific mortality than their Caucasian counterparts. This finding has been the source of much criticism and research

because of the poor quality of data at the older ages, especially for blacks (Preston, Elo, Rosenwaike, & Hill, 1996). But, even after careful corrections for data quality, the pattern persists (Hill, Preston, & Rosenwaike, 2000). Similar crossovers also have been found between other majority and minority populations and in other countries (Nam, 1995).

The conventional explanation is that the crossover is due to a mortality selection process. That is, compared to a more advantaged social group, a less advantaged population may experience higher mortality in the earlier childhood and adult ages, which could result in greater vitality and lower mortality at older ages (Johnson, 2000). The findings of Land, Guralnik, and Blazer (1994) are consistent with this explanation. Using a longitudinal panel study of individuals ages 65 and over, they found crossovers of both TLE and ALE for both males and females. That is, by age 85, African-American males and females were found to have longer life and active life expectancies than their Caucasian counterparts. After introducing controls for education, only small differences remained between African Americans and Caucasians in both TLE and ALE.

Recent research also has focused on the explanation of mortality differences between Hispanics and non-Hispanic whites. Most Hispanic groups, with the exception of Puerto Ricans, have overall mortality rates similar to those of Caucasians. But greater proportions of Hispanics live in poverty and lack health insurance (Elo & Preston, 1997; Hummer, Rogers, Amir, Forbes, & Frisbie, 2000). This inconsistency between the generally lower SES of Hispanics and their parity with Caucasians on mortality has been termed the *epidemiologic paradox* (Markides & Coreil, 1986). Explanations of this Hispanic mortality paradox have focused on the greater proportional presence of immigrants among Hispanics in the United States than among the non-Hispanic black or white populations. International migrants tend to be healthy and eager to succeed and are less likely to be frail or unmotivated (Rosenwaike, 1991). In addition, Hummer et al. (2000) found that immigrant and native Hispanics are less likely to smoke and drink than non-Hispanic blacks or whites. These differences in population composition and health behaviors account for much of the Hispanic mortality paradox. Palloni and Arias (2004) found that return migration of the sickest was particularly important for explaining the foreign-born Mexican mortality advantage.

## C. Socioeconomic Status

The inverse association between SES and the risk of ill health and mortality is one of the most firmly established patterns in the social distribution of morbidity and mortality. Evidence for older adults commences with this general pattern but also varies depending on the SES indicators and specific health outcomes examined.

The three measures of SES most often used in studies of adult morbidity and mortality are educational attainment (typically measured as years of schooling completed), income (typically measured as gross annual income or income adjusted for household size and composition), and, for the working age population, occupational prestige or status. Conceptually, however, SES dimensions also include community standing, power, and wealth (Moss & Krieger, 1995). Empirically, these are increasingly recognized by the incorporation of new measures of SES such as health insurance, credit card debt, food stamps and welfare receipt, childhood socioeconomic conditions, persistently low income and income insecurity, home ownership and other asset holdings, income inequality, and national-level economic swings (Becker & Hemley, 1998; Bond Huie

et al., 2002; Drentea & Lavrakas, 2000; Robert & House, 1996; Seccombe & Amey, 1995; Smith & Kington, 1997). Accounting for how these various dimensions of SES affect morbidity and mortality between the sexes, in different race/ethnic groups, at various ages, across cultures, and within other subgroups of the overall population is very much a continuing research problem. In absence of this, the effects of SES on morbidity and mortality outcomes can be understated.

Education has long been the most widely used indicator of SES in studies of adult morbidity and mortality (e.g., Elo & Preston, 1996; Kitagawa & Hauser, 1973) because educational attainment generally is completed relatively early in life; is usually easy to ascertain for large samples; has a substantial impact on other measures of SES, including income, occupational status, and wealth; and can be used as an SES indicator for elderly populations wherein most persons are retired. Education is strongly associated with a lower prevalence of chronic illness (House, Kessler, Herzog, Mero, Kinney, & Breslow, 1990) and lower levels of functional disability (Ferraro, 1993; Mutran & Ferraro, 1988). Education and income have been shown to have independent effects on changes in chronic conditions and disability during later life (Crimmins & Saito, 1993; House, Lepkowski, Kinney, Mero, Kessler, & Herzog, 1994; Rogers, Rogers, & Belanger, 1992). Strawbridge, Camacho, Cohen, and Kaplan (1993) reported that income is a significant predictor of functional declines for men but not women, which suggests an interaction effect between SES and sex on disability. SES has also been found to interact with age. The relationship between aging and health is stratified by education and income. Both cross-sectional and longitudinal data show that SES differences in health increase with age during adulthood, but diminish late in life (House et al., 1990, 1994).

As noted previously, differences in SES have been shown to be an important explanatory factor of sex and race/ethnic differentials in morbidity. In other words, SES explains or mediates the relationship between demographic factors and health (George, 1996). Maddox and Clark (1992) found that not only did education and income mediate the effects of sex on disability, but the relationship reversed after controlling for these two factors. This suggests that women who were equally advantaged in SES as men actually exhibited lower rates of functional disability. Although education and income do not explain away the African-American–Caucasian differences in functional disability, they partially mediate the effects of race (Clark & Maddox, 1992).

Research has found that educational differences in U.S. adult mortality remain graded and very wide (Rogers et al., 2000). The impacts of education may also have increased in recent decades (Pappas, Queen, Hadden, & Fisher, 1993; Preston & Elo, 1995).

Several mechanisms have been hypothesized to account for SES differences in adult morbidity and mortality. First, *differential exposure to stress* may have contributed to the observed social class differences in health and well-being (Turner, Wheaton, & Lloyd, 1995). This hypothesis suggests that systemic sources of stress such as chronic financial strains and negative life events are more prevalent among social groups in lower socioeconomic strata and expose individuals to increased risk of illness (Aneshensel, 1992). For example, individuals with lower occupational statuses and incomes often work in jobs that entail more exposure to physically demanding, emotionally stressful, or environmentally unsafe working conditions (Monson, 1986; Moore & Hayward, 1990), and are less able to afford safer housing in less dangerous neighbor-

hoods (Robert, 1999). Individuals with lower SES are also more likely to engage in risky health behaviors such as smoking, excessive drinking, and immoderate eating (House et al., 1994). By contrast, those with higher SES are more likely to engage in lifestyle choices and behaviors that decrease the effect of stress on risk of morbidity and mortality from diabetes, cardiovascular disease, various cancers, accidents, homicide, and many other causes of death (Rogers et al., 2000; Sickles & Taubman, 1997).

Two psychosocial risk factors that substantially explain the social stratification of aging and health are *amount and quality of social support*, and *social-psychological coping resources*. A large body of literature suggests social support not only has robust main effects on health, but also has the stress-buffering effects (George, 1996). Studies have also shown that sense of control, self-esteem, competence, and self-efficacy are related to better health and they mediate the relationship between social factors and health (George, 2001; House et al., 1994). Individuals of lower SES have been found to have fewer social relationships and support, lower self-esteem and mastery, and higher levels of chronic conditions and disability (House, Landis, & Umberson, 1988; House et al., 1994; Williams, 1990).

Third, SES differences in health and mortality can also be a result of *differences in access to and quality of health care*. High SES is associated with a greater access to health insurance and medical care. Although all individuals face some risk from disease or accidents, those with higher incomes and higher levels of education are more likely to promptly seek medical attention, receive better medical care, and comply with medicinal or therapeutic regimens.

Unlike sex and race/ethnicity, SES is not fixed at birth. Rather, SES can be affected by health status, especially during the working ages. The potential reciprocal relationship between SES and health outcomes makes causal interpretations of social status differences in health and mortality in later life somewhat ambiguous. There are two competing hypotheses of the causal dynamics between SES and health. The *selection, or "drift," hypothesis* argues that the association between SES and illness is a function of health-related downward mobility. This means that the presence of illness prevents individuals from obtaining or staying on the jobs or social positions that would maintain their SES, attract positive social relationships, and contribute to upward social mobility. According to this view, health problems or morbidity causes individuals to drift into lower SES groups or fail to jump out of low SES positions at rates comparable to those of healthy individuals. In contrast, the *social causation hypothesis* holds that social structure and processes are the causes of morbidity, and illnesses are inevitable consequences of inequality in the distributive system. It argues that the higher rates of illness in lower SES groups are due to the socioeconomic adversities that expose low SES individuals to higher levels of pathogenic conditions and provide fewer resources for coping with distress (Yu & Willliams, 1999). Although the weight of empirical evidence favors the social causation interpretation, recent research suggests that social selection and social causation may be operating simultaneously (Dooley, Prause, & Ham-Rowbottom, 2000; Ross & Mirowsky, 1995; Smith & Kington, 1997; Thoits & Hewitt, 2001). However, the precise interplay of these two underlying processes remains an important question for future work. We need prospective studies that attend to more careful delineation and specification of the causal models by which biological vulnerabilities combine with social adversities and resources to affect adult morbidity and mortality outcomes.

## IV. Conclusions and Future Research Directions

This chapter reviewed some major directions and findings from recent research on morbidity, disability, and mortality among adults and the elderly. Several conclusions and directions for important future research can be summarized.

First, during the last two decades of the twentieth century, the United States continued to exhibit shifts in the age distribution of both overall deaths and deaths from major degenerative diseases toward older ages. This is consistent with predictions from the fourth stage of the epidemiologic transition, the age of delayed degenerative diseases, as postulated by Olshansky and Ault (1986). Furthermore, the pattern of shifting age distributions of deaths likely has substantial inertia and may continue well into the twenty-first century, but this question merits future monitoring and research. Indeed, future research needs to focus on the extent of acceleration or deceleration of the shifting age distributions of deaths by race/ethnic group and SES. Also, if the shifts in the age distributions of deaths show acceleration or deceleration across the decades, this may provide important information on limits to the human life span.

Second, research on the dynamics of morbidity and mortality in medical demography shows that the age-dependence of mortality risk can be substantially reduced or explained by taking into account several measures of physiological functioning. That is, by maintaining physiological parameters such as blood pressure, body mass, and cholesterol at or near the optimal values for an individual's age, the growth of the force of mortality with increasing age can be substantially reduced. Additional studies of these dynamics are needed in the context of the new biomedical therapies that have been, and continue to be, developed in recent years. If the therapies have the effect of helping a larger fraction of elderly cohorts maintain their physiological parameters near the optimal values, this could reduce the age dependence of mortality and further raise life expectancy, which has implications for forecasts of the size and health status of the elderly population that are based on the medical demography model (Manton & Stallard, 1992). Continued monitoring and study also are needed of the impacts of cohort replacement on disability/mortality dynamics as earlier cohorts age out and are replaced by more recent cohorts.

Third, research in social demography, epidemiology, and medical sociology has greatly improved knowledge of how social, economic, and lifestyle/behavioral factors affect differentials in morbidity, disability, and mortality by sex, race/ethnicity, and SES. It is evident from this research that, as the SES and lifestyle/behavioral differences between the sexes and among race/ethnic groups increase or decrease, differentials in morbidity and mortality will correspondingly expand or decline. Research contributions have begun the task of mapping the specific behavioral and biological pathways through which these SES and lifestyle/behavioral factors have their impacts, but much more research is needed to fully identify these linkages.

## References

Anderson, R. N., & DeTurk, P. B. (2002). United States life tables, 1999. *National Vital Statistics Reports, 50*, 1–40.

Aneshensel, C. S. (1992). Social stress: Theory and research. *Annual Review of Sociology, 18*, 15–38.

Becker, C., & Hemley, D. (1998). Demographic change in the former Soviet Union during the transition period. *World Development, 26*, 1957–1977.

Bond Huie, S. A., Hummer, R. A., & Rogers, R. G. (2002). Individual and contextual risks of death among race and ethnic groups in the United States. *Journal of Health and Social Behavior, 43*, 359–381.

Carey, J. R. (1997). What demographers can learn from fruit fly actuarial models and biology. *Demography, 34*, 17–30.

Clark, D. O. (1996). The effect of walking on lower body disability among older blacks and whites. *American Journal of Public Health, 86*, 57–61.

Clark, D. O. (1997). U.S. trends in disability and institutionalization among older blacks and whites. *American Journal of Public Health, 87*, 438–442.

Clark, D. O., & Maddox, G. L. (1992). Racial and social correlates of age-related changes in functioning. *Journal of Gerontology: Social Sciences, 47B*, S222–S232.

Crimmins, E. M., & Saito Y. (1993). Getting better and getting worse: Transitions in functional status among older Americans. *Journal of Aging and Health, 5*, 3–36.

Crimmins, E. M., Saito, Y., & Ingegneri, D. (1997). Trends in disability-free life expectancy in the United States, 1970–90. *Population and Development Review, 23*, 555–572.

Dooley, D., Prause, J., & Ham-Rowbottom, K. A. (2000). Underemployment and depression: Longitudinal relationships. *Journal of Health and Social Behavior, 41*, 421–36.

Drentea, P., & Lavrakas, P. J. (2000). Over the limit: The association among health, race and debt. *Social Science and Medicine, 50*, 517–529.

Elo, I. T., & Preston, S. H. (1996). Educational differentials in mortality: United States, 1979–85. *Social Science and Medicine, 42*, 47–57.

Elo, I. T., & Preston, S. H. (1997). Racial and ethnic differences in mortality at older ages. In L. G. Martin & B. J. Soldo (Eds.), *Racial and ethnic differences in the health of older Americans* (pp. 10–42). Washington, DC: National Academy Press.

Ferraro, K. F. (1993). Are black older adults health-pessimistic? *Journal of Health and Social Behavior, 34*, 201–214.

Ferraro, K. F., Farmer, M. M., & Wybraniec, J. A. (1997). Health trajectories: Long-term dynamics among black and white adults. *Journal of Health and Social Behavior, 38*, 38–54.

George, L. K. (1996). Social factors and illness. In R. H. Binstock & L. K. George (Eds.), *Handbook of aging and the social sciences* (pp. 229–253). San Diego: Academic Press.

George, L. K. (2001). The social psychology of health. In R. H. Binstock & L. K. George (Eds.), *Handbook of aging and the social sciences* (pp. 217–237). San Diego: Academic Press.

Gross, P. A., Quinan, G. V., Rodstein, M., LaMontagne, J. R., Kaslow, R. A., Saah, A., Wallenstein, S., Neufield, R., Denning, C., & Gaerlan, P. (1988). Association of influenza immunization with reduction in mortality in an elderly population: A prospective study. *Archives of Internal Medicine, 148*, 562–565.

Guralnik, J. M., Land, K. C., Blazer, D., Fillenbaum, G. G., & Branch, L. G. (1993). Educational status and active life expectancy among older blacks and whites. *New England Journal of Medicine, 329*, 110–116.

Hill, M. E., Preston, S. H., & Rosenwaike, I. (2000). Age reporting among white Americans aged 85+: Results of a record linkage study. *Demography, 37*, 175–186.

Holmes, T., & Rahe, R. H. (1967). The Social Readjustment Rating Scale. *Journal of Psychosomatic Research, 1*, 213–218.

House, J. S., Landis, K., & Umberson, D. (1988). Social relationships and health. *Science, 241*, 540–545.

House, J. S., Lepkowski, J. M., Kinney, A. M., Mero, R. P., Kessler, R. C., & Herzog, A. R. (1994). The social stratification of aging and health. *Journal of Health and Social Behavior, 35*, 213–234.

House, J. S., Kessler, R. C., Herzog, A. R., Mero, R. P., Kinney, A. M., & Breslow, M. J. (1990). Age, socioeconomic status, and health. *The Milbank Quarterly, 68*, 383–411.

Hoyert, D. L., & Kung, H. C. (1997). Asian or Pacific Islander mortality, selected states, 1992. *Monthly Vital Statistics Reports, 46*, 1–64.

Hummer, R. A., Rogers, R. G., Amir, S. H., Forbes, D., & Frisbie, W. P. (2000). Adult mortality differentials between Hispanic subgroups and non-Hispanic whites. *Social Science Quarterly, 41*, 459–476.

Hummer, R. A. (1996). Black-white differences in health and mortality: A review and conceptual model. *The Sociological Quarterly, 37*, 105–125.

Johnson, N. E. (2000). The racial crossover in comorbidity, disability, and mortality. *Demography, 37*, 267–283.

Katz, S., & Akpom, C. A. (1976). A measure of primary sociobiological functions. *International Journal of Human Services, 6*, 493–508.

Kelley-Moore, J. A., & Ferraro, K. F. (2004). The black/white disability gap: Persistent inequality in late life? *Journal of Gerontology: Social Sciences, 59B*, S34–S43.

Kitagawa, E. M., & Hauser, P. M. (1973). *Differential mortality in the United States: A study in socioeconomic epidemiology.* Cambridge, MA: Harvard University Press.

Land, K. C., Guralnik, J. M., & Blazer, D. G. (1994). Estimating increment-decrement life tables with multiple covariates from panel data: The case of active life expectancy. *Demography, 31*, 297–319.

Lawton, M. P., & Brody, E. M. (1969). Assessment of older people: Self-maintaining and instrumental activities of daily living. *Gerontology, 9*, 179–186.

Leveille, S. G., Penninx, B.W.J.H., Melzer, D., Izmirlian, G., & Guralnik, J. M.. (2000). Sex differences in the prevalence of disability in old age: The dynamics of incidence, recovery, and mortality. *Journal of Gerontology: Social Sciences, 55B*, S41–S50.

Liao, Y., McGee, D. L., Cao, G., & Cooper, R. S. (1999). Black-white differences in disability and morbidity in the last years of life. *American Journal of Epidemiology, 149*, 1097–1103.

Maddox, G. L., & Clark, D. O. (1992). Trajectories of functional impairment in later life. *Journal of Health and Social Behavior, 33*, 114–125.

Manton, K. G. (1988). A longitudinal study of functional change and mortality in the United States. *Journal of Gerontology: Social Sciences, 43*, 153–S161.

Manton, K. G., Corder, L., & Stallard, E. (1993). Estimates of change in chronic disability and institutional incidence and prevalence rates in the U.S. elderly population from the 1982, 1984, and 1989 National Long Term Care Surveys, *Journal of Gerontology: Social Sciences, 48*, S153–S166.

Manton, K. G., & Land, K. C. (2000). Active life expectancy estimates for the U.S. elderly population: A multidimensional continuous-mixture model of functional change applied to completed cohorts, 1982–1996. *Demography, 37*, 253–265.

Manton, K. G., & Stallard, E. (1992). Projecting the future size and health status of the US elderly population. *International Journal of Forecasting, 8*, 433–458.

Manton, K. G., & Stallard, E. (1994). Medical demography: Interaction of disability dynamics and mortality. In L. G. Martin & S. H. Preston (Eds.), *Demography of Aging*, (pp. 217–278). Washington, DC: National Academy Press.

Manton, K. G., Stallard, E., & Corder, L. (1997). Changes in the age dependence of mortality and disability: Cohort and other determinants. *Demography, 34*, 135–157.

Manton, K. G., Stallard, E., & Singer, B. H. (1994). Methods of projecting the future size and health status of the U.S. elderly population. In D. A. Wise (Ed.), *Studies in the economics of aging* (pp. 41–77). Chicago: The University of Chicago Press.

Manton, K. G., Stallard, E., Woodbury, M. A., & Dowd, E. (1994). Time-varying covariates in models of human mortality and aging: Multidimensional generalizations of the Gompertz. *Journal of Gerontology: Biological Sciences, 49A*, B169–B190.

Markides, K. S., & Coreil, J. (1986). The health of Hispanics in the southwestern United States: An epidemiological paradox. *Public Health Reports, 101*, 253–265.

Mendes de Leon, C. F., Beckett, L. A., Fillenbaum, G. G., Brock, D. D., Branch, L. G., & Evans, D. A. (1997). Black-white differences in risk of becoming disabled and recovering from disability in old age: A longitudinal analysis of two EPESE populations. *American Journal of Epidemiology, 145*, 488–497.

Monson, R. R. (1986). Observations on the healthy worker effect. *Journal of Occupational Medicine, 28*, 425–433.

Moore, D. E., & Hayward, M. D. (1990). Occupational careers and mortality of elderly men. *Demography, 27*, 31–53.

Moss, N., & Krieger, N. (1995). Measuring social inequalities in health: Report on the conference of the National Institutes of Heath. *Public Health Reports, 110*, 302–305.

Mutran, E., & Ferraro, K. F. (1988). Medical need and use of services among older men and women. *Journal of Gerontology: Social Sciences, 43*, S162–S171.

Nagi, S. (1976). Epidemiology of disability among adults in the United States. *Milbank Memorial Fund Quarterly, 54*, 439–468.

Nam, C. B. (1995). Another look at mortality crossovers. *Social Biology, 42*, 133–142.

National Center for Health Statistics. (2004). *National Vital Statistics Report: United States Life Tables, 2001*, vol. 52. Hyattsville, MD: National Center for Health Statistics.

Oliver, M. L., & Shapiro, T. M. (1995). *Black wealth/white wealth: A new perspective on racial inequality*. New York: Routledge.

Olshansky, S. J., & Ault, A. B. (1986). The fourth stage of the epidemiological transition: The age of delayed degenerative diseases. *Milbank Memorial Fund Quarterly, 64*, 355–391.

Olshansky, S. J., Carnes, B. A., Rogers, R. G., & Smith, L. (1997). Infectious diseases: New and ancient threats to world health. *Population Bulletin, 52*, 1–48.

Omran, A. R. (1971). The epidemiologic transition: A theory of the epidemiology of population change. *Milbank Memorial Fund Quarterly, 49*, 509–538.

Palloni, A., & Arias, E. (2004). Paradox lost: Explaining the Hispanic adult mortality advantage. *Demography, 41*, 385–416.

Pampel, F. C. (2002). Cigarette use and the narrowing sex differential in mortality. *Population and Development Review, 28*, 7–104.

Pappas, G., Queen, S., Hadden, W., & Fisher, G. (1993). The increasing disparity in mortality between socioeconomic groups in the United States, 1960 and 1986. *New England Journal of Medicine, 329*, 103–109.

Pearlin, L. I., Lieberman, M. A., Menaghan, E. G, & Mullan, J. T. (1981). The stress process. *Journal of Health and Social Behavior, 22*, 337–356.

Pol, L. G., & Thomas, R. K. (1992). *The demography of health and health care*. New York: Plenum.

Preston, S. H., & Elo, I. T. (1995). Are educational differentials in adult mortality increasing in the United States? *Journal of Aging and Health*, 7, 476–496.

Preston, S. H., Elo, I. T. Rosenwaike, I., & Hill, M. (1996). African-American mortality at older ages: Results of a matching study. *Demography*, 33, 193–209.

Preston, S. H., Heuveline, P., & Guillot, M. (2001). *Demography: Measuring and modeling population processes*. Malden, MA: Blackwell.

Robert, S. A. (1999). Socioeconomic position and health: The independent contributions of community socioeconomic context. *Annual Review of Sociology*, 25, 489–516.

Robert, S. A., & House, J. S. (1996). SES differentials in health by age and alternative indicators of SES. *Journal of Aging and Health*, 8, 359–388.

Rockett, I. R. H. (1999). *Population and Health: An Introduction to Epidemiology*. Washington, DC: Population Reference Bureau.

Rogers, R. G. (1992). Living and dying in the USA: Sociodemographic determinants of death among blacks and whites. *Demography*, 29, 287–303.

Rogers, R. G., & Hackenberg R. (1987). Extending epidemiological transition theory: A new stage. *Social Biology*, 34, 234–243.

Rogers, R. G., Hummer, R., & Nam, C. (2000). *Living and dying in the USA*. New York: Academic.

Rogers, R. G., Hummer, R., & Krueger, P. M. (2005). Adult mortality. In D. L. Poston, Jr. & M. Micklin (Eds.), *Handbook of population* (pp. 283–309). New York: Springer.

Rogers, R. G., Rogers, A., & Belanger A. (1992). Disability-free life among the elderly in the United States: Sociodemographic correlates of functional health. *Journal of Aging and Health*, 4, 19–42.

Rosenberg, H. M., Maurer, J. D., Sorlie, P. D., Johnson, N. J., MacDorman, M. F., Hoyert, L., Spitler, J. F., & Scott, C. (1999). Quality of death rates by race and Hispanic origin: A summary of current research. *Vital and Health Statistics*, Series 2, No.128.

Rosenwaike, I. (1991). Mortality experience of Hispanic populations. In I. Rosenwaike (Ed.), *Mortality of Hispanic populations*. New York: Greenwood.

Ross, C. E., & Mirowsky, J. (1995). Does employment affect health? *Journal of Health and Social Behavior*, 36, 230–243.

Schoenbaum, M., & Waidmann, T. (1997). Race, socioeconomic status, and health: Accounting for race differences in health. *Journal of Gerontology*, 52B (Special issue), 61–73.

Seccombe, K., & Amey, C. (1995). Playing by the rules and losing: Health insurance and the working poor. *Journal of Health and Social Behavior*, 36, 168–181.

Sickles, R. C., & P. Taubman, P. (1997). Mortality and morbidity among adults and the elderly. In M. R. Rosenzweig & O. Stark (Eds.), *Handbook of population and family economics* (vol. 1A, pp. 559–643). Amsterdam: Elsevier.

Smith, J. P., & Kington, R. (1997). Demographic and economic correlates of health in old age. *Demography*, 34, 159–170.

Strawbridge, W. J., Camacho, T., Cohen, R. D., & Kaplan, G. A. (1993). Gender differences in factors associated with change in physical functioning in old age: A 6-year longitudinal study. *The Gerontologist*, 33, 603–609.

Thoits, P. A., & Hewitt, L. N. (2001). Volunteer work and well-being. *Journal of Health and Social Behavior*, 42, 115–131.

Turner, R. J., Wheaton, B., & Lloyd, D. A. (1995). The epidemiology of social stress. *American Sociological Review*, 60, 104–125.

Verbrugge, L. M., & Jette, A. M.. (1994). The disablement process. *Social Science and Medicine*, 38, 1–14.

Waldron, I. (1983). Sex differentials in human mortality: The role of genetic factors. *Social Science and Medicine*, 17, 321–333.

Willams, D. R. (1990). Socioeconomic differentials in health: A review and redirection. *Social Psychology Quarterly*, 53, 81–99.

Woodbury, M. A., & Manton, K. G. (1977). A random-walk model of human mortality and aging. *Theoretical Population Biology*, 11, 37–48.

Woodbury, M. A., & Manton, K. G. (1983). A theoretical model of the physiological dynamics of circulatory disease in human populations. *Human Biology*, 55, 417–441.

Yu, Y., & Williams, D. R. (1999). Socioeconomic status and mental health. In C. S. Aneshensel & J. C. Phelan (Eds.), *Handbook of the sociology of mental health* (pp. 151–166). New York: Kluwer Academic/Plenum Publishers.

Four

# Old Age Through the Lens of Family History

Carole Haber

Within the last 30 years, historians have discovered old age. In a sense, this recognition is ironic. In contrast to other life stages, old age did not need to be created; it has always been a recognized part of the life cycle. Whether portrayed as powerful and wise, or impoverished and debilitated, the old have been the subject of Western art, literature, and legislation, at least since the times of the ancient Greeks (Falkner & de Luce, 1992). Although until the twentieth century, individuals of advanced age generally comprised a relatively small demographic component of their societies, their impact on their communities often far exceeded their proportionately small numbers.

Why, then, did scholars fail to explore their history, while, since the 1960s, the new social history led them to examine the history of children and young adulthood through scores of monographs and articles? In part, this failure may have reflected the elderly's small numbers; in part, too, it may have been based on a shared assumption among historians that they already knew all that was important about old age in the past. This understanding, generally established through anthropological and sociological studies based on modernization theory, divided the history of the old into two broad periods. Scholars assumed that, in the preindustrial world, the old, though few in number, commanded great respect. Esteemed for their knowledge of the past, they were the admired possessors of cultural memory and tradition. With industrialization, however, the lives of the old changed radically. As their numbers and proportion of the population increased, their skills became of little use; technology rapidly replaced and outdated them. Moreover, their role in the extended family declined. Children and grandchildren deserted the family farm, leaving the old to face isolation and dependency. In this broad historical account, then, the modern-day old share little with their preindustrial counterparts. Where once powerful and important, they had now become all but obsolescent in the modern world.

During the last thirty years, however, a small, though growing, number of historians have come to challenge many of the assumptions that formed the basis of

*Handbook of Aging and the Social Sciences, Sixth Edition*

earlier accounts. These scholars clearly do not speak with one voice about the nature of old age in the past or the character of the elderly's experiences, but they have traced a far different history of growing old. By focusing on recent "history of the family" scholarship, this chapter highlights several of the important questions and approaches that historians have used in their study of old age. As we shall see, family history serves as an ideal theme through which to trace the evolution of historical research into the role of older people and beliefs about old age. In the late 1960s and early 1970s, key research on household structure, although not always focused directly on the old, first challenged scholars to understand the experience of the elderly by examining their demographic place in the family and the community. Such work was of central importance; it not only questioned earlier anthropological assumptions but also led scholars to begin specifically to explore the lives and families of the old as their central focus of study. By the late 1970s, and especially in the 1980s, this scholarship placed the old in their own historical framework. Generally, this work was based on demographic studies of Western Europe, colonial America, and the United States; moreover, it tended to focus on the role of the household head, who, most often, was an older man. Nonetheless, it revealed that the lives of the old and their families shared few characteristics with earlier depictions. By the 1990s, however, new research expanded the focus of the family history of old age in terms of geography, economics, and gender. Several scholars also began to link quantitative studies with the literary record left by the old themselves. By the beginning of the twenty-first century, then, historians had begun to establish a far more complex understanding of the role of the old and their place in their families and, by extension, their role in past societies.

# I. The Initial Interpretative Phase: Modernization and the Families of the Old

In his 1945 monograph, *The Role of the Aged in Primitive* Society, and again in 1960 in a chapter in the *Handbook of Social Gerontology*, Leo Simmons described what he perceived to be the influential position of the elderly in preindustrial cultures. Although he found variation among societies in their attitude toward their elderly members, he argued that, "in primitive societies, and among preliterate agrarian peoples well into historical times, an aged man or woman had a distinct advantage in experience, knowledge and wisdom" (Simmons, 1960, p. 82; Simmons, 1945). As the custodian of traditions, these individuals served as a link to the past; as the repository of needed skills and experiences, they possessed valued assets. "By the exercise of their knowledge, wisdom, experience, property rights, and religious or magical powers," Simmons wrote, "[the aged] have often played useful roles" (Simmons, 1945, p. 216).

Nowhere did this advantage seem more secure than within their own families. Here, the old served as esteemed patriarchs controlling the lives and resources of large, multigenerational families. Scholars assumed that in preindustrial societies, older persons' possession of valued land and knowledge ensured that they would be respected and obeyed among their own kin. Able to dictate the timing of their children's marriage and the distribution of needed assets, they exerted power well into advanced old age. Even within the medieval town, scholars such as Ernest Burgess argued, patriarchal-led families, although somewhat smaller, were the norm, consisting of several generations, including parents and children, grandparents, unmarried siblings, and other relatives (Burgess, 1945).

Modernization, however, appeared to have challenged the existence of such family networks, as it robbed the old of their value and control. With technological innovations, the skills of older people began to be labeled obsolete; as literacy increased, their memory of traditions was no longer valuable. Moreover, as mortality rates declined, their growing numbers diminished their distinctiveness or importance. As a result, where once the old had been respected and honored, with modernization, they were more likely to be seen as needy individuals in need of support and care. "Industrialization," asserted Burgess in 1960, "created the problems of aging in modern culture" (Burgess, 1960, p. 5). Other scholars emphatically agreed. "Changes in technology, the occupational system, urbanization and residential mobility, and the family," wrote Irving Rosow in 1965, "have all been harmful to old people" (Rosow cited by Cowgill, 1972, p. 9).

According to this interpretation, the negative impact of modernization was especially obvious within the older person's own families and led directly to the "disintegration of the extended family" (Burgess, 1960, p. 10). Although the agricultural system of labor supposedly relied on large kinship networks, industrialization seemed to favor the establishment of the nuclear household and the loss of status for the elderly. Without land, scholars argued, the old quickly became powerless; they possessed few assets with which to entice their offspring to remain with them as they aged. As a result, young adults often deserted the old, leaving them to suffer in isolation. "The status of the aged is high," concluded Cowgill and Holmes in *Aging and Modernization* in 1972, "in societies in which the extended form of family is prevalent and tends to be lower in societies which favor the nuclear form of the family and neolocal marriage" (Cowgill & Holmes, 1972, p. 322).

In this formulation, such scholars starkly contrasted "preindustrial times" with the period of industrial change. Once Western societies had undergone economic modernization, they argued, the old were displaced and despised. While widely accepted, this narrative, in fact, relied on little historical research; it tended to be based on ethnographic studies of nonindustrial cultures. Yet many social scientists argued that such studies not only provided insight into the family structure of these societies but also presented an accurate account of the role of family in the historical past. "It is legitimate to assume," wrote Burgess in 1945, "that in the prehistorical period, the familial structure resembled more or less that of contemporary primitive people. This is not merely an inference; it is supported by survivals found among many people, particularly among those of northern Europe at the dawn of their history" (p. 18).

## II. The Second Phase: The Cambridge Group and Its Followers

In the late 1960s, however, demographic studies into the history of the family began to produce a radically different view of the families, especially in Western Europe, colonial America, and the United States. In this research, the assumptions about the complex family were sharply challenged. Even in agricultural societies in this region, most historians found few three-generational families residing within the same household. Rather, despite the overwhelmingly agrarian economy of the societies, they argued that the nuclear household was, and continued to be, the predominate form of household structure.

The leader is this field was undoubtedly Peter Laslett. Under his direction in the late 1960s, the Cambridge Group for Population and Social Structure began to explore the demographic structure of households. Laslett and his colleagues looked particularly at the co-resident domestic group, that is, individuals who occupied the same household and generally shared the same location, kinship, and activity. For Laslett, the study of the household residence pattern was key. Although family members might live in close proximity to each other, their residence within the home created the household, the basic unit of study. In establishing this focus, Laslett differentiated among three different types of households. First, the *nuclear* or simple household consisted of "a married couple, a married couple with children or a widowed person with offspring," whose biological or marital links created a conjugal family unit. Second, the *extended* household was composed of a "conjugal family unit with the addition of one or more relatives other than offspring." Finally, he noted the possibility of a *multiple* family household, in which there were "two or more conjugal family units connected by kinship or marriage" (Laslett, 1972a, pp. 28–30). While adopting Laslett's notion of the nuclear and extended households, later historians generally focused on the most common form of the multiple household, the *complex* family, consisting (at the very least) of an aging couple with a married offspring. (As such, this chapter follows this form and refers to the position of the old in the *nuclear, extended*, or *complex* household.)

Although earlier studies had argued that before the onset of industrialization, most individuals lived in complex or, at the very least, large extended households, Laslett found that among families in Western Europe, colonial America, and the United States, little evidence supported these assertions. Rather, in an examination of 100 English communities between the sixteenth and nineteenth centuries, he discovered that in only 39 of 5843 households was a married child living with a spouse

and his or her married parents (Laslett, 1972b). In addition, his study not only specifically countered the argument that rural areas encouraged complex households but also directly contradicted the belief that these households were composed of large numbers of related individuals. According to Laslett's findings, between 1599 and 1901, mean household size in both rural and urban communities ranged only from 3.97 to 5.48, most households remaining rather constant at around 4.75 persons (Laslett, 1972b). Whatever the locale, over more than three centuries, the great majority of English individuals chose to reside in small, nuclear households.

In presenting these results, Laslett directly attacked the anthropological assertion that preindustrial households "resembled more or less that of contemporary primitive people." Declaring that the nuclear household was hardly the creation of industrial-urban change, he argued that the aging, preindustrial patriarch ruling over a large kinship network was little more than myth. "There is no sign," wrote Laslett, "of the large extended coresidential family group of the traditional peasant world giving way to the small, nuclear, conjugal household of modern industrial society . . . [T]he large joint or extended family seems never to have existed in common form" (Laslett, 1972b, p. 126).

In the 1970s, American scholars examining the demographic structure of colonial New England communities found similar results: the nuclear household remained the family structure of choice, regardless of the age of the male, household head. Like Laslett, they uncovered little evidence that the structure of the largely rural society encouraged the creation of complex households sheltering multiple generations of kin (Demos, 1972; Greven, 1972). As scholars such as Philip Greven and John Demos demonstrated, the possession of valued land in rural New England communities, rather than encouraging the establishment of multiple generations living in the same home, worked to solidify the continuation of the nuclear household (Demos, 1970, 1978; Greven, 1970). Given the large number of children born to the average family, and the surprisingly low mortality rate of the first generations, most individuals continued to raise young children well into middle age. Even in old age, they often had growing adolescents in their home. Landowning older men then ensured their status as the household head of a nuclear family by using their assets to control the timing of the departure of their maturing children. Fathers often delayed the transfer of needed resources to the youngest male heirs until their own deaths. In Andover, Massachusetts, for example, in 1670, Richard Barker permitted his eldest son to marry at age 27 and granted him a portion of his land to build a house. The other sons, however, were not so fortunate. Not until their father's death in 1693 did they gain their independence through the terms of their father's will. The eldest had been allowed to form his own family, but his siblings continued to reside with their father as part of the aging man's nuclear family (Greven, 1970).

As family historians and demographers associated with Laslett challenged the existence of complex families in Western Europe and American rural societies of the past, they also began to question the notion that industrialization was directly responsible for the "disintegration of the extended family" (Burgess, 1960, p. 10). Surprisingly, in fact, they discovered that although nuclear families predominated from the sixteenth through the nineteenth century, urban and industrial life was more likely to *increase*, rather than to *decrease*, the need and tendency for the married young to seek shelter with the old. Although somewhat contrary to traditional reasoning, the explanation for

this phenomenon was not difficult to understand: in rapidly industrializing cities, older people had valuable assets to share, not only with their unmarried children with whom they typically resided, but even with offspring who had matured and formed families of their own. Most clearly, the possession of a home was a prized resource that often created unexpected ties among generations.

In his study of Lancaster, England, Michael Anderson first noted the importance of complex households in the expanding nineteenth-century city. Urban-industrial life, Anderson noted, "increased the proportion of wage-earners families in which the parents and married children coresided" (Anderson, 1978, p. 43; Anderson, 1972, p. 225; Anderson, 1971). In Preston, Lancaster, in 1851, for example, only half of all couples without children (53%) occupied the entire house in which they lived. The other half chose to reside in a portion of the house, sharing their residence with lodgers or with kin, especially for the first few years of marriage (Anderson, 1971). Other studies of English life confirmed the increase in households that contained an older couple with a married offspring. In Nottinghamshire, in 1688, only 8% of the community's residents lived in complex households; by 1851, the proportion was 21%; in Cardington, Bedfordshire, from 1782 to 1851, the proportion rose from 7% to 20% (Ruggles, 1987).

One benefit of such residences was that elderly women could provide necessary child and domestic care that allowed the rest of the household to labor. Relying on the combined income of kin, families maximized their earnings by increasing the number of potential wage earners. Co-residence with aging parents clearly improved their ability to adapt to the economic demands of the city. According to Anderson, in Lancashire, in 1851, 29% of all women with a grandmother in the house and children under 10 were engaged in the labor force; without a grandmother in the home, the proportion fell to 12% (Anderson, 1978).

In studying family structure, American historians offered similar explanations for the rise in complex household structure often discovered in nineteenth-century cities. In the 1970s, several scholars noted the importance of the life cycle on the family structure of households (Chudacoff, 1978; Chudacoff & Hareven, 1978; Modell & Hareven, 1978). In contrast to the rural young who often delayed marriage until they could acquire their own land, young individuals in the city were likely to marry and share their first residence with their aging parents. In 1865, in Providence, Rhode Island, for example, 41% of all newlyweds lived in extended households, although only a total of 13.4% of all families were extended (Chudacoff, 1978). Through this arrangement, the newly married couple was able to obtain necessary shelter, whereas the old were assured support and financial aid. By combining their households, they joined the incomes and assets of multiple generations into a successful family economy (Haber & Gratton, 1993).

Not surprisingly, such complex arrangements were especially prevalent during times of financial crisis. Where economic expansion often led to the purchase of homes and autonomous households, tightening markets had the opposite effect. In the cities of Essex County, Massachusetts, for example, the Panic of 1873—one of the major recurring depressions of the nineteenth century—and the contraction of the housing market led a high proportion of young adults to seek shelter with their elders, who had been able to buy homes in earlier decades (Chudacoff & Hareven, 1978). Similarly, in Chilvers Coton, England, as the silk industry declined, adult children were more likely to reside in complex households with their married parents who already owned a home. Widowed parents, as well, increased the tendency to form extended households. In 1851, 6% of widowed men and 4% of widowed women lived with their children; by 1901, the proportions had risen to 10% and 14%, respectively (Quadagno, 1982).

In arguing for the dominance of nuclear families, the Cambridge Group made clear that this conclusion rested on demographic data from Western Europe and the United States. At the same time, Laslett and his colleagues called for cross-cultural comparisons, especially with Eastern Europe. In these areas, demographic evidence seemed to reveal that larger, complex households were often common and contrasted significantly with the Western European and American nuclear form (Hammel, 1972; Halpern, 1972; Laslett & Clarke, 1972; Wall, 2001).

Not everyone agreed, however, that complex families did not exist in significant parts of Western Europe. Laslett had directly attacked the presence of multi-generational families in rural Western Europe, finding them to be both demographic and culturally rare, but others claimed that such families were quite common. In 1871, sociologist Frederic Le Play had asserted that what he termed *stem* families, households containing a married child with his aging parents, were common in Europe. In contrast to Laslett's assertion that these families were rare indeed, in the 1970s, advocates of Le Play's position asserted that stem families could indeed be found in considerable number in parts of Western and Central Europe at specific times in families' life cycles (Laslett, 1972a; Berkner, 1972).

One of the strongest advocates for this position was undoubtedly Lutz K. Berkner. Writing in the *Journal of American History* in 1972, he declared that his study of the eighteenth-century peasant stem family in Waldviertel, Lower Austria, challenged Laslett's notion of the scarcity of such families in the past in Western culture. Berkner argued that his research led to two conclusions: "first, that the stem family did and does exist as an important part of the social structure in many parts of rural Western Europe, and second, that the stem family structure does not necessarily emerge from empirical studies of demographic statistics unless the developmental cycle of the family and household are taken into consideration" (Berkner, 1972, p. 399). In contrast to the nuclear families described by other historians, Berkner found that it was not uncommon for elderly rural Austrian homeowners to share their homes with a married child. Once the young couple took up residence in the home, the older couple officially retired and moved into a room annexed to the original house. This rearrangement was clearly more than spatial; it reflected a significant transformation in power and control. No longer the household head and spouse of the head, the older couple moved from a position of authority into one of relative dependence and withdrawal, while the young assumed management over the household.

Like those who had studied changing patterns in urban environments, Berkner emphasized that co-residence between the young and old was hardly a permanent condition. Rather, it was part of the ever-evolving life course of both sons and aging parents at a specific point in their lives. Berkner argued, therefore, that such transitory co-residence was not always caught by the broad census data used by the Cambridge School. Moreover, he contended that the impact of economics on family structure needed to be considered. For Austrian landowners, Berkner claimed, complex families were indeed common; for the landless peasant, there was little tendency or ability to shelter multiple generations.

## III. The New History of Old Age

For scholars specifically examining the history of old age, the debate on family structure raised important issues and concerns. Laslett and his colleagues had clearly challenged earlier beliefs about powerful patriarchal men ruling over multiple generations of kin. Subsequent research, both on the existence of complex and extended families in urban-industrial areas, and on the cyclical presence of stem families in places such as Austria and Eastern Europe, emphasized the possible diversity among the elderly's families in the past, and the dangers in making sweeping statements about the history of aging. In the 1980s and 1990s, these issues became central to a number of historians who turned their focus directly on the old and the variations in their experiences. If old age history could neither be explained as a radical decline from the status of preindustrial societies to the debasement of the urban-industrial world, nor as a uniform formation across time and place, what issues and ideas best explained the varied experiences of the old?

Berkner's assertion that the timing of life course as well as economics played a central role in family history most certainly had an impact on understanding the varied and complex history of old age. The research of the 1970s demonstrated that older people could not be grouped as a single entity, without regard to location, economics, or stage in the life cycle. Rather, historians who examined the old through their family structure and experience looked at a wide variety of factors, including gender, economics, and geography. These, they found, contributed to a complex understanding of aging in the past. Moreover, by exploring the actual words and beliefs of the old, they discovered that past assumptions about the displacement of the old or their isolation needed to be reevaluated. Moving beyond wide-ranging assumptions about the elderly, or portrayals based solely on broad quantitative data, they began to create a new history of the family and, in turn, of the role of the old in past societies.

## A. Gender

Basic to this reevaluation of family structure and old age was an assessment of the family role of the elderly woman. Most early portrayals of aging in the past focused on the older male as representative of the stage of life. According to social scientists, aging men had retained power through their possession of land and their valued knowledge; for family demographers, they generally maintained the role as household heads, despite their age or infirmity. One of Laslett's colleagues, Richard Wall, for example, noted that in seventeenth- and eighteenth-century rural English communities, as well as the more urban centers of Lichfield in 1692 and Stoke in 1701, men experienced little disruption in their family life, regardless of their advancing age. "For elderly men," Wall wrote, "the most likely co-resident was a spouse, followed in the case of Stoke and Lichfield by unmarried children. Co-residence with a married child was considerably rare. Even in the rural communities, only 10% of older men lived with a married child" (Wall, 1995, p. 90). For elderly men, this constancy in the nuclear family structure clearly persisted through time. Even as late as 1900, according to the U.S. census, 82% of all farm males age 60 and over listed themselves as head of household; only 13% lived as dependents in their children's homes (Haber & Gratton, 1993). Unless hampered by debility or severe impoverishment, they generally experienced little modification in their family arrangement. Well into old age, they remained head household, often retaining the support of their dependent offspring in the nuclear household.

The new histories of old age that examined the role of elderly women in the family, however, challenged this notion of stability and directly countered the two earlier assumptions about the status of the old in the past. The family lives of these older females, especially once they were widowed, neither followed the pattern of rural power and esteem that had been projected by social scientists, nor did they reflect the continued stability within the nuclear family assumed by some scholars. When family history was viewed from the perspective of these elderly women, the resulting histories looked remarkably different.

As historians of aging discovered, for aging women, unlike many of their male counterparts, rural societies hardly guaranteed family power and stability. As long as their husbands lived, old women generally occupied the role of spouse of the household head. Once their husbands died, however, elderly widows often experienced a radical change in their roles and responsibilities; their old age no longer ensured the power and esteem traditionally tied to the possession of land. Not uncommonly, their new status was spelled out in wills that passed the family farm to the next generation. At times, these provisions could be quite specific, designating which room the individual would occupy, the furniture she possessed, and even the livestock under her control (Demos, 1978; Shammas, Salmon, & Dahlin, 1987). By dictating that the offspring would receive their inheritance only if they provided for the widow, these documents ensured that the elderly woman would not be abandoned in her senescence.

The resulting co-residence, however, did not necessarily imply a great respect for age and directly countered the notion of the power of the old in preindustrial societies. In moving from the role of spouse of the household head to a dependent in her offspring's home, an aging woman clearly lost her status in the household. In 1804, for example, when Maine midwife Martha Ballard's husband was incarcerated, her son's family moved uninvited, and most unwanted, into her home. Now limited to one room, and no longer in control of the household, the 72-year-old midwife lamented her plight, finding her home in chaos and her daughter-in-law, Sally, to be rude and disrespectful. Sally was, wrote Ballard, "an inconsiderate or very impudent woman to treat me as shee (sic) does" (Ballard cited by Ulrich, 1990, p. 281). For such older women, advancing age hardly brought the honor and authority assumed to exist in preindustrial societies; rather, to be old was to face increasing dependence.

Ironically, at times, historians found that in preindustrial societies of the sixteenth and seventeenth century, the rural landowner elderly woman who sought to maintain her independence often placed herself in a most precarious position. In contrast to powerful older men who gained authority from property, elderly rural women with great wealth could attract suspicion and hostility. Rich widows were expected to marry or at least cede their economic decisions to male members of the family. Those who failed to do so flirted with social censure and even accusations of witchcraft. Such was the case of Katharine Harrison, the wealthiest individual in Wethersfield, Connecticut. Widowed in 1650, she refused to remarry and attempted to remain in control of her large estate. In turn, the community destroyed her property, maimed her livestock, and ultimately accused her of witchcraft. She finally escaped the wrath of her town by signing her property over to male guardians and fleeing to a neighboring colony. Harrison hardly received the respect and authority supposedly connected with wealthy old age. Rather, by remaining independent and beyond male control, she and women like her served

as a threat to the patriarchal system (Karlsen, 1987). European witchcraft accusations followed a similar pattern. Targeting women over age 50 who fell outside the support of a kinship network, these indictments were directed at widows who failed to age appropriately and threatened to destroy the stability of society (Bever, 1982).

As the rural family life of older women often conflicted with the assumptions of the past, so did their place in urban settings. Recent historical studies found a surprising result: elderly women often flocked to the cities where they could retain far greater independence than they had in rural settings. Here, they could find not only the necessary housing in which to reside, but the support of servants and boarders to provide for their needs (Premo, 1990). In 1768, for example, recently widowed Englishwoman Mary Delany, age 68, decided to move to Bath to establish an independent residence, an act applauded by her friends and neighbors. Similarly, in the eighteenth century, the townspeople in Abingdon, Oxfordshire, supported aged female household heads and approved of their decision to have a home of their own (Ottaway, 2001). In contrast to rural areas, the appearance of the elderly women in villages and cities did not appear to engender the hostility awarded to the large, landowning widow. Divorced from the large estate that had so protected the status of her husband, her role as an urban household head often provided her with community acceptance.

Such older women, obviously, lived out their final days in sharp contrast to the notion that little change occurred in the nuclear family as individuals aged. Even in rural areas in 1900 in the United States, although the majority of men maintained the status of household heads, census takers reported that only a minority, 44%, of older farmwomen retained their status as spouse of the head. With the deaths of the husbands, their lives were greatly transformed; a small proportion took over the headship of their own homes, but many became dependents of their kin or left the countryside entirely (Haber & Gratton, 1993).

These findings directly challenged the notion that rural life brought authority and respect to the old, and the urban setting ensured their powerlessness. For aging women, rural settings often meant that, unless married to the head of household or able to retain their own homes, they became dependents, reliant on the care of their heirs. In villages and cities, however, they were far more likely to exert the power associated with being in control of their own households. When viewed from the perspective of their last days, then, there seemed little evidence to support the notion that urbanization destroyed the power of the old, or that the elderly lived their entire lives in nuclear households. Historians who looked specifically at the lives of old women traced a very different narrative that emphasized the diversity of elderly women's experience. As seen through the experiences of these older individuals, old age history, even in Western Europe and the United States, was hardly a time of continuity within the nuclear household, or as a stage when rural life guaranteed unquestioned status and stability (Gratton & Haber, 1993; Haber, 1997; Haber & Gratton, 1993; Hussey, 2001; Ottaway, 2001; Premo, 1990; Thane, 2000, 2001).

## B. Economics

The new histories that focused on the elderly also revealed the important role economics play in creating a diverse history of old age. As early as 1972, both Berkner and Anderson had pointed to the significance of economic differences among the old. For Berkner, it was clear that retirement agreements between generations could be reached only by those who had property to share; few stem households existed among the poor or landless. Similarly, Anderson noted the key role of home ownership and wealth in encouraging complex households in urban areas. He concluded that such households were often impossible for the laboring class who lived near or at the poverty level and lacked valued resources to share. The inclusion of a dependent individual served only to weaken their ability to support their own nuclear family. Rather, in the nineteenth century, such household formation was much more common among the middle and upper classes. In Lancaster, England, in 1871, for example, more than 30% of all bourgeois families lived in extended households; for the unskilled the proportion was only 12% (Ruggles, 1987; Anderson, 1978).

The resulting focus on economics not only explained the variation among the families of the old but allowed historians to question why complex household formation rose in the late nineteenth century, only to decline in the course of the twentieth century. For early scholars, the decrease in the proportion of complex households had been a sign of older people's increasing obsolescence and disrespect. Assuming that preindustrial households had included multiple generations, they argued that the solitary household showed the uselessness of the old. The historical scholarship of the 1970s made clear that urban households were often more likely to include multiple generations than their rural counterparts. Why then, historians asked, did the tendency to co-reside decline in the twentieth century? Had earlier social scientists been correct? Was this a sign of disrespect?

In the 1980s and 1990s, studies in the variation in the economic status of the old and their families arrived at a very different answer. The rise and fall of complex households, historians such as

Steven Ruggles argued, were tied directly to the evolving economic status of the household. According to Ruggles, in the late nineteenth century, in both England and America, complex households were formed by those who were able to provide resources and shelter for multiple generations. In 1880, in Erie County, New York, for example, 25% of middle class families and 41.4% of families with servants lived in extended households, but only 17.2% of the unskilled formed such households (Ruggles, 1987). By the early twentieth century, however, new patterns of household residence became evident for both the middle and working class. In the United States, between 1900 and 1940, the proportion of older men who lived as dependents in their children's home declined from 16% to 11%; for women the percentage fell from 34% to 23% (Haber & Gratton, 1993). With increased wealth, middle-class families began to move away from complex and extended households. For the first time, both the old and their children had the resources necessary to establish separate households. At the same time, an increased number of working-class families included a dependent elder whose presence signaled their rising economic status (Ruggles, 1987). Like the middle class of an earlier era, they now acquired the resources necessary to bring a needy member into the household.

Similarly, as historians focused on economics to explain the diversity in households of the old in urban areas, they found it also played a central role in creating variations in the household structure of rural elders. In exploring the structure of rural families in Western Europe and the United States, historians found that complex households were most likely to be adopted when the sharecropping system of farming was in place. In parts of France and Italy, in contrast to England, higher proportions of the old lived in combined rural households in areas where share-

cropping and family contracts dominated. In 1871, for example, in Casalecchio di Reno, Italy, 40% of the people lived in complex households, and another 13% lived in extended families; only a minority, 43%, followed the pattern of the nuclear households (Kertzer and Karweit, 1995). In Southern France, as well, although the proportion of complex households was not as high, the economic system still led to large numbers of such households. French farmers often signed contracts that created complex households and co-residence with the old. In 1810, in Eguilles, France, at least 20% of all households included three generations (Troyansky, 1989). Yet even within a single country, such patterns were not universal but reflected the specific economic organization of the area. In France, in the mid-nineteenth century, the proportion of complex households ranged throughout the country, from 7% to 37%, depending on region; in Italy, at the same time, they varied from 8% to 44% (Wall, 2001).

Within the United States, diversity also existed among farm families based on their landholding system. For rural African Americans in post-bellum South, sharecropping created far more complex households than among their Caucasian counterparts. Landholders contracted with older men who agreed to share the labor with multiple generations of kin (Haber & Gratton, 1993). For those who owned their land outright, however, evolving inheritance patterns often decreased the likelihood that complex, or even extended, families would remain on the farm. Before the nineteenth century, farmers routinely guaranteed that they would be cared for in old age, by holding on to their land, or deeding it to their heirs with the provision of continued support. By the late nineteenth century, however, large numbers of rural property owners simply sold their farms before their own deaths and created their own retirement capital. In Bucks County, Pennsylvania, for example, in the colonial period, 87% passed their property to their heirs, but by the 1790s, the proportion had fallen to 71%. By 1890, this inheritance pattern was no longer dominant; less than a third chose to will their property to their heirs. Instead, they generally sold off their land, and moved to small towns or cities where they provided for their own final days (Shammas et al., 1987).

The motivation behind this behavior was not hard to understand. In addition to examining the economic basis for family patterns, historians of old age turned to diaries, letters, court cases and other qualitative materials. These documents were extremely important in allowing scholars to look beneath the broad demographic trends and "hear" the voice of both the old and their families. By linking economic data to qualitative sources, historians found that although shared households were often founded on rational calculations that allowed for the allocation of needed assets, they were generally based on necessity rather than desire. Even in eighteenth-century America and England, women who were financially able struggled to maintain their own homes apart from their children, while nineteenth-century aging couples often sold their farms and moved to small villages rather than become dependents in their children's homes (Hussey, 2001; Premo, 1990; Thane, 2000, 2001).

Without such financial resources, however, elderly individuals often had little alternative but to co-reside with their kin. As diaries, court records, and popular literature revealed, however, life within such residences was often far from ideal. In some cases, co-residence actually led to physical violence among family members, whereas other old people faced the unhappy prospect of being joylessly passed from dutiful child to dutiful child, always reliant on the goodwill of their

own offspring (Ryan, 1981; Abel, 1992). Even in parts of Europe where complex families were more common, combined households did not necessarily lead to peaceful coexistence. In examining the combined households of Austria, Berkner (1972) noted that, "The retiring peasants of Waldviertel had no illusions about the tranquility of future relations with their children" (p. 402). Within such households, both generations often resented the presence of the other and struggled to exert control. By the early twentieth century, in fact, Berkner found that Austrian popular literature acknowledged the conflicts inherent in these arrangements. In 1926, a local folklorist wrote, "The 'Old Ones' don't like the daughter-in-law or the way the young ones run the farm. The 'Young Ones' in return don't always quietly accept the grumblings of the 'Old Ones' and once a strained relationship has developed, it usually cannot be overcome" (Rauscher, cited by Berkner, p. 402).

Such sentiments were also expressed throughout England and the United States. By the late nineteenth and early twentieth century, social commentators often criticized the complex household, finding the arrangement to be destructive to the well-being of both the young and old. In 1885, for example, Englishman Samuel Butler wrote, "I find more unhappiness comes from . . . the attempt to prolong family connection unduly and to make people hang together artificially who would never naturally do so . . . And the old people do not really like it so much better than the young" (Butler, cited by Ruggles, 1987, p. 3). Individuals who reflected on their own family situation agreed with this characterization. Only five years after the Austrian folklorist found little of value in the kinship arrangement, an American author expressed similar concerns. Writing in *Harper's*, she declared, "I took it for granted that a grandmother or grandfather should live in the house of nearly every one of my playmates. Soon I came to take it for granted, also that these homes should be full of friction. The association of grandparents with friction took such a hold in my mind that I called myself lucky because my own were dead" (Anonymous, 1931, p. 715). In her own maturity, however, the writer found herself faced with the need to provide shelter to her own aging mother. Able financially to accept her needy parent into her home, yet unable to provide a separate residence, she dutifully accepted her obligation. As the author made clear, however, if she had sufficient resources, or her mother was guaranteed financial support, they would both have chosen to establish separate households.

The discovery of such ideas radically changed the explanation for the increasing tendency of the old to live apart from the children. Rather than being a sign of disrespect and obsolescence as early theorists had projected, several historians argued that this modern pattern reflected the fulfillment of longstanding desires. In the early twentieth century, with increasing wealth, growing numbers of middle-class individuals in the United States and Western Europe finally had the resources to support the creation of independent households (Ruggles, 1987; Haber & Gratton, 1993). The Great Depression challenged the economic basis of such homes and forced individuals back into co-residence, but the passage and expansion of federal pensions provided the assurance that resources would be available to support nuclear households. As a result, the majority of elderly individuals no longer resided with their children (Korbin, 1976). In the United States, in 1900, more than 60% of all individuals over 65 lived with at least one of their offspring; by 1962, the proportion had decreased to 25% and by 1975, it dropped to only 14% (Smith, 1982). In the United Kingdom, in 1911, only 8% of all older

men and 9% of all older women lived alone. By 1985, it had risen markedly to 20% for men and 47% for older women (Thane, 2001.) Such individuals now had the income and economic security to support their independent households.

## C. Global Perspectives

These findings served to explain both the diversity in households of the elderly and the trend toward independent residences. To a great extent, however, this research rested on models based largely on the United States and Europe. These studies obviously highlighted the diversity among the families of older people, and the importance of demography, culture, and economics on family structure, but many of the countries studied shared similar histories and traditions. Recently, therefore, historians of aging have begun to expand their focus to explore whether trends and patterns discerned in the West have resonated in other parts of the world. Looking especially at aging in East Asia, they have found that such cross-cultural perspectives add greatly to an understanding of the history of the elderly.

In many East Asian countries, even contemporary residential patterns of family life of older individuals contrast greatly with Western trends. Whereas in the United States, for example, by 1988, three-fourths of all older people lived alone or with their spouse, and only 14% resided with a child or children, in Thailand, the proportion of the elderly who lived apart from their children was only 10%; more than three-fourths of all older individuals continued to share households (Hermalin, Ofstedal, & Chang, 1996). The East, therefore, appears to retain a very different approach to the family structure and roles of the old.

Historians have found, in fact, that unlike England or the United States, in the twentieth century, complex families continued to be important forms of family organization; historically, they both provided assistance for the old and guaranteed linear descent. Thus, in contrast to England in the seventeenth and eighteenth century, in which only 2% of individuals lived as the parent of the household head, in Japan, in 1920, when the first national census was taken, the corresponding figure was 26% (Saito, 2001). Moreover, these households were not simply a transition stage for young, childless couples before they established their own homes, as was often the case in the West. Nearly a quarter of the residences included both the parent of the household and the grandchildren of the elder. In addition, unlike the Austrian households of the eighteenth century, the combined residences did not signify the passing of power from the older generation to the young adult. Although the aging male householder might "retire" and contractually pass headship to the young, the older generation did not immediately lose their authority over their households. For years to come, they still demanded the filial piety and obedience of the young (Wakao, 2001).

Yet historians have also discovered that, in the East, these patterns are hardly stable. In recent decades significant changes in the family structure of the old have occurred throughout the region. In Taiwan, for example, from 1976 to 1989, the proportion of older adults who lived with a married child declined from about two-thirds to a little more than half, and the percentage living alone or with their spouse rose from under 9% to nearly 23% (Knodel, Chayovan, & Siriboon, 1996). In Japan, since World War II, the predominance of the complex family has also been eroding. Even within a decade, this change had become noticeable: between 1980 and 1990, the proportion of older individuals who co-resided with married children declined from 53% to 42%, and the percentage living alone or with only

their spouse increased from 28% to nearly 37% (Morioka, 1996).

Scholars have pointed to a number of factors to explain this trend. As in the West, economic, demographic, and cultural changes have combined to challenge traditional family structure. With increasing urban and industrial growth, large numbers of individuals no longer lived on the farm. In Taiwan, for example, while one-fourth of the population was urban in 1949, the proportion had risen to three-fourths by 1988 (Knodel et al., 1996). Throughout East Asia, higher education and employment opportunities have led women into the workforce, rather than remaining at home and providing assistance to the their in-laws. The economic growth of the region has also created resources that serve to support the establishment of separate households. Moreover, legal and cultural changes have contributed to the evolution of family structure. In Japan, for example, complex households had traditionally been reinforced by the nineteenth-century Meiji Civil Code, which placed great emphasis on a linear continuation of the family and enforced support of the old by the co-resident offspring. In revising the Civil Code in 1947, the government decreed that all offspring, rather than the individual who resided with the old, were responsible for their care and support. This change, according to Kiyomi Morioka, "relieved the eldest son of the duty to live together with his parents" (Morioka, 1996, p. 271). Rather than shared residences being seen as a happy model, they have begun to take on a negative connotation. As in the West, individuals increasingly acknowledge that they would prefer to live in the independent household (Morioka, 1996).

## III. A Research Agenda

Work in the history of the family over the last 30 years has clearly challenged earlier assumptions about the role of the elderly in their kinship networks. As such research has shown, the family life of older people is marked by change and diversity. Scholars can no longer present the narrative as a simple tale of modernization, delineated by a preindustrial and an industrial phase. Nor can they describe the resulting history as a linear decline from authority and respect to disrespect and obsolescence. Rather, factors such as economics, gender, demography, and culture have combined to shape a stage of life characterized by significant variations. In different parts of the world, and even within a single country or region, the lives of the old within their own families have varied greatly. Although in the nineteenth century, the elderly African-American sharecropper, the village widow, the retired Austrian farmer, and even the Chinese mother-in-law may all have attained great age, their experiences in the last stage of life were hardly uniform. The nature of their final years reflected their own individual histories and desires, as well as their gender, ethnicity, economics, and culture. Historians must examine the common threads among these older individuals, even as they recognize and explore the vast differences.

This complexity, therefore, underscores the need and direction of future research. In tracing a broad history of old age, scholars must continue to determine how social forces, such as economics, demography, gender, and ethnicity, affected the lives of the old. At the same time, they must connect these factors with qualitative sources that reflect the desires of older individuals and their families. Such an approach is clearly not easy. In rescuing the elderly from a simplistic past by both exploring their differences and hearing their unique voice, historians cannot simply rely on a single individual or even a group as representative of the entire stage. Rather, they must confront the diversity inherit in the aging population and deal with its intricacies. The

recent cross-cultural studies have only emphasized how complicated this research agenda may be. Challenging scholars to look more closely at the convergence between culture, demographics, and economics, such studies have raised important questions about the impact of current developments, including those on public policy, on kinship, and household structure. This research not only allows historians to ask what is distinctive about a particular country or region but also provides an opportunity to examine the impact of specific cultural ideas and beliefs on more broadly shared social and economic trends. In the future, then, the work of historians has the promise to contribute to a meaningful and multifaceted understanding of what it was like for men and women in the past—of different classes, regions, ethnicities, and cultures—to experience the realities of growing old.

## References

Abel, E. (1992). Parental dependence and filial responsibility in the nineteenth century: Hial Hawley and Emily Hawley Gillespie, 1884–1885. *The Gerontologist, 32*, 519–526.

Anderson, M. (1971). *Family structure in nineteenth-century Lancashire.* London: Cambridge University Press.

Anderson, M. (1972). Household structure and the industrial revolution: Mid-nineteenth century Preston in comparative perspective. In P. Laslett (Ed.), *Household and family in past time* (pp. 215–235). Cambridge: Cambridge University Press.

Anderson, M. (1978). Family, household and the industrial revolution. In M. Gordon (Ed.), *The American family in social-historical perspective* (2nd ed., pp. 38–50). New York: St. Martin's Press.

Anonymous. (1931). Old age intestate. *Harper's,* 715.

Berkner, L. K. (1972). The stem family and the developmental cycle of the peasant household: An eighteenth-century Austrian example. *The American Historical Review, 77,* 398–418.

Bever, E. (1982). Old age and witchcraft in early modern Europe. In P. Stearns (Ed.), *Old age in preindustrial society* (pp. 150–190). New York: Holmes & Meier.

Burgess, E. W. (1945). *The family, from institution to companionship*. New York: American Book Company.

Burgess, E. W. (1960). Aging in western culture. In E. W. Burgess (Ed.), *Aging in western society* (pp. 3–28). Chicago: University of Chicago Press.

Chudacoff, H. (1978). Newlyweds and family extension: The first stage of the family cycle in Providence, Rhode Island, 1864–1865 and 1879–1880. In T. Hareven & M. Vinovskis (Eds.), *Family and population in nineteenth-century America* (pp. 179–205). Princeton, NJ: Princeton University Press.

Chudacoff, H., & Hareven, T. (1978). Family transition in old age. In T. Hareven (Ed.), *Transitions: The family and life course in historical perspective* (pp. 217–243). New York: Academic Press.

Cowgill, D. (1972). A theory of aging in cross-cultural perspective. In D. Cowgill & L. Holmes (Eds.), *Aging and modernization* (pp. 1–13). New York: Appleton-Century-Crofts.

Cowgill, D., & Holmes, L. (1972). Summary and conclusion: The theory in review. In D. Cowgill & L. Holmes (Eds.), *Aging and modernization* (pp. 305–323). New York: Appleton-Century-Crofts.

Demos, J. (1970). *A little commonwealth: Family life in Plymouth colony*. New York: Oxford University Press.

Demos, J. (1972). Demography and psychology in the historical family study. In P. Laslett (Ed.), *Household and family in past time* (pp. 561–569). Cambridge: Cambridge University Press.

Demos, J. (1978). Old age in New England. In M. Gordon (Ed.), *The American family in social-historical perspective* (2nd ed., pp. 220–256). New York: St. Martin's Press.

Falkner, T., & de Luce, J. (1992). A view from antiquity: Greece, Rome, and elders. In T. Cole, D. D. Van Tassel, & R. Kastenbaum (Eds.), *Handbook of the humanities of aging* (pp. 3–39). New York: Springer Publishing Co.

Gratton, B., & Haber, C. (1993). In search of "intimacy at a distance": Family history from the perspective of elderly women. *Journal of Aging Studies, 7,* 183–194.

Greven, P. (1970). *Four generations: Population, land and family in colonial Andover*. Ithaca, NY: Cornell University Press.

Greven, P. (1972). The average size of families and households in the Province of Massachusetts in 1764 and in the United States in 1970: An overview. In P. Laslett (Ed.), *Household and family in past time* (pp. 545–560). Cambridge: Cambridge University Press.

Haber, C. (1997). Widows, witches, wives and workers: The historiography of elderly women in America. In J. Coyle (Ed.), *Handbook on women and aging* (pp. 29–40). Westport, CT: Greenwood Press.

Haber, C., & Gratton, B. (1993). *Old age and the search for security*. Bloomington: Indiana University Press.

Halpern, J. M. (1972). Town and countryside in Serbia in the nineteenth century. In P. Laslett (Ed.), *Household and family in past time* (pp. 401–427). Cambridge: Cambridge University Press.

Hammel, E. A. (1972). The zadruga as process. In P. Laslett (Ed.), *Household and family in past time* (pp. 335–374). Cambridge: Cambridge University Press.

Hermalin, A., Ofstedal, M. B., & Chang, M.-C. (1996). Types of support for the aged and their providers in Taiwan. In T. Hareven (Ed.), *Aging and generational relations: Life-course and cross-cultural perspectives* (pp. 179–216). New York: Aldine de Gruyter.

Hussey, S. (2001). "An inheritance of fear": Older women in the twentieth-century countryside. In L. Botelho & P. Thane (Eds.), *Women and ageing in British society since 1500* (pp. 187–206). Harlow, England: Longman Press.

Karlsen, C. (1987). *The devil in the shape of a woman*. New York: Norton.

Kertzer, D. I., & Karweit, N. (1995). The impact of widowhood in nineteenth-century Italy. In D. Kertzer & P. Laslett (Eds.), *Aging in the past: Demography, society and old age* (pp. 229–248). Berkeley: University of California Press.

Knodel, J., Chayovan, N., & Siriboon, S. (1996). Familial support and the life course of Thai elderly and their children. In T. Hareven (Ed.), *Aging and generational* relations: Life-course and cross-cultural perspectives (pp. 217–240). New York: Aldine de Gruyter.

Korbin, F. (1976). The fall in household size and the rise of the primary individual in the United States. Demography, 13, 127–138.

Laslett, P. (1972a). Introduction: the history of the family. In P. Laslett (Ed.), Household and family in past time (pp. 1–89). Cambridge: Cambridge University Press.

Laslett, P. (1972b). Mean household size in England since the sixteenth century. In P. Laslett (Ed.), Household and family in past time (pp. 125–158). Cambridge: Cambridge University Press.

Laslett, P., & Clarke, M. (1972). Houseful and household in an eighteenth-century Balkan city. In P. Laslett (Ed.), Household and family in past time (pp. 375–400). Cambridge: Cambridge University Press.

Modell, J., & Hareven, T. (1978). Urbanization and the malleable household. In M. Gordon (Ed.), The American family in social-historical perspective (2nd ed., pp. 51–68). New York: St. Martin's Press.

Morioka, K. (1996). Generational relations and their changes as they affect the status of older people in Japan. In T. Hareven (Ed.), Aging and generational relations: Life-course and cross-cultural perspectives (pp. 263–280). New York: Aldine de Gruyter.

Ottaway, S. (2001). The old woman's home in eighteenth-century England. In L. Botelho & P. Thane (Eds.), Women and ageing in British society since 1500 (pp. 111–138). Harlow, England: Longman Press.

Premo, T. (1990). Winter friends: Women growing old in the new republic, 1785–1835. Urbana, IL: University of Illinois Press.

Quadagno, J. (1982). Aging in early industrial England. New York: Academic Press.

Ruggles, S. (1987). Prolonged connections: The rise of the extended family in nineteenth-century England and America. Madison, WI: University of Wisconsin Press.

Ryan, M. (1981). The cradle of the middle class. Cambridge: Cambridge University Press.

Saito, O. (2001). Two forms of stem family system in one country?: The evidence from Japan's first national census. In R. Wall, T. Hareven, & J. Ehmer (Eds.), Family his-tory revisited: Comparative perspectives (pp. 331–349). Newark, DE: University of Delaware Press.

Simmons. L. W. (1945). The role of the aged in primitive society. New Haven: Yale University Press.

Simmons, L. W. (1960). Aging in preindustrial societies. In C. Tibbitts (Ed.), Handbook of social gerontology (pp. 62–91). Chicago: University of Chicago Press.

Shammas, C., Salmon, M., & Dahlin, M. (1987). Inheritance in America. New Brunswick, NJ: Rutgers University Press.

Smith, D. S. (1982). Historical change in the household structure of the elderly in economically developed societies. In P. Stearns (Ed.), Old age in preindustrial society (pp. 248–273). New York: Holmes & Meier.

Thane, P. (2000). Old age in English history. Oxford: Oxford University Press.

Thane, P. (2001). Old women in twentieth century Britain. In L. Botelho & P. Thane (Eds.), Women and ageing in British society since 1500 (pp. 207–231). Harlow, England: Longman Press.

Troyansky, D. (1989). Old age in the old regime. New York: Cornell University Press.

Ulrich, L. T. (1990). The life of Martha Ballard based on her diary, 1785–1812. New York: Random House.

Wakao, Y. (2001). A comparative perspective on rural families in Japan from the early modern period until the middle of the nineteenth century. In R. Wall, T. Hareven, & J. Ehmer (Eds.), Family history revisited: comparative perspectives (pp. 311–330). Newark, DE: University of Delaware Press.

Wall, R. (1995). Elderly persons and members of their household in England and Wales from preindustrial times to the present. In D. Kertzer & P. Laslett (Eds.), Aging in the past: Demography, society, and old age (pp. 81–106). Berkeley: University of California Press.

Wall, R. (2001). The transformation of the European family across the centuries. In R. Wall, T. Hareven, & J. Ehmer (Eds.), Family history revisited: comparative perspectives (pp. 217–241). Newark, DE: University of Delaware Press.

## Five

# Internal and International Migration

Charles F. Longino, Jr., and Don E. Bradley

Scholarship on later-life migration has grown considerably over the past decade, owing largely to new studies on international migration coming from Europe and elsewhere. This chapter, therefore, is divided primarily into two parts, one reviewing internal migration in the United States, and the other international migration.

## I. Internal Migration

### A. Conceptual Models

The 1990s and early 2000s saw a steady advancement of conceptual models in the study of later-life migration. They do not compete directly with one another, but instead have different types of starting points: the migration decision process, the life course, and place identity.

### 1. The Migration Decision Models

Attempts to understand the dynamics of general migration began in the late nineteenth century with a paper presented at the Royal Statistical Society of London by E. G. Ravenstein (1885), which was then elaborated and formalized by Everett Lee (1966) some 70 years later. In this formulation, the origin and destination of the migrant have attractions and repulsions (pushes and pulls). There is a strong tendency in migration research to attempt to infer the motivation of the migrant from studying the characteristics of the places they leave or those to which they move (Plane & Heins, 2003). For example, in aggregate, origins have lower average winter temperatures than destinations, and higher costs of living; both are pushes. Rural areas in the Southeast United States that have consistently attracted older migrants tend to have mild climates, to be growing economically, and to have lower taxes. They tend to be coastal or mountainous and many are adjacent to metropolitan areas (Serow, 2001; Walters, 2002). Purely aggregate geographical research, however, is declining. The better decision models today include both place characteristics and personal attributes and often in creative and useful combinations (Cutchin, 2001).

*Handbook of Aging and the Social Sciences, Sixth Edition*

Wiseman (1980) delineated person-environment adjustment processes by which older adults decide whether or not and where to move. Wiseman argued that moves are triggered by push-and-pull factors, such as climate, environmental hassle level, or cost of living, and facilitated or hampered by indigenous filters such as personal resources or the housing market. There are also feedback loops in Wiseman's model. People who do not decide to move, or cannot successfully choose a destination, may adjust to their present location through various mechanisms to avoid feeling trapped there. Furthermore, over time, migration outcomes that initially are improvements, generate new pushes and pulls that may eventually trigger another move.

Haas and Serow (1993) elaborated on the Wiseman model, fitting it to the circumstance of the recently or nearly retired amenity-seeking migrant. They added to the model "remote thoughts" or daydreams about moving (Furstenberg, 2002; Krout, Moen, Holmes, Oggins, & Bowen, 2002) that precede the formal process, and the information sources that make the actor aware of push-pull factors. Whether, where, and when to migrate may be a three-phase decision-making process that can occur in any order (DeJong, 1999; Hays & Longino, 2002; Schiamberg & McKinney, 2003; Watkins, 1999).

*2. The Life-Course Models.*

Rossi (1955) may have been the first to carefully analyze age and mobility, showing that younger people move for many reasons related to their need to establish educational, work, and family statuses. It was just a matter of time until Rossi's approach was extended to later-life mobility that is related to retirement and health (Warnes, 1992; Plane and Heins, 2003).

Litwak and Longino (1987) were the first to present a developmental context

for the patterns of older interstate migration that are now commonly reported in demographic studies. They argued that retirement and health change, over time, put older people under pressures to make three basic types of moves. The first type involves persons who are recently retired; these are often "amenity-driven moves" (Newbold, 1996). A second type includes persons who are experiencing moderate forms of disability (Longino, Jackson, Zimmerman, & Bradsher, 1991; Miller, Longino, Anderson, James, & Worley, 1999), a situation often compounded by widowhood (Bradsher, Longino, Jackson, & Zimmerman, 1992). Movement toward family members is one result (Silverstein, 1995; Silverstein and Angelelli, 1998). Researchers often refer to these as "assistance moves." A third type is an institutional move when health problems overwhelm the capability of the family to care for older relatives in the community.

DeJong, Wilmoth, Angel, & Cornwell (1995) and Hays & Longino (2002) argued effectively that not only poor health but reduced social affiliation, economic insecurity, and functional limitations can motivate a move in later life. The life-course model merely arranges some of these motivations around a type of move.

*3. The Place Identity Models*

A final conceptual framework emerging during the 1990s is what has been referred to in the literature as the place identity model (Cuba, 1989; Cutchin, 2001). There are some migrants who never put down roots but remain emotionally tied to their former communities. Some of them have problems changing from being a vacationer to being a permanent resident after they arrive in their destination communities. And some put on an "ageless self" identity when joining the ranks of the active retirees in their new communities (McHugh, 2000, 2003). This social psychological approach has brought a whole new dimension to understanding migration and migrants, and deserves greater study.

## B. Patterns of Migration in the United States

One way of describing migration destinations is to compare the numbers of individuals who moved to different states or counties, ranking the states or counties that received the largest proportions. In 1940, and since 1960, the U.S. Census has asked where one lived exactly five years before the census: in the same house, in another county in the same state, in another state, or abroad. Using this five-year item, the numbers and proportions of interstate and intrastate migrants can be compared over time. Interstate migration has held very steady for migrants age 60 and older, at 4.0% to 4.6% over five years (Longino & Bradley, 2003). Short distance migration within states has declined over the past half century for persons of all ages. Census micro-data are handy for making such comparisons. All U.S. census micro-data files contain a sample of individual census records (with identifiers removed). Because the data are not aggregated, these files allow the researcher to create new custom-designed tabulations. There is a drawback when using micro-data, however, because counties are clustered together so that no county containing fewer than 100,000 persons can be separately identified. These units are called PUMAs (public use micro-data areas).

### 1. Substate Destinations

Using the 2000 census micro-data files, the top 100 counties or county groups have been ranked in terms of net interstate migration. In this ranking, Florida contains 31 of these destinations for interstate migrants, in keeping with its longstanding status as the leading migration destination

for older migrants. Palm Beach County ranks second. Nationally, the leading sub-state destinations are located in coastal, mountain, and desert counties across the United States, from seaside Maine and Cape Cod in Massachusetts to the Puget Sound in Washington and coastal Oregon. Maricopa County, Arizona (Phoenix), and Clark County, Nevada (Las Vegas), rank first and third nationally, respectively, and are the leading substate destinations in the West. Riverside County, California (Palm Springs), ranks 28th and is California's only entry on the list.

Although the Sunbelt is generally the dominant regional destination, there is greater variety than is commonly assumed. Ocean County, New Jersey, for example, has consistently received enough retirees from New York and Pennsylvania to keep it among the top 100 interstate destinations for several decades.

Regional destinations attract migrants primarily from adjacent states. Examples are Cape Cod, Massachusetts, the New Jersey shore, the Pocono Mountains of northeastern Pennsylvania, all located outside the Sunbelt. Other locations in the Appalachian Mountains and the Ozark region of Missouri and Arkansas are in the noncoastal Sunbelt. Southern and western Nevada and areas in the Pacific Northwest are all retirement areas of strong regional attraction and are frequently cited in retirement guides as good places to retire (Savageau, 2000).

### 2. State Destinations

One of the defining characteristics of interstate retirement migration is that the migrants coming from many states are concentrated in only a few destinations, a result of highly focused flows into certain states. In 2000, over half of older migrants, 54% (compared to 56% in 1990), arrived in just 10 states, having lived in other states five years before.

Florida dominates the scene, having attracted from one-fifth to a quarter of all interstate migrants over 60 in all five census decades from 1960 to 2000.

A new phenomenon occurred in the 1985–1990 migration period. There was a small, gradual, decrease in the proportion of migrants received by the major destination states, with a gentle spreading out of the flows (as compared with earlier migration periods).

As Table 5.1 shows, the proportion of total migration going to the leading two destination states, Florida and California, has declined each decade since 1980, California losing its second place ranking in 2000 to a much less populous state, Arizona. Although the losses for Florida and California were relatively small, the trend is clear and persistent. Underscoring the reality of this change, these declines are particularly noticeable because the numbers of interstate migrants leveled off between 1990 and 2000, causing the numbers, as well as the proportions, of migrants into Florida and California to drop between the past two censuses. It would be wrong, however, to predict the demise of Florida as the leading destination for retired migrants on the basis of these trends. It still attracts more later-life migrants than Arizona, California, and Texas combined.

### 3. Origins of Interstate Migrants

The 100 counties in 2000 sending the largest numbers of interstate migrants to other states were the comparatively populous metropolitan or suburban counties, led by Los Angeles County, California, and Cook County, Illinois. Not surprisingly, the majority (58) of these counties or county groups were from outside the Sunbelt. The surprise is that the remaining 42 are located in the states that attract the most interstate migrants. Thirteen are located in Florida. These Florida counties receive far more inter-

state migrants than leave them for counties outside of Florida. However, migrants of retirement age do leave Florida and other Sunbelt states, a point often missed by media accounts of retirement migration. Indeed, Florida ranks third, below only New York and California, on the list of major sending states. Counterstream and return migration help to explain outmigration from the major receiving states. They are both discussed later in this chapter.

When the 100 leading origin counties (or county groups) are examined, they are nearly all metropolitan or suburban counties (Longino, 1995). This fact may help to explain why interstate migrants like to move to counties that have a lower cost of living, are less congested, and are more scenic, but counties nonetheless that are either metropolitan counties themselves or are not far from metropolitan counties (e.g., Dade and Hillsborough counties in Florida and Maricopa County in Arizona) and can support important aspects of the migrants' former metropolitan lifestyles.

### C. "Migration" to Nursing Homes

In the life-course theoretical model, the final type of move is a move away from informal care by family members and others to institutional care. Research on movement for institutional care is a promising new area of migration research. It typically includes all migrants, those moving across county lines in the same state, as well as those moving from a different state. McAuley, Pecchioni, and Grant (1999) used a conceptual framework based on both the migration theory and the long-term care decision process. These researchers compared the distance of the move and characteristics of migrants who moved from other communities into Virginia nursing homes. Most moved from within state. The data indicated that scarcity of supply (i.e., low availability of nursing home beds) in the

**Table 5.1.**
Ten States Receiving Most In-Migrants Age 60+ in Five-Year Periods Ending in 1960, 1970, 1980, 1990, and 2000

| Rank | 1960 State | 1960 # | 1960 % | 1970 State | 1970 # | 1970 % | 1980 State | 1980 # | 1980 % | 1990 State | 1990 # | 1990 % | 2000 State | 2000 # | 2000 % |
|---|---|---|---|---|---|---|---|---|---|---|---|---|---|---|---|
| 1 | FL | 208,072 | 22.3 | FL | 263,200 | 24.4 | FL | 437,040 | 26.3 | FL | 451,709 | 23.8 | FL | 401,052 | 19.1 |
| 2 | CA | 126,883 | 13.6 | CA | 107,000 | 9.9 | CA | 144,880 | 8.7 | CA | 131,514 | 6.9 | AZ | 134,183 | 6.4 |
| 3 | NJ | 36,019 | 3.9 | AZ | 47,600 | 4.4 | AZ | 94,600 | 5.7 | AZ | 98,756 | 5.2 | CA | 127,693 | 6.1 |
| 4 | NY | 33,794 | 3.6 | NJ | 46,000 | 4.3 | TX | 78,480 | 4.7 | TX | 78,117 | 4.1 | TX | 101,446 | 4.8 |
| 5 | IL | 30,355 | 3.3 | TX | 39,800 | 3.7 | NJ | 49,400 | 3.0 | NC | 64,530 | 3.4 | NC | 77,720 | 3.7 |
| 6 | AZ | 29,571 | 3.2 | NY | 32,800 | 3.0 | PA | 39,520 | 2.4 | PA | 57,538 | 3.0 | GA | 63,120 | 3.0 |
| 7 | OH | 27,759 | 3.0 | OH | 32,300 | 3.0 | NC | 39,400 | 2.4 | NJ | 49,176 | 2.6 | NV | 62,155 | 3.0 |
| 8 | TX | 26,770 | 2.9 | IL | 28,800 | 2.7 | WA | 35,760 | 2.2 | WA | 47,484 | 2.5 | PA | 60,082 | 2.9 |
| 9 | PA | 25,738 | 2.8 | PA | 28,600 | 2.7 | VA | 35,720 | 2.1 | VA | 46,554 | 2.4 | NJ | 54,425 | 2.6 |
| 10 | MO | 20,308 | 2.2 | NY | 25,300 | 2.3 | NY | 34,920 | 2.1 | GA | 44,475 | 2.3 | VA | 53,776 | 2.6 |
| **Total Interstate Migrants** | 931,012 | | | 1,079,200[1] | | | 1,622,120[2] | | | 1,901,105 | | | 2,096,841 | | |
| **% of Total in Top 10 States** | 60.7 | | | 60.4 | | | 59.5 | | | 56.3 | | | 54.3 | | |

Source: Authors' calculations, based on U.S. Census Bureau Public Use Micro-data samples weighted to provide 100% population estimates.
[1] This figure was derived by extrapolating from a 1-in-100 sample. The actual census  count was 1,094,014.
[2] This figure was derived by extrapolating from a 1-in-40 sample. The actual census  count was 1,654,000.

county of origin is a push factor in the move. Additionally, nursing homes in Virginia with religious affiliations were more likely to attract admissions from other counties, resulting from, presumably, loyalty to church sponsorship. Stoller and Perzynski (2003) expanded this notion by showing that respondents in their study were more likely to mention nursing home placement as part of their planning for long-term care if they had been geographically mobile and if they were identified with and involved in an ethnic community.

Furthermore, older persons who become more seriously disabled are especially likely to move, although their moves may be short-term rather than long-term moves (Miller et al., 1999). Moreover, Walters (2002) observed that severely disabled migrants are more likely than other older migrants to exit those locations with inadequate nursing home facilities. Finally, Colsher & Wallace (1990) studied older rural residents, comparing their anticipated and actual relocations. Comparing institutional and noninstitutional moves, they found a high proportion of health-related moves in both categories. In some ways, those not moving to institutions were in poorer physical and mental health. Although it is a mistake to think that all health-related moves late in life are to institutions, it is equally false to assume that only the healthy move.

## D. Migration Selectivity

"Who moves among the elderly?" was the title of the first comprehensive census analysis of the population characteristics of older mover types (Biggar, 1980). Biggar's article made a very strong statement, showing that there were distinctive profiles among the various elderly mobility categories (nonmovers, local movers, intrastate migrants, and interstate migrants). Local movers (in contrast

to nonmovers) had lower average incomes, and a higher proportion were living dependently with others. Interstate migrants were younger, more often married, more likely to live in their own homes, and had higher average incomes and education than persons in the other mobility categories.

Walters (2002) reminded us that it is fairly common for studies to include personal attributes of migrants and seek to infer mobility motivation from them. Hazelrigg and Hardy (1995) extended Biggar's work by comparing the income characteristics of older migrants with nonmigrant age peers at their destinations and finding that the migrants were economically better off. They attributed this to the tendency of migrants to move to locations with a somewhat lower cost of living than at their origin. Cost of living and income are higher in large cities. Second, some important selectivity factors are at work. Moving is costly, and this tends to screen out those who cannot afford to make a move. Further, amenity migrants tend to move soon after retirement, before there is any decay in their retirement income relative to more recent retirees.

The study of migration selectivity seems disjointed and incomplete apart from theoretical frameworks. In Wiseman's (1980) migration decision model, for example, if life transitions, such as divorce, death of spouse (Chevan, 1995), children leaving home and, of course, retirement, are likely triggers for migration among people in their fifties and sixties, then one could expect to find a higher proportion of persons with these experiences "selected" into the ranks of the migrants. The same would be true for previous travel experience. In Lee's (1966) push-pull model, economic and health resources are viewed as "intervening obstacles" that could hinder or facilitate mobility. Pulls from the destination could include climate, cost of living, and even the tax structure (Serow, 2003; Duncombe, Robbins, & Wolf, 2003).

## E. Cyclical Migration

Three cyclical patterns of interstate migration have been identified in the United States over the last 20 years. They are seasonal migration, counterstream migration, and return migration.

### 1. Seasonal Migration

The Census Bureau does not attempt to directly measure seasonal migration; however, there have been several useful local surveys. Survey results (McHugh & Mings, 1991) have identified Arizona seasonal migrants as overwhelmingly Caucasian, retired, healthy, and married couples largely in their sixties. These are characteristics associated, in other studies, with amenity migration. McHugh and Mings (1991) were the first to document the up until then assumed fact that the colder the climate, the more likely retirees are to migrate seasonally. United States retirees in states along the Canadian border have a greater propensity to migrate seasonally than those in states located farther south.

Is seasonal migration only a precursor to a permanent move? It seems to depend on the balance between their ties to places and persons at origin and destination, and the shift in these ties over time, in keeping with Lee's push-pull model. The vast majority of seasonal migrants, perhaps 80%, apparently do not relocate permanently. They extend or shorten their visits, and they finally end their extended series of visits when their health forces them to do so. Arizona seasonal migrants tend to adjust to health decrements over time, reducing the number of side trips and giving up their recreational vehicles in favor of rented lodging during their seasonal trips (McHugh & Mings, 1994).

McHugh, Hogan, and Happel (1995) found that seasonal migration often occurs in stages, beginning with vacationing in midlife and leading to longer stays in the retirement years. When those who moved to Arizona only for the winter were combined with those who left in the summer and those who moved within Arizona seasonally, Hogan & Steinnes (1998) estimated that one-fourth of older persons in the state fall into one of these categories!

Apparently, seasonal migration generates its own lifestyle and culture. Once having adopted the lifestyle, seasonal migration is likely to last for several years, finally interrupted, and reluctantly terminated.

### 2. Counterstream Migration

When the state-to-state streams of older migrants were studied, using 1980 census data, researchers were not surprised to find paired exchanges of migrants between states that they called streams and counterstreams. These paired exchanges are an expected part of the migration landscape. Furthermore, the researchers found that a higher proportion of the migrants who were somewhat older, on average, were more often widowed and living dependently with relatives among those who had moved in counterstreams than in streams (Litwak & Longino, 1987). There are many first-time movers in the counterstreams, too, even from popular destinations.

Using 1990 census data, and comparing the 50 largest pairs of streams and counterstreams, three geographical patterns were found (Longino, 1995). The first is exchanges between Florida and some of its major "partners": New York, Ohio, Pennsylvania, Michigan, Illinois, Massachusetts, Connecticut, Indiana, Virginia, Maryland, and Wisconsin. The streams were into Florida, of course, with counterstreams in the opposite direction.

The second geographical pattern is exchanges between California and adjacent or regional states: Arizona, Washington, Oregon, Nevada, and Texas. The smaller counterstreams in this pattern are back to California!

The third pattern, also regional, is the Mid-Atlantic exchange system. It includes streams out of New York to three adjacent states, Pennsylvania, New Jersey, and Connecticut, with counterstreams back to New York. These three exchange patterns held in the 2000 census.

These findings led to the speculation that counterstreams contain large proportions of returning migrants who had moved at an earlier time to a popular destination and are later returning to the state from which they came. This speculation was bolstered by data showing the large proportions of migrants in counterstreams who were returning to their states of birth (Longino, 1995).

### 3. Return Migration (to One's State of Birth) Over Time

For older people nationally, return migration as a proportion of total migration is on the decline. One-fifth (20.3%) of older migrants in 1970 were returning to their states of birth. Fewer (18.6%) returned in 1980 and fewer still (17.5%) in 1990, leveling off at 17.5% in 2000.

*Ethnic enclave settlement and return migration* of African Americans to the South and Southwest involves a historical work cycle. Industrial states recruit workers from rural parts of the country. Over time, however, return migration streams develop that carry some of the retired workers back to their states of birth.

In this context, it is not surprising to find that a majority of African-American migrants age 60 and older are moving into the southern states. Nor is it surprising to

find that return migration rates are high among these migrants (Longino & Smith, 1991). It is too early in the process of industrial recruitment of Hispanics to see high rates of return migration among Hispanics from Illinois and Michigan to the Southwest. However, projecting from the African-American work and retirement migration patterns, it would not be surprising to find such a development in the future.

There are two additional types of return migration discussed in the literature. The first is *provincial return migration*, a subset of amenity migration. It consists of life-style-motivated movers who are choosing to move to their states of birth. They are younger, slightly better educated, more affluent, and far more often married than return migrants in general. The second type, *counterstream return migration*, discussed in the previous section, is a subset of *assistance migration*, a move undertaken to gain assistance in activities of daily living. Interregional migrants, returning to their states of birth in the Northeast and Midwest, fit the aggregate description of counterstream return migration, and interregional migrants to the South and the Southwest fit the aggregate description of provincial return migration (Longino & Serow, 1990).

### F. Migration impact

### 1. Economic Impact

The decade of the 1990s began with a spate of articles considering the economic impact of retirees at their destination. A sizable amount of annual income is transferred to and from states as a result of interstate migration. This money tends to concentrate, of course, in the major destination states (Longino & Crown, 1990; Crown & Longino, 1991; Sastry, 1992; Serow, Friedrich, & Haas, 1992). Unfortunately a comprehensive measure of consumer spending is not included in the census micro-data files. Income, in these studies, is a proxy for consumer spending.

During the same period, 515 rural counties, where the older population was growing through migration, outperformed nonmetropolitan area averages for job growth (Reeder & Glasgow, 1990; Glasgow, 1991), ostensibly a result of retiree consumer spending. Hodge (1991) reported data supportive of this analysis in his study of smaller communities in the province of British Columbia, Canada, as did Bennett (1992, 1993, 1996) in his studies of high-amenity retirement counties on the Atlantic seaboard. Deller (1995) used a regional economic model to simulate the impact of a policy of retirement recruitment on the state of Maine, showing a significant beneficial short-run economic impact on employment.

## 2. Local Political Activism and Support for Public Services

The positive economic impact must be balanced against a *negative* effect for public school financing. Local voting studies have tended to examine the results of local school budget referenda. Using the results of school district bond elections in Florida, Button (1992) and MacManus (1997) found that a higher percentage of older residents and voters in a school district are associated with lower support for schools. This finding is consistent with recent research by Simonsen and Robbins (1996), who found that citizens and senior citizens, in particular, were much less supportive of public services that they do not expect to use, including schools. We do not mean to imply that only older citizens, or the migrants among them, vote against school bonds. Younger persons without children and those who send their children to private and parochial schools tend to do the same.

## 3. Impact on Community Social Structure and Values

Longino (1990) argued that retirement enclaves in rural counties tend to be worlds unto themselves, relatively unattached to local social structure. McHugh, Gober, & Borough (2002) called them "common interest developments." Cuba (1992) even argued that on Cape Cod, the distinguishing characteristics of older migrants make them susceptible to being treated as outsiders by nonmigrants and younger migrants. This pattern is also seen with international migrants, discussed later in this chapter.

Later studies have seen migrants as proactive change agents in their communities. Rowles and Watkins (1993), for example, provided case studies of three contrasting Appalachian communities at different stages of development as retirement destinations (emergence, recognition, restructuring, and saturation). This study is refreshingly insightful because it analyzes retirement migration in a broader social context. For example, middle-class retirees are likely to band together to protect the environmental ambiance of the community. Chambers of Commerce trying to recruit both retirees and industry to their community could find the retirees actively opposing industrial development on environmental grounds.

## II. Late-Life International Migration

An emerging body of research examines international mobility among older adults. The discussion to follow borrows from Litwak and Longino's (1987) model, introduced previously, to draw a distinction between *international assistance migration* (i.e., family-based international moves motivated by moderate disability or negative life circumstances) and *international amenity migration* (i.e., international moves motivated by life-style considerations). In addition, our review reflects the importance of cyclical international migration among older adults, particularly return migration (Blakemore, 1999).

## A. International Assistance Migration

### 1. Why Do They Move?

Most contemporary later-life international migrants to the United States join children who have become citizens (Treas, 1997). Adult children migrating out of a region often leave parents behind with no one to care for them as they grow old and infirm. Joining children working abroad is one resolution to this problem (van der Geest, Mul, & Vermeulen, 2004).

Older *refugees* who accompany younger family members constitute an additional source of international assistance migration; political upheaval and persecution generate out-migration pressures on both young and old. Under these circumstances international mobility is often traumatic and disorderly, such that refugees are unprepared for their new lives. Economic and social adjustment to the receiving society is especially difficult for older refugees and their families who may, for example, have been forced to leave assets and loved ones behind. (Detzner,1996; Weinstein-Shr & Henkin 1991).

### 2. How Do They Adjust on Arrival?

Angel and Angel, in Chapter 6 of this volume, describe serious obstacles to economic and social adjustment confronting later-life international migrants, especially those arriving from countries in the developing world where citizens possess limited occupational skills. Long-term economic dependence on younger family members is suggested by a range of studies indicating that age at immigration is inversely related to the likelihood of living independently.

Yet, relatively high rates of family co-residence among later-life immigrants probably reflect both necessity and cultural preference. Multivariate analyses demonstrate that the inverse relationship between age at immigration and co-residence persists despite controls for duration of residence, English ability, education, income, and health among other factors considered (Angel, Angel, & Markides, 2000; Glick, 2000; Wilmoth, DeJong, & Himes, 1997).

Immigrants face many challenges of social and cultural adjustments. Among immigrants, those arriving late in life may suffer relatively high rates of depression (Angel & Angel 1992; Black, Markides, & Miller 1998). Second language acquisition may be particularly difficult for immigrants arriving late in life (Stevens, 1999). Poor language skills, in turn, may undermine adjustment to the receiving society. For example, the ability to form supportive friendships outside the family depends in part on facility in the language of the host society, and social isolation among immigrant elders appears to have negative mental health implications (Krause & Goldenhaar, 1992; Litwin 1995, 1997).

Linguistic difficulties similarly constrain access to services, most notably health care (Strumpf, Glicksman, Goldber-Glen, Fox, & Logue, 2001). Where medical professionals that speak the immigrants' native language are unavailable, older immigrants may be forced to rely on their children or grandchildren to serve as intermediaries and translators (Chappell & Lai, 1998; Remennick & Ottenstein-Eisen, 1998).

Communication difficulties with health care professionals may be compounded by cultural differences. By way of illustration, assistance migrants arriving from lesser developed countries often recognize the technical superiority of Western medicine but report dissatisfaction with physicians who do not practice medicine in the accustomed manner. For example, Emami, Benner, and Ekman's (2001) older Iranian respondents found the less authoritative manner assumed by Swedish doctors compared to their Iranian counterparts disconcerting. In addition, the culturally defined meaning of health and aging may differ substantially between sending and receiving societies. A fatalistic attitude toward physical decline, for instance, may inhibit health-seeking behaviors and the adoption of healthy habits (Remennick & Ottenstein-Eisen, 1998; Torres, 2001). Immigrant patients may avoid drawing of blood (Yee, 1992) and blend prescribed treatment regimens with traditional remedies (Chappell & Lai, 1998).

Because assistance immigrants are often highly dependent on younger family members, immigration can lead to a shift in the household balance of power, frequently generating intergenerational conflict. In regions where assistance immigrants typically originate, adult children are expected to provide for and revere their aging parents (Kim, Kim, & Hurh, 1991; Weinstein-Shr & Henkin, 1991). In immigrant households, however, adult children who are relatively assimilated into the new culture are unlikely to consult parents who do not understand the host society very well (Treas & Mazumdar, 2002). Moreover, traditional obligations are difficult to enforce in industrial receiving societies where young adults do not depend on inheriting land from their parents but command independent income streams (Kim, Kim, & Hurh, 1991). Consequently, older parents may feel disappointed by the failure of younger family members to offer them the reverence and service they had anticipated (Detzner, 1996).

Despite forfeiting influence and respect within their families, older immigrants often make essential contributions to their households, providing childcare, performing household chores, and preserving the family's cultural heritage (Treas & Mazumdark, 2002). Declining health and increased dependency on younger family members, however, may generate further tension as the intergenerational balance of exchange is disrupted (Slonim-Nevo, Cwikel, Luski, Lankry, & Shraga, 1995).

## B. International Amenity Migration

An established literature examines the seasonal flow of Canadians to Florida, highlighting distinctive features generated by national differences in health care systems (Marshall, Longino, Tucker, & Mullins, 1989) and by geographical diversity of flows composed of francophones and anglophones (Tucker, Mullins, Beland, Longino, & Marshall, 1992). A more recently emerging literature documents the flow of amenity migrants from developed nations to less developed nations. Recent collaborative efforts have examined Northern European retirees across a range of destinations in Southern Europe (Casado-Diaz, Kaiser, & Warnes, 2004), and a handful of studies have looked at North Americans in Mexico (Truly, 2002).

### 1. Who Are They and Why Do They Move?

Increased long-distance mobility among older adults partly reflects broad societal changes (e.g., earlier retirement and increased longevity). In particular, an evident increase in amenity moves across international boundaries (Warnes, 2001) reflects higher rates of international experience owing to (1) the globalization of labor markets, (2) the expansion of international tourism, and (3) improved transportation infrastructures. In addition, the emergence of the European Union and the democratization of Southern Europe have removed barriers to property ownership and voting rights for expatriate retirees (King, Warnes, & Williams, 2000), and the North American Free Trade Agreement (NAFTA) has permitted North Americans in Mexico access to familiar products and services (Truly, 2002).

Consistent with the discussion of amenity-seeking migration presented previously, international amenity immigrants identify the climate, a slower pace of life, and lower cost of living as key pull factors (Casado-Diaz, Kaiser, & Warnes, 2004; Huber & O'Reilly, 2004). However, some expressed dissatisfaction with their homeland as a push factor motivating relocation (Buller & Hoggart, 1994; Truly, 2002). Amenity immigrants typically report previous vacation experience in the destination region (Rodriguez, Fernandez-Mayoralas, & Rojo, 1998). At the same time, economic or other types of linkages between sending and receiving countries may generate work and family-related ties leading amenity immigrants to a particular destination (King & Patterson, 1998; Warnes & Patterson, 1998).

As might be expected, amenity immigrants are typically relatively healthy and affluent, though some North American retirees may relocate to Mexico out of financial necessity (Truly 2002; Otero 1997). In addition, amenity immigrants often report substantial international experience before retirement (King, Warnes, & Williams, 2000). Despite these general observations, for any given destination (1) the amenities offered condition the type of in-migrants attracted (King & Patterson, 1998) and (2) the earliest arrivals tend to be well-educated professionals with relatively advanced ability in the local language (Huber & O'Reilly, 2004).

### 2. How Do They Adjust on Arrival?

Existing literature suggests generally high levels of satisfaction among Northern European amenity immigrants. In terms of the adjustment process, being able to access local services is of course critical; however, a more thoroughgoing integration into the host community is often neither necessary nor desired. Limited linguistic skills rarely present a great problem, partly because amenity immigrants often settle in international tourist destinations where their own language has become the *lingua franca* (King et al., 2000; Casado-Diaz et al., 2004).

Northern European amenity migrants report a satisfying social life within linguistically bounded communities, but interaction with local populations is often quite limited (Huber & O'Reilly, 2004). Class differences between the relatively affluent expatriates and the local older population may further constrain interaction (Rodriguez et al., 1998). The character of expatriate social life varies across retirement destinations. For example, compared to their counterparts in tourist destinations along Spain's Mediterranean Coast, British retirees in Tuscany rarely participate in expatriate clubs, a result of dispersed settlement in the countryside and longstanding individual ties to the region (King et al., 2000).

Maintaining contact with friends and family at home, in the case of Northern European amenity immigrants, is partly accomplished by means of regular return trips, often on a seasonal basis. Additionally, retirement to a tourist destination often encourages visits from family members and friends that some describe as a mixed blessing. Professional/managerial and former military retirees receive a relatively large number of visitors, though in general the frequency of visits declines over time (Huber & O'Reilly, 2004; Casado-Diaz et al., 2004).

For Northern European amenity immigrants in Southern Europe, regulations governing access to public health care are quite complex and reflect not only European Union policies but also laws within, and reciprocal agreements between, sending and receiving nations. To ensure access to adequate health care, most migrants rely at some level on private insurance to compensate for deficiencies in local public health systems and many take specific steps to retain access to public health care in their native countries (e.g., regular return visits) (Dwyer, 2001; King et al., 2000).

Less is known about the adjustment of North American amenity migrants in Central and South America. Mexico's Lake Chapala region has attracted North Americans since the late 1880s. Otero (1997) reports limited language ability in a local sample of migrants and finds that those least capable in Spanish typically settle in areas with larger populations of English speaking retirees. These enclaves appear to be somewhat insulated from the broader host society. Truly (2002) argues that the lack of modern amenities has historically constrained settlement to a select group of culturally adaptable immigrants but that NAFTA and the arrival of multinational corporations such as Wal-Mart have been associated with the emergence of a new type of North American, even less interested in interacting with Mexican culture and traditions.

## C. International Return and Cyclical Migration

### 1. Returning Labor Force Immigrants

The available literature on international return migration of older adults focuses on labor force migrants returning from more-developed to less-developed regions. Return migration on retirement may be unavoidable where maintaining legal residence depends on employment (Blakemore, 1999). On the other hand, return migration may be part of a retirement strategy, where immigrants take advantage of the enhanced purchasing power of government- or employer-spon-

sored pensions in their communities of origin (Duleep, 1994).

Overlooked in this literature is the experience of retirees returning to developed nations after careers abroad (e.g., Foreign Service officers or missionaries). Our own analysis of data from the 2000 census suggests that of the estimated 370,000 adults 60 and older moving into the United States from abroad between 1995 and 2000, roughly 27% were natives. Notably, among these home comers, some 40% percent are 75 or older who, rather than returning immediately on dropping out of the labor force, may be making an assistance move after spending a portion of their retirement abroad.

### 2. Returning Assistance Immigrants

Excluding refugees, adjustment difficulties experienced by international migrants may prompt a return. Return migration may be particularly likely among those recently arrived who have retained strong ties to the sending community. A return is less likely, however, where the sending region offers a particularly low standard of living (Treas, 1997), or where supportive family and co-ethnic ties are available in the host society (Blakemore, 1999). Some older adults may cycle between their native communities and the homes of adult children living abroad (Treas & Mazumdar, 2004).

### 3. Returning Amenity Immigrants

Among international amenity immigrants, permanence of settlement varies substantially. Seasonal return migration, for example, is quite common (Casado-Diaz et al., 2004). Responses by British retirees to hypothetical triggering events suggest a reluctance to abandon homes in Southern Europe, though this varies across destinations depending on locally available services and support (Warnes,

King, Williams, & Patterson, 1999). Multi-site interview data suggest that return migration is by no means uncommon and is typically precipitated by the death of a spouse, disabling illness, or financial problems (Casado-Diaz et al., 2004; Dwyer, 2001). Even where desired, however, the capacity to return may be constrained. As a result of shifting housing markets, for instance, expatriate retirees may be able to sell their homes only if they are willing to take a loss (Buller & Hoggart, 1994).

## III. Future Research Priorities

The knowledge gained during the 1990s and early 2000s in the study of internal and international migration were substantial. Studies pertaining to the distribution of the older population are necessarily related to policy issues, especially those concerning health and social services. Economic development has been added to that list over the last 15 years. As the baby boom generation matures, these issues will increase in importance.

The basic patterns of migration now have been explored. No doubt these will be updated and refined in the future. But the topic that offers the greatest opportunity for research advances is that of migration selectivity. The availability of large, national panel studies, such as the Health and Retirement Survey at the University of Michigan, make it possible now to develop causal models that predict both migration decisions or anticipations and actual mobility behavior.

Migration that is related to early retirement will become visible for the first time in the next decade simply because the early retirees will be baby boomers, thus boosting their numbers. And there will be a high level of anticipation and speculation about the geographical distribution and migratory behavior of this large cohort as it crosses the line into retirement in the following decade (Haas and Serow, 2002; Golant, 2002; Longino, 1995). Finally, also because of the impending retirement of baby boomers, economic development issues are likely to increase in both importance and research viability during the first decade of the twenty-first century.

## References

Angel, J. L., & Angel, R. J. (1992). Age at migration, social connections and well-being among elderly Hispanics. *Journal of Aging and Health, 4*, 480–499.

Angel, J. L., Angel, R. J., & Markides, K. S. (2000). Late life immigration, changes in living arrangements, and headship status among older Mexican-origin individuals. *Social Science Quarterly, 81*, 389–403.

Bennett, D. G., (1992). The impact of retirement migration on Carteret and Brunswick counties, N.C. *North Carolina Geographer, 1*, 25–38.

Bennett, D. G. (1993). Retirement migration and economic development in high-amenity, nonmetropolitan areas. *The Journal of Applied Gerontology, 12*, 466–481.

Bennett, D. G. (1996). Implications of retirement development in high-amenity non-metropolitan coastal areas. *The Journal of Applied Gerontology, 15*, 345–360.

Biggar, J. D. (1980). Who moved among the elderly, 1965–1970: A comparison of types of older movers. *Research on Aging, 2*, 73–91.

Black, S. A., Markides, K. S., & Miller, T. Q. (1998). Correlates of depressive symptomatology among older community-dwelling Mexican Americans: The Hispanic EPESE. *The Journals of Gerontology, 53B*, S198–S208.

Blakemore, K. (1999). International migration in later life: Social care and policy implications. *Aging and Society, 19*, 761–774.

Bradsher, J. E., Longino, C. F., Jr., Jackson, D. J., & Zimmerman, R.S. (1992). Health and geographic mobility among the recently widowed. *Journal of Gerontology: Social Sciences, 47*, S261–S268.

Buller, H., & Hoggart, K. (1994). *International counterurbanization: British migrants in* rural France. Aldershot and Brookfield, VT.: Avebury

Button, J. W. (1992). A sign of generational conflict: The impact of Florida's aging voters on local school and tax referenda. *Social Science Quarterly, 73*, 786–797.

Casado-Diaz, M. A., Kaiser, C., & Warnes, A. M. (2004). Northern European retired residents in nine Southern European areas: Characteristics, motivations and adjustments. *Ageing and Society, 24*, 353–381.

Chappell, N. L., & Lai, D. (1998). Health care service use by Chinese seniors in British Columbia, Canada. *Journal of Cross-Cultural Gerontology, 13*, 21–37.

Chevan, A. (1995). Holding on and letting go. *Research on Aging, 17*, 278–302.

Colsher, P. L., & Wallace, R. B. (1990). Health and social antecedents of relocation in rural elderly persons. *Journal of Gerontology: Social Sciences, 45*, S32–S38.

Crown, W. H., & Longino, C. F., Jr. (1991). State and regional policy implications of elderly migration. *Journal of Aging and Social Policy, 3*(1/2), 185–207.

Cuba, L. J. (1989). Retiring from vacationland: From visitor to resident. *Generations, 13*(2), 63–67.

Cuba, L. J. (1992). *The Cape Cod retirement migration study: A final report to the National Institute on Aging*. Wellesley, MA: Wellesley College.

Cutchin, M. P. (2001). Deweyan integration: Moving beyond place attachment in elderly migration theory. *International Journal of Aging and Human Development 52*(1), 29–44.

DeJong, G. F. (1999). Choice processes in migration behavior. In K. Pandit & S. D. Withers (Eds.), *Migration and restructuring in the United States* (pp. 273–293). Lanham, MD: Rowan and Littlefield.

DeJong, G. F., Wilmoth, J. M., Angel, J. L., & Cornwell, G. T. (1995). Motives and the geographic mobility of very old Americans. *Journal of Gerontology: Social Sciences, 50B*, S395–S404.

Deller, S. C. (1995). Economic impact of retirement migration. *Economic Development Quarterly, 9*(1), 25–38.

Detzner, D. (1996). No place without a home: Southeast Asian grandparents in refugee families. *Generations, 20*(1), 45–49.

Duleep, H. O. (1994). Social security and the emigration of immigrants. *Social Security Bulletin, 57*(1), 37–52.

Duncombe, W., Robbins, M., & Wolf, D. A. (2003). Place characteristics and residential location choice among the retirement-age population. *Journal of Gerontology: Social Sciences, 58B*, S244–S252.

Dwyer, P. (2001). Retired EU migrants, health-care rights and European social citizenship. *Journal of Social Welfare and Family Law, 23*, 311–327.

Emami, A., Benner, P., & Ekman, S. (2001). A sociocultural health model for late-in-life immigrants. *Journal of Transcultural Nursing, 12*(1), 15–24.

Furstenberg, A. (2002). Trajectories of aging: imagined pathways in later life. *International Journal of Aging and Human Development, 55*(1), 1–24.

Glasgow, N. L. (1991). A place in the country. *American Demographics, 13*(3), 24–30.

Glick, J. E. (2000). Nativity, duration of residence and the life course pattern of extended family living in the USA. *Population Research and Policy Review, 19*, 179–198.

Golant, S. M. (2002). Deciding where to live: The emerging residential settlement patterns of retired Americans. *Generations, 26*(11), 66–73.

Haas, W. H., III, & Serow, W. J. (1993). Amenity retirement migration process: A model and preliminary evidence. *The Gerontologist, 33*, 212–220.

Haas, W. H., III, & Serow, W. J. (2002). The baby boom, amenity retirement migration, and retirement communities: Will the golden age of retirement continue? *Research on Aging, 24*(1), 150–164.

Hays, J. C., & Longino, C. F., Jr. (2002). Florida migration in the AHEAD study, 1993–1995: A note on the flight of the oldest retirees. *Research on Aging, 24*, 473–483.

Hazelrigg, L. E., & Hardy, M. A. (1995). Older adult migration to the Sunbelt: Assessing income and related characteristics of recent migrants. *Research on Aging, 17*, 209–234.

Hodge, G. (1991). The economic impact of retirees on smaller communities. *Research on Aging, 13*(1), 39–54.

Hogan, T. D., & Steinnes, D. N. (1998). A logistic model of the seasonal migration decision for elderly households in Arizona and Minnesota. *The Gerontologist, 38,* 152–158.

Huber, A., & O'Reilly, K. (2004). The construction of Heimat under conditions of individualized modernity: Swiss and British elderly migrants in Spain. *Ageing and Society, 15,* 325–353.

Kim, K. C., Kim, S., & Hurh, W. M. (1991). Filial piety and intergenerational relationship in Korean immigrant families. *International Journal of Aging and Human Development, 33,* 233–245.

King, R., & Patterson, G. (1998). Diverse paths: The elderly British in Tuscany. *International Journal of Population Geography, 4,* 157–182.

King, R., Warnes, A. M., & Williams, A. (2000). *Sunset lives: British retirement migration to the Mediterranean.* New York: Berg.

Krause, N., & Goldenhaar, L. M. (1992). Acculturation and psychological distress in three groups of elderly Hispanics. *Journal of Gerontology: Social Sciences, 47B,* S272–S288.

Krout, J. A., Moen, P., Holmes, H. H., Oggins, J., & Bowen, N. (2002). Reasons for relocation to a continuing care retirement community. *The Journal of Applied Gerontology, 21,* 236–256.

Lee, E. S. (1966). A theory of migration. *Demography, 3,* 147–157.

Litwak, E., & Longino, C. F., Jr. (1987). Migration patterns among the elderly: A developmental perspective. *The Gerontologist, 27,* 266–272.

Litwin, H. (1995). *Uprooted in old age: Soviet Jews and their social networks in Israel.* Westport, Connecticut: Greenwood Press.

Litwin, H. (1997). The network shifts of elderly immigrants: The case of Soviet Jews in Israel. *Journal of Cross-Cultural Gerontology, 12,* 45–60.

Longino, C. F., Jr. (1990). Geographical distribution and migration. In R. H. Binstock & L. K. George (Eds.), *Handbook of Aging and the Social Sciences,* (3rd ed., pp. 45–63). San Diego, CA: Academic Press.

Longino, C. F., Jr. (1995) *Retirement migration in America.* Houston: Vacation Publications.

Longino, C. F., Jr., & Bradley, D. E. (2003). A first look at retirement migration trends in 2000. *The Gerontologist, 43,* 904–907.

Longino, C. F., Jr., & Crown, W. H. (1990). Retirement migration and interstate income transfers. *The Gerontologist, 30,* 784–789.

Longino, C. F., Jr., Jackson, D. J., Zimmerman, R. S., & Bradsher, J. E. (1991). The second move: Health and geographic mobility. *Journal of Gerontology: Social Sciences, 46,* S218–S224.

Longino, C. F., Jr., & Serow, W. J. (1990). Regional differences in the characteristics of elderly return migrants. *Journal of Gerontology: Social Sciences, 47,* S38–S43.

Longino, C. F., Jr., & Smith, K. J. (1991). Black retirement migration in the United States. *Journal of Gerontology: Social Sciences, 46,* S125–S132.

MacManus, S. (1997). Selling school taxes and bond issues to a generationally diverse electorate: Lessons from Florida referenda. *Government Finance Review,* April, 17–22.

Marshall, V. W., Longino, C. F., Jr., Tucker, R. D., & Mullins, L. G. (1989). Health care utilization of Canadian snowbirds: An example of strategic planning. *Journal of Aging and Health, 1,* 150–168.

McAuley, W. J., Pecchioni, L., & Grant, J. (1999). Admission-related migration by older nursing home residents. *Journal of Gerontology: Social Sciences, 54B,* S125–S135.

McHugh, K. E. (2000). The ageless self? Emplacement of identities in Sun Belt retirement communities. *Journal of Aging Studies, 14,* 103–115.

McHugh, K. E. (2003). Three faces of ageism: Society, image, and place. *Ageing and Society, 23,* 165–185.

McHugh, K., Gober, P., & Borough, D. (2002). The Sun City Wars: Chapter 3. *Urban Geography 23*(7): 627–648.

McHugh, K. E., Hogan, T. D., & Happel, S. K. (1995). Multiple residence and cyclical migration: A life course perspective. *Professional Geographer, 47,* 251–267.

McHugh, K. E., & Mings, R. C. (1991). On the road again: Seasonal migration to a Sunbelt metropolis. *Urban Geography, 12,* 1–18.

McHugh, K. E., & Mings, R. C. (1994). Seasonal migration and health care. *Journal of Aging and Health, 6,* 111–122.

Miller, M. E., Longino, C. F., Jr., Anderson, R. T., James, M. K., & Worley, A. S. (1999). Functional status, assistance, and the risk of a community-based move. *The Gerontologist, 39,* 187–200.

Newbold, K. B. (1996). Determinants of elderly interstate migration in the United States, 1985–1990. *Research on Aging, 18,* 451–476.

Otero, L. M. Y. (1997). U.S. retired persons in Mexico. *American Behavioral Scientist, 40,* 914–922.

Plane, D. A., & Heins, F. (2003). Age articulation of U.S. inter-metropolitan migration flows. *The Annals of Regional Science, 37,* 107–130.

Ravenstein, E. G. (1885). The laws of migration. *Journal of the Royal Statistical Society, 48,* 167–227.

Reeder, R. J., & Glasgow, N. L. (1990). Nonmetro retirement counties' strengths and weaknesses. *Rural Development Perspectives, 6*(2), 12–17.

Remennick, L. I., & Ottenstein-Eisen, N. (1998). Reaction of new Soviet immigrants to primary health care services in Israel. *International Journal of Health Services, 28,* 555–574.

Rodriguez, V., Fernandez-Mayoralas, G., & Rojo, F. (1998). European retirees on the Costa del Sol: A cross-national comparison. *International Journal of Population Geography, 4,* 183–200.

Rossi, P. H. (1955). *Why families move: A study in the social psychology of urban residential mobility.* Glencoe, IL: Free Press.

Rowles, G. D., & Watkins, J. F. (1993). Elderly migration and development in small communities. *Growth and Change, 24,* 509–538.

Sastry, M. L. (1992). Estimating the economic impacts of elderly migration: an input-output analysis. *Growth and Change, 23*(1), 54–79.

Savageau, D. (2000). *Retirement places rated.* New York: Macmillan.

Schiamberg, L. B., & McKinney, K. G. (2003). Factors influencing expectations to move or age in place at retirement among 40 to 65 year olds. *The Journal of Applied Gerontology, 22*(1), 19–41.

Serow, W. J. (2001). Retirement migration counties in the Southeastern United States: geographic, demographic, and economic correlates. *The Gerontologist, 41,* 220–227.

Serow, W. J. (2003). Economic consequences of retiree concentrations: A review of North American studies. *The Gerontologist, 43,* 897–903.

Serow, W. J., Friedrich, K., & Haas, W. H. (1992). Measuring the economic impact of retirement migration: The case of Western North Carolina. *The Journal of Applied Gerontology, 11*(2), 200–215.

Silverstein, M. (1995). Stability and change in temporal distance between the elderly and their children. *Demography, 32*(1), 29–45.

Silverstein, M., & Angelelli, J. J. (1998). Older parents' expectations of moving closer to their children. *Journal of Gerontology: Social Sciences, 53,* S153–S163.

Simonsen, W., & Robbins, M. (1996). Does it make any difference anymore? Competitive versus negotiated municipal bond issuance. *Public Administration Review, 56*(1), 57–64.

Slonim-Nevo, V., Cwikel, J., Luski, H., Lankry, M., & Shraga, Y. (1995). Caregiver burden among three-generational immigrant families in Israel. *International Social Work, 38,* 191–204.

Stevens, G. (1999). Age at immigration and second language proficiency among foreign-born adults. *Language in Society, 28*(4), 555–578.

Stoller, E. P., & Perzynski, A. T. (2003). The impact of ethnic involvement and migration patterns on long-term care plans among retired Sunbelt migrants: Plans for nursing home placement. *Journal of Gerontology: Social Sciences, 58*(6), S369–S376.

Strumpf, N. E., Glicksman, A., Goldber-Glen, R. S., Fox, R. C., & Logue, E. H. (2001). Caregiver and elder experiences of Cambodian, Vietnamese, Soviet Jewish, and Ukranian refugees. *International Journal of Aging and Human Development, 53,* 233–252.

Torres, S. (2001). Understandings of successful aging in the context of migration: The case of Iranian immigrants in Sweden. *Ageing and Society, 21,* 333–355.

Treas, J. (1997). Older immigrants and U.S. welfare reform. *International Journal of Sociology and Social Policy, 17*(9/10), 8–33.

Treas, J., & Mazumdar, S. (2002). Older people in America's immigrant families: Dilemmas of dependence, integration, and isolation. *Journal of Aging Studies, 16,* 243–258.

Treas, J., & Mazumdar, S. (2004). Kinkeeping and caregiving: Contributions of older people in immigrant families. *Journal of Comparative Family Studies,* 35(1), 105–122.

Truly, D. (2002). International retirement migration and tourism along the Lake Chapala Riviera: Developing a matrix of retirement migration behavior. *Tourism Geographies,* 4(3), 261–281.

Tucker, R. D., Mullins, L. C., Beland, F., Longino, C. F., Jr., & Marshall, V. W. (1992). Older Canadians in Florida: A comparison of Anglophone and Francophone seasonal migrants. *Canadian Journal on Aging, 11,* 281–297.

van der Geest, S., Mul, A., & Vermeulen, H. (2004). Linkages between migration and the care of frail older people: Observations from Greece, Ghana, and The Netherlands. *Ageing and Society, 24,* 431–450.

Walters, W. H. (2000). Types and patterns of later-life migration. *Geografiska Annaler,* 82B(3). 129–147.

Walters, W. H. (2002). Place characteristics and later-life migration. *Research on Aging,* 24(2), 243–277.

Warnes, A. M. (1992). Migration and the life course. In T. Champion & T. Fielding (Eds.), *Migration Processes and Patterns* (pp. 175–187). London: Belhaven Press.

Warnes, A. M. (2001). The international dispersal of pensioners from affluent countries. *International Journal of Population Geography, 7,* 373–388.

Warnes, A. M., King, R., Williams, A. M., & Patterson, G. (1999). The well-being of British expatriate retirees in Southern Europe. *Ageing and Society, 19,* 717–740.

Warnes, A. M., & Patterson, G. (1998). "British retirees in Malta: Components of the cross-national relationship." *International Journal of Population Geography, 4,* 113–133.

Watkins, J. F. (1999). Life course and spatial experience: A personal narrative approach in migration studies. In K. Pandit & S. Davies-Wiothers (Eds.), *Migration and restructuring in the United States* (pp. 294–312). Boulder, CO: Rowan and Littlefield.

Weinstein-Shr, G., & Henkin, N. Z. (1991). Continuity and change: Intergenerational relations in Southeast Asian refugee families. *Marriage and Family Review, 16,* 351–367.

Wilmoth, J., DeJong, G. F., & Himes, C. L. (1977). Immigrant and non-immigrant living arrangements among America's White, Hispanic, and Asian elderly population. *International Journal of Sociology and Social Policy,* 17(9/10), 57–82.

Wiseman, R. F. (1980). Why older people move. *Research on Aging, 2,* 141–154.

Yee, Donna L. (1992). Health care access and advocacy for immigrant and other under-served elders. *Journal of Health Care for the Poor and Underserved, 2,* 448–464.

Six

# Diversity and Aging in the United States

Ronald J. Angel and Jacqueline L. Angel

## I. Population Diversity and the Pact Between the Generations

At the beginning of the twenty-first century, the population of the United States is socially, demographically, and culturally almost unrecognizably different than it was at the beginning of the twentieth century. In 1900, the nation was still being populated by immigrants from Europe, and most Americans still lived in small towns and on farms (Portes & Rumbaut, 1990). Urban Americans, many of whom had recently arrived, found good jobs in construction and manufacturing building a new and dynamic society. Individuals and families provided for themselves, and the care of poor and elderly people was still the responsibility of families and local communities. The New Deal and Social Security lay in the future. Today the nation is vastly richer, most Americans live in large cities, manufacturing jobs are rapidly moving overseas, and the state has assumed an increasing share of the responsibility for the poor and the elderly population. The

New Deal redefined the pact between the generations long before most Americans who are alive today were even born.

But perhaps the biggest difference today, and the one that provides the motivation for this chapter, is the fact that a growing number of Americans do not trace their lineage to Europe. For the last few decades, immigration has originated primarily in the nations of Asia and Latin America, and the result is a vastly changed cultural landscape (He, 2002). Today, Spanish-language television and radio can be heard even in the heartland and in places that until recently were known for a parochial xenophobia. Although the majority of Americans are still white and non-Hispanic, Americans of African, Asian, and Latin origin have far higher fertility rates, and by the middle of this century one in two Americans will be a member of one of these groups (U.S. Census Bureau, 2004a). Individuals from Latin America and Asia, most of whom are citizens but some of whom are not, are redefining the cultural landscape of California and Texas and becoming important political constituencies in

*Handbook of Aging and the Social Sciences, Sixth Edition*

94

other states as well (Hayes-Bautista, 2004). Higher fertility means that the Hispanic population is relatively young. One in four non-Hispanics is under the age of 18, but one in three Hispanics is that young (Reed & Ramirez, 1998). Although the Hispanic population will remain younger than the non-Hispanic white population for the foreseeable future, the number of older Hispanics, and the proportion of the older population that they represent, will increase in the years to come (Guzmán, 2001).

This fact brings us to a core theme of our discussion. The nation faces major challenges in financing the retirement and health care needs of the baby-boom generation. Although addressing such problems will be painful in the short term, the crisis is historically unique and limited. As the baby boomers pass from the scene, so will the crisis. A far more serious potential problem arises from the ethnic and racial overlay to the age grading of our society. Although the population over the age of 65 is growing more racially and ethnically diverse, the fact that minority populations will remain young means that well into the twenty-first century, the racial and ethnic composition of different age strata will vary dramatically. In the future the younger age strata will be disproportionately minority and the older strata disproportionately non-minority with non-Hispanic whites remaining in the majority even by the year 2050 (U.S. Census Bureau, 2003a).

The ethnic diversity of the United States results from a history of changing immigration and the arrival of new citizens from very different parts of the world. The majority non-Hispanic white population that defined the nation came from the various nations of Europe in different waves. The Africans who were brought as slaves represented many different peoples, each with distinct cultures, religions, and languages (Franklin

& Moss, 1999). More recently, the ethnic diversity of the U.S. population stems from both high levels of immigration from Latin America and Asia and the high fertility rates of those groups (Angel & Hogan, 2004). Along with Latinos, Americans of Asian origin are changing the faces of states such as California and Texas. Unfortunately, the space available for this chapter does not allow us to deal with the social and demographic reality of the many different Asian nationalities, nor are comparable data sources on Asians available. As a consequence, although we present some statistics for Asians as a single category, in what follows we focus primarily on the demographic, socioeconomic, and cultural characteristics of Latinos and African Americans, the nation's oldest and, until recently, largest minority group.

## II. The Ethnic Age Grading of the Population

Figure 6.1 dramatically illustrates the extent of ethnic age grading of the population in Texas in 2000. Texas has a large Mexican-origin population, but it serves as a useful example of trends that are affecting the nation as a whole (U.S.

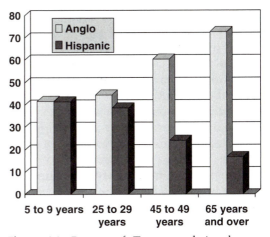

**Figure 6.1** Percent of Texas population by age group and ethnicity, 2000.

Census Bureau, 2003b). At the time of the last census, 41% of the population of Texas between five and nine years old was Hispanic, but only 42% was non-Hispanic white. At the other end of the age distribution, only about 17% of Texans over the age of 65 were Hispanic, whereas nearly 73% of that age group was non-Hispanic white. Arizona, Colorado, California, New Mexico, and Texas have historically had large Mexican-origin populations, but more recently Mississippi, Tennessee, North Carolina, and other states that had almost no Mexican-origin residents in previous decades have experienced rapid growth in the Mexican-origin and other Hispanic populations as these groups seek economic opportunities and take jobs for which no other workers are available (Suro & Singer, 2002). In 1990, approximately 85% of all immigrants from Mexico settled in California, Texas, and Illinois, but by 2000 that figure had declined to 68% as more recent Mexican immigrants moved to areas not traditionally associated with Mexican immigration (American Immigration Law Foundation, 2002).

The implications for the composition of the future labor force are obvious. By the year 2040, well over half of the Texas labor force will be Hispanic and another 8% will be African American (Murdock, 2004). Although Texas may represent an extreme case because of the size of the state's Hispanic population, in most of the rest of the country the working age population will be disproportionately minority in the relative short term. This fact has profound implications for the pact between generations. In 1945, there were approximately 40 workers for each retiree; by the year 2003 there were slightly more than three workers supporting each retired American (Social Security Administration, 2004a). In the future the number of workers supporting each retiree is expected to decline even further to two by 2030 (Social Security

Administration, 2004a). If Social Security remains a pay-as-you-go system in which the support of the retired population comes directly from the paychecks of those who are still working, those workers will have to contribute a larger fraction of their income in Social Security and Medicare taxes (Bongaarts, 2004). If one of those two workers is a minority American who, because of educational and other disadvantages in youth, is restricted to a low-wage occupation, he or she will not have the resources nor likely be willing to shoulder the burden of supporting a disproportionately privileged non-Hispanic white elderly population (Lee, 1997).

A few simple statistics readily illustrate the problem. Approximately 80% of Hispanic men 16 years and over are in the labor force, the highest participation rate of any racial or ethnic group (Grenier & Cattan, 2000). Yet as Table 6.1 shows, among Hispanics 22 to 30 years old, the period of the life course after which the vast majority of schooling has been completed, educational attainment remains particularly low for Hispanics. Far fewer Hispanics than non-Hispanic whites receive education beyond high school. The situation is even worse for the foreign born, fewer than half of whom have graduated from high school. Only 59.1% of non-Hispanic blacks have some college or more compared with 69.2% of non-Hispanic whites. Unless the educational level of this population increases extensively and rapidly, the working age population of the future will be characterized by low productivity and low income.

These lower educational levels and the large number of recent immigrants among Hispanics and Asians translate into lower household incomes for young working age families. Almost two-thirds (62.3%) of recent Hispanic immigrants and more than half (52.8%) of Asian immigrants between the ages of 22 and 30 report annual household incomes of less

**Table 6.1**

Educational Attainment for Persons 22–30 Years in the United States by Race and Hispanic Ethnicity: 2003
(Weighted percentages)

| | Hispanic | | Non-Hispanic Asian | | Non-Hispanic Black | Non-Hispanic White |
|---|---|---|---|---|---|---|
| | Entry Past 1984 | Native-born | Entry Past 1984 | Native-born | | |
| 0–11 Years | 54.5% | 23.4% | 4.7% | 0.0% | 8.5% | 3.8% |
| High School Graduate | 30.8% | 37.0% | 14.2% | 13.7% | 32.5% | 27.0% |
| Some College or more | 14.8% | 39.6% | 81.1% | 86.3% | 59.1% | 69.2% |

Source: Authors calculations from http://dataferrett.census.gov; *Current Population Survey Annual Demographic Survey: March Supplement, 2003.*

than $20,000. Less than one-third (29.2%) of non-Hispanic whites in this age range report incomes that low (U.S. Census Bureau, 2004b). These young minority workers are clearly in no position to pay the taxes that the nation will require to support the elderly population and provide for all of the other needs of the nation (Henkin & Kingson, 1998–1999).

These data make it clear that the potential for serious intergenerational conflict fueled further by racial and ethnic tensions is far more than just a dramatic scenario that might be used to make a rhetorical point; it is quite real. For numerous reasons, states with relatively large elderly populations spend slightly less on children than states with smaller elderly populations (South, 1991). It is imperative, therefore, that we remain aware of the potential social and political consequences that the dramatic changes in demographic and cultural composition of the population could bring about.

## III. Culture and Diversity

By cultural diversity we are of course referring to people's nation of origin and the language and other cultural heritage they bring with them. Some years ago Richard Alba, a keen observer of

American ethnicity, observed that, as large-scale European immigration was a thing of the past and because these groups had been here for generations, distinctions between Americans of European origin had all but disappeared. Today, differences between individuals of English, German, French, and other nationalities have been replaced by a common American cultural identity (Alba, 1990). There can be little doubt that distinctions among Americans of European origin are less obvious or socially significant than distinctions between European-origin Americans as a whole and African Americans, Asians, and Latinos. In addition to representing minority groups, Americans who trace their origins to Asia and Latin America differ significantly among themselves. Latinos with roots in the Caribbean differ from those who emigrated from Mexico or those who have lived in the American Southwest since it was part of Mexico. Cuban Americans are largely political refugees, whereas Mexican Americans are economic immigrants. Those who move from Puerto Rico to the mainland are U.S. citizens who arrive with all of the rights and privileges that that status entails.

Latinos at least share a common core language. Asians, on the other hand, not only come from a broad range of nations, but they speak a wide variety of languages including Chinese, Japanese, Vietnamese, Cambodian, Hindi, and others. In addition to linguistic variation, differences among and between Latinos and Asians arise from the fact that the different nationalities immigrated under different political circumstances, sometimes arriving as political refugees, and they settled in different parts of the country that offered varying occupational opportunities. In 2002, Mexican Americans accounted for slightly more than half of Hispanics in the United States 65 and older (Angel & Hogan, 2004). Because of its proximity to Mexico and the fact that the states of the Southwestern United States were part of Mexico, Mexican-origin people have historically been concentrated in the Southwest, although today they are fanning out across the country (Suro & Singer, 2002). Los Angeles, with more than 1 million residents of Mexican origin, has the largest Mexican-origin population in the country; Chicago, with more than a half-million Mexican-origin residents, was second in 2000 (U.S. Census Bureau, 2003b). Cuban Americans, who represent less than 4% of the total U.S. Hispanic population but who have lower fertility than other Hispanic groups and are an older population, made up 17% of the total Latino population over age 65 (U.S. Census Bureau, 2003c). Hispanics from Central and South America, other Spanish-speaking countries, and the Dominican Republic make up about 20% of the older Latino population (U.S. Census Bureau, 2003c).

During the first half of the twenty-first century, Asian Americans will represent a larger proportion of the population over 65 than they do today, and they will be highly diverse in terms of population characteristics such as age, immigration, and geographic location (Chan, 1991). Individuals of Chinese, Filipino, and Japanese origin make up almost three-

fourths (70%) of the elderly Asian population. The peak immigration period for these groups was in the nineteenth and early twentieth centuries. As a result, a large fraction of elderly individuals in these groups have lived their entire lives in the United States, often in ethnic enclaves. Although in 1980 there were relatively few of the "new Asian immigrants" among the total Asian population, that situation is changing rapidly (Takaki, 1998). Today Vietnamese and Cambodians make up 8% of the total Asian elderly population, and Koreans and Asians from other nations make up the remaining 22%. Of particular interest is that since 1970, Asians have comprised the largest percentage (43.5%) of the elderly immigrant population (He, 2002).

## IV. Health of the Elderly Minority Population

Now that we have reviewed some of the racial and ethnic characteristics of the older population, let us examine some of their health indicators beginning with life expectancy. Life expectancy at birth has increased for all racial and ethnic groups and there seems to be no end in sight (U.S. Census Bureau, 2003d). Based on Census Bureau projections, life expectancy at birth for both men and women will increase dramatically in the future (U.S. Census Bureau, 2000). Yet important racial and ethnic differences that seem to favor Hispanics will persist (Hayward, Warner, & Crimmins, 2003). From 1999 to 2050, life expectancies are projected to increase on average from 74.7 to 81.1 years for non-Hispanic white men, from 68.4 to 78.5 for African-American men, and from 77.2 to 83.0 years for Hispanic men (U.S. Census Bureau, 2000). Women, who already live longer than men, will live even longer and, again, all racial and ethnic groups will participate in the increase (Elo & Preston,

1997). Yet group differences will remain that will favor Hispanics. Between 1999 and 2050, life expectancy at birth for women is projected to increase from 80.1 to 86.4 years for non-Hispanic white women; from 75.1 to 84.6 years for African-American women; and from 83.7 to 88.4 years for Hispanic women (U.S. Census Bureau, 2000).

Life expectancy at age 65 has risen dramatically for all racial and ethnic groups and will continue to do so, especially for women. Based on Census Bureau projections, by the year 2050 non-Hispanic white women who reach 65 can expect to live an additional 22.7 years, reaching their ninth decade of life (Day, 1996). Hispanic women will live even longer, an additional 27.9 years. Even African-American females who survive to age 65 are expected to live into their mid-eighties. There is, of course, a down side to greater longevity. Because of their longer life spans, women are more likely than men to suffer serious, protracted illnesses and functional incapacity requiring long-term care (Verbrugge, 1989).

In addition to differing in life expectancy at birth and at age 65, racial and ethnic groups differ in the most common causes of death (Hayward, Crimmins, Miles, & Yang, 2000). After the age of 65, African Americans are more likely than non-Hispanic whites to die from heart disease, cancer, diabetes, and stroke (Anderson, 2002). Older Hispanics, on the other hand, have lower death rates than African Americans and non-Hispanic whites from these diseases, with the exception of diabetes (Anderson, 2002). Longer life increases the probability that women will develop osteoporosis, a major cause of frailty, fractures, and functional incapacity in old age. Certain data indicate that hip fractures are more common among white women than among African-American or Hispanic women (Manton & Stallard, 1997). Explanations for the possible racial variation in the incidence of hip fracture and the rate of onset of osteoporotic changes include differences in bone density at menopause (possibly resulting from early differences in nutrition, physical activity, and body mass) and possible differences in the postmenopausal production of sex and parathyroid hormones (Manton & Stallard, 1997).

Racial and ethnic differences in morbidity and mortality, then, are more complex than one might initially imagine. Although African Americans have higher rates of illness and death from most causes, except perhaps for osteoporosis, Hispanics as a whole, and Mexican Americans in particular, have quite favorable mortality experiences, even though their socioeconomic profile is similar to that of African Americans. The reasons for these counterintuitive morbidity and mortality patterns remain unclear and require further investigation. The Mexican-American mortality advantage has been characterized as a paradox and has puzzled epidemiologists for years. Mexican-American mortality rates for heart disease, cancer, and cerebrovascular disease are lower than one would expect for a group with a generally low socioeconomic profile, and they are far more favorable than that of similarly disadvantaged non-Hispanic whites (Palloni & Arias, 2004). These mortality differences among groups from the same social strata raise the possibility that genetic factors contribute to mortality advantages, as well as to disadvantages among groups. As of yet data concerning the genetic component of group differences in mortality and morbidity are only suggestive, and much more research is necessary to disentangle what is probably a complex and interactive set of biological, cultural, and social class factors (Hayward et al., 2000). As we note later, group differences in patterns of diabetes and its sequelae suggest some intriguing possible genetic links among ethnic factors, morbidity, and its lethality.

Most explanations for the potential Hispanic mortality advantage, though, focus on social, cultural, genetic, and health care system factors. Many observers, for example, have speculated that there is some protective factor associated with Mexican culture that we as yet do not fully understand (Rumbaut, 1997). Traditional family support systems may protect health (Bagley, Angel, Dilworth-Anderson, Liu, & Schinke, 1995). Even demographics may play a role. Hispanics have larger families than non-Hispanics, and numerous writers have suggested that Hispanic culture inculcates strong norms concerning family loyalty, traditional family values, and mutual support in its members. Although there is little hard evidence for this health-protective aspect of the Hispanic family, larger families may translate into more effective social support systems, more adaptive health behaviors, and less depression (Bagley et al., 1995). In the Cuban-origin elderly community, the stresses and emotional strains that accompany migration to the United States may well be counteracted by the fact that Cubans have re-created their culture of origin in Miami's Little Havana (Angel & Angel, 1992).

An intriguing possible genetic component in group differences in morbidity and mortality is suggested by the fact that, despite their generally favorable mortality experience, Mexican-origin individuals suffer from high rates of diabetes (e.g., Yong-Fang, Mukaila, Markides, Ray, Espino, & Goodwin, 2003). Estimates from a variety of studies reveal older Mexican Americans have particularly high rates of non-insulin-dependent (type 2) diabetes (Harris et al., 1998). Even after controlling for sociodemographic risk factors, including sex, age, level of education, marital status, immigrant status, and living arrangements, Mexican Americans with diabetes face a higher risk of chronic conditions such as heart disease, stroke, hypertension, circulation and foot problems, obesity, impaired vision, and limitations in activities of daily living than those reported for other groups (Black, Ray, & Markides, 1999). In addition, the epidemiological evidence indicates a great deal of co-occurring depression among older Mexican Americans with diabetes (Black, 1999).

Data also suggest that Mexican Americans are at higher risk of death from diabetes-related complications at earlier ages than non-Hispanic whites (Bastida, Cuellar, & Villas, 2001). Once again, the fact that the higher diabetes-related morbidity among Mexican Americans cannot be entirely explained by socioeconomic factors or obesity leads to the speculation that genetic factors may be involved, possibly reflecting the high degree of American Indian admixture in at least the Mexican-origin population, and the fact that Native Americans suffer from extremely high rates of diabetes (Diehl & Stern, 1989). In light of the complexity of the genetic/environment nexus, though, identifying the underlying causes of these perplexing patterns of lower overall mortality among certain Hispanic groups and higher death rates from certain causes clearly requires new studies that deal with biological, socioeconomic, and cultural factors simultaneously.

Because of the importance of public health and health care to overall health levels, one cannot, of course, ignore the potential role of health system factors in explaining racial and ethnic differences in morbidity and mortality. As we have documented, African Americans have higher rates of mortality from all causes, largely because these conditions are diagnosed later and treated less aggressively than among non-Hispanic whites (Li, Malone, & Daling, 2003). Many studies suggest that system-level factors are a major explanation for higher diabetes-related mortality among Mexican Americans. Among Mexican Americans a diagnosis of diabetes is often delayed so that by the time the disease is discovered, it has done significant damage (Wu, Haan, Liang, Ghosh, Gonzalez, & Herman, 2003). Older Mexican Americans with diabetes often go untreated or undertreated for years in service-poor areas such as South Texas (Bastida et al., 2001). The fact that Mexican Americans of all ages are less likely than non-Hispanic whites to have private health insurance, including Medigap plans, may well contribute to later diagnosis and less aggressive treatment (Angel, Angel, & Markides, 2002).

Of course life expectancy and mortality patterns do not tell the whole story. Increasing life expectancies have inevitably given rise to a concern with the quality of the added years. A growing body of evidence reveals that African Americans suffer higher rates of functional limitations and disability than non-Hispanic whites (Kelley-Moore & Ferraro, 2004) and that they enjoy fewer disability-free years than non-Hispanic whites (Hayward & Heron, 1999). Based on self-reports, older Mexican Americans suffer from more functional limitations and experience more disability than non-Hispanic whites of similar ages (Angel & Angel, 1997). Twice as many African Americans (11.8%) and Hispanics (11.2%) as non-Hispanic whites (5.5%) report that they have problems carrying out basic activities of daily living (U.S. Census Bureau, 2003e). Again, the extent to which these differences reflect genetic or social factors remains unclear. As we have noted, given the complex interaction between genes and environment, the reality is that they probably reflect both.

Elderly Mexican Americans also fare somewhat worse in comparison to non-Hispanic whites and African Americans in terms of limitations in instrumental activities of daily life (IADL) such as shopping, preparing meals, and driving. Data from a longitudinal study of Mexican Americans 65 and older at the time of the first interview indicate that elderly Mexican Americans, and especially elderly Mexican-American women, experience substantially more IADL disabilities than both non-Hispanic whites and African Americans (Angel & Angel, 1997; Angel, Angel, McLelland, & Markides, 1996). Instrumental activities include cognitively and socially complex tasks, such as driving and managing finances. Many immigrant women never learn to do either, so high rates of IADL disability among Hispanics may reflect experience rather than cognitive or functional incapacity.

## V. Income and Wealth: The Sources of Retirement Security

Despite their increasing life expectancies, the economic situations of the African-American and Hispanic elderly populations have not improved greatly relative to that of non-Hispanic whites and large fractions of both groups face serious economic insecurity in retirement (Shea, Miles, & Hayward, 1996). This economic insecurity results from a lifetime of labor force disadvantage and the inability to build a nest egg during the working years (Crystal & Shea, 1990). Individuals who spend their lives in low-wage service sector jobs are unable to save for retirement, and the jobs in which they work rarely offer health or retirement benefits (Crystal & Shea, 2003). Even with minimal Social Security and Medicare, these individuals are at serious risk of poverty and inadequate medical care in old age (U.S. Census Bureau, 2004b).

After the passage of the Social Security Act, poverty among the elderly declined dramatically. Between 1959, when the official U.S. Government poverty index was established, and 2000, poverty rates among the elderly fell by over two-thirds, from 35% to 10% (U.S. Census Bureau,

2001). Even with Social Security, though, the household income of a substantial fraction of older minority Americans falls below the poverty line (Kijakazi, 2001). In 2002, one-third of Hispanic (32.7%) and of African-American (33.3%) persons over the age of 65 reported incomes below 125% of poverty; 65% of Hispanic women and 56.7% of African-American women over 65 who were living alone reported incomes this low (U.S. Census Bureau, 2004b). Today Social Security is the only source of income for approximately one-fifth of elderly Americans (Social Security Administration, 2004b). Older minority households are particularly dependent on Social Security, as they have little wealth and few other sources of income (Hendley & Bilimoria, 1999). Without Social Security income, nearly two-thirds of older African Americans and Hispanics would sink into poverty (Hendley & Bilimoria, 1999). One-third of elderly African Americans and Hispanics depend completely on Social Security for their retirement income compared with only 16% of older non-Hispanic whites (Hendley & Bilimoria, 1999).

For older individuals a middle class existence depends on a private pension (Wise, 1996). A private pension represents an important part of a package that includes Social Security benefits and income from assets (Crystal & Shea, 2003). Without income from a private pension, an older individual's economic security remains precarious, as the maximum monthly Social Security benefit for an individual in 2003 was $1,741 (Social Security Administration, 2004b), and most individuals receive much less. In November 2004, the average payment was only $929.40 (Social Security Administration, 2004c). According to data from the Survey of Consumer Finances, 53.7% of non-Hispanic white households owned retirement accounts in 1998, but only 32.1% of nonwhite or

Hispanic households were vesting in such plans (Aizcorbe, Kennickell, & Moore, 2003). This low rate of pension plan participation by minority households means that the economic security of a large proportion of older minority Americans rests on a single pillar and they face a high risk of an inadequate retirement income (Honig, 2000).

## VI. Age at Immigration

For Hispanics and Asians, immigration remains a core demographic phenomenon that is a major engine propelling the diversity we have documented. Immigration, though, is a complex process, both for the immigrant and for the receiving society into which he or she must incorporate (Bean, Berg, & Van Hook, 1996). A large and growing body of research shows that the age at which an individual immigrates makes a great difference in the extent and success of his or her material and psychological incorporation (e.g., Angel, Buckley, & Sakamoto, 2001). Children quickly learn the language and customs of the host society. Some may be handicapped in their social mobility by the limited resources of their parents, but for most young immigrants the new country truly means a new and better life.

For those individuals who immigrate in midlife or beyond, on the other hand, the experience of immigration is often traumatic, as they are uprooted from the familiar surroundings in which they grew up and thrust into a new culture in which they have to learn a new language, new customs, and the requirements of a new set of social institutions (Salgado de Snyder & Diaz-Guerrero, 2003). Not all are able to do so and many remain trapped in the no-man's-land of the person who fits in nowhere. Except for doctors, scientists, and other highly trained professionals, older immigrants arrive with few high demand skills, and if they find work at all it is often in services or manual labor (DeFreitas, 1991). Many have spent their lives toiling in the fields or in harsh, dangerous conditions for very low pay because working conditions outside the United States, especially for emigrants from the developing world, are usually poor. The combination of a lifetime of physically demanding work and poor remuneration means that older immigrants arrive with few resources and face serious challenges in incorporation. Individuals who immigrate in mature adulthood or later in life face particularly difficult problems in assimilation and acculturation, and many never really succeed. With low incomes and relatively few years in which to work, they are simply unable to save much for retirement and, like low-skill native workers, they are unlikely to be offered jobs with health or retirement benefits.

Consequently, these older Mexican-American immigrants often remain dependent on their families because they do not qualify for government programs (Angel, Angel, Lee, & Markides, 1999; Binstock & Jean-Baptiste, 1999). Recent immigration and welfare reform legislation imposes the requirement that an immigrant's sponsor must agree to provide complete support to the person they sponsor for five years (Angel, 2003). During that time the immigrant is ineligible for most public programs. The burden of having to support an older immigrant parent no doubt discourages some families from bringing their aging parents from the home country (Friedland & Pankaj, 1997).

## VII. Medical Care, Living Arrangements, and Long-term Care

The introduction of Medicare in 1965 represented a major benefit for the elderly. Although the United States is the only industrialized nation that does not offer universal access to health care to all of its citizens, those over the age of 65 receive fairly comprehensive health coverage through Medicare. Before Medicare many older individuals, especially those with low incomes, could not afford medical care (Hoffman, 2001). The poor depended on charitable care and their families or assumed crushing medical debt. Unfortunately, although the Medicare program is hugely expensive, it does not cover all health-related costs that the elderly incur (see Chapter 21).

Almost all citizens 65 and older are covered by Medicare or some other government health plan (U.S. Census Bureau, 2004c). Some data suggest that a small fraction of Hispanics (approximately 5%) may not participate, perhaps because they are non-citizens (Angel et al., 2002). Yet the data also reveal major differences in the ownership of supplemental Medigap insurance that covers the costs of what Medicare does not pay. In 2001, approximately 69% of non-Hispanic whites had supplemental Medigap plans, but only 38% of African Americans and 25% of Hispanics reported owning such plans (National Center for Health Statistics, 2004). In the case of serious chronic illness, individuals who do not have supplemental coverage are often unable to afford prescription drugs and other care they need. They must spend their limited resources for other purposes.

For the destitute elderly, Medicaid serves as the Medigap plan of last resort, and it pays the Medicare premiums and other costs that are not covered. Because elderly Hispanics and African Americans have lower average incomes than non-Hispanic whites, they are more likely to rely on Medicaid for this purpose (Lamphere & Rosenbach, 2000). Such individuals are deemed to be "dual eligibles," as they qualify for both Medicare and Medicaid. Such dual eligibility reflects the economic marginality associated with minority group status.

Smaller families, geographic mobility, cultural change, and the increasing necessity for younger women to work means that in the future, even among Hispanics, the family will, in all likelihood, play less of a role in caring for the elderly than it has in the past (Villa & Aranda, 2000). Yet because of the fact that many older minority individuals have few resources and often lack adequate retirement incomes that might allow them to buy personal care services, their need for family care will remain high (Angel et al., 1999). Largely because they have no alternative, elderly African Americans and Latinos, especially women, are more likely than non-Hispanic whites to live with their children (Himes, Hogan, & Eggebeen, 1996).

Yet in spite of their supposed greater "familism" and greater economic need, many older individuals do not live with their children even when they suffer significant declines in health (Worobey & Angel, 1990). Older African Americans and Latinos, like older non-Hispanic white individuals, remain in their own homes even after their spouse has died (Burr, 1990). Nursing homes are clearly an option of last resort for all groups (Mui, Choi, & Monk, 1998). African Americans enter nursing homes at a higher rate than other racial and ethnic groups (Angel & Hogan, 2004). Hispanics, on the other hand, are far less likely than other racial and ethnic groups to use nursing homes (Angel & Hogan, 2004). Hispanics are also less likely than non-Hispanic whites to use in-home health care services (Wallace, Levy-Storms, & Ferguson, 1995).

Many observers have speculated as to the reasons for the low use of nursing homes among Hispanics, especially Mexican Americans. These include a lack of culturally appropriate homes and cultural norms that place pressure on children to keep their aging parents at home (Torres-Gil & Villa, 1993). Other factors, including the inability to pay for acceptable nursing home care, no doubt also influence decisions about living arrangements later in life (Himes et al., 1996). Depleting a spouse's meager resources may strike an elderly minority couple as an unacceptable option (Angel & Angel, 1997). In addition, many older African Americans live in communities with few high-quality long-term care facilities (Mor, Zinn, Angelelli, Teno, & Miller, 2004). For whatever reason, including cultural norms, the unacceptability of drawing on their families' resources, or not wanting to resort to Medicaid, older Hispanic individuals seem to find nursing homes an unacceptable living arrangement until there is simply no alternative (Angel et al., 1996).

# VIII. Conclusion

The New World, including the United States, has become ever more ethnically and racially diverse since the first Europeans arrived in the fifteenth century. Cultural homogeneity was historically confined to tribal societies, or small provinces and regions defined by mountain ranges or other geological barriers that kept people separated and in their own culturally and linguistically unique worlds. Exploration and the mass migration of peoples put an end to that isolation, and the nations of the New World have been defined from their founding by cultural and ethnic mixing, a process that has rarely been peaceful. What has changed in the last century is the color of that diversity. The European immigrants who in earlier eras were the often rejected and reviled newcomers are today's old stock Americans. The new arrivals speak various versions of Spanish and a wide range of Asian languages and dialects. America's dynamic cities have always been a mosaic of cultures and languages, and newspapers, magazines, and books written in dozens of languages have been readily available. Despite the conflicts that often accompany it, immigration is what has given our nation its dynamic vitality and unique strength.

Today the United States is moving rapidly into a period in which the majority white population will become the minority. Other groups, religions, and creeds will change and enrich an already rich mélange of cultures. If we were not aware of the importance of understanding cultural differences before September 11, 2001, Americans now realize that we do not live in isolation from the rest of the world and the great oceans that have protected us before are easily crossed. Americans need to study and understand cultural differences and other languages just as the Europeans, who have had little choice, have done for centuries. The benefits of a more sophisticated understanding of culture, both domestically and internationally, are clear. The failure to understand other cultures and world views isolates one from important and potentially enlightening differences of opinion. As we have argued, the failure to appreciate the importance of ethnicity runs the risk of introducing a dimension of racial and ethnic strife into what could be serious age-based conflicts in the decades to come.

Today's ethnic minorities will be tomorrow's majority in many states, and they will make up a major part of the labor force in the nation as a whole. As we have become acutely aware, the changing ethnic composition of the population will be accompanied by a rapid and extensive aging of the population. Within the next decade the baby boom generation will begin arriving at retirement age and the number of retired Americans will increase dramatically. As we have shown, the working age population that will support them will be increasingly African American and Latino. Everyone's welfare, therefore, depends on the productivity of those groups. If these groups are confined to the low-paying service sector, yet another dimension based on race and ethnicity will be introduced into our structures of social inequality. That the productive potential of a large segment of the future labor force might be undermined by poor health and low educational levels has profound implications for older, as well as younger, Americans.

As the population at large changes in color and nation of origin, the elderly will also become more heterogeneous in terms of language proficiency, education, occupational attainment, migration history, income, and wealth. Based on the differences in income and wealth we have documented, inequality will almost inevitably increase in the years to come. As the baby boom generation arrives at retirement age, benefit cuts that will almost inevitably be necessary will have their most serious impact on African Americans and Latinos, and especially African-American and Latino women, because so many depend on Social Security alone for their economic security (Herd, 2005). In the future minority elderly individuals will find themselves particularly dependent on Medicaid.

The groups we have dealt with differ in many important respects that will affect their economic, housing, and medical care needs in old age. When and how each group arrived and the degree of their economic and social incorporation will determine their health, wealth, social support, and the social and health services they are likely to need and use (Borjas, 1994; Palloni, Soldo, & Wong, 2002). Some groups, especially immigrant adults, face serious barriers to health care, and especially preventive care, because they lack a usual source of care or health insurance (Wallace & Gutierrez, 2004). Although Medicare has eliminated many disparities among elderly Americans, differences in access to high-quality health and long-term care services persist into old age. The demographic processes and changes in the cultural composition of each age stratum that we have touched on in this chapter, then, have profound implications for all age groups and for the demands that the elderly will place on our health care system and on other formal and informal sources of support. Understanding the implications of all of these changes represents a new and important research agenda for the foreseeable future.

## References

Aizcorbe, A. M., Kennickell, A. B., & Moore, K. B. (2003). Recent changes in U.S. family finances: Evidence from the 1998 and 2001 Survey of Consumer Finances. *Federal Reserve Bulletin*, January, 1–32.

Alba, R. D. (1990). *Ethnic identity: The transformation of white America*. New Haven: Yale University Press.

American Immigration Law Foundation. (2002). *Mexican immigrant workers and the U.S. economy*. Retrieved December 15, 2004, from http://www.ailf.org/pubed/pe_0902.asp.

Anderson, R. N. (2002). Deaths: Leading causes for 2000. *National Vital Statistics Reports*, 50(16), Table 1. Washington, DC: National Center for Health Statistics.

Angel, J. L. (2003). Devolution and the social welfare of elderly immigrants: Who will bear the burden? *Public Administration Review*, 63, 79–89.

Angel, J. L., & Angel, R. J. (1992). Age at migration, social connections, and well-being among elderly Hispanics. *Journal of Aging and Health*, 4, 480–499.

Angel, J. L., Angel, R. J., McLelland, J. L, & Markides, K. S. (1996). Nativity, declining health, and preferences in living arrangements among elderly Mexican Americans: Implications for long-term care. *The Gerontologist*, 36, 464–473.

Angel, J. L, Buckley, C. J., & Sakamoto, A. (2001). Duration or disadvantage? Exploring nativity, ethnicity, and health in midlife. *Journal of Gerontology: Social Sciences*, 56, S275–284.

Angel, J. L., & Hogan, D. P. (2004). Population aging and diversity in a new era. In K. E. Whitfield (Ed.), *Closing the gap: Improving the health of minority elders in the new millennium* (pp. 1–12). Washington, DC: The Gerontological Society of America.

Angel, R. J., & Angel, J. L. (1997). *Who will care for us? Aging and long-term care in multicultural America*. New York: New York University Press.

Angel, R. J., Angel, J. L., Lee, G. Y., & Markides, K. S. (1999). Age at migration and family dependency among older Mexican immigrants: Recent evidence from the Mexican American EPESE. *The Gerontologist*, 39, 59–65.

Angel, R. J., Angel, J. L., & Markides, K. S. (2002). Stability and change in health insurance among older Mexican Americans: Longitudinal evidence from the Hispanic Established Populations for Epidemiologic Study of older adults. *American Journal of Public Health*, 92, 1264–1271.

Bagley, S. P., Angel, R. J., Dilworth-Anderson, P., Liu, W., & Schinke, W. (1995). Adaptive health behaviors among ethnic minorities. *Health Psychology*, 14, 632–640.

Bastida E., Cuellar, I., & Villas, P. (2001). Prevalence of diabetes mellitus and related conditions in a south Texas Mexican American sample. *Journal of Community Health and Nursing*, 18, 75–84.

Bean, F. D., Berg, R. R., & Van Hook, J. V. (1996). Socioeconomic and cultural incorporation and marital disruption among Mexican Americans. *Social Forces*, 75, 593–617.

Binstock, R. H., & Jean-Baptiste, R. (1999). Elderly immigrants and the saga of welfare reform. *Journal of Immigrant Health*, 1, 31–40.

Black, S. A. (1999). Increased health burden associated with co-morbid depression in older diabetic Mexican Americans: Results of the Hispanic EPESE. *Diabetes Care*, 22, 56–64.

Black, S. A., Ray, L. A., & Markides, K. S. (1999). The prevalence and health burden of self-reported diabetes in the Mexican American elderly: Findings from the Hispanic EPESE. *American Journal of Public Health*, 89, 546–552.

Bongaarts, J. (2004). Population aging and the rising cost of public pensions (Working Paper No. 185, Policy Research Division). New York: Population Council.

Borjas, G. J. (1994). The economics of immigration. *Journal of Economic Literature, 32*, 1667–1717.

Burr, J. A. (1990). Race/sex comparisons of elderly living arrangements: Factors influencing institutionalization of the unmarried. *Research on Aging, 12*, 507–530.

Chan, S. (1991). *Asian Americans: An interpretive history*. Boston, MA: Twayne Publishers.

Crystal, S., & Shea, D. G. (1990). Cumulative advantage, cumulative disadvantage, and inequality among elderly people. *The Gerontologist, 30*, 437–443.

Crystal, S., & Shea, D. G. (2003). Prospects for retirement resources in an aging society. In S. Crystal & D. G. Shea (Eds.), *Focus on economic outcomes in later life: Public policy, health, and cumulative advantage* (pp. 271–281). New York: Springer.

Day, J. C. (1996). Life expectancy at age 65 by race, Hispanic origin, and sex: 1995 to 2050. Population projections of the United States by age, sex, race, and Hispanic origin, 1995 to 2050. *Current Population Reports*, P25–1130, Appendix B-2. Washington, DC: U.S. Census Bureau.

DeFreitas, G. (1991). *Inequality at work: Hispanics in the U.S. labor force*. New York: Oxford University Press.

Diehl, A. K., & Stern, M. P. (1989). Special health problems of Mexican-Americans: Obesity, gallbladder disease, diabetes mellitus, and cardiovascular disease. *Advances in Internal Medicine, 34*, 79–96.

Elo, I. T., & Preston, S. H. (1997). Racial and ethnic differences in mortality at older ages. In L. G. Martin & B. J. Soldo (Eds.), *Racial and ethnic differences in the health of older Americans* (pp. 10–43). Washington, DC: National Academy Press.

Franklin, J. H., & Moss, Jr., A. (1999). *From slavery to freedom: A history of African Americans*, 8th ed. New York: McGraw Hill Publishing Company.

Friedland, R. B., & Pankaj, V. (1997). *Welfare reform and elderly legal immigrants*. Washington, DC: National Academy on Aging.

Grenier, G. J., & Cattan, P. (2000). Latino immigrants in the labor force: Trends and labor market issues. In S. M. Pérez (Ed.), *Moving up the economic ladder: Latino workers and the nation's future prosperity* (pp. 88–123). Washington, DC: National Council of La Raza.

Guzmán, B. (2001). *The Hispanic population: Census 2000 brief C2KBR/01-3* (Table 3). Washington, DC: U.S. Census Bureau.

Harris, M. I., Flegal, K. M., Cowie, C. C., Eberhardt, M. S, Goldstein, D. E., Little, R. R., Wiedmeyer, H. M., & Byrd-Holt D. D. (1998). Prevalence of diabetes, impaired fasting glucose, and impaired glucose tolerance in U.S. adults: The Third National Health and Nutrition Examination Survey (NHANES) 1988–1994. *Diabetes Care, 21*, 518–524.

Hayes-Bautista, D. E. (2004). *La nueva California: Latinos and California society, 1940–2040*. Berkeley, CA: The University of California Press.

Hayward, M. D., Crimmins, E. M., Miles, T., & Yang, Y. (2000). The significance of socioeconomic status in explaining the racial gap in chronic health conditions. *American Sociological Review, 65*, 910–930.

Hayward, M. D., & Heron, M. (1999). Racial inequality in active life among adult Americans. *Demography, 36*, 77–91.

Hayward, M. D., Warner, D. F., & Crimmins, E. M. (2003). Toward a better understanding of racial/ethnic differences in active life expectancy. (Paper presented at the International Network on Health Expectancy and the Disability Process, Guadalajara, Mexico, May 5–7).

He, W. (2002). The older born foreign-born population in the United States: 2000. *Current Population Reports, P23–211*. Washington, DC: U.S. Bureau of the Census.

Hendley, A. A., & Bilimoria, N. F. (1999). Minorities and social security: An analysis of racial and ethnic differences in the current program. *Social Security Bulletin, 62*(2), 59–64.

Henkin, N., & Kingson, E. (1998–99). Advancing an intergenerational agenda for the twenty-first century. *Generations, 22*, 99–105.

Herd, P. (2005). Reforming a breadwinner welfare state: Gender, race, class and Social Security Reform. *Social Forces, 83*, 1365–1394.

Himes, C. L., Hogan, D. P., & Eggebeen, D. J. (1996). Living arrangements among minority elders. *Journal of Gerontology: Social Sciences, 51B*, S42–S48.

Hoffman, B. (2001). *The wages of sickness: The politics of health insurance in progressive America*. Chapel Hill: University of North Carolina Press.

Honig, M. (2000). Minorities face retirement: Worklife disparities repeated? In B. Hammond, O. S. Mitchell, & A. Rappaport (Eds.), *Forecasting retirement needs and retirement wealth* (pp. 235–252). Philadelphia, PA: University of Pennsylvania Press.

Kelley-Moore J. A., & Ferraro, K. F. (2004). The black/white disability gap: Persistent inequality in later life? *Journal of Gerontology: Social Sciences, 59*, S34–43.

Kijakazi, K. (2001). *Women's retirement income: The case for improving Supplemental Security Income* (paper presented at the Institute for Women's Policy Research Annual Conference). Retrieved December 15, 2004, from http://www.cbpp.org/6-8-01socsec.htm.

Lamphere, J., & Rosenbach, M. L. (2000). Promises unfulfilled: Implementation of expanded coverage for the elderly poor. *Health Services Research, 35*, 207–217.

Lee, R. (1997). *Public costs of long life and low fertility: Will the baby boomers break the budget?* Center for Economics and Demography of Aging, Berkeley, CA: University of California. Retrieved December 15, 2004, from University of California at Berkeley Resource Center on Aging Web site: http://socrates.berkeley.edu/~aging /Lee.html.

Li, C. I., Malone, K. E., & Daling, J. R. (2003). Differences in breast cancer stage, treatment, and survival by race and ethnicity. *Archives of Internal Medicine, 163*, 49–56.

Manton, K. G., & Stallard, E. (1997). Health and disability differences among racial and ethnic groups. In L. G. Martin & B. J. Soldo (Eds.), *Racial and ethnic differences in the health of older Americans* (pp. 43–105). Washington, DC: National Academy Press.

Mor, V., Zinn, J., Angelelli, J., Teno, J. M., & Miller, S. C. (2004). Driven to tiers: Socioeconomic and racial disparities in the quality of nursing home care. *The Milbank Quarterly, 82*, 227–256.

Mui, A. C., Choi, N. G., & Monk, A. (1998). *Long-term care and ethnicity*. Westport, CT: Auburn House.

Murdock, S. H. (2004). *Population change in Texas: Implications for human and socioeconomic resources in the 21st century*. Slide 30. San Antonio, TX: Texas State Data Center, The University of Texas at San Antonio.

National Center for Health Statistics. (2004). *Health, United States: 2003*. Retrieved December 15, 2004, from the National Center for Health Statistics Web site: http://www.cdc.gov/nchs/data/hus/tables/2003/03hus130.pdf.

Palloni, A., & Arias, E. (2004). Paradox lost: Explaining the Hispanic adult mortality advantage. *Demography, 41*, 385–415.

Palloni, A., Soldo, B. J., & Wong, R. (2002). Health status and functional limitations in a national sample of elderly Mexicans (paper presented at the Population Association of America Conference, Atlanta, May).

Portes, A., & Rumbaut, R. G. (1990). *Immigrant America: A portrait*. Berkeley, CA: University of California Press.

Reed, J., & Ramirez, R. R. (1998). The Hispanic population in the United States: March 1997 (Update). *Current Population Reports*. (P20–511), Washington, DC: U.S. Bureau of the Census.

Rumbaut, R. G. (1997). Paradoxes and orthodoxies of assimilation. *Sociological Perspectives, 40*, 483–511.

Salgado de Snyder, V. N., & Diaz-Guerrero, R. (2003). Enduring separation: The psychological consequences of Mexican migration to the United States. In L. L. Adler & U. P. Gielen (Eds.), *Migration: Immigration and emigration in international perspective* (pp. 143–157). Westport, CT: Praeger.

Shea, D. G., Miles, T., & Hayward, M. (1996). The health-wealth connection: Racial differences. *The Gerontologist, 36*, 342–349.

Social Security Administration (2004a). *The 2004 Annual Report of the Board of Trustees of the Federal Old-Age and Survivors Insurance and Disability Insurance Trust Fund*, Table IV.B2. Retrieved December 15, 2004, from the Social Security Administration Actuarial Resources Web site:http://www.ssa.gov/OACT/TR/TR04/IV_LRest.html#wp178448.

Social Security Administration. (2004b). *Social Security basic facts*. Retrieved December 15, 2004, from the Social Security Administration Press Office Web site: http://www.ssa.gov/pressoffice/basicfact.htm.

Social Security Administration (2004c). *Monthly statistical snapshot: Social security benefits*. November 2004, Table 2. Retrieved January 27, 2005, from the Social Security Administration Press Office Web site: http://www.ssa.gov/policy/docs/quickfacts/stat_snapshot/#table2.

South, S. J. (1991). Age structure and public expenditures on children. *Social Science Quarterly, 72*, 661–675.

Suro, R., & Singer, A. (2002). *Latino growth in metropolitan America: Changing patterns, new locations*. Washington, DC: The Brookings Institution.

Takaki, R. (1998). *Strangers from a different shore: A history of Asian Americans*. New York: Penguin.

Torres-Gil, F., & Villa, V. (1993). Health and long-term care: Family policy for Hispanic aging. In M. Sotomayor & A. Garcia (Eds.), *Elderly Latinos: Issues and solutions for the 21st century* (pp. 45–58). Washington, DC: National Hispanic Council on Aging.

U.S. Census Bureau. (2000). *Projected life expectancy at birth by race and Hispanic origin, 1999 to 2100*. Table C. Retrieved December 15, 2004, from U.S. Census Bureau Web site: www.census.gov/population/documentation/twps0038/tabC.txt.

U.S. Census Bureau. (2001). *Income and poverty: 2000*. Retrieved December 15, 2004, from U.S. Department of Commerce, Economics and Statistics Administration Web site: http://www.census.gov/Press Release/www/2001/PressBri.pdf.

U.S. Census Bureau. (2003a). *Statistical abstract of the United States, 2002* (122nd edition). Washington, DC. Table No. 17, Resident Population by Race, Hispanic Origin Status, and Age—Projections: 2005 and 2010. Retrieved December 15, 2004, from U.S. Census Bureau Web site: http://www.census.gov/prod/2003pubs/02statab/pop.pdf.

U.S. Census Bureau. (2003b). Cities with 250,000 or more inhabitants in 2000: Hispanic and non-Hispanic groups: 2000. *Statistical Abstract of the United States: 2003*, Table no. 33. Retrieved December 20, 2004, from U.S. Census Bureau Web site: http://www.census.gov/prod/2004pubs/03statab/pop.pdf.

U.S. Census Bureau (2003c). Social and economic characteristics of the Hispanic population: 2002. *Statistical Abstract of the United States: 2003*, Table 46. Retrieved December 15, 2004 from U.S. Census Bureau Web site: http://www.census.gov/prod/2004pubs/03statab/pop.pdf.

U.S. Census Bureau. (2003d). Selected life table values: 1979 to 2001 (No. 106. Vital Statistics). *Statistical Abstract of the United States: 2003*. Washington, DC: Government Printing Office.

U.S. Census Bureau. (2003e). Persons 65 years old and over with limitations of activity caused by chronic conditions. No. 196. *Statistical Abstract of the United States*. Washington, DC. Government Printing Office.

U.S. Census Bureau. (2004a). *Projected population of the United States, by race and Hispanic origin: 2000 to 2050*. Retrieved December 22, 2004, from U.S. Census Bureau Web site: http://www.census.gov/ipc/www/usinterimproj/natprojtab01a.pdf

U.S. Census Bureau. (2004b). Age and sex of all people, family members and unrelated individuals iterated by income-to-poverty ratio and race. *Annual Demographic Survey*: March supplement, POV01. Retrieved December 15, 2004, from U.S. Census Bureau Web site: http://ferret.bls.census.gov/macro/032003/pov/new01_125.htm.

U.S. Census Bureau. (2004c). *Health insurance coverage status and type of coverage by selected characteristics: 2003*. Retrieved December 15, 2004, from U.S. Census Bureau Web site: http://ferret.bls.census.gov/macro/032004/health/h01_001.htm

Verbrugge, L. M. (1989). The twain meet: Empirical explanations of sex differences in health and mortality. *Journal of Health and Social Behavior, 30*, 282–304.

Villa, V. M., & Aranda, M. P. (2000). The demographic, economic, and health profile of older Latinos: Implications for health and long-term care policy and the Latino family. *Health and Human Services Administration, 23*, 1611–1680.

Wallace, S. P., & Gutierrez, V. F. (2004). *Mexican immigrants lack health services in the United States.* Retrieved December 15, 2004, from ttp://releases.usnewswire.com/GetRelease.asp?id=36965

Wallace, S. P., Levy-Storms, L., & Ferguson, L. R. (1995). Access to paid in-home assistance among disabled elderly people: Do Latinos differ from non-Latino whites? *American Journal of Public Health, 85,* 970–975.

Wise, D. A. (Ed.). (1996). *Advances in the economics of aging.* Chicago, IL: The University of Chicago Press.

Worobey, J. L., & Angel, R. J. (1990). Functional capacity and living arrangements of unmarried elderly persons. *Journal of Gerontology: Social Sciences, 45,* S95–S101.

Wu, J. H., Haan, M. N., Liang, J., Ghosh, D., Gonzalez, H. M., & Herman, W. H. (2003). Diabetes as a predictor of change in functional status among older Mexican Americans: A population-based cohort study. *Diabetes Care, 26,* 314–319.

Yong-Fang K., Mukaila, R. A., Markides, K. S., Ray, L. A., Espino, D. V., & Goodwin, J. S. (2003). Inconsistent use of diabetes medications, diabetes complications, and mortality in older Mexican Americans over a 7-year period: Data from the Hispanic Established Population for the Epidemiologic Study of older adults. *Diabetes Care, 26,* 3054–3060.

Seven

# Social Networks and Health

Jennifer L. Moren-Cross and Nan Lin

## I. Social Structure and Health

### A. Introduction and Purpose

A compelling body of research has accumulated indicating that social structure affects health (e.g., Lin & Peek, 1999; Lin, Ye, & Ensel, 1999; Marmot, Kogevinas, & Elston, 1987; Pearlin, 1989; Ross & Wu, 1995; Turner & Marino, 1994; Turner, Wheaton, & Lloyd, 1995). This research has been pursued along two lines of social structure, one based on the socioeconomic hierarchy and the other on social networks, including social integration and social support. The purpose of this chapter is to examine health among older adults through the latter form of social structure, social networks, which will be covered in four major sections. The first section briefly distinguishes the social network approach from social support and social integration. In the second section, we review the development of social network scholarship and propose a typology of social network properties. We review empirical evidence on social networks and health among older adults in

the third section, noting both the contributions such work has provided, as well as questions left unanswered. Finally, in the fourth section, we provide conclusions and point out several promising research areas concerning health and social networks, including the life course framework, the Internet, and biological pathways.

Underpinning these sections are several contentions that are elaborated throughout the chapter: (1) research on social relationships and health will benefit from being explicitly embedded in a social network framework; (2) to advance this line of research, investigators should seek to understand how the structure of social networks gives rise to social capital, and how network structure and social capital affect health; and (3) this line of research can benefit from a life course perspective.

### B. Social Networks, Social Integration, and Social Support

Although several scholars have noted over the years that "social network," "social integration," "social support,"

*Handbook of Aging and the Social Sciences, Sixth Edition*

and related concepts are used inter-changeably, and sometimes metaphori-cally, without rigorous attention to their theoretical and operational meanings (e.g., Berkman & Glass, 2000; House, Umberson, & Landis, 1988), current research is still beset by this problem. In this chapter, we echo the call to improve clarity when doing research in these areas. These concepts are, of course, intertwined and often interdependent, but here we discuss features that gener-ally distinguish them.

Social networks encompass *interrela-tions among individuals*. A social net-work is a set of nodes (i.e., usually individuals in the case of health out-comes) that are tied to one another by types of relations between them (Hall & Wellman, 1985). "The strength of social network theory rests on the testable assumption that the social structure of the network itself is largely responsible for determining individual behavior and attitudes by shaping the flow of resources which determine access to opportunities and constraints on behavior" (Berkman & Glass, 2000, 141–142). The "social struc-ture of the network itself" to which Berkman and Glass refer has many prop-erties such as the ones detailed in a typology later in the chapter. Social inte-gration is a concept that *attaches the individual to the larger social structure*. Some have even broadly defined social integration as the opposite of social isolation (e.g., Seeman, 1996). Moreover, social integration carries with it the notion that social structure shapes the individual, but there is little attention to the reverse of this—how the individual affects the structure. Social support, in contrast, deals with an *individual draw-ing upon others or resources from the whole (received social support), or even the mere perception that one can do so (perceived social support)*—the latter of which is more strongly associated with psychological distress (e.g., Wethington

& Kessler, 1986). Received and perceived social support may be further classified into types, including emotional, informa-tional, and/or instrumental (e.g., House & Kahn, 1985). This chapter focuses exclu-sively on social networks.

## II. The Network Approach

### A. Historical Development

Although Durkheim (1857/1951) pur-ported a relationship between social rela-tionships and health more than a century and a half ago, it is interesting to note that the "network approach" is a contemporary development from the earlier part of the twentieth century, gaining greater atten-tion during the past few decades (Marsden, 1990). Much current social network analy-sis descends from Jacob Moreno's (1934) sociometric models developed in the 1930s. Using a Gestalt psychology frame-work, he created sociograms (groups iden-tified as dots connected by lines) to demonstrate relationship dynamics among people. Subsequently, several developments in the 1950s advanced the network approach, including Festinger and colleagues' (Festinger, Schachter, & Back, 1950) work on physical propinquity and friendship formation, as well as Newcomb's (1956) research on interper-sonal agreement and attraction. At the same time, the research of Barnes (1954) and Bott (1957) on social networks broke the mold of anthropological work that was based on traditional categories defined by kinship, residence, and class (Berkman & Glass, 2000). The social network approach enabled these British anthropologists to study the structural characteristics of human interrelations outside such bounded groups.

### B. Two Types of Network Approaches

Two broad approaches are used in net-work analysis. The first approach is *egocentric* or *personal networks* (Hall & Wellman, 1985). This method samples individuals or entities and examines their networks' characteristics, such as the composition and structure, extending from a focal person—the ego or a respondent. This is the most common approach used in health-related research and is the focus in this chapter. The second network approach studies the *entire network of a specified population—the network saturation method.* That is, once a population is identified, information is collected on who is connected to whom within that population, and characteristics about those individuals or entities. An advantage of this method is that one can simultaneously examine the parts of a social system, as well as the social system itself (Hall & Wellman, 1985).

Berkman (1985) noted that in the 1970s, epidemiologists began to observe that some people were *protected* from social upheavals such as rapid social change, social disorganization, and the effects of mobility because of factors related to social and community ties (e.g., Antonovsky, 1974; Cassel, 1976; Nuckolls, Cassel, & Kaplan, 1972). At the same time, others (e.g., Berkman & Syme, 1979; Jenkins, 1971) were pressing harder to better understand how some aspects of social networks could be *harmful*. These researchers sought more refined measures of social networks to better understand both the mechanisms involved and the outcomes. A breakthrough in this area was the discovery that social isolation was associated with adverse social and health outcomes (Berkman, 1985). These lines of inquiry were the starting points for contemporary investigations on social networks as both buffering agents and/or stressor(s). House and colleagues (1988, p. 543) were among the first to contend that a broader theory is needed tying social relationships to health; a theory that must clearly link (1) the existence of social relationships, (2) the formal structure of those relationships (e.g., den-

sity, reciprocity), and (3) the content of those relationships (e.g., social support). We concur with this argument and discuss later how social capital theory meets these conditions.

## C. A Typology of Social Network Properties

It is important to develop a typology of social network properties because it assists in systematically reviewing the literature and identifying gaps. More important, such a typology provides a theoretical and measurement framework from which to draw. We organize social network properties along three broad dimensions: (1) network features, (2) location features, and (3) resource features (Table 7.1).

The *network features* refer to characteristics related to the distribution and connection of individuals in the network (i.e., nodes/ties). For instance, density indicates the degree to which individuals are interconnected as measured by the actual number of direct ties in the individual's network relative to the number of possible ties. Size of the network is another indicator of network composition, and a very common measure used in the study of health and social networks. Size simply refers to the number of individuals directly and/or indirectly connected within a specified network. Size and density have no reference to personal and social characteristics concerning the ties. Homogeneity-heterogeneity, on the other hand, refers to the degree to which the ties are alike or different on a specified characteristic, such as race/ethnicity or socioeconomic status. Demographic characteristics could also include race/ethnicity and socioeconomic status, but the focus would be on the distribution of those characteristics in the network.

*Location features* refer to relationships among ties within the network. For instance, degree indicates the extent

**Table 7.1**
Typology of Social Network Properties

| Type | Definition |
|---|---|
| **Network Features** | |
| Density | Extent individuals are connected (measured by the actual number of direct ties in the ego's network relative to the number of possible ties) |
| Size | Number of individuals directly and/or indirectly connected within a specified network |
| Homogeneity | Extent that ties are alike or different on a specified characteristic, such as race/ethnicity or socioeconomic status |
| Demographics | Descriptive, aggregate indicators of demographic characteristics of the network, such as the proportion of a particular race/ethnicity, or the mean income |
| **Location Features** | |
| Degree | Extent to which one member of the network is tied to others |
| Strength of Tie | Whether connection between two ties is strong or weak |
| Frequency | How often two ties interact |
| Duration | How long two ties have known one another |
| Intimacy | Perceived emotional attachment of one tie to another |
| Multiplexity | Number of relationships between two particular ties, such as whether they are friends, as well as neighbors |
| Reciprocity | Extent to which resources are both received and given |
| Reachability | Average number of ties necessary to link any two members of the network |
| **Resource Features** | |
| Social Capital | Resources embedded in a network that are accessed and/or mobilized in purposive actions. These can be material or emotional. |

to which one member of the network has direct ties to others. Strength of tie refers to whether the connection between two members is strong or weak, as perceived by ego or inferred by the investigator. For example, one's spouse is commonly considered a strong tie by researchers. Frequency indicates how often ties interact—daily, weekly, monthly, and so on. Duration indicates the length of time two ties have been connected. The perceived emotional attachment of one tie to another represents intimacy. Multiplexity refers to the number of relationships between two particular ties, such as whether they are friends, as well as neighbors, as well as co-workers. Reciprocity reflects the extent to which resources are received and given between ego and a tie. The average number of ties needed to link any two members of the network indicates the degree of reachability.

Finally, *network properties* can be classified according to their resource features. The main property here is social capital, which is defined as ". . . resources embedded in a social structure that are accessed and/or mobilized in purposive actions" (Lin, 2001, p. 29). These resources can be material or emotional. A substantial body of literature exists on material and emotional resources conceived as social support related to health; much less research is based on social capital theory. The difference is that research on social capital explicitly embeds the resources in a social network structure. That is, resources are modeled as mediators between the social network structure and health outcome. This permits us to understand the type(s) of social structure that generates resources related to health outcomes.

## III. Review of Social Network Properties and Health

Durkheim (1857/1951) is cited as the classic scholar who examined social relationships and health because of his seminal research associating indicators of social integration with suicide. Although Durkheim never formally defined social integration, it is inferred that he considered this to be both attachment to and regulation by social groups. Much time passed before social relationships and health became a prominent research topic in sociology. Indeed, it is only recently that research examining the associations between social relationships and health and well-being became a mainstay of the sociology of health and illness (Peek & Lin, 1999). Most of the research to date on social relationships and health, however, has examined social integration and social support, with much less focusing on the structure of social networks.

Transitioning into older adulthood is associated with age-graded normative changes in the structure and function of social networks that may impact health. For instance, van Tilburg (1998) found that although the total network size remains the same over time, the number of close relatives increases and the number of friends decreases. Moreover, older adults have less social contact compared to younger adults (e.g., Due, Holstein, Lund, Modvig, & Avlund, 1999; van Tilburg, 1998). Regarding resources embedded in social networks, research suggests that as one ages, there is an increase in the amount of instrumental support received with a concomitant increase in the amount of emotional support given (e.g., van Tilburg, 1998).

In this section, we review empirical evidence related to social network proper-ties and health among the older adult population. Ideally, research on social networks and health would address the full range of social network properties; however, this has often not been the case. Research is available about some network properties and health among older adults such as network size, some demographic characteristics, frequency of contact, and reciprocity; but many aspects have been largely, if not wholly, neglected (e.g., homogeneity, degree, reachability). Therefore their salience for health outcomes for this population remains to be demonstrated. In addition, even among the properties studied, research is often limited to a single health outcome. Thus, additional research is needed on virtually all network properties.

### A. Size

Network size is the most commonly studied network property related to health. Research on older adults has examined how network size relates to a variety of outcomes including mental and physical health, disability and physical functioning, cognitive ability, and mortality. The broad premise usually underlying such studies is that larger networks afford one more resources, and thus, result in better health outcomes—but this has not been supported in all empirical investigations (e.g., Haines & Hurlbert, 1992). Size generally indicates the total number of members in ego's network, but this obviously can be (and has been) operationalized in numerous ways. For example, in a study not only including older adults but also adults of all ages, Haines and Hurlbert (1992) used a name generator to estimate network size, and then assessed how size relates to stress, social support, and distress. The name generator listed nine relational contents (e.g., helping with household tasks, engaging in social activities) and asked respondents to identify all the ties they had pertaining to each one. On average, the respondents identified 18.5 ties, ranging from 2 to 67. Although social network size is positively related to distress for women, this relationship becomes nonsignificant when stress is added as a mediator. In other words, social networks indirectly affect distress through levels of stress. Surprisingly, size was not related to levels of social support, a finding discussed further later.

Using a similar name generator approach on survivors of Hurricane Andrew in Louisiana, Haines, Beggs, and Hurlbert (2002) examined relationships between social network properties (e.g., size), social support, and distress. They found that size indirectly affects distress through social support rather than stress. Both studies found that size only indirectly affects psychological distress. But Haines and Hurlbert (1992) found that size matters because larger networks predispose women to more life events (including events that happened to network members) that increased distress levels. In contrast, Haines and colleagues (2002) found that people with larger networks reported more social support after the hurricane, which in turn mitigated distress levels. Lin, Ye, and Ensel (1999), using an upstate New York sample, found that larger social networks were significantly related to perceived instrumental support, perceived expressive support, and actual instrumental support. Moreover, social network size was directly and indirectly related to psychological distress. Again, support resources served as a mediator between size of networks and depressive symptoms. The measure of network size used by Lin and colleagues is somewhat confounded with the frequency of interaction, as it was operationalized as the number of *weekly* contacts rather than just contacts in general. Doing so is not uncommon in the health literature (e.g., Avlund, Lund, Holstein, Due, Sakari-Rantala, &

Heikkinen, 2004; Bowling & Browne, 1991; Zunzunegui, Alvarado, Del Ser, & Otero, 2003). Additional research is needed to disentangle the precise network properties and mechanisms at work.

Finally, examining a sample of London adults 85 years and older, Bowling and Browne (1991) found that network size (measured as "significant" ties who interact at least monthly) is significantly and negatively correlated with depressive and anxiety symptoms; however, when covariates are added to the model, social network size becomes nonsignificant. More specifically, they disaggregated the total network size into proportions of relatives, friends, and confidants (so that network size is confounded with composition). Although number of confidants was significantly related to depressive and anxiety symptoms with only network variables in the model, the relationship becomes nonsignificant after adjusting for health. Clearly, more research is needed to further disentangle this complex picture—particularly among older adults.

In addition to mental health outcomes, researchers also have investigated the relationships between social networks and older adults' cognitive functioning. In samples of Spanish (Zunzunegui et al., 2003) and Baltimore (Holtzman, Rebok, Saczynski, Kouzis, Doyle, & Eaton, 2004) older adults, social network size is related to cognitive functioning, controlling for baseline cognitive functioning and other covariates. More specifically, Zunzunegui and colleagues (2003) found that the number of relatives seen at least monthly is a significant predictor of cognitive functioning, holding constant multiple measures of social integration and social engagement. Of interest, they also found that neither having friends nor the number of relatives contacted by telephone at least monthly was associated with cognitive functioning. Thus, something about having many face-to-face interactions with relatives is associated with better cognitive functioning. Again, this measure of network size is confounded with both composition and frequency. More research is needed to unravel the precise mechanisms that account for this relationship. What type of social capital is generated by seeing many relatives in person, as opposed to phone contacts and having friends? In the Baltimore sample, Holtzman and colleagues (2004) also found that changes in network size over 12 years are related to cognitive functioning, net of cognitive functioning and network size at baseline. Specifically, they found that larger networks at baseline and networks that grow in size over time are protective for maintaining cognitive functioning levels.

Research also has shown that social network size is related to the onset of disability among older adults. Using the MacArthur Studies of Successful Aging, investigators have shown a relationship between baseline social network size characteristics and functional disability onset two and seven years later (Seeman, Bruce, & McAvay, 1996; Unger, McAvay, Bruce, Berkman, & Seeman, 1999, respectively). More specifically, Seeman and colleagues (1996) found that, among men, having more close ties to children is significantly protective against disability onset, which is operationalized here as activities of daily living (ADLs). This relationship does not hold for women, nor did they find that total network size, number of close relatives, number of close friends, or number of visual contacts is significantly related to disability onset for either gender. Again, the network size measure is confounded with other social network properties—namely, aspects of strength of tie and intimacy because the ties are specified as "close." Of interest, although Unger and colleagues (1999) found that the number of social ties is not related to change in Nagi

Impairment Scores in a bivariate correlational analysis, they are significantly related in multivariate models. Moreover, they found that the effect of social ties on disability change over seven years is contingent on gender and baseline physical performance. Although social ties significantly affect disability levels for both genders, the effects are stronger among men. Social ties also are especially protective for those with low baseline levels of physical performance compared to those with higher levels (Unger et al., 1999).

Using eight waves of annual data from the New Haven EPESE, Mendes de Leon and colleagues (Mendes de Leon, Glass, Beckett, Seeman, Evans, & Berkman, 1999) found that not only do larger social networks protect against the onset of disability, but they also facilitate recovery. In particular, having larger networks (in total and of relatives) significantly mitigates the development of ADL disability. And larger networks (in total, of relatives, and of friends) predict recovery from disability. However, they do not find significant associations between larger children or confidant networks and disability onset or recovery. As with other studies reviewed here, the measures of social network size are confounded with aspects of social network frequency and geography, so future research will have to parse out these properties' specific effects on disability outcomes. Further, it is interesting to note that Mendes de Leon and colleagues (1999) did not find any significant relationships between any of these measures of network size and disability onset and recovery measured by the Rosow-Breslau disability scale.

Research also has examined the converse of this relationship: whether physical functioning and health status affect network size (Stoller & Pugliesi, 1991). These authors found that changes in network size are not predicted by baseline physical or functional health status. It is relevant to note that the measure of network size used in this study is con-founded with social resources because it is operationalized as the number of helpers available to the older adult.

Finally, many early studies examined the effect of social bonds on mortality (e.g., Berkman & Syme, 1979). Although much of this work failed to differentiate social support from the structural compo-nents of social networks (Berkman, 1985), recent work on mortality has been more precise. For example, in studies using the number of children as an indicator of social network size (size is confounded with composition), results have been mixed. Walter-Ginzburg, Blumstein, Chetrit, and Modan (2002) found that, among older Israeli Jews, number of liv-ing children is significantly related to risk of 8-year mortality in models that only include measures of the social network, social support, and social engagement. This relationship becomes nonsignifi-cant, however, when sociodemograhpic and health covariates are added to the model. Others found that number of chil-dren is particularly protective for women over the age of 70 compared to younger women, but is not related to men's mor-tality risk (Tucker, Schwartz, Clark, & Friedman, 1999). These authors also report that number of siblings does not matter for either gender's survival. Clearly more research is needed investi-gating whether social network size is related to mortality.

## B. Frequency

A variety of health outcomes related to network frequency have been explored among older adults, that is, how fre-quently ego interacts with network mem-bers. As observed for social network size, research finds mixed results on the rele-vance of social network frequency for mortality risk. In a Japanese sample, Sugisawa, Liang, and Liu (1994) found that frequency of contact with children,

relatives, and friends (combined) is not significantly related to survival. Similarly, frequency of contact with chil-dren is apparently not related to mortality risk among Israeli Jews (Walter-Ginzburg et al., 2002); however, research shows that frequency does matter for survival among Swedish women, but not in expected ways. Swedish women live longer if they are seldom or never visited by their children, or do not have any chil-dren compared to women who are visited at least once a month (Gustafsson, Isacson, & Thorslund, 1998). Further, the frequency of children visits is unrelated to Swedish men's mortality, and the fre-quency of visits by other relatives is not associated with either gender's survival.

Results also are not consistent when various physical health indicators have been examined. In the Japanese sample, Sugisawa et al. (1994) did not find a sig-nificant relationship between the com-bined frequency of contact with children, relatives, and friends with measures of smoking, self-rated health, or number of chronic conditions. In Moncton, Canada, a city characterized as having a diversi-fied economy and being well integrated into its surrounding community, fre-quency of contact with friends is associ-ated with self-rated health among older adults, but family and children frequency are nonsignificant (Zunzunegui, Kone, Johri, Beland, Wolfson, & Bergman, 2004). In contrast, in the more socioeconomi-cally deprived Hochelaga Maisonneuve, Canada, frequency of contact with chil-dren and family is significant, but friends are less important.

Lennartsson (1999) also separated fre-quency of contact with children, rela-tives, and friends in an investigation on older Swedish adults. Results demon-strate that children frequency is not related to any of the three physical health outcomes examined (self-rated health, circulatory problems, and respiratory peak flow); however, frequency of contact with relatives and friends is related to respiratory peak flow. Having no contact with friends and lacking siblings or other relatives significantly increases the odds of low peak flow. In addition, Lennartsson (1999) found that no contact with friends is significantly associated with mental health problems. In a nationally representative American sample, however, Musick and Wilson (2003) found that frequency of interaction with friends and relatives is not related to depressive symptoms. There is some evidence that frequency of contact with social ties is protective against disability. Sugisawa et al. (1994) found that visits with friends, family, and children is associated with less functional disability, net of sociodemograhpic, health, and social network covariates. In the same vein, Avlund and colleagues (2004) found that people who have less than weekly telephone contact with children and friends have greater functional decline.

There is even less research on the frequency of interaction with social ties than on network size. Nor do the findings paint a coherent picture. Thus, the relevance of frequency of social ties for health in late life is tenuous; at this point additional research will have to determine if and how it matters.

## C. Composition

Many studies reviewed here include measures of size or frequency that are confounded with the composition of social ties. For example, numerous studies measure network size as number of children or friends, rather than as the complete social network. Consequently, some of the effects of social network composition are intertwined with those findings. Examining the proportion of kin in social networks in samples that included young and older adults, Haines and Hurlbert (1992) and Haines and colleagues (2002) found little support for

effects on psychological distress. Some evidence, however, suggests that having a network with proportionally more men exacerbates psychological distress in the context of a post-hurricane disaster (Haines et al., 2002). In the same study, having a greater or lesser proportion of ties who completed high school is not related to psychological distress. Peek and Lin (1999) also investigated the effects of kin composition on psychological distress, but their measure is confounded with social resources because it is the proportion of kin in the perceived support network. Nonetheless, they found that a higher proportion of kin indirectly (but not directly) mitigates psychological distress among adults 60 years and older.

Mendes de Leon and colleagues (1999) also found that the composition of ties is predictive of disability development and recovery. Having more relative ties is associated with less disability onset and more recovery, whereas a larger friend network is only associated (positively) with recovery. Both children and confidant networks were unrelated to either disability onset or recovery.

## D. Other Social Network Properties

Beyond network size, frequency, and composition, several other network properties have received limited attention in research on older adults' health. For example, Ramos and Wilmoth (2003) found that older Brazilian adults have fewer depressive symptoms when there is more reciprocity in their relationships. And others have found no relationship between psychological distress and other network properties, including density and tie content multiplexity (Haines & Hurlbert, 1992), as well as mean closeness of ties and relationship duration (Haines et al., 2002). The dearth of research on these network properties makes generalizations about their contributions to older adult health infeasible at this time.

## E. Composite Measures of Social Networks

Several studies use an index or latent construct with multiple indicators of the social network, rather than separate measures of network properties. In these studies, it is difficult to parse out specific properties' effects; nonetheless they provide valuable information on social networks and health. An example is the Berkman-Syme index, which includes marital status, friend and relative contacts, church membership, and participation in group activities (Berkman & Syme, 1979). Using this index, Eng, Rimm, Fitzmaurice, and Kawachi (2002) found that those with fewer social ties experienced greater risks of mortality caused by accidents, suicide, and all-cause mortality. The Berkman-Syme index also has been used to study stroke outcomes among older adults. Findings indicate that stroke victims with more social ties have better physical functioning and are less likely to be institutionalized six weeks after hospital discharge (Colantonio, Kasl, Ostfeld, & Berkman, 1993).

Alternatively, Ferraro, Mutran, and Barresi (1984) created a social network latent construct that included indicators of intimacy, friendship network integration, and frequency of interaction. They found that better social networks predict better subsequent health among older adults. Finally, Litwin (2003), using a cluster analysis, created five social-network types to investigate physical activity among Israeli retirees: diverse, neighbors, friends, family, and restricted networks. He demonstrates that being embedded in a diverse social network is more advantageous in terms of physical activity compared to all other types of social networks. Those in restricted or exclusively family networks participated in the least physical activity.

## F. Social Capital

As stated previously, although there are differences among social capital, social support, and social integration, the boundaries are not always clear. Using Lin's (2001, p. 29) definition of social capital, ". . . resources embedded in a social structure that are accessed and/or mobilized in purposive actions," some research that meets the definition is not identified as "social capital" research (e.g., Haines & Hurlbert 1992; Haines et al., 2002; and so on). We claim that the indicators of social resources in some of these studies can be conceived as social capital given the definition above and we briefly summarize selected findings. We argue that social capital consists of social resources (instrumental or expressive) that are explicitly embedded in social networks. As noted earlier, social capital theory fulfills the conditions put forth by House and colleagues (1988) for a broader theory linking social relationships and health. Social capital theory contends that social capital (the "content of social networks" to which House and colleagues referred) comprises the resources embedded in a social network (Lin, 2001). Further, it is argued that we must understand what it is about the structure of the network (e.g., size, frequency, reciprocity) that gives rise to this social capital. Finally, putting all of this together, the goal is to comprehend how mental and physical health are affected by the structure of social networks and the social capital they engender.

Surprisingly, of all the network properties Haines and Hurlbert (1992) examined (including network size, content multiplexity, density among alters, geographic range, work range, mean tie strength, sex range, and proportion kin), they found barely a handful of significant associations with men and women's various forms of social support (i.e., social capital) (including instrumental support, companionship, and emotional aid). This leads the authors to state, "we found no evidence that, at the general social network level, a predominance of strong ties yields access to social support" (Haines & Hurlbert, 1992, p. 264). This is surprising because it is expected that those with more network ties will have more social resources (e.g., House et al., 1988; Lin, 2001). Other studies of psychological distress (e.g., Haines et al., 2002; Lin et al., 1999), however, reported opposite results. Haines and colleagues' research on a sample of Hurricane Andrew survivors in Louisiana demonstrates that more network ties are associated with more social capital (or social support as the authors call it here), which mitigated distress. A possible explanation for these discrepant findings is that the 2002 study examined hurricane survivors, and the support measures were targeted at hurricane-related assistance (i.e., having "enough people to help them in the preparation and recovery phases of Hurricane Andrew [instrumental support]" and "enough people to talk to about the storm in its preparation and recovery phases [expressive support])" (Haines et al., 2002, p. 278).

But, Lin and colleagues (1999) examined this process outside the context of a natural disaster. In their representative local sample, they demonstrate that (1) social network size exerts independent negative effects on depressive symptoms and (2) social capital, such as perceived and actual instrumental and expressive support, partially mediate the effects of network size on psychological distress. Perceived expressive support is particularly robust.

Evidence also is mixed regarding the process of social networks, social capital, and disability outcomes among older adults. For instance, Mendes de Leon and colleagues (1999) found that emotional support has no direct or indirect effects on disability onset, but instrumental support has significant direct effects and marginally acts as a mediator of network size. Neither instrumental nor emotional support (i.e., social capital) directly or indirectly affects recovery from disability.

Unfortunately, although a number of other studies include variables on both social network properties and social support, models testing whether social support is a product of social network structure, as well as testing direct and indirect effects of social support on health outcomes among older adults, were not reported. As a consequence of this and the limited research on this topic, we are left with a poor understanding of how social network structure (i.e., network properties) is related to social capital and health outcomes, despite a strong theory that predicts relationships among these constructs (e.g., House et al., 1988; Lin, 2001). This is an important literature gap to be filled by future research.

## IV. Conclusions and Directions for Future Research

Much has been covered in this chapter, including distinguishing the social network approach from social integration and social support, briefly reviewing the historical development of social network theory, proposing a typology of social network properties, and reviewing the empirical evidence concerning social networks and health among older adults. As a broad summary, it is clear that social networks affect mental and physical health. What is lacking, however, is a coherent picture of the mechanisms through which this occurs. There are three main reasons for this:

1. There is not enough research examining the effects of social networks on health outcomes. Among the most

neglected topics are examination of the full range of relevant health outcomes and tests of social capital as a mediator of the relationships between social network properties and health.

2. In research to date, variations in the conceptualization and measurement of network characteristics make comparisons across studies difficult. A benefit of the variety of measures is that many are creative and elucidate previously unexplored aspects of social networks, but a drawback is that we are left with too little evidence about specific network properties to understand when and how they operate.

3. Much of the current evidence is based on samples that are not nationally representative. In addition, much of this research has not adequately addressed selection (e.g., selective mortality), an especially important issue in studies of older adults.

Consequently, more research on physical and mental health among older adults needs to be based on a social network framework, in which specific network properties (such as those in Table 7.1) are examined. In addition, more research that evaluates how and when social networks give rise to social capital, and how this affects health among older adults, is needed. To comprehensively assess the impact of social networks on health, multiple indicators of network properties must be included.

A. Life Course

Research on mental and physical health and social networks will be advanced by incorporating a life course perspective. Most research on social networks and health to date has viewed social networks as static over the life course (Falk, Hanson, Isacsson, & Ostergren, 1992; van Tilburg, 1998 for initial efforts). There has been an implicit assumption that findings yielded by a snapshot picture of the effects of social networks on health will be largely true irrespective of time periods, age, history, and intergenerational context. These assumptions may not be valid and deserve theoretical, as well as empirical, attention. Incorporating a life course perspective will enrich this research topic by making the findings more dynamic and representing life processes more accurately.

Conceptualization and operationalization of social networks should move from only examining the effects of social structure (i.e., the network properties) on health to resources embedded in social networks, a point made several times in this chapter. Put in dynamic perspective, such research will determine who has access to social capital related to health, as well as the health effects of mobilizing such social capital. Social capital theory and research proposes that investment in members of the social network is critical to obtain instrumental and expressive resources upon which to act (Lin, 2001). Thus, in future investigations, research designs should pay more attention to social capital in networks. One example is use of the position generator methodology (for its development see Lin & Dumin, 1986). Recent developments using this methodology, sampling hierarchal positions or social resources (e.g., van der Gaag & Snijders, 2004), present exciting possibilities for rigorous research related to social capital and health. Compared to prior methods, these newer developments are less biased toward strong ties. The name generator methodology discussed earlier in the chapter samples network ties based on relational contents (e.g., helping with household tasks), which predominantly captures strong ties. In contrast, the position generator methodology samples hierarchal positions (e.g., Do you have a senator/janitor/factory worker as an acquaintance or friend?), so strong and weak ties are identified.

Addressing these issues, we can begin to articulate how social capital is related to health across the life course. In the older population, for example, demographic and economic role changes would be expected to change the resources embedded in social networks. We predict that retirement and disengagement from the labor market reduces social capital through work ties. Expressive, and especially instrumental, functions of social networks should be reduced among work peers. And chiefly among women (because of their longer average survival), the loss of a spouse, and possibly the subsequent loss of these womens' ties to their husbands' ties, would reduce instrumental and expressive resources. Detailed studies of role-related loss of social capital will help to identify predictable deficiencies among older adults' health-related resources. Such research also will also offer important information about compensation for resource loss through other networks (e.g., agencies or help groups, use of the Internet). Integrating social network theory and the life course framework will highlight the dynamic role social relationships play in health. Here, we have sketched out only a few of the possibilities for such a research agenda.

## B. The Internet

Given the explosion of Internet use in modern societies, it is important to determine whether older adults' social networks developed through the Internet affect health. Lin (2001) supported the notion that cybernetworks are a form of social capital; however, other researchers disagree on whether the time spent on the Internet leads to social isolation or the accumulation of social capital (e.g., DiMaggio, Hargittai, Neuman, & Robinson, 2001; Wellman & Haythornthwaite 2001). Some evidence demonstrates displacement—that Internet users will

displace face-to-face interaction resulting in less socializing and time spent outside the home. Other research, however, shows no displacement of socializing time with Internet time (e.g., DiMaggio et al., 2001). And at least one study reports that Internet socializing is associated with higher levels of offline socializing (Miyata, 2001), indicating that usage may be associated with proclivities toward sociability and extroversion (DiMaggio et al., 2001).

Support groups in online communities provide an anonymous forum for exchanging advice, information, and support (e.g., Drentea & Moren-Cross, 2005; Miyata, 2001). Users interact often to check on and help one another; related web sites are sources of support and information. Based on Lin's (2001) definition of social capital, a support group clearly provides social capital in that it is an embedded community activated for purposeful action. We are unaware of any research examining older adults' online social networks and health, but a recent, nationally representative study by the Kaiser Family Foundation (2005) suggests that such research would be useful. This study reports that fewer than one-third of persons 65 years and older have ever been online, but that more than two-thirds of those 50 to 64 have. They also found that 21% of the older group has sought health information online, compared to 53% of the younger group. Examining the effects of Internet use on the health of older adults will become increasingly important as more computer-literate younger cohorts grow older.

## C. Getting Under the Skin

Elucidating the ways social networks affect health by identifying specific network properties is one way of examining mechanisms, but how social networks "get under the skin" to affect health outcomes also is important. Allostatic load refers to the "wear and tear" the body experiences as a consequence of cycles of reactions to stress and returning to homeostasis over the life course (McEwen & Seeman, 1999). Allostatic load is multidimensional, including blood pressure, urinary norepinephrine and epinephrine, urinary cortisol, serum cholesterol, high-density lipoprotein, and others (Seeman, Singer, Ryff, Love, & Levy-Storms, 2002), Recent technological advances make it possible (albeit expensive) to measure allostatic load in large-scale surveys.

Even more recent are attempts to relate social relationships to allostatic load and subsequent health. In a study of two cohorts of older adults, Seeman and colleagues (2002) found that better social relations are associated with lower allostatic load. This line of research represents a compelling opportunity to demonstrate how the structural arrangements in which people are embedded manifest into changes at the physiological level. Moreover, anchoring this research agenda in a life course framework will help us to understand how social networks, effects on allostatic load cumulate through the life course, resulting in different levels of health during late life.

## References

Antonovsky, A. (1974). Conceptual, methodological problems in the study of resistance resources and stressful life events. In B. S. Dohrenwend & B. P. Dohrenwend (Eds.), Stressful life events: Their nature and effects (pp. 245–258). New York: Wiley.

Avlund, K., Lund, R., Holstein, B. E., Due, P., Sakari-Rantala, R., & Heikkinen, R. (2004). The impact of structural and functional characteristics of social relations as determinants of functional decline. Journal of Gerontology: Social Sciences, 59B, S44–S51.

Barnes, J. A. (1954). Class and communities in a Norwegian island parish. Human Relations, 7, 39–58.

Berkman, L. F. (1985). The relationship of social networks and social support to morbidity and mortality. In S. Cohen & S. L. Syme (Eds.), Social support and health (pp. 241–262). New York: Academic Press, Inc.

Berkman, L. F., & Glass, T. (2000). Social integration, social networks, social support, and health. In L. F. Berkman & I. Kawachi (Eds.), Social epidemiology (pp. 137–173). Oxford: Oxford University Press.

Berkman, L. F., & Syme, S. L. (1979). Social networks, host resistance and mortality: A nine-year follow-up study of Alameda County residents. American Journal of Epidemiology, 109, 186–204.

Bott, E. (1957). Family and social network. London: Tavistock Press.

Bowling, A., & Browne, P. (1991). Social networks, health, and emotional well-being among the oldest old in London. Journal of Gerontology: Social Sciences, 46, S20–S32.

Cassel, J. (1976). The contribution of the social environment to host resistance. American Journal of Epidemiology, 104, 107–123.

Colantonio, A., Kasl, S. V., Ostfeld, A. M., & Berkman, L. F. (1993). Psychosocial predictors of stroke outcomes in elderly population. Journal of Gerontology: Social Sciences, 48, S261–S268.

DiMaggio, P., Hargittai, E. S., Neuman, W. R., & Robinson, J. P. (2001). Social implications of the Internet. Annual Review of Sociology, 27, 307–336.

Drentea, P., & Moren-Cross, J. L. (2005). Social capital and social support on the web: The case of an Internet mother site. Sociology of Health and Illness, 27, forthcoming.

Due, P., Holstein, B., Lund, R., Modvig, J., & Avlund, K. (1999). Social relations: Network, support and relational strain. Social Science and Medicine, 48, 661–673.

Durkheim, E. (1857/1951). Suicide: A study in sociology. Glencoe, IL: Free Press.

Eng, P. M., Rimm, E. B., Fitzmaurice, G., & Kawachi, I. (2002). Social ties and change in social ties in relation to subsequent total and cause-specific mortality and coronary heart disease incidence in men. American Journal of Epidemiology, 155, 700–709.

Falk, A., Hanson, B. S., Isacsson, S., & Ostergren, P. (1992). Job strain and mortality in elderly men: Social network, support and influence as buffers. American Journal of Public Health, 82, 1136–1139.

Ferraro, K. F., Mutran, E., & Barresi, C. M. (1984). Widowhood, health, and friendship support in later life. *Journal of Health and Social Behavior, 25*, 246–259.

Festinger, L., Schachter, S., & Back, K. (1950). *Social pressures in informal groups.* New York: Harper & Row.

Gustafsson, T. M., Isacson, D. G. L., & Thorslund, M. (1998). Mortality in elderly men and women in a Swedish municipality. *Age and Ageing, 27*, 585–593.

Haines, V. A., Beggs, J. J., & Hurlbert, J. S. (2002). Exploring the structural contexts of the support process: Social networks, social statuses, social support, and psychological distress. In J. Levy & B. Pescosolido (Eds.). *Social networks and health*, volume 8 (pp. 269–292). Stamford, CT: JAI Press.

Haines, V. A., & Hurlbert, J. S. (1992). Network range and health. *Journal of Health and Social Behavior, 33*, 254–266.

Hall, A., & Wellman, B. (1985). Social networks and social support. In S. Cohen & S. L. Syme (Eds.), *Social support and health* (pp. 23–41). New York: Academic Press, Inc.

Holtzman, R. E., Rebok, G. W., Saczynski, J. S., Kouzis, A. C., Doyle, K. W., & Eaton, W. W. (2004). Social network characteristics and cognition in middle-aged older adults. *Journal of Gerontology: Psychological Sciences, 59B*, P278–P283.

House, J. S., & Kahn, R. L. (1985). Measures and concepts of social support. In S. Cohen & S. L. Syme (Eds.), *Social support and health* (pp. 83–108). New York: Academic Press, Inc.

House, J. S., Umberson, D., & Landis, K. R. (1988). Structures and processes of social support. *Annual Review of Sociology, 14*, 293–318.

Jenkins, C. D. (1971). Psychological and social precursors of coronary disease. *New England Journal of Medicine, 284*, 244–255.

Kaiser Family Foundation. (2005). e-Health and the elderly: How seniors use the Internet for health—survey. Retrieved February 6, 2005, from htpp://www.kkf.org/entmedia/entmedia011205pkg.cfm

Lennartsson, C. (1999). Social ties and health among the very old in Sweden. *Research on Aging, 21*, 657–681.

Lin, N. (2001). *Social capital.* Cambridge: Cambridge University Press.

Lin, N., & Dumin, M. (1986). Access to occupations through social ties. *Social Networks, 8*, 365–385.

Lin, N., & Peek, M. K. (1999). Social networks [au 6] and mental health. In A. Horwitz & T. L. Scheid (Eds.), *A handbook for the study of mental health: Social contexts, theories, and systems* (pp. 241–258). Cambridge University Press.

Lin, N., Ye, X., & Ensel, W. M. (1999). Social support and depressed mood: A structural analysis. *Journal of Health and Social Behavior, 40*, 344–359.

Litwin, H. (2003). Social predictors of physical activity in later life: The contribution of social-network type. *Journal of Aging and Physical Activity, 11*, 389–406.

Marmot, M. G., Kogevinas, M., & Elston, M. A. (1987). Social/economic status and disease. *Annual Review of Public Health, 8*, 111–135.

Marsden, P. (1990). Network data and measurement. *Annual Review of Sociology, 16*, 435–463.

McEwen, B. S., & Seeman, T. (1999). Protective and damaging effects of mediators of stress: Elaborating and testing the concepts of allostasis and allostatic load. In N. E. Adler, M. Marmot, & B. S. McEwen (Eds.), *Socioeconomic status and health in industrial nations: Social, psychological and biological pathways* (pp. 30–47). New York: New York Academy of Sciences.

Mendes de Leon, C. F., Glass, T. A., Beckett, L. A., Seeman, T. E., Evans, D. A., & Berkman, L. F. (1999). Social networks and disability transitions across eight intervals of yearly data in the New Haven EPESE. *Journal of Gerontology: Social Sciences, 54B*, S162–S172.

Miyata, K. (2001). Social support for Japanese mothers online and offline. In B. Wellman & C. Haythornthwaite (Eds.), *The Internet in everyday life* (pp. 520–548). Malden, MA: Blackwell Publishers Ltd.

Moreno, J. (1934). *Who shall survive?* New York: Beacon Press.

Musick, M. A., & Wilson, J. (2003). Volunteering and depression: The role of psychological and social resources in different age groups. *Social Science and Medicine, 56*, 259–269.

Newcomb, T. M. (1956). The prediction of interpersonal attraction. *American Psychologist, 11*, 575–586.

Nuckolls, K. B., Cassel, J. C., & Kaplan, B. H. (1972). Psychosocial assets, life crisis, and prognosis of pregnancy. *American Journal of Epidemiology, 95*, 431–441.

Pearlin, L. I. (1989). The sociological study of stress. *Journal of Health and Social Behavior, 30*, 241–256.

Peek, M. K., & Lin, N. (1999). Age differences in the effects of network composition on psychological distress. *Social Science and Medicine, 49*, 621–636.

Ramos, M., & Wilmoth, J. (2003). Social relationships and depressive symptoms among older adults in southern Brazil. *Journal of Gerontology: Social Sciences, 58B*, S253–S261.

Ross, C. E., & Wu, C. (1995). The links between education and health. *American Sociological Review, 60*, 719–745.

Seeman, T. (1996). Social ties and health: The benefits of social integration. *Annals of Epidemiology, 6*, 442–451.

Seeman, T. E., Bruce, M. L., & McAvay, G. J. (1996). Social network characteristics and onset of ADL disability: MacArthur studies of successful aging. *Journal of Gerontology: Social Sciences, 51B*, S191–S200.

Seeman, T. E., Singer, B. H., Ryff, C. D., Love, G. D., & Levy-Storms, L. (2002). Social relationships, gender, and allostatic load across two age cohorts. *Psychosomatic Medicine, 64*, 395–406.

Stoller, E. P., & Pugliesi, K. L. (1991). Size and effectiveness of informal helping networks: A panel study of older people in the community. *Journal of Health and Social Behavior, 32*, 180–191.

Sugisawa, H., Liang, J., & Liu, X. (1994). Social networks, social support, and mortality among older people in Japan. *Journal of Gerontology: Social Sciences, 49*, S3–S13.

Tucker, J. S., Schwartz, J. E., Clark, K. M., & Friedman, H. S. (1999). Age-related changes in the associations of social network ties with mortality risk. *Psychology and Aging, 14*, 564–571.

Turner, R. J., & Marino, F. (1994). Social support and social structure: A descriptive epidemiology. *Journal of Health and Social Behavior, 35*, 193–212.

Turner, R. J., Wheaton, B., & Lloyd, D. A. (1995). The epidemiology of social stress. *American Sociological Review, 60*, 104–125.

Unger, J. B., McAvay, G., Bruce, M. L., Berkman, L., & Seeman, T. (1999). Variation in the impact of social network characteristics on physical functioning in elderly persons: MacArthur studies of successful aging. *Journal of Gerontology: Social Sciences, 54B*, S245–S251.

Van der Gaag, M., & Snijders, T. (2004). Proposals for the measurement of individual social capital. In H. Flap & B. Völker (Eds.) *Creation and returns of social capital: A new research program* (pp. 199–218). New York: Routledge.

van Tilburg, T. (1998). Losing and gaining in old age: Changes in personal network size and social support in a four-year longitudinal study. *Journal of Gerontology: Social Sciences, 53B*, S313–S323.

Walter-Ginzburg, A., Blumstein, T., Chetrit, A., & Modan, B. (2002). Social factors and mortality in the old-old in Israel: The CALAS study. *Journal of Gerontology: Social Sciences, 57B*, S308–S318.

Wellman, B., & Haythornthwaite, C. (2001). The Internet in everyday life. In B. Wellman & C. Haythornthwaite (Eds.) *The Internet in everyday life* (pp. 3–41). Malden, MA: Blackwell Publishers Ltd.

Wethington, E., & Kessler, R. C. (1986). Perceived support, received support, and adjustment to stressful life events. *Journal of Health and Social Behavior, 27*, 78–89.

Zunzunegui, M., Alvarado, B. E., Del Ser, T., & Otero, A. (2003). Social networks, social integration, and social engagement determine cognitive decline in community-dwelling spanish older adults. *Journal of Gerontology: Social Sciences, 58B*, S93–S100.

Zunzunegui, M. V., Kone, A., Johri, M., Beland, F., Wolfson, C., & Bergman, H. (2004). Social networks and self-rated health in two French-speaking Canadian community dwelling populations over 65. *Social Science and Medicine, 58*, 2069–2081.

## Eight

# Converging Divergences in Age, Gender, Health, and Well-Being
## Strategic Selection in the Third Age

Phyllis Moen and Donna Spencer

One can think of the life course as a series of role transitions and trajectories as people move through their biographies, entering one role, exiting another over time (Elder, 1994; George, 1996; Giele & Elder, 1998; Mortimer & Shanahan, 2003). The subject matter of life course research is typically patterns of continuity and change in roles, relationships, health, identity, and attainment. The focus can be on discerning and examining patterns such as the incidence, timing, duration, or ordering of roles (Han & Moen, 1999a, 1999b; Hogan, 1978; Macmillan & Eliason, 2003; Moen & Han, 2001) or on the determinants and outcomes of various patterns, including health and well-being (Moen, 2003; Moen, Dempster-McClain, & Williams, 1989; Pavalko & Artis, 1997; Pavalko & Smith, 1999). But where do these patterns come from?

The life course also captures the historical times and cultural dynamics in which biographies unfold, the uneven rates of social and institutional change, and the complex interplay between biography and history. In fact, the life course approach developed in response to an effort to understand the implications of social change on individual lives—events such as immigration (Thomas & Znaniecki, 1918–1920) and the Great Depression (Elder, 1974). Life course research thus emphasizes the ecological embeddedness of lives in social structure and social change, capturing the biographies of people as they strategically respond to institutional regimes, changing circumstances, and unchanging exigencies.

The life course itself is constructed through cultural beliefs about the ways lives should play out, along with institutionalized age-graded expectations and sequences built into roles and rules (Mayer & Tuma, 1990). It is a product of primarily twentieth-century policies and practices developed around education, employment, and retirement (Kohli, 1986). This is readily apparent in the work of Matilda White Riley (Riley,

Supported by the Alfred P. Sloan Foundation, #2002-6-8 and NIH, U01 HD051256-01

Kahn, & Foner, 1994), who emphasizes the age segregation that is built in to roles and relationships in terms of age-related expectations, obligations, and possibilities. Riley also introduced the important concept of *structural lag*, as policies and practices shaping the life course frequently lag behind changing social realities. This highlights the *age-graded* lock-step regimen, the shared understandings and taken-for-granted rules, roles, relationships, resources and risks appropriate or available at different ages and life stages. But the social organization of the life course is *gender-graded* as well, typically producing diverging life courses for men and women, even though they may begin life with similar backgrounds and abilities (Han & Moen, 1999b, 2002; Moen, 1996a, 1996b, 2001; Moen & Roehling, 2005). That the life course is socially constructed means that it is *reconstructed* from time to time, especially in light of dramatic shifts in the larger social fabric of society. Consider "adolescence," for example, a stage of the life course that came to be distinct from childhood and adulthood only in the early years of the twentieth century (Shanahan, 2000), in part a result of universal public education.

We believe a new stage is now emerging in the twenty-first century life course, resulting from a confluence of demographic, technological, economic, and ideological changes transforming the very nature of the later life course. This stage was first discussed in the 1970s and 1980s in France, in conjunction with Universities of the Third Age, designed for the enrichment of pensioners. The notion of a new life stage was also promoted in Great Britain and the United States by Peter Laslett (1989). The *third age* is viewed as distinct from both the second age (adulthood) and the fourth age (old age). Most commonly it is depicted as the longevity bonus of extra years of vitality between retirement and old age.

Some define this life stage as a particular age period, such as from age 65 to 75. Others refer to a time of life before old age but beyond retirement (Bass, 2000; Laslett, 1989). We define it more as a time of transition, *midcourse* between the career- and family-building tasks associated with adulthood, but before any debilitating infirmities associated with old age (Moen, 2003). In our view, the third age incorporates the period before and after retirement, roughly the fifties, sixties, and seventies. Sorensen (forthcoming) makes the case that the third age is not a recent phenomenon. What is new is the fact that being "sixty-something" is no longer equated with old age.

Both the emerging third age and the key status passage in this life stage—retirement—are undergoing social transformations that are literally rewriting the scripts about later life choices and chances in contemporary society. Both are now *incomplete institutions* (Moen & Altobelli, forthcoming; see also Cherlin, 1978 for a discussion of incomplete institutions). As such, they offer insights into the twin and often uneven processes of social change—changing lives and changing institutions.

In this chapter we focus on both the micro (changing biographical) and the macro (changing social organizational) aspects of this new period of the life course. We argue that (1) taken-for-granted age-graded and gender-graded constellations of roles, risks, and relationships effectively frame real and perceived options in the third-age years; (2) these institutionalized arrangements are outdated, given concurrent demographic, labor market, technological, and economic changes; (3) this is producing a confluence of ambiguity, uncertainty, and ambivalence about retirement and life after retirement, promoting reflective processes of *strategic selection*, with current cohorts "making up" the third-age years as they move through them; and (4) all of this plays out in a *converging divergence*, in that age and gender are now less apt to define the expectations of people approaching or living in their fifties, sixties, and seventies. The term *convergence* invokes processes of increasing similarity (in, for example, roles or health) as men and women age. *Divergence* points to widening within- and between-gender disparities, as a consequence in part of processes of cumulative advantages for men (as in income, pensions) and cumulative disadvantages for (many) women as they move through their life courses. We combine both concepts to capture the growing heterogeneity by age and by gender in the strategic selections and opportunity structures of men and women, especially in the years around retirement, the third-age years.

## I. Age- and Gender-Graded Role Constellations

The third age is really outside of what Mayer (1986, p. 167) describes as institutional careers: the orderly flow of persons through segmented institutions. A number of life course scholars (e.g., Chudacoff & Hareven, 1979; Kohli, 1986; Mayer, 1986; Moen, 1994, 2003; Moen & Roehling, 2005; Riley, 1987; Riley & Riley, 1989) have pointed to occupational careers as providing the organizational blueprint for the life course, which begins with a period of education, followed by years of productive work, and then retirement (Kohli, 1986; Riley, 1987; Riley & Riley, 1989). In this formulation, retirement is equivalent to the passage to old age, a transition moving older adults outside the productive sphere of society. But the emerging third-age concept differentiates retirement, along with the years preceding and following it, from conventional notions of old age.

Most age-graded policies and practices in American society developed in terms of the lock-step, occupational career path, a career mystique promising hard work, long hours, and continuous employment as the ticket to the good life. The lock-step career mystique bolsters the notion as well of a retirement mystique, golden years of continuous, full-time leisure as an end in itself (see Moen & Roehling, 2005). The age-graded life course legitimizes the occurrence, timing, and sequencing of expected role transitions, especially around education, employment, and retirement, but also around family transitions (such as marriage, parenthood) and social welfare (Social Security and Medicare in the United States, but more forms of welfare supports in Europe). Such institutionalization effectively standardized individuals' biographical pacing, that is, the nature, timing, and sequencing of their social roles. Consider the age-graded institutionalization of education. In the United States virtually everyone ages 6 to 16 (and increasingly to 18) is a student, enrolled in and attending school. This student role permeates young people's identities, the ways others respond to them, their social location in society, and the organization of their days, weeks, and years.

In the post-World War II economic boom, retirement from paid work was similarly institutionalized; most workers eligible for Social Security at 65 retired if they could afford to do so. Since then, retirement has become a "natural" component of life.

This "expected life course" is so embedded in American institutions and ways of thinking that it is hard to see this role sequence as only a relatively recent, twentieth-century invention. Moreover, life course expectations are in the process of being reformulated, as retirement becomes a blurred transition, with considerable heterogeneity in its timing and in how lives are lived after retirement (Kim & Moen, 2001; Moen & Altobelli, forthcoming). These changes are establishing the groundwork for differentiating the third age from the fourth age of old age.

Men and women come to the third age by different routes. As Daily (1998) observed, "The history of work and retirement is really the story of men's work and retirement" (p. 1). Women's life paths, on the other hand, have tended to be neither orderly nor neatly segmented. Women have always been more apt to move in and out of education, employment, and community roles, often in conjunction with changing family care obligations and/or accommodating their husbands' job-related moves. Constrained options in men and women's life paths, along with gender stereotypes that exist in American society (Lorber & Moore, 2002), can contribute to a lifetime of cumulative advantage for some (mostly educated, Caucasian, middle-class men) and a lifetime of cumulative disadvantage for others (mostly women, but also minorities, immigrants, and the poorly educated; see Hardy & Shuey, 2000; Heath, Ciscel, & Sharp, 1998; Lopata, 1994; Moen, 1996a, 1996b, 1998; O'Rand, 1996). As women have sought equality in educational and employment opportunities, they have tried to accommodate to this prevailing model of men's life course while simultaneously pursuing the housework and care work traditionally allocated to them. This has resulted in women's restricted occupational participation and advancement.

More fruitful than a view of the life course as simply the accumulation of advantages and disadvantages may be a control cycles model of *strategic selection* (Figure 8.1), as men and women adapt to their changing circumstances by shifting either their roles or their role enactments.

Strategic selection as a process takes place in a structural and cultural environment legitimating and even necessitating some choices, and not others. For example, men are more likely than women to follow the conventional career mystique (Moen & Roehling, 2005) embedded in the American Dream of the bootstrap path to success. Thus men almost uniformly work for pay (often more than full time) on a continuous basis, from the time they complete their schooling until they retire, and, increasingly, are working for pay even after retirement from their "career jobs." Women also follow gendered scripts, typically as the major care providers of children, as well as ailing or infirm spouses, parents, and other relatives, both as young adults and also throughout their life course. Such unpaid care work increasingly occurs simultaneously with women's paid work. Another example is that women tend to retire in conjunction with their husbands' retirement, while men tend to make their retirement decisions independently (Moen, Sweet, & Swisher, 2005; Smith & Moen, 1998). The processes of strategic selection produce and perpetuate gender differences in roles, relationships, resources and risks at all life stages, including the third age (e.g., Mirowsky, 1996; Moen, Fields, Quick, & Hofmeister, 2000; Moen & Wethington, 1999; O'Rand & Henretta, 1999; Settersten, 1997).

More generally, then, the concept of career evokes the temporal nature of life course processes. We use the concept to capture employment trajectories, as well as trajectories of identity, health, and well-being leading to and through the third age. Scholars have usefully applied the career concept to the constellation and dynamics of health—and health disparities—at all stages of the life course (Clipp, Pavalko, & Elder, 1992; Moen & Chermack, 2005; Pavalko & Smith, 1999). George (1996), for example, noted the need for a temporal understanding of mental health. Viewing health across the life span is important, as continuities can exist across adolescence, early and middle adulthood, and the third age (see, for example, Wink, forthcoming).

The career concept is thus central to understanding the existing age- and

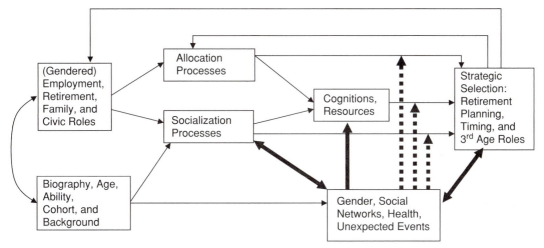

**Figure 8.1**  The gendered process of strategic selection in the third age: planning, timing, and living retirement.

gender-graded life course, as well as the emerging third-age life stage that is challenging these existing templates. It can be a fruitful concept for examining cultural schema and scripts around gender and age, work and retirement, because occupational careers are at the intersection of microlevel (individual and family) and macrolevel (e.g., political, demographic, medical, and economic) phenomena. Studying the occupational, retirement, caregiving, and civic engagement paths and passages of men and women forces attention to the embeddedness of health, age, and gender in the social fabric of lives, institutions, and changing societal landscapes. But conventional expectations are often outdated, given the increasingly wide variations in men and women's roles, behaviors, and relationships at all ages. Hence, we propose processes of *converging divergences* by both age and gender, especially among men and women in their fifties, sixties, and seventies, who may or may not be employed, married, retired, grandparents, or well-off in terms of income or health.

## II. The Third Age and Retirement: Institutions and Role Constellations in Flux

The traditional occupational blueprint of careers and the life course is at odds with the emergence of the third age. Consider how three common experiences in the third-age years—paid work, retirement, and caregiving for infirm family members—are being transformed by unprecedented medical and technological advances, along with demographic, economic, and policy shifts (Aneshensel, 1999; Aneshensel, Pearlin, & Schuler, 1993; Barrett, 2000; Moen, 1994, 1998, 2003; Riley, Foner, & Waring,1988).

The emergence in the early twenty-first century of the third age as a life stage between prime adulthood and old age is similar to the emergence in the early twentieth century of adolescence as a distinctive period between childhood and adulthood; both are consequences of a confluence of social forces (Shanahan, 2000). The third age represents a shifting life chronology emanating from multiple layers of change: demographic changes in labor force participation and longevity; organizational changes in fundamental institutions (such as school, work, and retirement); changing technologies including pharmaceutical advances for managing chronic health conditions; a global information economy replacing more physically strenuous manufacturing jobs with occupations in the service-sector; and (slower) changes in governmental policies and practices affecting age-graded incentives and constraints around paid work, unpaid and paid civic engagement, education, training, health insurance, and Social Security eligibility and benefits.

One of the principal forces defining the third age is the uncertainty spawned as a by-product of today's global economy. Neither age nor gender now provides the job security that was taken as a "given" for (mostly male) employees with seniority in the thriving, post-war 1950s economy. Job guarantees, along with guarantees of a "living" wage, are historical relics of a world and an economy that no longer exist. New technologies, an international workforce, and a never-ending story of mergers, buyouts, acquisitions, and bankruptcies mean that many 50-somethings find themselves retired or unemployed unexpectedly (Moen & Roehling, 2005). The institution of retirement is also in disarray, no longer a single, one-way, irreversible exit from a traditional, continuous, and cumulative occupational career. Accordingly, we refer to this new stage less by age markers (e.g., 65 to 75 years old) but more as a series of shifts, a time over a period of years or even decades when people begin thinking about and moving from their main career job to and through retirement and into "second acts," (that is, paid and unpaid activities beyond retirement), but not yet experiencing the infirmities associated with old age (Moen, 2003; Moen & Altobelli, forthcoming)

Another major demographic shift crucial to understanding the emerging third age has been women's increased labor force participation, and consequently their increased participation in the retirement transition. Historical events, such as the women's movement, the shift to first a service and now a global economy, and concomitant policy responses, have transformed women and men's education, employment, and family experiences (Bradburn, Moen, & Dempster- McClain, 1995; Elman & O'Rand, 1998a, 1998b; Farkas & O'Rand, 1998; Moen, 1994, 2003; Townsend, 2002), meaning that many aspects of women and men's life patterns are becoming more similar. As a case in point, women are increasingly retiring from their own career jobs, and couples increasingly face the reality of two retirement exits, "his" and "hers" (Han & Moen, 1999a, 1999b). This is the first time in history when retirement is no longer almost exclusively a male status passage.

Thus far we have depicted life in the third age as resulting from a confluence of historical forces producing what have become outdated institutional arrangements. But women and men's life courses are also products of their individual choices and prior biographies. The concept of *adaptive strategies* has long been a staple in life course research (Elder, 1974; Moen & Wethington, 1992). It refers to both customary responses to particular circumstances (e.g., age- and gender-related scripts) and to ad hoc responses to the dislocations associated with biographical chance events and large-scale social change. Drawing on Carstensen's (1995) theory of socioemotional selectively and Baltes and Baltes' (1990) theory of successful aging (including selection, optimization, and compensation), we propose that individuals also engage in selective role entries, exists, and modifications when old scripts no longer fit real-life exigencies. We term this process *strategic selection* (Figure 8.1). It is in times of multidimensional social change, such as what we are observing around the retirement transition, that what are typically invisible processes of allocation, socialization, and selection become visible. The complexity and contingent nature of women's life paths, along with historical changes in gender norms and the broader opportunity structure, are encouraging scholars to examine more critically previously taken-for-granted arrangements in the form of segmented institutions designed around men's lives, but affecting both men and women, institutional convoys producing an age-and-gender-segmented life course.

As purposive actors, women and men are making strategic choices about role and relationship involvement as they move through the decades of their fifties, sixties, and seventies. In doing so they create the biographical pacing (e.g., Han & Moen, 1999a, 1999b) of their later adulthood: the timing, sequencing, and duration of roles in their third age. These decision processes of strategic selection and biographical pacing are more self-reflective precisely because the third age, and increasingly retirement itself, are *incomplete institutions*. The taken-for-granted scripts that do exist are ill-fitting at best. In this way the current generation of retirees and the baby boom cohort approaching their 60s are in the process of creating new patterns for life in the space between what have been to date the "main acts" of adulthood (career- and family-building) and the frailties of old age.

Still, even deliberative choices are bound by a logic based on existing options, cumulative contingencies, and historical and biographical circumstances described in the preceding sections. Careers are what Pearlin (1988, p. 259) describes as "durable arrangements that serve to organize experience over time," what we term "institutional convoys." Men and women come to the third age from different paths. It is precisely this experience that affects how third-age individuals see and define their circum-

stances and act to preserve or change them.

One example of the converging divergences (by age and by gender) in the third age is in differences, not only in the timing of retirement by gender, but also in the wide variation in that timing and the contingencies shaping it. In a study of older adults ages 50 to 72, Dentinger and Clarkberg (2002) examined the relationship between caregiving and retirement timing, with a particular eye toward gender and how it may moderate the relationship. They found that men in this third-age sample are similar to women in providing some informal care. In fact, "most men had been caregivers at one time, and men … shouldered the caregiving responsibilities only 10% less of the time than did women" (p. 875). However, the men and the women differed in their retirement behavior in response to such caregiving responsibilities: while there is "a tendency for women to stay at home to provide time-consuming care to one or more ill, aged, or otherwise disabled friend or family member, … men respond to loved one's needs for support by delaying their retirement … [which] means that men are shouldering the financial burden associated with disability" (pp. 875–876). The authors call attention to the similarity between this pattern and that earlier in the life course related to the informal care of infants. Another important finding from Dentinger and Clarkberg's study has to do with the relevance of the nature of the relationship between the caregiver and care recipient. Caring for a spouse, for instance, had the most potent impact on retirement timing. Women in the sample taking care of their husbands were five times more likely to retire than women who were not caregivers. Men providing care to their wives, however, were only half as likely to retire. The authors conclude that " … caregiving responsibilities may contribute to more strongly sex-segregated gender roles during the retirement years" (p. 876).

Another study of retirement timing by Zimmerman, Mitchell, Wister, and Gutman (2000) used a political economy of aging perspective to argue that "socially-structured patterns of gender inequality related to women's multiple roles across the life course affect patterns of retirement timing" (p. 109). Using a sample of 275 retired and preretired women, 45 years or older, the authors tested two hypotheses: that (1) main predictors of actual retirement timing are related to women's place in paid and unpaid work (e.g., timing of spouse's retirement, family care responsibilities, health-related reasons, adequate income), and (2) preretirees do not expect these factors to be related to their retirement timing. The authors found support for both hypotheses. Health and stress, family caregiving responsibilities, and the timing of their spouse's retirement were all significant predictors of actual retirement, suggesting considerable heterogeneity (divergence) in this status passage.

Biographical experiences leading up to retirement may not only have implications for why and when people retire, but what they expect out of this life stage as well. Timmer, Bode, and Dittmann-Kohli (2003), using data from the 1996 German Aging Study, found that men and women between the ages of 40 and 85 differed in the type of gains they expect during later adulthood, with women more likely to anticipate making more time for themselves. The authors hypothesize that these gender differences occur because earlier points along men and women's life courses entail the exclusion of different activities, leading to "different wishes to make up for earlier chances" (p. 6). Another study, based on longitudinal data of 113 61-year-old women who graduated from the same college in California, found a vision of the third age as an opening of possibility: More than 80% of the participants saw retirement as a "a time to enjoy life," "a time to do things you haven't done before," and "a time to do what you want" (Helson & Cate, forthcoming).

Biographical experiences shape perceived options in the third age, but they also serve to define the resources and conditions men and women bring with them to this life stage. Sewell (1992) makes the point that "structure," the noun, always implies "structuring," the verb. This suggests that the social organization of paid work, unpaid household and care work, and retirement serve "to structure" virtually all aspects of both men and women's lives in the years leading up to and through the third age, directly and indirectly, but in different ways, at different times, and with different consequences. Such consequences have included the differential power, status, and earnings men and women have accrued as a result of a life course defined by the occupational career. Health insurance, pensions, unemployment insurance, disability insurance, and Social Security all rest on the edifice of the male lock-step life course. Given this gendered character of the contemporary life course, Americans moving toward the third-age years have experienced both enduring and age-related income, power, and health disparities between men and women, especially minority women (see, for example, Combs, 2002; Jackson, Brown, & Faison, forthcoming). The third age as an identifiable phase may be new, but it remains embedded in existing gender and age scripts, even if these scripts are increasingly outdated, producing disparate personal resources for those in their fifties, sixties, and seventies.

## III. Converging Divergences in the Third Age: Consequences of Obsolete Age- and Gender-Graded Constellations

We focus on disparities in psychological resources (including perceived personal control and life satisfaction) as well as in emotional and physical health and well-being, even as we hypothesize both a narrowing of gender differences (convergence) and a widening of within-gender and within-age group differences (divergence) in the third-age years. The existing literature rarely invokes the language of the third age; nevertheless, we review findings related to people typically moving to or through the retirement years, specifically those in their fifties, sixties, and seventies.

## A. Psychological Resources

The term *biographical pacing* (Han & Moen, 1999a, 1999b; Moen & Han, 2001) captures perceptions of choice and control. The notions of control cycles (Elder, 1985; Moen & Yu, 2000) and capital (human, cultural, social, economic) are important factors in understanding the distribution of health and well-being by gender, age, and the interactions between the two. Gaps between resources and needs (claims or expectations) occur both on the home and work or community fronts, with individuals and families at more or less risk at various life stages. Demands at home in the third age include caregiving for parents, spouses, siblings, grandchildren, and disabled children; housework; and personal care. Demands related to work or community roles include long work hours, low income, shift work, job insecurity, arduous (physical or mental) job conditions, or for the retired, the absence of routines, clear identities, and integrative roles. Resources can include human/cultural capital (education, autonomy, flexibility, initiative), social capital (family, friends, community ties, co-worker relationships, supportive supervisor), and economic capital (income, job security). Another concept, *perceived control*, captures individuals' sense of mastery, their feeling that they are in charge of their lives.

Despite the stresses built in to managing paid work and unpaid care work (described previously), a growing body of research points to the positive physical and psychological impacts, for women as well as men, of employment. This is especially true under working conditions that promote a sense of control (e.g., Adelman, Antonucci, Crohan, & Coleman, 1990; House, Stecher, Metzner, & Robbins, 1986; Lennon, 1994; Ross & Mirowsky, 1995; Schieman, 2002; Sorenson & Verbrugge, 1987), with unstable work conditions related to poor health (Hibbard & Pope, 1993; Jahn, Becker, Jöckel, & Pholabeln, 1995). Men tend to be more apt than women to have jobs with greater degrees of discretion and flexibility; they also tend to have higher levels of personal mastery (perceived control over their lives) and are more apt than women to plan for the future (e.g., Ross & Mirowsky, 2002). Both mastery and planning have been linked to life satisfaction (Prenda & Lachman, 2001).

Ross and Mirowsky (2002) have made an important contribution to the understanding of gendered dimensions of perceived control. Using 1995 and 1998 data from adults (18 years and older) who participated in the survey of Aging, Status and Sense of Control, these authors tested hypotheses that men report higher overall perceived personal control than women, that these gender differences in control are more pronounced in older age groups, and that age differences in the relationship between gender and personal control can be explained by education, work, economic conditions, and health. Summarizing the extant literature regarding the impact of these factors on personal control, the authors argue that older women, characterized by lower levels of education, inconsistent paid employment, and poor health, are likely to be at a "dual disadvantage" (p. 128). Results of their cross-sectional and longitudinal analyses support all of their hypotheses with one exception. The authors found that education, a history of full-time employment, household income, and physical functioning do help to explain the age-based relationship between gender and perceived control, but other factors (work fulfillment, fairness of domestic labor, economic hardship, and self-reported health) do not. Overall, the authors emphasize a divergence in age between men and women in personal control: "Although men's and women's social roles may be similar in older age, their lives were different in earlier years. Men's socioeconomic advantages and women's disadvantages cumulate through life, producing large disparity in older men's and older women's levels of personal control. Older age represents a summation of experiences over the life course, not merely one's current state" (p. 142). Fernandez-Ballesteros, Zamarron, and Ruiz (2001) also found education and income to be the most important predictors of life satisfaction among a sample of Spanish men and women 65 years and older.

In terms of resources, Danigelis and McIntosh (2001) examined gender differences in monetary and nonmonetary resources related to the financial satisfaction among people 65 to 96 years old in the United States, emphasizing the importance of these resources in empowering older people with a real or imagined sense of control. Overall, based on data from the Americans' Changing Lives Panel Study, the authors report a tendency for nonmonetary resources to be significant for women in their sample but not for men. The second most important predictor for men, however, was nonmonetary, and for women, the second most important predictor of financial satisfaction was monetary. In terms of nonmonetary sources, for men, lowered control was indicated by loss of another person in the household, his wife, whereas in the case of women, lowered control was

within the individual herself, as measured by number of chronic ailments. In conclusion, the authors argued that the evidence provides additional support for Moen's (1996a) assertion that status and role changes illustrate "the ways in which gender cross-cuts the experience of aging in contemporary American society" (p. 172).

## B. Emotional Well-Being

Life satisfaction and sense of control are important for other outcomes of interest in the third age as well. In a study of adults 60 to 84 years old residing in a North Carolina county, Jang, Haley, Small, and Mortimer (2002) observed that mastery, social networks, and support moderate the relationship between disability and depression, concluding that these resources help to "buffer the adverse consequences of disability" (p. 811). Although gender was not found to be a significant covariate, the authors did not analyze separate models and did not include interaction terms to further assess gender differences in this relationship.

Schieman, Van Gundy, and Taylor (2002) attempted to "unpack" (p. 261) the well-documented negative relationship between age and depression by assessing the personal and social conditions that are linked to this association and the factors that suppress it. Multivariate analyses were performed using longitudinal data from approximately 700 disabled and 850 nondisabled adults (both men and women) living in 10 counties in a region in Ontario. Respondents' ages ranged from 24 to 92 years, with an average of 58. Calling on both stress process and socioemotional selectivity theories and encouraging "study of the variation in the objective and subjective situations of people's lives across the age span" (p. 275), the authors included measures within their models for age, gender, employment, education, economic hardship, religiosity, positive and negative interpersonal exchanges, self-rated health, and personal mastery. In discussing their results, the authors distinguished between the "age as decline" (p. 275) and "good old age" (p. 277) views of aging, the former concentrating on losses with age (e.g., health or mastery) and the latter emphasizing gains (e.g., economic, socioemotional). They find that less economic hardship and interpersonal conflict are positively associated with fewer depressive symptoms. Physical impairment and a lower sense of mastery, however, tend to suppress the negative association between age and depression. Gender differences in this suppression, however, were not discussed.

Participation in new activities, "an essential developmental task for the third age" (Timmer & Aartsen, 2003, p. 644), may be positively associated with psychological resources as well. Analyzing data collected from adults between 61 and 75 years old who were participants in the most recent phase (1998/1999) of the Longitudinal Aging Study of Amsterdam, these authors examined five components of mastery (self-esteem, control, and three aspects of self-efficacy: initiative, persistence, and effort to follow through) and their relevance for individuals' participation in education and volunteer activities. The women in the sample were more likely to engage in educational activities (this is in line with what research on participation in Universities of the Third Age has said; see, for example, Yenerall, 2003), whereas the men were more likely to participate in volunteer activities. Although self-esteem and control were not found to be significant predictors of participation in either activity, aspects of self-efficacy (initiative for educational activities and persistence for volunteer work) were. According to Grafova, McGonagle, and Stafford (forthcoming), good health is an important predictor of volunteering among third agers.

## C. Physical Health and Functioning

Age, gender, and health are all biological circumstances, but they are also socially constructed (Bem, 1999; Lorber & Moore, 2002; Moen, 2001; Rosenfield, 1999; West & Zimmerman, 1987). And each is related to the other, such that women tend to live longer than men (at birth, their life expectancy in the United States is 5 years longer) but typically experience more stress and poorer health along the way (Crimmins & Saito, 2001; Jans & Stoddard, 1999; Kessler et al., 1994; Lorber & Moore, 2002; Mirowsky, 1996). And a greater proportion of women's lives are lived with disability (Robine, Romieu, & Cambois, 1997). Based on a review of the literature documenting that women spend a greater proportion of their lives with significant disability, Laditka and Laditka (2002) suggested that higher rates of disability among women may well reflect a process of disability accumulation over their life course.

Forthofer, Janz, Dodge, and Clark (2001) empirically compared the relevance of self-esteem, stress, and social support with that of sociodemographic and clinical factors for the physical and psychological functioning of older adults inflicted with heart disease. Their sample consisted of approximately 700 men and women 60 years or older enrolled in an evaluation of a program specifically for people with heart disease in four Midwestern hospitals. Multivariate analyses reveal that self-esteem and stress are more predictive (than the other explanatory variables) of the maintenance or improvement in functioning. Self-esteem plays an especially protective role for women. Low stress is positively related to physical functioning for both men and women, but it was a risk factor only for men in terms of their psychological functioning.

That women's paid work trajectories have not been "conventional" (or marked by continuous, stable employment in the years between education and retirement) is something that Marshall, Clarke, and Ballantyne (2001) discussed in their study of the effects of instability in the retirement transition on health. These authors call attention to the changing institution of retirement and the greater instability associated with it (e.g., early retirements, contingent and nonstandard work, self-employment), questioning whether such instability impacts men and women's health and well-being in different ways. Because instability has been more typical of women's labor force participation than men's, they hypothesize that greater instability in retirement is associated with poorer health outcomes, especially for men. In their analyses of survey data from a sample of retired employees (average age, 51 years) of a communications company in Canada, the authors found that both subjective and objective measures of instability are related to psychological measures of health and well-being. Both men and women who experienced unemployment periods after retirement were more likely to report lower life satisfaction, and the effects of such unemployment were especially negative for women. At the same time, multiple periods of post-retirement employment were related to greater stress for both men and women, although (for women only) this relationship was moderated by whether the respondent had retired for health reasons. This study provides evidence of a negative relationship between retirement instability and health and that the associations differ for men and women.

## IV. A Converging Divergence?

The life course has been institutionalized around periods of rapid social change, such as industrialization, urbanization, and bureaucratization. We have argued that the early twenty-first century is also a time of large-scale social transformations, producing new life course shifts, culminating in a "third age" around the retirement years but before old age infirmities. The cultural scripts associated with two fundamental social markers—age and gender—are being rewritten, as are the institutions (e.g. family, retirement, work) in which they play out.

The literature we have reviewed shows that one way that gender and age "matter" for health and well-being in the third-age years is in the *differences in men and women's life course biographies*. Health disparities reflect men and women's different locations in the social fabric of roles, resources, relationships, and risks at different ages and stages. We have drawn on the career concept to underscore both the temporal aspects of existing historical and institutional "givens," in the form of social policies, and dramatic social transformations in longevity, scientific and medical advances, the economy, and the labor market. Both existing institutional arrangements and social transformations set aggregate baseline parameters around women and men's health risks and resilience. These external influences constitute the gendered contexts in which health-related experiences and behaviors take place. It is important, therefore, to examine cohort variations in the third-age progression of men and women.

Educational, labor market, retirement, and other social policies in the middle of the twentieth century produced a convergence in the age-graded, lock-step life course that became the blueprint of the "normal" biography. Thus, the standardization of the lock-step life course fashioned a normative path—a career mystique and a retirement mystique—permeating individual, as well as cultural, prescriptions and expectations (Moen & Roehling, 2005). This convergence in the age-graded life course produced sharp age divergences, especially in the division by retirement, effectively coupling "productivity" with "employment," and "retirement" with "old age." This blueprint was gender-graded as well, again emblematic of men's, not women's, expectations and experiences.

Health paths and passages to and through the third age reflect the dynamic interplay between institutions and individual lives, with the occupational career as a fundamental organizing force shaping perceived control, health-related resources (e.g., health insurance, income, retirement, pensions), risks (e.g., layoffs, stress, burnout, injuries), behaviors (e.g., retirement, civic engagement), and health outcomes. The studies we reviewed provide examples of how past age and gender divisions, although increasingly obsolete, continue to shape the resources of men and women traversing the third age. The evidence suggests that the occupational career, retirement, and family care constitute institutional arrangements that perpetuate gendered disparities in access to important resources for this life stage, even as there is growing evidence of within-gender and within-age group divergences. An obvious example is the differential resources available to older men and women (Laurence & Weinhouse, 1997; Lorber & Moore, 2002; O'Rand & Henretta, 1999).

A second process shaping health in the third age *reflects changing mechanisms and pathways for both men and women.* For example, Scheiman's (2002) study of 18- to 55-year-old adults living in Toronto found "although men realize greater economic rewards from education, women seem to acquire greater intrapersonal rewards from such structural advantages" (p. 640). Structural advantages include education, job autonomy, and nonroutinized work. Rewards include sense of mastery, self-esteem, and fewer depression symptoms. Another example: studies show that engaging in employment

can be a source of health and well-being for men and women (Barnett, 1995; Barnett & Brennan, 1997; Barnett, Brennan, & Marshall, 1994). But employment also creates strains and overloads, especially for women, given their typical responsibilities for family care work (Hochschild, 1989; Menaghan, 1989; Moen, 2003; Roxburgh, 1996; Simon, 1995; Thoits, 1986).

The weight of the evidence, however, suggests that women and men's paths are becoming more similar as the lock-step path unravels in the face of the growing heterogeneity of the workforce and the globalization of the economy. Gender may well become less salient in light of the push toward equality of opportunity in many sectors of society. For example, the proportion of women earning bachelor's degrees now exceeds that of men. Unprecedented numbers of American women are now in corporate boardrooms, in the military, and serving as managers, professionals, engineers, physicians, college professors, etc. This gain in equality of opportunity has positive implications for health and life expectancy: education, for example, is positively related with longer, healthier lives regardless of gender (Laditka & Laditka, 2002).

## V. Summary

The deinstitutionalization of careers paths and retirement, along with evolving gender and age norms, are creating increasing flexibility in social roles for both men and women at all phases of the life course. This deinstitutionalization is producing a period of life with few shared norms and as yet few clear-cut possibilities, what some scholars call a "third age" around the time of cessation of one's career job but before the frailties of old age. The push for gender equality, along with a confluence of other experiences, options, and social forces—demographic, economic, technological, legislative, and cultural—have transformed women and men's lives over the past 50 years and are producing a growing pool of healthy, educated, and skilled men and women in this third age, at risk of being on the sideline of society. Given the absence of taken-for-granted scripts, men and women moving toward this life phase must be self-reflexive, making intentional choices (what we term *strategic selection*) about employment, retirement, civic engagement, caregiving, and other behaviors, roles, and relationships. The third age represents a time of increased heterogeneity by age and gender, a time of converging divergences. Nevertheless, men and women in the third age are products of past age- and gender-graded institutions and norms. People in, or moving toward, this emerging life stage bring with them existing disparities and outmoded scripts about age and gender, producing asymmetries in power, resources, needs, and preferences (Sorensen, forthcoming). Thus women and men approach this life stage from different angles and with different resources. The possibilities of achieving Riley's (1987) age-integrated society, and with it a gender-integrated society, may become increasingly feasible in the third age, depending on how new institutional arrangements develop, but also on whether the prior life paths of men and women become more equitable.

## References

Adelman, P., Antonucci, T., Crohan, S., & Coleman, L. (1990). A causal analysis of employment and health in midlife women. *Women and Health, 16,* 5–20.

Aneshensel, C. (1999). Mental illness as a career: sociological perspectives. In C. Aneshensel & J. Phelan (Eds.), *Handbook of the sociology of mental health* (pp. 585–603). New York: Kluwer Academic/Plenum Publishers.

Aneshensel, C., Pearlin, L., & Schuler, R. (1993). Stress, role captivity, and the cessation of caregiving. *Journal of Health and Social Behavior, 34,* 54–70.

Baltes, P., & Baltes, M. (1990). Psychological perspectives on successful aging: The model of selective optimization with compensation. In P. Baltes & M. Baltes. (Eds.), *Successful aging: Perspectives from the behavioral sciences* (pp. 1–34). New York: Cambridge University Press.

Barnett, R. (1995). Change in job and marital experiences and change in psychological distress: A longitudinal study of dual-earner couples. *Journal of Personality and Social Psychology, 69,* 839–850.

Barnett, R., & Brennan, R. (1997). Change in job conditions, change in psychological distress, and gender: A longitudinal study of dual-earner couples. *Journal of Organizational Behavior, 18,* 253–274.

Barnett, R., Brennan, R., & Marshall, N. (1994). Gender and the relationship between parent role quality and psychological distress. *Journal of Family Issues, 15,* 229–252.

Barrett, A. (2000). Marital trajectories and mental health. *Journal of Health and Social Behavior, 41,* 451–464.

Bass, S. (2000). Emergence of the third age: toward a productive aging society. *Journal of Aging and Social Policy, 11*(2/3), 7–17.

Bem, S. (1999). Gender, sexuality, and inequality: When many become one, who is the one and what happens to the others? In P. Moen, D. Dempster-McClain, & H. Walker (Eds.), *A nation divided: diversity, inequality, and community in American society* (pp. 70–86). Ithaca, NY: Cornell University Press.

Bradburn, E., Moen, P., & Dempster-McClain, D. (1995). Women's return to school following the transition to motherhood. *Social Forces, 73,* 1517–1551.

Carstensen, L. (1995). Evidence for a life span theory of socioemotional selectivity. *Current Directions in Psychological Science, 4*(5), 151–156.

Cherlin, A. (1978). Remarriage as an incomplete institution. *The American Journal of Sociology, 84*(3), 634–650.

Chudacoff, H., & Hareven, T. (1979). From the empty nest to family dissolution: Life course transitions into old age. *Journal of Family History, 4*(1), 69–83.

Clipp, E., Pavalko, E., & Elder, G. (1992). Trajectories of health: In concept and empirical pattern. *Behavior, Health, and Aging, 2,* 159–179.

Combs, Y. (2002). Midlife health of African-American women: Cumulative disadvantage as a predictor of early senescence. *Social Inequalities, Health, and Health Care Delivery, 20,* 123–135.

Crimmins, E., & Saito, Y. (2001). Trends in health life expectancy in the United States, 1970–1990: Gender, racial, and educational differences. *Social Science and Medicine, 52,* 1629–1641.

Daily, N. (1998). *When baby boom women retire.* Westport, CT: Praeger Publishers.

Danigelis, N., & McIntosh, B. (2001). Gender's effect on the relationships linking older Americans' resources and financial satisfaction. *Research on Aging, 23,* 410–428.

Dentinger, E., & Clarkberg, M. (2002). Informal caregiving and retirement timing among men and woman: Gender and caregiving relationships in later midlife. *Journal of Family Matters, 23,* 857–879.

Elder, G. (1974). *Children of the Great Depression.* Chicago: University of Chicago Press.

Elder, G. (1985). *Life course dynamics: Trajectories and transitions, 1968–1980.* Ithaca, NY: Cornell University Press.

Elder, G. (1994). Time, human agency, and social change: Perspectives on the life course. *Social Psychology Quarterly, 57,* 4–15.

Elman, C., & O'Rand, A. (1998a). Midlife work pathways and educational entry. *Research on Aging, 20,* 475–505.

Elman, C., & O'Rand, A. (1998b). Midlife entry into vocational training: A mobility model. *Social Science Research, 27,* 128–158.

Farkas, J., & O'Rand, A. (1998). The pension mix for women in middle and late life: More evidence of the changing employment relationship. *Social Forces, 76,* 1007–1032.

Fernandez-Ballesteros, R., Zamarron, M., & Ruiz, M. (2001). The contribution of socio-demographic and psychosocial factors to life satisfaction. *Ageing and Society, 21,* 25–43.

Forthofer, M., Janz, N., Dodge, J., & Clark, N. (2001). Gender differences in the associations of self-esteem, stress, and social support with functional health status among older adults with heart disease. *Journal of Women and Aging, 13*(1), 19–37.

George, L. (1996). Social factors and illness. In R. Binstock & L. George (Eds.), *Handbook of aging and the social sciences* (4th ed., pp. 229–252). San Diego, CA: Academic Press.

Giele, J., & Elder, G. (1998). *Methods of life course research: Qualitative and quantitative approaches.* Thousand Oaks, CA: Sage Publications.

Grafova, I., McGonagle, K., & Stafford, F. (forthcoming 2006). Functioning and well-being in the third age, 1986–2001. In J. James, & P. Wink (Eds.), *The crown of life: Dynamics of the early post-retirement period.* New York: Springer.

Han, S-K., & Moen, P. (1999a). Work and family over time: A life course approach. *The Annals of the American Academy of Political and Social Science, 562,* 98–110.

Han, S-K., & Moen, P. (1999b). Clocking out: Temporal patterning of retirement. *American Journal of Sociology, 105,* 191–236.

Han, S-K., & Moen, P. (2002). Coupled careers: Pathways through work and marriage in the United States. In H.-P. Blossfield & S. Drobnic (Eds.), *Careers of couples in contemporary societies: From male breadwinner to dual earner families* (pp. 201–231). Oxford, UK: Oxford University Press.

Hardy, M., & Shuey, K. (2000). Pension decisions in a changing economy: Gender, structure and choice. *Journal of Gerontology: Social Sciences, 55B,* S271–S277.

Heath, J., Ciscel, D., & Sharp, D. (1998). The work of families: The provision of market and household labor and the role of public policy. *Review of Social Economy, 56,* 501–521.

Helson, R., & Cate, R. (forthcoming). Late middle age: Transition to the third stage. In J. James & P. Wink (Eds.), *The crown of life.* New York: Springer.

Hibbard, J., & Pope, C. (1993). Health effects of discontinuities in female employment and marital status. *Social Science and Medicine, 36,* 1099–1104.

Hochschild, A. (1989). *The second shift.* New York: Avon Books.

Hogan, D. (1978). The variable order of events in the life course. *American Sociological Review, 43,* 573–586.

House, J., Stecher, V., Metzner, H., & Robbins, C. (1986). Occupational stress and health among men and women in the Tecumseh community health study. *Journal of Health and Social Behavior, 27*, 62–77.

Jackson, J., Brown, E., & Faison, N. (forthcoming). The work and retirement experiences of aging black Americans. In J. James & P. Wink, P. (Eds.), *The crown of life: Dynamics of the early post-retirement period.* New York: Springer.

Jahn, I., Becker, U., Jöckel, K-H., & Pohlabeln, H. (1995). Occupational life course and lung cancer risk in men: Findings from a socio-epidemiological analysis of job-changing histories in a case-control study. *Social Science and Medicine, 40*, 961–975.

Jang, Y., Haley, W., Small, B., & Mortimer, J. (2002). The role of mastery and social resources in the associations between disability and depression in later life. *Gerontologist, 42*, 807–813.

Jans, L., & Stoddard, S. (1999). *Chartbook on women and disability in the United States: An InfoUse Report.* Washington, D.C.: U.S. National Institute on Disability and Rehabilitation Research. http://www. infouse. com/disabilitydata/ © 1996–1999 InfoUse.

Kessler, R., McGonagle, K., Zhao, S., Nelson, C., Hughes, M., Eshelman, S., Witchen, H., & Kendler, K. (1994). Lifetime and 12-month prevalence of DSM-III-R psychotic disorders in the United States: Results from the national comorbidity survey. *Archives of General Psychiatry*, 518–519.

Kim, J., & Moen, P. (2001). Moving into retirement: Preparation and transitions in late midlife. In M. Lachman (Ed.), *Handbook of midlife development* (pp. 487–527). New York: John Wiley & Sons.

Kohli, M. (1986). The world we forget: A historical review of the life course. In V. Marshall (Ed.), *Later life: The social psychology of aging* (pp. 271–303). Beverly Hills, CA: Sage.

Laditka, S., & Laditka, J. (2002). Recent perspectives on active life expectancy for older women. In S. Laditka (Ed.), *Health expectations for older women: International perspectives* (pp. 163–184). New York: Haworth Press, Inc.

Laslett, P. (1989). *A fresh map of life: The emergence of the third age.* Cambridge, MA: Harvard University Press.

Laurence, L., & Weinhouse, B. (1997). *Outrageous practices: How gender bias threatens women's health.* New Brunswick, NJ: Rutgers University Press.

Lennon, M. C. (1994). Women, work, and well-being: The importance of work conditions. *Journal of Health and Social Behavior, 35*, 235–247.

Lopata, H. (1994). *Circles and settings: Role changes of American women.* Albany, NY: SUNY Press.

Lorber, J., & Moore, L. (2002). *Gender and the social construction of illness.* New York: Roman and Littlefield.

Macmillan, R., & Eliason, S. (2003). Characterizing the life course as role configurations and pathways: A latent structure approach. In J. Mortimer & M. Shanahan (Eds.), *Handbook of the life course* (pp. 529–554). New York: Kluwer Academic/ Plenum Publishers.

Marshall, V., Clarke, P., & Ballantyne, P. (2001). Instability in the retirement transition: Effects on health and well-being in a Canadian study. *Research on Aging, 23*, 379–409.

Mayer, K. U. (1986). Structural constraints on the life course. *Human Development, 29*, 163–170.

Mayer, K., & Tuma, N. (1990). *Event history analysis in life course research.* Madison: University of Wisconsin Press.

Menaghan, E. (1989). Role changes and psychological well-being: Variations in effects by gender and role repertoire. *Social Forces, 67*, 693–714.

Mirowsky, J. (1996). Age and the gender gap in depression. *Journal of Health and Social Behavior, 37*, 362–380.

Moen, P. (1994). Women, work and family: A sociological perspective on changing roles. In M. Riley, R. Kahn, & A. Foner (Eds.), *Age and structural lag: The mismatch between people's lives and opportunities in work, family, and leisure* (pp. 151–170). New York: John Wiley & Sons.

Moen, P. (1996a). Gender, age and the life course. In R. Binstock & L. George (Eds.), *Handbook of aging and the social sciences* (4th ed., pp. 171–187). San Diego, CA: Academic Press, Inc.

Moen, P. (1996b). A life course perspective on retirement, gender, and well-being. *Journal of Occupational Health Psychology, 1,* 131–144.

Moen, P. (1998). Recasting careers: Changing reference groups, risks and realities. *Generations, 22,* 40–45.

Moen, P. (2001). The gendered life course. In L. George & R. Binstock (Eds.), *Handbook of aging and the social sciences* (pp. 179–196). San Diego, CA: Academic Press, Inc.

Moen, P. (2003). *It's about time: Couples and careers.* Ithaca, NY: Cornell University Press.

Moen, P., & Altobelli, J. (forthcoming). Strategic selection as a retirement project: Will Americans develop hybrid arrangements? In J. James & P. Wink (Eds.), *The crown of life: Dynamics of the early post-retirement period.* New York: Springer.

Moen, P., & Chermack, K. (forthcoming). Gender disparities in health: Strategic selection, careers, and cycles of control. *Journal of Gerontology, Series B 2005,* Vol 60B.

Moen, P., Dempster-McClain, D., & Williams, R. (1989). Social integration and longevity: An event history analysis of women's roles and resilience. *American Sociological Review, 54,* 635–647.

Moen, P., Fields, V., Quick, H., & Hofmeister, H. (2000). A life course approach to retirement and social integration. In K. Pillemer, P. Moen, E. Wethington, & N. Glasgow (Eds.), *Social integration in the second half of life* (pp. 75–107). Baltimore: The Johns Hopkins Press.

Moen, P., & Han, S-K. (2001). Reframing careers: Work, family, and gender. In V. Marshall, W. Heinz, H. Kruger, & A. Verma (Eds.), *Restructuring work and the life course* (pp. 424–445). Ontario: University of Toronto Press.

Moen, P., & Roehling, P. (2005). *The career mystique: Cracks in the American dream.* Boulder, CO: Rowman & Littlefield.

Moen, P., Sweet, S., & Swisher, R. (forthcoming). Embedded career clocks: The case of retirement planning. In R. Macmillan (Ed.). *The structure of the life course: Standardized? individualized? differentiated? (Advances in Life Course Research, vol. 9, 237–265.* New York: Elsevier.

Moen, P., & Wethington, E. (1992). The concept of family adaptive strategies. *Annual Review of Sociology, 18,* 233–251.

Moen, P., & Wethington, E. (1999). Midlife development in a life course context. In S. Willis & J. Reid (Eds.), *Life in the middle* (pp. 3–23). San Diego, CA: Academic Press.

Moen, P., & Yu, Y. (2000). Effective work/life strategies: Working couples, work conditions, gender, and life quality. *Social Problems, 47*(3), 291–326.

Mortimer, J., & Shanahan, M. (2003). *Handbook of the life course.* New York: Kluwer Academic/Plenum Publishers.

O'Rand, A. (1996). The precious and the precocious: Understanding cumulative disadvantage and cumulative advantage over the life course. *The Gerontologist, 36,* 230–238.

O'Rand, A., & Henretta, J. (1999). *Age and inequality: Diverse pathways through later life.* Boulder, CO: Westview Press.

Pavalko, E., & Artis, J. (1997). Women's caregiving and paid work: Causal relationships in late mid-life. *Journal of Gerontology: Social Sciences, 52B,* S1–S10.

Pavalko, E., & Smith, B. (1999). The rhythm of work: Health effects on women's work dynamics. *Social Forces, 77,* 1141–1162.

Pearlin, L. (1988). Social structuring and social values: The regulation of structural effects. In H. O'Gorman (Ed.), *Surveying social life* (pp. 252–264). Middletown, CT: Wesleyan University.

Prenda, K., & Lachman, M. (2001). Planning for the future: A life management strategy for increasing control and life satisfaction in adulthood. *Psychology and Aging, 16,* 206–216.

Riley, M. (1987). On the significance of age in sociology. *American Sociological Review, 52,* 1–14.

Riley, M., Foner, A., & Waring, J. (1988). Sociology of age. In N. Smelser (Ed.), *Handbook of Sociology* (pp. 243–290). Newbury Park, CA: Sage.

Riley, M., Kahn, R., & Foner, A. (1994). *Age and structural lag: Society's failure to provide meaningful opportunities in work, family, and leisure.* New York: Wiley and Sons, Inc.

Riley, M., & Riley, J. (1989). The lives of old people and changing social roles. *The Annals of the American Academy of Political and Social Science, 503,* 14–28.

Robine, J., Romieu, I., & Cambois, E. (1997). Health expectancies and current research. *Reviews in Clinical Gerontology, 7,* 73–81.

Rosenfeld, R. (1999). Splitting the difference: Gender, the self, and mental health. In C. Aneshensel & J. Phelan (Eds.), *Handbook of the sociology of mental health* (pp. 209–224). New York: Kluwer Academic/Plenum Publishers.

Ross, C., & Mirowsky, J. (1995). Does employment affect health? *Journal of Health and Social Behavior, 36*, 3(Sept), 230–243.

Ross, C., & Mirowsky, J. (2002). Family relationships, social support, and subjective life expectancy. *Journal of Health and Social Behavior, 43*, 469–489.

Roxburgh, S. (1996). Gender differences in work and well-being: Effects of exposure and vulnerability. *Journal of Health and Social Behavior, 37*, 265–277.

Schieman, S. (2002). Socioeconomic status, job conditions, and well-being: Self-concept explanations for gender contingent effects. *The Sociological Quarterly, 43*, 627–646.

Schieman, S., Van Gundy, K., & Taylor, J. (2002). The relationship between age and depressive symptoms: A test of competing explanatory and suppression influences. *Journal of Aging and Health, 14*(2), 260–285.

Settersten, R. (1997). The salience of age in the life course. *Human Development, 40*, 257–281.

Sewell, W. (1992). A theory of structure: Duality, agency, and transformations. *American Journal of Sociology, 98*, 1–29.

Shanahan, M. (2000). Pathways to adulthood in changing societies: Variability and mechanisms in life course perspective. *Annual Review of Sociology, 26*, 667–692.

Simon, R. (1995). Gender, multiple roles, role meaning, and mental health. *Journal of Health and Social Behavior, 36*, 182–194.

Smith, D., & Moen, P. (1998). Spouse's influence on the retirement decision: His, her, and their perceptions. *Journal of Marriage and the Family, 60*, 734–744.

Sorensen, A. (forthcoming). The demography of the third age. In J. James & P. Wink (Eds.), *The crown of life: Dynamics of the early post-retirement period.* New York: Springer.

Sorenson, G., & Verbrugge, L. (1987). Women, work, and health. *Annual Review of Public Health, 8*, 235–251.

Thoits, P. (1986). Multiple identities: Examining gender and marital status differences in distress. *American Sociological Review, 51*, 259–272.

Thomas, W. I., & Znaniecki, F. (1918–1920). *The Polish peasant in Europe and America.* Chicago: University of Chicago Press.

Timmer, E., & Aartsen, M. (2003). Mastery beliefs and productive leisure activities in the third age. *Social Behavior and Personality, 31*(7), 643–656.

Timmer, E., Bode, C., & Dittmann-Kohli, F. (2003). Expectations of gains in the second half of life: A study of personal conceptions of enrichment in a lifespan perspective. *Ageing and Society, 23*, 3–34.

Townsend, N. (2002). *The package deal: Marriage, work, and fatherhood in men's lives.* Philadelphia, PA: Temple University Press.

West, C., & Zimmerman, D. (1987). Doing gender. *Gender and Society, 1*(2), 125–151.

Wink, P. (forthcoming). Everyday life in the third age. In J. James & P. Wink (Eds.), *The crown of life: Dynamics of the early post-retirement period.* New York: Springer.

Yenerall, J. (2003). Educating an aging society: The university of the third age in Finland. *Educational Gerontology, 29*, 703–716.

Zimmerman, L., Mitchell, B., Wister, A., & Gutman, G. (2000). Unanticipated consequences: A comparison of expected and actual retirement timing among older women. *Journal of Women and Aging, 12*(1/2), 109–128.

# Nine

# Stratification and the Life Course
## Life Course Capital, Life Course Risks, and Social Inequality

Angela M. O'Rand

Patterns of inequality within and between cohorts and their consequences for life course outcomes, including mortality, health, and economic well-being over the life span, have always been core concerns of research on aging. However, recent trends in the relationship between social inequality and health disparities, coupled with improved databases for studying inequality across time, societal level, and countries, have pushed this issue to the forefront. Major demographic and structural changes have generated several trends across societies, including: population aging (e.g., Fogel & Costa, 1997; Vaupel & Lundstrom, 1994); increased earnings and income inequality in societies with diverse welfare systems (Gottschalk & Smeeding, 1997; Gustafsson & Johansson, 1999); persistent, if not widening, social inequalities in health in spite of advances in medical technology (Marmot, Bobak, & Smith, 1995; Wilkinson, 1986, 1996); and shifts away from social welfare policies toward individualized and market-centered strategies for income- and health-maintenance (Poland, Coburn, Robertson, & Eakin,

1998). Aside from the putatively positive effects of recent increased levels of national wealth and economic progress on general health and well-being (Pritchett & Summers, 1996), growing economic and social inequalities between and within populations appear to be yielding divergent patterns in health and well-being (Link & Phelan, 1995).

This chapter offers a broad review of the relationship of stratification to the life course. It begins with a review of evolutionary theories of the organization of the human life course. These theories offer the foundation for understanding the importance of patterns of fertility, parental investment in childhood, and intergenerational transfers of resources for unequal patterns of human well-being and survival. Then, it summarizes the state of our knowledge of the sequential processes of cumulative advantage and adversity that begin in infancy and childhood and accumulate as biographies diverge. The approach hangs on the extension of two linked concepts: *life course capital* and *life course risk*. Both serve to simplify the multidimensional

*Handbook of Aging and the Social Sciences, Sixth Edition*

and temporally complex processes by which stratification emerges over time within populations.

An argument for the application of the concept of life course capital was introduced in greater detail in the last edition of this chapter (O'Rand, 2001). Life course capital is conceptualized as multiple stocks of resources that can be converted and exchanged to meet human needs and wants. Along these lines, I argued that it is useful to examine interdependent forms of life course *capital*, including human capital, social capital, psychophysical capital (mental and physical health), and personal capital (self-esteem, efficacy, and identity). Arguably, these multiple forms of life course capital (and probably others) interact across the life course to condition the emergence of divergent pathways of economic attainment and health maintenance. Life course risks, on the other hand, present both opportunities for the accumulation of forms of life course capital and challenges to the acquisition and maintenance of life course capital over time. They emanate from structural sources, principally from sequentially contingent exposures to adverse conditions and/or resource opportunities that begin in childhood and extend across the life course. Hence, the framework for studying stratification and the life course rests on three general concepts:

- *The life course*, defined as the interdependent and variable sequences of social statuses across life domains (education, family, work, wealth, health, leisure, etc.) over the life span.
- *Life course capital*, defined as interdependent stocks of resources across life domains that are accumulated and/or dissipated over the life course in the satisfaction of human needs and wants.
- *Life course risks*, defined as the differential likelihoods of exposure to adverse conditions (disadvantages) or structural opportunities (advantages)

for the accumulation, protection, or depletion of forms of life course capital.

# I. Life Course Capital: Evolutionary and Social Origins

The human life course is shaped by the interaction of bio-evolutionary and social processes. Its length, quality, and social organization reflect "a lifetime of reciprocal exchanges between person (including biological makeup) and context" (Shanahan, Hofer, & Shanahan, 2003, p. 599). However, childhood origins, including heritable and environmental variations, may have formative and perhaps *fateful* influences on subsequent person-environment interactions (Elo & Preston, 1992). One reason provided by evolutionary theory for the long-range effects of childhood on longevity and general well-being in adulthood is the long period of development and dependence of children on adults, especially their parents (but also including the educational system in modern societies that acts as a custodial institution in child development). During the protracted period of childhood dependence from in utero to the transition to adulthood, children undergo sustained but highly variable physical and cognitive development that probably establishes baseline vitality and capabilities extending through the life course. Recent revisions of evolutionary theory discussed later emphasize this argument.

The central concern of evolutionary theories of aging is the explanation of senescence or age-specific mortality across species. The classical theory linked continued survival to remaining lifetime fertility with age (e.g., Hamilton, 1966; Medawar, 1952). The core hypothesis is that because declining lifetime fertility contributes less to reproductive fitness (and population equilibrium), survival also declines. The restricted emphasis on fertility alone as the driving mechanism, however, ignores the importance of post-birth investment in children for survival to a given age, especially in species with relatively longer periods of juvenile development. A revision that takes account of this omission in classical theory has been proposed by Ronald D. Lee (2003), who argues that the level of investment in developing children is as, if not more, important as births per se for explaining senescence in social species. Investment in children requires continuing transfers from parents and other adults including post-reproductive females (e.g., grandmothers). In addition, "the force of selection against mortality should rise with juvenile age" (2003, p. 9637), as parental investment enables development and survival. Deaths later in the course of childhood development, however, are more costly for parents who have made such investments and lost the opportunity to produce more children or to invest more in surviving children and thus enhance the survival of the latter to later ages.

This revision of classical evolutionary theory is consistent with evolutionary anthropology, which is the study of human life histories. Evolutionary anthropologists argue that the human life history is a product of the co-evolution of the human brain and its capacity for intelligence with four other distinctively human characteristics: a long life span; a relatively extended period of juvenile dependence on parents; the male role in the reproductive process that includes the provisioning of females and their offspring; and the support of reproduction by older post-reproductive individuals, particularly post-menopausal females (Kaplan, Hill, Lancaster, & Hurtado, 2000). They propose that these distinctive traits were evolutionary responses to a dietary shift toward higher quality food sources that are harder to acquire. The shift required the acquisition of higher levels of knowledge, skills, and physical-mental coordination that, in turn, required significant investments in childhood development.

Accordingly, following revised theories of senescence and evolutionary anthropology social patterns related to the extended early developmental phase of the human life course, longevity well past reproductive ages (especially among females), and intergenerational flows of resources from older to younger members of the population are founded on evolutionary processes centered on the accumulation, conservation, conversion, and transmission of resources or forms of life course capital that enable survival. Advanced technologies at the turn of the twenty-first century may have amplified these evolutionary processes. Life expectancy has increased and has been accompanied by declines in morbidity (Fogel & Costa, 1997; Manton, Stallard, & Corder, 1997). The educational phase of the life course into what we formerly defined as adulthood (Bernhardt, Morris, Hancock, & Scott, 2001; Elman & O'Rand, 2004) now extends well past the actual assumption of adult roles. And, the expansion of multigenerational caregiving and resource transfers over the entire life course and across three or more generations (Bengtson & Silverstein, 1993) are now prominent features of human lives in contemporary advanced societies.

These average tendencies, however, mask considerable heterogeneity and inequality across subgroups of the population. Some subpopulations (but not all) benefit from longer, more advantageous periods of education that afford them greater success in modern economies. And, multigenerational transfers take on different forms (e.g., monetary, temporal) and exchange values depending on the relative fortunes of succeeding generations. Consequently, economic status, life expectancy, and patterns of morbidity and mortality are highly variable and highly correlated. In the United States, socioeconomically disadvantaged groups still live shorter lives with higher risks for more years spent in poor health than their more advantaged counterparts. Hayward and Heron (1999) reported that, although Caucasian and Asian groups have longer lives with fewer years lived in poor health, African Americans and Native Americans suffer relatively more from extended periods with chronic illness. Mortality rates are highest among African Americans until the oldest ages. Similarly, although women live longer than men across socioeconomic and ethnic status groups, a socioeconomic gradient of morbidity and mortality differentiates them as well (McDonough, Williams, House, & Duncan, 1999; Ross & Bird, 1994). The correlations between socioeconomic status (SES) and health among women match men's. In addition, women's longer lives are associated with higher risks for extended suffering from often multiple chronic and acute disabilities (Verbrugge & Jette, 1994) that survival curves of active life expectancy can mask (Verbrugge, 1991). Race and class stratification of the fortunes of the U.S. population across the life course ends with the highest levels of inequality among older adults (Smeeding, 1997) that are correlated with patterns of ill health (Smith & Kington, 1997a, 1997b).

## II. Forms of Life Course Capital: A Brief Review

Unequal parental (and societal) investment in the early life course contributes significantly to unequal fortunes across the life course. The processes by which this occurs are complex and cumulative, but the application of the concept of "capital" for this purpose has been adopted elsewhere (Coleman, 1990; Institute of Medicine, 2003; Lin, 1999; O'Rand, 2001; Rosen, 1998). The multiple interdepend-

ent forms of capital that cumulate over the life course include these.

*Human capital* (referred to as *HC* hereafter) is usually measured as years of education or schooling and experience in the workforce (see Becker, 1964; Schulz, 1961, for classical definitions). The accumulation of HC through extended acquisition of valued skills and knowledge and participation in the paid labor force is now considered to be *a primary mechanism* of social inequality within cohorts, although its specific influences over time are yet to be clearly specified. HC influences income streams, access to income and health insurance, and wealth accumulation that, in turn, affect the ongoing well-being of individuals and their capacities to support themselves and their families and to invest in their offspring.

*Psychophysical capital (PPC)* can be considered the stock of health, or physical and psychological well-being accumulated across the life course. Perhaps the longest tradition of life-course research has addressed this topic. It spans several theoretical traditions.

First, biological theories of senescence address the relative importance of random damage from environmental insults and genetic/developmental processes underlying the aging process (see Cristofalo, Tresini, Francis, & Volker, 1999, for a general review). Some current thinking assumes that both developmental/genetic processes and random damage interact over the life span to produce diverse trajectories of physical and mental health and senescence (Fogel & Costa, 1997; Vaupel & Lundstrom, 1994).

Second, stress theories of aging emphasize the homeostatic processes by which physiological and related psychological well-being, respectively, are maintained. Physiological stress theories address how the human nervous system responds to environmental insults (Finch & Seeman, 1999). In this tradition, homeostatic resiliency constitutes a physiological stock, which the body acts to maintain; exposure to diverse environmental insults (risks) over time can deplete this stock. Psychological and social psychological stress theories address how personal and social resources (such as education, social support, and selected psychosocial traits) mediate and moderate the effects of stress on physical and mental health (Pearlin, 1999).

Third, *social capital* (SC) is the stock of direct and indirect social relationships that can be mobilized to advantage (or disadvantage) by individuals (Lin, 1999). Whereas HC focuses on economic investment in the individual, SC focuses on the social integration of the individual in systems of social relationships of varying economic and social value. Social relationships of varying salience exist within families and within friendship, professional, and other community networks. They can be positive and negative in their effects on diverse outcomes including economic attainment and health. As such, SC is a noneconomic stock of social relationships that can substitute for other forms of capital to support status attainment and health or to diminish them (Berkman, 1984; Elder, George, & Shanahan, 1996).

*Personal capital* (PC) links the individual as perceiver and actor to his/her environment. Cumulative efficacy (Bandura, 1995) and competence (Clausen, 1993) in the performance of social roles and in the successful negotiation of stressful life events (Elder, George, & Shanahan, 1996) over the life course build a stock of personal capital. Identity theory (e.g., Thoits, 1991) subsumes these elements of personal stock at its core, as it argues that the accumulation of role-identities (self-evaluations of efficacy and competence relative to cultural expectations) is the foundation of self-esteem, which in turn is found repeatedly to be positively correlated with psychological and physical health. Theories of the disablement

process express the dynamics among economic, health, social, and personal capital as a "gap between personal capability and environmental demand" (Verbrugge & Jette, 1994, p. 1). Chronic and acute conditions can deplete resiliency and accumulate into patterns of comorbidity. Personal and environmental factors can exacerbate or ameliorate these conditions. Besides medical interventions, significant environmental factors that can abate or even fend off disablement include socioeconomic status and its correlates (e.g., human capital, access to health insurance and medical care), social capital (e.g., personal assistance, social support, social integration), and *personal capital* (e.g., resiliency, positive affect, self-confidence, and locus of control). The disablement process imposes costs on all forms of capital and is accelerated or decelerated by relative access to different stocks of resources.

Another form of life course capital has gained recent attention in the stratification literature. *Cultural capital* (CC) refers to levels of proficiency in dominant, socially valued codes and practices, including linguistic, aesthetic, and interaction styles that are rewarded in the educational system and wider society and serve directly to enhance HC and PC and possibly indirectly to enhance economic and health status (Bourdieu, 1977; Mohr & DiMaggio, 1995).

## III. Childhood: The First Life Course Risks in the Development of Life Course Capital

The cumulative acquisition of life course capital is conditioned by life course risks that are confronted from birth until death (Crosnoe & Elder, 2004; Werner & Smith, 2001). The first life course risks are attached to social origins, when the unequal provision of physical, social, and economic resources by parents to their children conditions lifelong patterns of inequality (Hertzman, 1999). The relationship between parental social and economic resources and children's health status and human capital achievement is well established. It begins with differential rates of neonatal and infant mortality, if not earlier in parents' lives, across racial and economic classes. Deemed the "first injustice" by Gortmaker (1997), the life course risks of infant mortality and neonatal mortality are negatively correlated with parental resources. The African American/Caucasian ratio of infant mortality rates was approximately 2.5/1.0 in 2000, presenting an approximate 25% increase since 1980. The increase in this "survival disadvantage" has been linked to average lower birth weights among African Americans (pointing to in utero origins of survival risks; see Elo & Preston, 1992) and related higher risks for respiratory distress syndrome as a major cause of infant death linked to race (Frisbie, Song, Powers & Street, 2004). According to Frisbie and colleagues (2004), a major source of this disparity is unequal access to health care innovations that reduce the risks of infant mortality. Another source of inequality of parental investment in prenatal, neonatal, and infant care is related, on average, to socioeconomic resources but is most strongly tied to poverty or near poverty and social exclusion from mainstream institutional resources (Lichter, 1997).

As mentioned previously, an early marker of infant health is birth weight. This is an indicator of maternal health behavior or the prenatal environment. Its study also provides the strategic opportunity to explore the relationship between SES and health at a point in the life course when issues of causal directionality (i.e., endogeneity) are seemingly less murky. Conley and Bennett (2000) used intergenerational data from the Panel Study of Income Dynamics between 1968 and 1992 to ask two questions: Does the SES of the mother during pregnancy affect her chances of having a low-birth-weight baby after controlling for her own birth weight, the father's birth weight and other unobserved, family-related factors? And does birth weight affect adult life chances after controlling for mother's SES at birth? Siblings are compared using family fixed-effects models. They found that maternal SES during pregnancy (measured as an income-to-needs ratio) is unrelated to infant birth weight, but that low birth weight predicts lower educational attainment of the child controlling for other factors, including gender, race, mother's education, and parents' birth weights. Excluded from these controls were subsequent, intervening indicators of forms of life course capital such as family SES at adolescence, time-varying family social capital, and trajectories of psychophysical capital. Also, the fixed-effects design (comparing siblings) accounts for variations within families rather than between families, thus masking the potential influence of variations in parents' SES. Hence, the study did not sufficiently adjudicate the self-imposed problem of causal ordering, but it found associations that support the argument of the interdependence of forms of life course capital.

Postnatal childhood adversity related to poor nutrition or poverty has been found to have serious formative implications for subsequent acquisition of human capital and maintenance of health. Lynch, Kaplan, and Salonen (1997) examined data from the Kuopio Ischaemic Heart Disease Risk Factor Study, a study of Finnish men with retrospective information on their family SES at age 10 and their own educational and occupational attainments. They found a high correlation between childhood and adult socioeconomic status. Also, a number of detrimental health behaviors (smoking, poor diet, alcohol abuse), psychosocial characteristics such as depression, hostility and hopelessness, and heart disease in adulthood were positively associated with lower SES in childhood. Similar omissions of intervening life course events and transitions in their models result again in a partial test of the causal ordering of SES and health, but the strong association over time among multiple forms of capital is upheld.

Resources for the support and nurturance of children's health are challenged by economic adversity, which can also create family distress that further depletes parents' capacities to protect or enhance their children's general well-being (Wickrama, Lorenz, & Conger, 1997). Health-related behaviors such as regular bedtimes, seat belt use, and home-prepared meals, and others are often sacrificed in these environments (Case, Lubotsky, & Paxson, 2002). More important, however, economic adversity in childhood is correlated with unsafe and unhealthy living environments and limited access to health care and support structures for the maintenance of good health (Frisbie et al., 2004).

After these initial "injustices" in early childhood, inequality in parental investment continues throughout middle childhood and adolescence, leading to clearly diverging levels of educational achievement among young adults. Economic hardship in childhood has been associated repeatedly with lower educational attainment, lower occupational status, employment instability and lower wage attainment, poorer physical and mental health, and higher mortality rates in adulthood (e.g., Bernhardt et al., 2001; Elman & O'Rand, 2004; Kaplan, Turrell, Lynch, Everson, Helkala, & Alonen, 2001; Kuh & Davey Smith, 1997; Warren & Hauser, 1997).

In this regard, McLanahan (2004) argued that two trajectories of parental investment have developed during the "second demographic transition" since 1960 and produced growing inequality among children. The second demographic transition has been distinguished by increased employment among women (and especially mothers of young children), delayed fertility and marriage, increased cohabitation, higher divorce rates, and nonmarital childbearing (Lesthaeghe, 1995). But these major trends have converged to produce two distinct trajectories or streams of parenting. The first consists of patterns of delayed childbearing among women with higher levels (and durations) of education, market employment, and marriage. These resources, which translate into money and time for children, afford their offspring greater advantages in the attainment of higher education, social skills and social capital, and other benefits (such as better health). The second trajectory is defined by patterns of lower educational attainment among women with higher rates of divorce and nonmarital childbearing. This is a more adverse parenting sequence that produces fewer resources, and frequent losses of resources, for children whose life chances are seriously constrained. Childhood poverty is an increasingly common experience within this trajectory (Lichter, 1997).

The timing of economic adversity during childhood is possibly another specific mechanism of relative cumulative disadvantage. Duncan, Yeung, Brooks-Gunn, and Smith (1998) corroborated earlier studies by documenting parental SES effects on educational attainment, especially among the poorest groups, using sibling models. They found that economic deprivation earlier rather than later in childhood has particularly severe effects on learning and performance in school. Later deprivation, on the other hand, appears to influence behavioral problems more than educational attainments *per se*.

*Cultural capital (CC)* in the developmental environment throughout childhood and adolescence may also condition later economic achievement and health.

A long tradition of research has established the importance of "enriched learning environments" (Duncan et al., 1998) for childhood and adolescent achievement. These environments are characterized not only by more economic resources but also by more social and cultural resources associated with the amount and quality of parental time spent with children, direct adult involvement (including non-parental adults) with child socialization, access to so-called "highbrow" cultural capital in elaborated forms of artistic, verbal/linguistic and abstract skills and knowledge, and styles of parenting that build PC and encourage responsible independence (see classic study by Kohn & Schooler, 1983).

Two competing hypotheses frame research in this area. The first is the cultural reproduction thesis, associated with Bourdieu (1977), which proposes that the unequal distribution of cultural capital leads to the reproduction of inequality. Cultural capital is passed from generation to generation. A study by Lareau (2002) followed in the cultural reproduction tradition. She conducted field observations of 88 children between 8 and 10 years old and their families between 1989 and 1997. She identified two class-related styles of parenting with different outcomes in children's expectations of themselves. Both African-American and Caucasian middle-class parents exercised what Lareau refers to as "concerted cultivation." This parenting style fostered routines of daily organized activities such music lessons and sports participation, extensive verbal interactions between parents and children, and a sense of connectivity. Lower-class parenting, on the other hand, followed a style of "accomplishment of natural growth," a pattern that may attend to the basic physical needs of children but is accompanied by limited verbal interactions between parents and children and leaves nonschool activities up to the children themselves.

This pattern implicates lower parental resources and investments in children. The outcomes for children's expectations of themselves (their personal capital) is that those reared in middle-class environments develop a sense of "entitlement," while those raised in lower-class environments develop a sense of "constraint."

The second hypothesis proposes that access to cultural capital in childhood increases chances for mobility across generations (Mohr & DiMaggio, 1995). Here studies tend to focus more on variations in children's participation in various high-status cultural activities in and out of school rather than on their parents' characteristics. One such study used longitudinal data from the Surveys of Public Participation in the Arts between 1982 and 1992 (Aschaffenburg & Maas, 1997). The results were that parents' and children's cultural capital, respectively, exert independent effects on later educational outcomes, with the latter effects tending to support a cultural mobility argument.

# IV. Challenges to Linking Childhood Origins to Adult Outcomes

The enduring effects of class origins on economic and health outcomes later in life remain problematic subjects of research in some respects. Few longitudinal studies collect sufficient information on class origins or childhood health. Those that do usually rely on respondents' recollections of a limited set of parental or early household characteristics, such as parents' education and occupation or welfare receipt. Efforts to correct these limitations by the addition of more indicators of childhood living conditions (Elo, 1998; Hayward & Gorman, 2004) or by accounting for the measurement error introduced by such data (O'Rand & Hamil-Luker, 2005) are under way. In addition, recently initiated longitudinal studies based on samples of children and adolescents are collecting more detailed information on social origins, including SES, health, and lifestyle data on both parents and children (e.g., the National Longitudinal Study of Adolescent Health).

These efforts to link childhood to adult economic and health outcomes are guided by the mounting evidence that economic adversity is a "fundamental cause" of poor health and premature death over the life course (Link & Phelan, 1995; Phelan, Link, Diez-Roux, Kawachi, & Levin, 2004). The core of the fundamental cause argument is that lower socioeconomic status is a health risk that operates above and beyond inherited vulnerabilities. Those with sufficient capital are able to protect themselves from preventable health risks; those without resources are not. The prenatal and postnatal childhood environments are the earliest exposures to health risk, with probable long-term latent effects on adulthood (Barker, 1992; Hertzman, 1999). Subsequent SES experiences via educational, occupational, familial, or other pathways may mediate early childhood adversity, but are more likely to reflect and perhaps amplify unequal origins (O'Rand & Hamil-Luker, 2005).

# V. Life Course Risks After Childhood: Variant Opportunities and Deviant Setbacks

Educational attainment appears to be the pivotal life course transition for predicting later well-being in adulthood (Reynolds & Ross, 1998; Ross & Wu, 1995). Yet, its pivotal role in life course stratification has yet to be fully explicated. Unquestionably, its role is complex and resides at several levels of explanation.

First, education acts to reproduce or amplify childhood origins. The long traditions of human capital and status attainment research have demonstrated that educational attainment strongly reflects childhood origins (Warren & Hauser, 1997) and can, in fact, amplify the impact of social origins on later adult outcomes including wage attainment (Elman & O'Rand, 2004) and health (O'Rand & Hamil-Luker, 2005). Heritable and environmental elements of the childhood risks discussed earlier affect cognitive and social development patterns, which come to be evaluated, defined, and often reinforced in educational institutions. Research in this tradition also suggests that the effects of education are strongest at career entry and diminish over time when unmeasured family background influences are taken into account (see Warren, Hauser, & Sheridan, 2002, using sibling data from the Wisconsin Longitudinal Study). Hence, educational attainment bears and transmits the effects of childhood risks that are themselves complex and not well studied in life course research, but intervening adult pathways have independent and mediating effects on adult SES outcomes.

Second, educational experiences vary considerably in the United States, so much so that a simple designation of "years of schooling" masks widespread inequalities in the content and quality of education (Gamoran & Mare, 1989) and in the resources provided to educational institutions (Condron & Roscigno, 2003).

Third, the labor market premium placed on different "credentials" (diplomas and degrees) assigns a qualitative meaning to types of education that has consequences for inequality above and beyond the level of attainment itself (Elman & O'Rand, 2004). The U.S. labor market since the 1970s has placed a higher and higher premium on postsecondary educational credentials. Yet, fewer than one-third of cohorts born since World War II have finished college (Bernhardt et al., 2001; Hughes & O'Rand, 2004). The explanation of this trend is a matter of considerable dispute, in a debate that pits a technologically-based skill argument against a price competition argument (Levy, 1998). Whichever explanation eventually prevails, the consequences of these patterns for the turn of the century include high levels of wage inequality (Gottschalk & Smeeding, 1997), noncoverage and under-coverage of families by health insurance (Institute of Medicine, 2003), and increasing health disparities across age, class, and race/ethnic groups (Hayward, Crimmins, Miles, & Yu, 2000; House, Lepkowski, Kinney, Mero, Kessler, & Herzog, 1994; Robert & House, 2000; Williams, Mourney, & Warren, 1994).

Nevertheless, despite these reasonable concerns the robust association of educational attainment with adult economic status and, in turn, with health over the life course has invited interpretation. The principal argument is that education provides the foundation for the accumulation of life course capital (Reynolds & Ross, 1998; Ross & Wu, 1995). As human capital, it influences occupational attainment, employment stability, and earnings. As social capital, it facilitates social integration and widens networks of social support. And as personal and health capital, it promotes a higher sense of efficacy and control that encourages more beneficial and positively reinforcing health behaviors and lifestyles. These forms of life course capital develop as interdependent and mutually reinforcing processes over time.

## VI. Variant Adult Pathways to Inequality: Patterns of Disadvantage and Advantage

The idea of cumulative advantage/disadvantage has become attached, implicitly or explicitly, to the longitudinal study of variability and stratification over the life course (Dannefer, 1987, 2003). It originated as a Mertonian framework to study

processes of professional recognition and reward in science (see O'Rand, 2002, for a summary of these origins). Hence, it was formulated to apply to quasi-economic, Pareto-optimal situations in which inequality emerges in a population over time and is biased in the direction of initial inequalities. Stratification occurs as the advantaged minority accumulates a growing disproportionate share of the rewards in a system. As the minority gets richer, the majority gets relatively (but not necessarily absolutely) poorer.

This idea has been applied explicitly to the study of economic stratification within aging cohorts. Education-dependent wage and retirement income inequality in middle-age and older populations supports the cumulative advantage argument. Using the National Survey of Households and Families to track the educational careers and wage outcomes of Baby Boomers, Elman and O'Rand (2004) found that early completion of postsecondary degrees is tied to earlier childhood advantage and later wage advantage. Delayed patterns of degree attainment do not compensate absolutely for early disadvantages. Bernhardt and her colleagues (2001) found similar patterns in two cohorts from the National Longitudinal Studies. They follow the "divergent paths" within cohorts born between 1946 and 1953 and 1958 and 1965, respectively, until they reached age 30 to 37. They found that less than one-third of these cohorts finished college, that succeeding cohorts took relatively longer to complete schooling, and that many worked while returning for additional education. Correlated with these patterns were increases in job instability and wage inequality within and across cohorts. Early postsecondary credential attainment and early job-shopping followed by stable employment among those with lower credential attainment were associated with economic advantage at midlife. Finally, Crystal and Waehrer (1996) found increasing income inequality with age across cohorts and tied retirement income inequality to earlier educational-, earnings-, and pension-attainment patterns, although they also identify complex patterns of upward and downward mobility tied to both cumulative and short-term factors.

The processes of cumulative advantage and cumulative disadvantage, however, are probably quite different. Cumulative disadvantage (also referred to as cumulative hardship and cumulative adversity in the literature) implies strong path dependence in the life course. This path dependence is anchored in early disadvantage, which exerts a gravity that constrains subsequent economic attainment and health maintenance. Poorer social origins increase the sequential risks of lower educational attainment, lower economic status in adulthood, and poorer health or earlier mortality. Thus, cumulative disadvantage connotes a chain of life course "insults" (Hayward & Gorman, 2004). The most compelling evidence for this conceptualization occurs in studies of severe health disparities. For example, early and sustained poverty has been shown repeatedly to predict higher rates of disability and mortality in later life (Lynch, Kaplan, & Shema, 1997). This pattern is especially pronounced among African Americans (Smith & Kington, 1997a, 1997b). Higher rates of hypertension and associated cognitive decline have been observed in this group (Rodgers, Ofstedal & Hertzog, 2003). In particular, the association between midlife high blood pressure (i.e., systolic blood pressure) and late life cognitive function is established (Launer, Masaki, Petrovich, Foley, & Havlik, 1995). Although these disparities are not yet fully understood, genetic and environmental risks (including prenatal and postnatal social factors) are believed to interact with adult experiences of discrimination to produce these outcomes,

following expectations from stress theory (Williams et al., 1994).

Throughout this discussion of life course processes of stratification so far, references to the general implications of these processes for economic inequality and health disparities in later life have been noted. Early life inequalities initiate trajectories of inequality extending from educational attainment to socioeconomic inequality in adulthood. In turn, economic inequality in adulthood is highly correlated with health disparities especially apparent in the distribution of some chronic health conditions and cause-specific mortality rates in late adulthood; however, some inconsistent findings require further specification. For example, overall mortality rates have been shown to be more directly associated with adult economic, lifestyle, and health statuses than with childhood conditions (see for example, Hayward and Gorman, 2004, using National Longitudinal Survey of Older Men, 1966–1990). Yet, the connections among childhood, adulthood, and late-life health and mortality connected with specific chronic conditions and causes of death are only beginning to be studied. Recent studies along these lines suggest that the etiologies of some health conditions are more readily traceable to heritability and childhood environments and their cumulative impact on adult statuses and behaviors than others (Galobardes, Lynch, & Davey Smith, 2004).

One area of study along these lines focuses on cardiovascular diseases, the most common (and among the most preventable) cause of death in the United States. These diseases have been tied to the effects of cumulative stress and allostatic load over the life course. Their link to childhood socioeconomic conditions is now established in the literature (e.g., Leon & Ben-Shlomo, 1997). One of these studies has found specifically that childhood adversity has severe enduring effects on high risks for heart attack (O'Rand & Hamil-Luker, 2005). A longitudinal study of trajectories of heart attack risk following Health and Retirement Study respondents between 1992 and 2002 found that childhood SES disadvantage and childhood poor health increase the risks for early high heart attack risk, after controlling for the intervening effects of early and late adulthood statuses such as educational attainment, household income, and health behaviors related to smoking, obesity, and poor exercise. The extension of such analyses to other adult diseases tied to long-term life chances and lifestyles is only in the beginning stages.

Another area of study focuses on cognitive decline in middle and old age, which appears to be linked to life course disadvantages associated with SES and race/ethnicity mentioned earlier. Although more contentious, this literature is building on early observations that prenatal and postnatal environments affect cognitive capacities (specifically IQ) (Scarr, 1992) leading to inequalities that grow as demands for cognitive performance (information processing and the accumulation of new knowledge) become more complex. The logic of the argument is that unequal resources (or stocks of life course capital in all forms; for example, psychophysical, human, and cultural) produce unequal opportunities for (or obstructions to) the maintenance of cognitive well-being.

In sum, cumulative processes of stratification set individuals on different pathways of relative advantage or disadvantage. Early advantage increases access to beneficial opportunity structures, but considerable heterogeneity develops within aging cohorts as encounters with potentially fortunate, derailing, or deflecting life course risks emerge (Bernhardt et al., 2001; Crystal & Waehrer, 1996). Alternatively, early disadvantage may increase the likelihood of persistent disadvantage in a path dependent pattern.

## VII. Deviant Setbacks in the Life Course: Criminal Records

As noted previously, the life course literature tends to focus on normative and variant patterns of development, with a recent but more limited consideration of highly adverse or deviant patterns. The latter, however, are receiving more attention as these patterns become more prevalent in the population and as data permit their observation. Adverse childhood conditions related to poverty, family distress, and poor health provide only one area of study in this regard. The impact of criminal records on life course outcomes is another area of growing interest.

Nontrivial trends in the life course of Americans include the increased levels of risk for arrest and incarceration, especially among subgroups of younger populations over the last few decades. After the turn of the twenty-first century, more than 2 million adults were incarcerated in the United States annually, most of whom were in young adulthood, with approximately one-half million released each year (Pager, 2003). This trend has led some researchers to argue that incarcerations are becoming a new stage of the life course (Pettit & Western, 2004). Criminal records are major setbacks in the life course; they are typically barriers to successful transitions to adult statuses, particularly employment and marriage. And, as employment (as human capital) and marriage (as social capital) are highly correlated with economic and health outcomes in adulthood, criminal records are among the most disadvantaged status characteristics in the population (Western, 2002).

The age-crime curve has received attention from life course researchers. Specifically, the processes whereby young criminal offenders desist from crime have been examined. Sampson and Laub's (e.g., 1990, 1993, 1996) innovative analyses of the Glueck data introduced this area of research and have spawned considerable interest. This body of work has examined how the formation of social bonds that increase life course capital increases the likelihood of desistance. These bonds primarily include employment, military service, and marriage. They are effectively "turning points" in these young lives (Uggen, 2000), at which their opportunities for accumulating life course capital improve and their likelihood of desistance is optimized. There is also evidence that these turning points cumulate over time and build life course capital (Laub, Nagin, & Sampson, 1998). Although Sampson and Laub study delinquents and nondelinquents who came from common experiences of childhood poverty, a considerable literature has linked criminal careers to disadvantaged childhood conditions (Sampson & Laub, 1993; Wilson, 1987). Hence, early life course trajectories are not only a matter of variable educational attainment but also of lives deflected (perhaps permanently) from the normative adult life course with higher risks for poverty, disease, and early death; however, we know far less about the health outcomes of incarceration and having a criminal record. Surveys of the noninstitutionalized population, of course, exclude those incarcerated. Also, the incarcerated are protected from possible exploitation by the research process and thus remain invisible in much social science research addressing diverse questions related to the life course.

# VIII. Conclusions: The Retrenchment of Equalizing Institutions and Life Course Stratification

The growth of income inequality and increased trends in health disparities are not the products of individual fate or random opportunity. They are associated with long-term structural shifts in the economy and with changing welfare institutions. In the environment of managed competition that predominated in the United States in the post-World War II period until the mid-1970s, market and welfare institutions complemented each other in ways that operated to expand public education at the secondary and postsecondary levels, promote employment stability, decrease wage inequality, and provide "safety nets" for dependent and vulnerable populations (Levy, 1998). Occupational welfare programs including health insurance and pension plans reached large portions of the working population and their families. Public programs, especially those associated with Social Security and Medicare, expanded coverage to wider segments of the dependent and the vulnerable (e.g., older people, children, displaced homemakers). Although inequality hardly disappeared, market and government institutions operated to spread risks across large populations using private and public welfare institutions.

Since the 1970s, the trend has been away from these arrangements and toward more risk-bearing by individuals, especially in the employment system (Shuey & O'Rand, 2004). Price competition and globalization processes have weakened the employment relationship and eroded the ethos of social insurance. Risks devolved to workers and their families are evident in changing education, health insurance, and pension institutions. Educational policies have increasingly shifted toward an ideology of choice apparent in the spread of private and charter schools and proposals to offer educational vouchers. Health insurance since the mid-1980s has become a highly stratified system of access to health care in which premium and co-payment costs have been linked to quality of service. And, pensions have moved steadily toward individualized retirement accounts (defined contribution plans) that place full responsibility on workers to defer earnings as market investment and release employers from the financial liability once associated with defined benefit plans. Even Social Security reforms include proposals to devolve risk and move from an ideology of social insurance to one of wealth accumulation.

Implications of these changes for stratification are self-evident. The previous Keynesian complementarity of market and welfare institutions provided some equalization of outcomes. Current arrangements and their emphasis on individualization appear to move in the opposite direction.

The future of the life course is contingent on these changing institutional arrangements. The educational institution is pivotal to stratification processes in wealth and health. Indeed, this institution, along with the family, is critical to childhood and adolescent development; it serves an important custodial role from both social and evolutionary vantage points. Investments in children are formative and enduring. They begin with unequal parental investments. Adding to this, origins are unequally enriching and, in some cases, deteriorating educational institutions and the increased prevalence of incarceration in selected disadvantaged subgroups of the population. We have not documented the full implications of inadequate schools and early criminal records and incarceration for the later life course, especially for health outcomes and mortality, but we should expect that they extend another long arm into future lives.

Employment institutions are also critical as potentially equalizing structures, although the growing evidence, particularly from longitudinal cohort comparisons like those conducted by Bernhardt and her colleagues (2001), is that inequality is growing because work histories and related family histories confront high risks for instability and disruption that increase the likelihood of decline and loss of income and disease onset. Workplace safety nets are disappearing and individual and family responsibility is rising for protection against normal and unexpected life course risks.

Stratification remains at the heart of life course studies. It has illuminated processes of economic attainment and health disparity. It has also raised many questions regarding the "fundamental causes" of these disparities. These causes lie at the intersection of institutional structures and individual biographies and require the integration of both levels of analysis in theory-building and in empirical research.

## References

Aschaffenberg, K., & Maas, I. (1997). Cultural and educational careers: The dynamics of social reproduction. *American Sociological Review, 62*, 573–587.

Bandura, A. (1995). *Self-efficacy: The exercise of control*. New York: Freeman.

Barker, D. (1992). *Fetal and infant origins of adult disease*. London: BMJ Publishing Group.

Becker, G. (1964). *Human capital* (2nd ed.). New York: Columbia University Press.

Bengtson, V. L., & Silverstein, M. (1993). Families, aging and social change: Seven agendas for 21st century researchers. In G. Maddox & M. P. Lawton (Eds.), *Kinship, aging and social change*, Vol. 13, Annual Review of Gerontology and Geriatrics (pp. 15–38). New York: Springer.

Berkman, L. F. (1984). Assessing the physical health effects of social networks and social support. *Annual Review of Public Health, 5*, 413–432.

Bernhardt, A., Morris, M., Handcock, M. S., & Scott, M. A. (2001). *Divergent paths: Economic mobility in the new American labor market*. New York: Russell Sage.

Bourdieu, P. (1977). Cultural reproduction and social reproduction. In J. Karabel & A. H. Halsey (Eds.), *Power and ideology in education* (pp. 487–511). New York: Oxford University Press.

Case, A., Lubotsky, D., & Paxson, C. (2002). Economic status and health in childhood: The origins of the gradient. *American Economic Review, 92,* 1308–1334.

Clausen, J. A. (1993). *American lives: Looking back at the children of the Great Depression.* New York: Free Press.

Coleman, J. S. (1990). *Foundations of social theory.* Cambridge MA: Harvard University Press.

Condron, D., J., & Roscigno, V. J. (2003). Disparities within: Unequal spending and achievement in an urban school district. *Sociology of Education, 76,* 18–36.

Conley, D. & Bennett, N. G. (2000). Is biology destiny? Birth weight and life chances. *American Sociological Review, 65,* 458–467.

Cristofalo, V. J., Tresini, M., Francis, M. K., & Volker, C. (1999). Biological theories of senescence. In V. Bengtson & K. W Schaie (Eds.), *Handbook of theories on aging.* (pp. 98–112). New York: Springer.

Crosnoe, R., & Elder, G. H., Jr. (2004). From childhood to the later years: Pathways of human development. *Research on Aging, 26,* 1–33.

Crystal, S., & Waehrer, K. 1996. Later life economic inequality in longitudinal perspective. *Journal of Gerontology: Social Sciences, 51B,* S307–S318.

Dannefer, D. (1987). Aging as intracohort differentiation: Accentuation, the Matthew effect and the life course. *Sociological Forum, 2,* 211–236.

Dannefer, D. (2003). Cumulative advantage/disadvantage and the life course: Cross-fertilizing age and social science theory. *Journal of Gerontology: Social Sciences, 58B,* S327–S337.

Duncan, G. J., Yeung, W. J., Brooks-Gunn, J., & Smith, J. R. (1998). How much does childhood poverty affect the life chances of children? *American Sociological Review, 63,* 406–423.

Elder, G. H., Jr., George, L. K., & Shanahan, M. J. (1996). Psychosocial stress over the life course. In H. B. Kaplan (Ed.), *Psychosocial stress: Perspectives on structure, theory, life course, and methods* (pp. 247–292). Orlando FL: Academic Press.

Elman, C., & O'Rand, A. M. (2004). The race is to the swift: Socioeconomic origins, adult education and economic attainment. *American Journal of Sociology, 110,* 123–160.

Elo, I. T. (1998). *Childhood conditions and adult health: Evidence from the health and retirement study.* Population Aging Research Center Working Paper 98–03, University of Pennsylvania.

Elo, I. T., & Preston, S. H. (1992). Effects of early life conditions on adult mortality: A review. *Population Index, 58,* 186–212.

Finch, C. E., & Seeman, T. E. (1999). Stress theories of aging. In V. Bengtson & K. W Schaie (Eds.), *Handbook of theories on aging.* (pp. 81–97). New York: Springer.

Fogel, R. W., & Costa, D. L. (1997). A theory of technophysio evolution, with some implications for forecasting population, health care costs, and pension costs. *Demography, 34,* 49–66.

Frisbie, W. P., Song, S.-E., Powers, D. A., & Street, J. A. (2004). The increasing racial disparity in infant mortality: Respiratory distress syndrome and other causes. *Demography, 41,* 773–800.

Galobardes, B., Lynch, J. W., & Davey Smith, G. (2004). Childhood socioeconomic circumstances and cause-specific mortality in adulthood: Systematic review and interpretation. *Epidemiologic Reviews, 26,* 7–21.

Gamoran, A., & Mare, R. D. (1989). Secondary school tracking and educational inequality: Compensation, reinforcement or neutrality? *American Journal of Sociology, 94,* 1146–1183.

Gortmaker, S. L. (1997). The first injustice: Socioeconomic disparities, health services, technology, and infant mortality. *Annual Review of Sociology, 23,* 147–170.

Gottschalk, P., & Smeeding, T. M. (1997). Cross-national comparisons of earnings and income inequality. *Journal of Economic Literature, 35,* 633–687.

Gustafsson, B., & Johansson, M. (1999). What makes income inequality vary across countries? *American Sociological Review, 64,* 585–605.

Hamilton, W. D. (1966). The moulding of senescence by natural selection. *Journal of Theoretical Biology, 12,* 12–45.

Hayward, M. D., Crimmins, E. M, Miles, T. P., & Yu, Y. (2000). The significance of socioeconomic status in explaining the racial gap in chronic health conditions.

*American Sociological Review, 65,* 910–930.

Hayward, M. D., & Gorman, B. K. (2004). The long arm of childhood: The influence of early-life social conditions on men's mortality. *Demography, 41,* 87–107.

Hayward, M. D., & Heron, M. (1999). Racial inequality in active life expectancy among adult Americans. *Demography, 36,* 77–91.

Hertzman, C. (1999). The biological embedding of early experience and its effects on health in adulthood. *Annals of the New York Academy of Sciences, 896,* 85–95.

House, J. S., Lepkowski, J. M., Kinney, A. M., Mero, R. P., Kessler, R. C., & Herzog, A. R. (1994). The social stratification of aging and health. *Journal of Health and Social Behavior, 35,* 213–234.

Hughes, M. E., & O'Rand, A. M. (2004). *The lives and times of the baby boom. Census 2000 Monograph.* New York Russell Sage Foundation/Washington DC: Population Reference Bureau.

Institute of Medicine. (2003). *Hidden costs, value lost: Uninsurance in America.* Washington DC: National Academy Press.

Kaplan, G. A., Turrell, G., Lynch, J. W., Everson, S. A., Helkala, E.-L., & Alonen, J. (2001). Childhood socioeconomic position and cognitive function in adulthood. *International Journal of Epidemiology, 31,* 256–263.

Kaplan, H., Hill, K., Lancaster, J., & Hurtado, A. M. (2000). A theory of human life history evolution: Diet, intelligence and longevity. *Evolutionary Anthropology, 9,* 1–30.

Kohn, M. L., & Schooler, C. (1983). *Work and personality: An inquiry into the impact of social stratification.* Norwood NJ: Ablex.

Kuh, D., & Davey Smith, G. (1997). *A life course approach to chronic disease epidemiology.* New York: Oxford University Press.

Laub, J. H., Nagin, D. S., & Sampson, R. J. (1998). Trajectories of change in criminal offending: Good marriages and the desistance process. *American Sociological Review, 63,* 225–238.

Launer, L. J., Masaki, K., Petrovich, H., Foley, D., & Havlik, R. J. (1995). The association between midlife blood pressure levels and late-life cognitive function: The Honolulu-Asia aging study. *Journal of the American Medical Association, 274,* 1846–1852

Lareau, A. (2002). Invisible inequality: Social class and childrearing in black and white families. *American Sociological Review, 67,* 747–776.

Lee, R. D. (2003). Rethinking the evolutionary theory of aging: Transfers, not births, shape senescence in social species. *Proceedings of the National Academy of Sciences, 100,* 9637–9642.

Leon, D., & Ben-Shlomo, Y. (1997). Preadult influences on cardiovascular disease and cancer. In D. Kuh & Y. Ben-Shlomo (Eds.), *A life course approach to chronic disease epidemiology* (pp. 45–77). New York: Oxford University Press.

Lesthaeghe, R. (1995). The second demographic transition in western countries: An interpretation. In K. O. Mason & A.-M. Jensen (Eds.), *Gender and family change in industrialized countries* (pp. 17–62). Oxford, UK: Clarendon Press.

Levy, F. (1998). *The new dollars and dreams: American incomes and economic change.* New York: Russell Sage.

Lichter, D. T. (1997). Poverty and inequality among children. *Annual Review of Sociology, 23,* 121–145.

Lin, N. (1999). Social networks and status attainment. *Annual Review of Sociology, 25,* 467–487.

Link, B. G., & Phelan, J. (1995). Social conditions as fundamental causes of disease. *Journal of Health and Social Behavior, 36,* 80–94.

Lynch, J. W., Kaplan, G. A., & Salonen, J. T. (1997). Why do poor people behave poorly? Variation in adult health behaviors and psychosocial characteristics by stages of the socioeconomic lifecourse. *Social Science and Medicine, 44,* 809–819.

Lynch, J. W., Kaplan, G. A., & Shema, S. J. (1997). Cumulative impact of sustained economic hardship on physical, cognitive, psychological and social functioning. *The New England Journal of Medicine, 337,* 1889–1895.

Manton, K. G., Stallard, E., & Corder, L. (1997). Changes in the age dependence of mortality and disability: Cohort and other determinants. *Demography, 34,* 135–157.

Marmot, M., Bobak, M., & Smith, G. D. (1995). Explanations for social inequalities in health. In B. C. Amick, III, S. Levine, A. R. Tarlov, & D. C. Walsh (Eds.), *Society and health* (pp. 172–210). New York: Oxford University Press.

McLanahan, S. (2004). Diverging destinies: How children are faring under the second demographic transition. *Demography, 41*, 607–627.

McDonough, P., Williams, D. R., House, J. S., & Duncan, G. J. (1999). Gender and the socioeconomic gradient in mortality. *Journal of Health and Social Behavior, 40*, 17–31.

Medawar, P. B. (1952). *An unsolved problem in biology*. London: Lewis.

Mohr, J., & DiMaggio, P. (1995). The intergenerational transmission of cultural capital. *Research in Social Stratification and Mobility, 14*, 167–200.

O'Rand, A. M. (2001). Stratification and the life course: The forms of life course capital and their interdependence. In R. B. Binstock & L. K. George (Eds.), *Handbook of aging and the social sciences* (5th ed., pp. 197–213). San Diego, CA: Academic Press.

O'Rand, A. M. (2002). Cumulative advantage theory in life course research. In S. Crystal & D. Shea (Eds.), Economic outcomes in later life: Public policy, health and cumulative advantage. *Annual Review of Gerontology and Geriatrics, 22* (Special Issue), 14–30.

O'Rand, A. M., & Hamil-Luker, J. (2005). Processes of cumulative adversity linking childhood disadvantage to increased risk of heart attack across the life course. *Journal of Gerontology: Social Sciences, 60* (Special Issue), 117–124.

Pager, D. (2003). The mark of a criminal record. *American Journal of Sociology, 108*, 937–975.

Pearlin, L. I. (1999). The stress process revisited: reflections on concepts and their interrelationships. In C. S. Aneshensel & J. C. Phelan (Eds.), *Handbook of the sociology of mental health* (pp. 395–415). New York: Plenum.

Pettit, B., & Western, B. (2004). Mass imprisonment and the life course: Race and class inequality in U.S. incarceration. *American Sociological Review, 69*, 151–169.

Phelan, J., Link, B. G., Diez-Roux, A., Kawachi, I., & Levin, B. (2004). "Fundamental causes" of social inequalities in mortality: A test of theory. *Journal of Health and Social Behavior, 45*, 265–285.

Poland, B., Coburn, D., Robertson, A., & Eakin, J. (1998). Wealth, equity and health care: A critique of a "population health" perspective on the determinants of health. *Social Science and Medicine, 46*, 785–798.

Pritchett, L., & Summers, L. H. (1996). Wealthier is healthier. *Journal of Human Resources, XXXI*, 841–867.

Reynolds, J. R., & Ross, C. E. (1998). Social stratification and health: Education's benefit beyond economic status and social origins. *Social Problems, 45*, 221–247.

Robert S. A., & House, J. S. (2000). Socioeconomic inequalities in health: An enduring sociological problem. In C. E. Bird, P. Conrad, & A. M. Fremont (Eds.), *Handbook of medical sociology* (5th ed., 79–97). Upper Saddle River, NJ: Prentice Hall.

Rodgers, W. L., Ofstedal, M. B., & Hertzog, A. R. (2003). Trends in scores on tests of cognitive ability in the elderly U.S. population, 1993–2000. *Journals of Gerontology B: Social Sciences, 58*, S338–S346.

Rosen, S. (1998). Human capital. In P. Newman (Ed.), *The new Palgrave dictionary of economics and the law* (Vol. 2, pp. 681–690). London: Macmillan.

Ross, C. E., & Bird, C. (1994). Sex stratification and health lifestyle: Consequences for men's and women's perceived health. *Journal of Health and Social Behavior 35*, 161–178.

Ross, C. E., & Wu, C. (1995). The links between education and health. *American Sociological Review, 60*, 719–745.

Sampson, R., & Laub, J. H. (1990). Crime and deviance over the life course: The salience of adult social bonds. *American Sociological Review, 55*, 609–627.

Sampson, R., & Laub, J. H. (1993). *Crime in the making: Pathways and turning points through life*. Cambridge MA: Harvard University Press.

Sampson, R., & Laub, J. H. (1996). Socioeconomic achievement in the lives of disadvantaged men: Military service as a turning point, circa 1940–1965. *American Sociological Review, 61*, 347–367.

Scarr, S. (1992). Developmental theories for the 1990s: Development and individual differences. *Child Development, 63*, 1–19.

Schulz, T. W. (1961). Investment in human capital. *American Economic Review, LI*, 1–17.

Shanahan, M. J., Hofer, S. M., & Shanahan, L. (2003). Biological models of behavior and the life course. In J. T. Mortimer & M. J. Shanahan (Eds.), *Handbook of the life course* (pp. 597–622). New York: Kluwer Academic/Plenum.

Shuey, M. M., & O'Rand, A. M. (2004). New risks for workers: Pensions, labor markets and gender, *Annual Review of Sociology, 30,* 453–477.

Smeeding, T. (1997). *Reshuffling responsibilities in old age: The United States in comparative perspective.* Working Paper No. 153, Luxembourg Income Study. Syracuse NY: Syracuse University, Maxwell School of Citizenship and Public Affairs.

Smith, J. P., & Kington, R. S. (1997a). Demographic and economic correlates of health in old age. *Demography, 34,* 159–170.

Smith, J. P., & Kington, R. S. (1997b). Race, socioeconomic status, and health late in life. In L. G. Martin & B. Soldo (Eds.), *Racial and ethnic difference in the health of older Americans* (pp. 105–162). Washington DC: National Academy Press.

Thoits, P. A. (1991) On merging identity theory and stress research. *Social Psychology Quarterly, 54,* 101–112.

Uggen, C. (2000). Work as a turning point in the life course of criminals: A duration model of age, employment and recidivism. *American Sociological Review, 67,* 529–546.

Vaupel, J. W., & Lundstrom, H. (1994). Prospects for a longer life expectancy. In D. Wise (Ed.), *Studies in the economics of aging* (pp. 79–94). Chicago: University of Chicago Press.

Verbrugge, L. M. (1991). Survival curves, prevalence rates, and dark matters therein. *Journal of Aging and Health, 3,* 217–236.

Verbrugge, L. M., & Jette, A. M. (1994). The disablement process. *Social Science and Medicine, 38,* 1–14.

Warren, J. R., & Hauser, R. M. (1997). Social stratification across three generations: New evidence from the Wisconsin longitudinal study. *American Sociological Review, 62,* 561–572.

Warren, J. R., Hauser, R. M., & Sheridan, J. (2002). Occupational stratification across the life course: Evidence from the Wisconsin longitudinal study. *American Sociological Review, 67,* 432–455.

Werner, E. E., & Smith, R. S. (2001). *Journeys from childhood to midlife: Risk, resilience and recovery.* Ithaca NY: Cornell University Press.

Western, B. (2002). The impact of incarceration on wage mobility and inequality. *American Sociological Review, 67,* 526–546.

Wickrama, K. A. S., Lorenz, F., & Conger, R. (1997). Parental support and adolescent physical health: A latent growth curve analysis. *Journal of Health and Social Behavior, 38,* 149–163.

Wilkinson, R. G. (Ed.). (1986). *Class and health: Research and longitudinal data.* London: Tavistock.

Wilkinson, R. G. (1996). *Unhealthy societies— The afflictions of inequality.* London: Routledge.

Williams, D. R., Mourney, R. L., & Warren, R. C. (1994). The concept of race and health status in America. *Public Health Reports, 109,* 26–41.

Wilson, W. J. (1987). *The truly disadvantaged.* Chicago IL: University of Chicago Press.

## Part Three

# Social Factors
# and
# Social Institutions

# Ten

# Intergenerational Family Transfers in Social Context

Merril Silverstein

A voluminous literature has emerged on the topic of intergenerational transfers within families. This research has gone well beyond the microeconomics of financial transfers to include time and labor transfers as well. Broadly defined, transfers refer to the intergenerational conveyance of resources from one generation to another. Much of the empirical literature on intergenerational relations in aging families investigates how generations are of assistance to each other but do not necessarily conceptualize these transactions as transfers per se (e.g., caregiving). The term *transfers* has a discernible meaning in the social sciences, and signals that a particular perspective is being taken. The literature on intergenerational family transfers specifically focuses on the structure and process of voluntary allocations of *valued resources* of money (cash and in-kind goods), time (labor services), and space (housing) across generational boundaries. This review focuses primarily on the transfer of resources that are explicitly conceptualized as exemplifying costs (to the sending generation) and benefits (to the receiving generation).

The study of intergenerational family transfers is gaining salience in the wake of globalization and the impending aging of national populations. In economically developed nations, policies that shift risk from public (government) to private (family) institutions are being followed with concern about the burden that families may experience when public transfer programs are under siege. The developing world is facing a different set of concerns that revolve around the possibility that rapid economic development will threaten traditional filial arrangements of mutual aid between generations. Policies intended to foster development are increasingly guided by global institutions, such as the World Bank, that have begun to take local family culture and transfer patterns into account when adopting strategies to allocate aid (The World Bank Group, 2005). In most nations of the world, declining fertility rates, increasing divorce rates, and changing gender roles are realigning the stock and flow of intergenerational transfers, causing anxiety over the continued viability of the family as a form of social

*Handbook of Aging and the Social Sciences, Sixth Edition*

insurance for its dependent members. To the extent that changes in social, economic, and political institutions have altered the incentive structure for intergenerational transfers and the relative wealth between generations, it has become ever more important to understand the socially situated motivations behind transfer behaviors, and the cross-generation metabolism—the ebb and flow—of transfers over the life span.

This review discusses emerging theoretical, conceptual, and empirical models of intergenerational transfers within the following thematic sections: (1) altruism, power, and reciprocity in family systems; (2) public-private interfaces; (3) corporate and mutual aid models; and (4) normative-moral perspectives.

## I. Altruism, Power, and Reciprocity in Family Systems

A transfer between generations, at its simplest level, is a dyadic affair, the transaction of goods and services between two individuals or households. Dyadic transfers are increasingly recognized as being nested within a complex network of related individuals that compose the family system. Implicit in the systems formulation is the notion that the family is a social organization that strives toward equilibrium by redistributing resources to where they are most needed (Klein & White, 1996). Particularly in societies with few public supports, family members are often intertwined in a web of mutually supportive transfers that ideally optimize the satisfaction of both personal and collective family needs.

Becker (1991) essentially relied on such a systemic model when developing the foundational principles for the modern field of household and family economics. In Becker's model, transfers are most efficient when an altruistic "dictator" allocates resources to where they will do the most good. For example, parents are vested in promoting the welfare of their children because producing high-quality children enhances the overall quality of the family unit over which the altruist presides. Based on this notion, Becker notoriously proposed the "rotten child" hypothesis, where even a putatively selfish child will make a transfer to his or her parent with the reasonable expectation that such a transfer maximizes the family's utility from which all members, including the "rotten child," will likely benefit.

Becker's emphasis on altruistic motivations ignited scholarly debates in family economics concerning the role of altruism as a guiding force behind the transfer of resources across generations. Evidence generally supports a model of transfers characterized by intergenerational altruism—where the transfer of money from richer to poorer individuals in the extended family provides evidence of altruistic tendencies. For instance, McGarry and Schoeni (1997) showed that adult children in the lowest income category were more than 50% more likely than those in the highest income category to receive a money transfer from their older parents. However, tests of altruistic motivations have provided mixed results, in large part, because the concept of altruism has been variously defined, and because evidence of its existence is necessarily inferred from behavior. Altonji, Hayashi, and Kotlkoff (1992), for example, found no evidence of what might be called "pure" altruism in their analysis of consumption patterns and extended family income. Because money transfers did not completely compensate for consumption inequalities across generations, transfers were not considered redistributive by the strict definition used by the researchers. Nor did the same team of scholars find that parents and children pooled resources to any great degree; upward and downward transfers that flowed to more needy generations tended to be small in absolute size (Altonji, Hayashi, & Kotlikoff, 1997, 2000).

That transfers are redistributive, but not strongly so, leads to consideration of constraints on altruistic tendencies that may result from strategic decisions by parents to temper provisions based on social considerations such as fear of inducing dependence in children, anticipation of envy among siblings, or worry about irresponsible consumption. The altruist is continuously at risk of being manipulated into providing more transfers than would be necessary to ensure the well-being of the recipient. For instance, needy adult children who make no effort to accumulate their own resources may exploit altruistic parents in a behavior known as *shirking*. Thus, even an altruistic provider may act strategically by tying transfers to a particular purpose or outcome, or by restricting the flow of transfers until shirking ceases (Gatti, 1999; Kotlikoff, Razin, & Rosenthal, 1990; Pollak, 1988).

Scholars have challenged Becker's corporate-altruistic model of family transfers on the grounds that his theory rests on the unsustainable assumption that preferences of the family head perfectly represent the preferences of other family members. Research finds that even when parents and children share the same goals, they make strategic decisions based on different sets of constraints and available alternatives. For instance, an older parent may prefer to receive care from a married adult daughter with children of her own. As care propensities tend to be lower among adult children who have competing family demands (Pezzin & Schone, 1999), however, this older parent may have little choice but to receive care from a less preferred, and possibly less willing, unmarried child, or move into an institution. In another example, wealthier children, for whom opportunity costs are higher, may be more likely to discharge their filial duty

to frail parents by purchasing formal services than by giving of their time (Altonji et al., 2000; Couch, Daly, & Wolf, 1999), a strategy that may or may not conform to parental expectations of what constitutes an appropriate response.

Most notable among Becker's critics are scholars who stress the importance of bargaining power in how family decisions are resolved. The decision by children to provide care to frail older parents is modeled within a game theoretical framework that takes into account conflicting interests and preferences among adult children, and between parents and children (Lundberg & Pollak, 2001; Pezzin & Schone, 1999; Pollak, 1988). In this framework, co-residence and the provision of care are decided in a two-stage process. First, parents and children must make a joint decision regarding co-residence based on an understanding of each other's intentions. Second, the allocation of care responsibilities is made under the constraints of the bargaining positions dictated by the living arrangement chosen. For example, Pezzin, Pollak, and Schone (2004) described the case of a daughter who invites a parent into her household with the understanding that a sister will help out from afar. After such a move, bargaining power weakens for the co-resident sister and strengthens for the non–co-resident sister, who is safe in the knowledge that the parent will not likely be evicted. One possible outcome is that the non–co-resident sister may not provide the support promised (a "free-rider" problem), or be reluctant to provide money knowing that the co-resident sister would also benefit from such a transfer. Thus, transfer decisions can be seen as the outcome of the strategic deliberations of multiple family members that take into account the anticipated preferences, actions, and bargaining power of others in the family system.

Recognizing that power differentials may be used as leverage to strategically exact resources from others in the family, Bernheim, Shleifer, and Summers showed that parents may use the threat of withholding a bequest to obtain assistance or attention from their children. In a recent test that supported this model, Caputo (2002) found that children tended to provide money transfers to parents who had surplus capital available for bequests. However, bequests, unlike in inter-vivo transfers, have strongly gravitated toward a norm of equal distribution (McGarry, 1999; Wilhelm, 1996), potentially undercutting their coercive power over children.

Much of the evidence supporting the role of power in determining intergenerational transfers comes from less developed societies, where family farming is the dominant mode of production. Older parents who control arable land may use their control of those assets to demand resources from children (Cox, 1987). The strong obligation to provide care to elders in rural areas is thought to derive from the bargaining power that land ownership confers on the elderly (Caffrey, 1992; Stark, 1995; Tsuya & Martin, 1992), the legacy of which is still seen in rural regions of developed nations (Groger, 1992; King, Silverstein, Elder, Bengtson, & Conger, 2004; Silverstein, Burholt, Wenger, & Bengtson, 1998). In societies suffering under chronic abject poverty, adult children may use their scarce resources for the betterment of their children rather than devote them to elderly parents who have few assets to share and whose dependence has become a burden (Aboderin, 2004). An alternative explanation relies on nonpecuniary motivations of children with wealthier parents. Studies in several Asian nations suggest that in the absence of elderly parents' economic dependence on children, the quality of the parent-child relationship improves, thus increasing the willingness of children to provide support (Chow, 1993; Ng, Phillips, & Lee, 2002).

Theories of intergenerational transfers that emphasize exchange share the premise that social relationships are governed by a norm of reciprocity—the expectation that a social debt should be repaid (Gouldner, 1960; Molm & Cook, 1995). Family members transfer valued resources to others to attract resources of equal or greater value, a perspective rooted in rational choice theory (Becker, 1974), as well as theories of moral economy and small group cohesion (Homans, 1950; Mauss, 1967; Whitbeck, Simons, & Conger, 1991).

Point-in-time empirical tests of intergenerational reciprocity in the United States are equivocal about whether older parents receive instrumental services from children in exchange for providing financial support to them. Several investigations have shown such a relationship (Caputo, 2002; Cox & Rank, 1992), but others have not (Altonji et al., 1997; McGarry & Schoeni, 1997). Cross-sectional research designs may fail to detect reciprocal transfers, however, because family members in more developed nations tend to assist each other intermittently, and reciprocation may be lagged by many years. Reciprocation need not be immediate or made in units equivalent to the initial investment for the exchange to be considered balanced over the long term (Hollstein & Bria, 1998). Research examining long-term serial patterns of intergenerational exchange found that parents who provided financial assistance to their young-adult children tended to receive more social support from them in old age (Henretta, Hill, Li, Soldo, & Wolf, 1997; Silverstein, Conroy, Wang, Giarrusso, & Bengtson, 2002). In a more general test of reciprocity as a motive for transfers, Ikkink, Van Tilburg, and Knipscheer (1999) used data from adult children in the Netherlands to show that the perception of reciprocity—the sense that they were repaying an earlier parental transfer—was a defining feature of those who provided social support to their older parents.

It has become increasingly clear, however, that motivations for transfers are mixed and not easily distinguished. For instance, Stark and Falk (1998) considered altruism and reciprocity to be a false dichotomy; altruistic transfers typically trigger gratitude from the recipient, the value of which is dependent on the emotional closeness of the relationship. Indeed, it has long been known that the strength of emotional bonds between parents and children is positively correlated with the volume of intergenerational transfers between them (Rossi & Rossi, 1990; Silverstein, Parrott, & Bengtson, 1995; Whitbeck, Simons, & Conger, 1991). Sloan, Zhang, and Wang (2002) noted that emotional and transactional approaches to transfers are virtually inseparable; time-for-money exchanges are as consistent with the principle of reciprocity as they are with "double-sided" altruism, where each generation makes transfers for the gratitude they elicit from the other. The blurred distinction between altruistic and self-interested motivations is further highlighted by the notion that providing support is also an act of "demonstration"; adult children may benevolently support their older parents, at least partially, to demonstrate to their offspring that providing parental support is an important duty of children, a form of child socialization from which they eventually hope to benefit (Cox & Stark, 1992).

Divorce and remarriage, as naturally occurring life events, provide a good test of the social basis for intergenerational transfers. Numerous studies have found that parental divorce weakens or severs the flow of upward and downward transfers of money and time between parents and their biological adult children, and that parental remarriage does the same between stepparents (mostly fathers) and their stepchildren (Amato, Rezac, &

Booth, 1995; Aquilino, 1994; Furstenberg, Hoffman, & Shesthra, 1995; Hogan, Eggebeen, & Clogg, 1993; Pezzin & Schone, 1999; Silverstein & Bengtson, 1997; Spitze & Logan, 1992). Divorce has been shown to disrupt transfer flows by weakening normative beliefs about intergenerational responsibility (Ganong & Coleman, 1998) and by reducing opportunities for interaction and the development of emotional cohesion between generations (Aquilino, 1994).

The impact of divorce on intergenerational transfers is greater on fathers, who typically do not receive primary custody of their children. Furstenberg, Hoffman, and Shesthra (1995) found that a shortfall in the amount of money divorced fathers contributed to child support did not compensate for the negative effect that separation had on support received from children later in life, essentially rejecting an economic basis for their support deficit. This suggests that lower intergenerational transfer rates to divorced fathers are also a function of their diminished investments of time and emotion in their natural children. In terms of downward transfers within stepfamilies, Pezzin and Schone (1999) found that fathers were not sensitive in responding to the needs of stepchildren, concluding from this that empathetic altruism was not a relevant social force in the stepfamilies of fathers. The age of children when the stepparent entered the family may be an important mitigating factor, however, under the assumption that sharing more time together in a common household allows the stepfather to better integrate into his new family.

Research on the transfer behaviors of grandparents tends to attribute their contributions to the family in terms of altruism and self-sacrifice. Indeed, grandparents who intervene to raise grandchildren in response to parental crises and incapacities often do this at great cost to their material, physical, and psychological well-being (Minkler, Fuller-Thomson,

Miller, & Driver, 2000; Minkler & Roe, 1993). Contemporary studies documenting the extraordinary efforts of grandparents as caregivers is consistent with theories from evolutionary biology positing that human longevity resulted from the favorable selection of able grandparents who could better ensure the survival of their grandchildren (Hawkes, O'Connell, Jones, Alvarez, & Charnov, 1998). The importance of downward transfers from grandparents has also been recognized under more ordinary circumstances, especially in their provision of childcare to working parents. Nationally, grandparents provided an estimated $17 to $29 billion annually in unpaid supervision and care of their grandchildren (Bass & Caro, 1996). Cardia and Ng (2003) found that parents who received childcare services from grandparents improved their economic status by increasing their paid labor force participation and avoiding formal childcare costs. On the other hand, direct money transfers from grandparents had little economic effect because such assistance reduced the amount of time that parents worked in the paid labor force.

Direct transfers of money from grandparents to their grandchildren are not uncommon. A study of three-generation families in France found that one-third of grandparents provided a financial transfer to at least one adult grandchild (Attias-Donfut, 2003). More than half of the grandchildren in this study provided supportive services to their grandparents, suggesting that flows of assistance are reciprocal. It is likely that grandparents will become more important to their grandchildren if recent fertility declines cause grandparents to compete ever more vigorously for the attention of fewer available grandchildren in their families (Uhlenberg, 2005).

Grandparents play a crucial role in maintaining the economic viability of families in many developing nations (Hermalin, Roan, & Perez, 1998). It is common for grandparents in rural China to act as surrogate parents when their adult children migrate to find work in urban areas (Chen, Short, & Entwisle, 2000; Sando, 1986). Childcare provided by grandparents allows adult children to seek out more promising labor markets and provide greater remittances in return (Agree, Biddlecom, Chang, & Perez, 2002; Yang, 1996). Grandparents are often key figures for maintaining family well-being in regions of the world wracked by disaster, war, and famine. The World Bank, for instance, in developing an action strategy for providing economic aid to the most dire regions, notes that in Africa, "AIDS orphans are often raised on the meager incomes of their grandparents, which makes it crucial to. . . start focusing on the provision of intra-family support mechanisms." (The World Bank Group, 2005).

## II. Public-Private Interfaces

Intergenerational transfers need to be understood within the context of national and international political economies. Most Western governments have sought to reduce their commitment to their elderly populations and shift more responsibility to older individuals and their families (O'Rand, 2003). Under pressures of globalization and the expansion of free-market trade, the role of government in providing for its most vulnerable citizens has weakened (Estes, 2003; Phillipson, 2003). The question of whether private transfers will compensate for retractions in government benefits is at the heart of current debates about how risk and responsibility for old age security will be allocated.

Recent literature on intergenerational transfers has illuminated the linkage between direct transfers between generations in the family and indirect transfers between age groups in the population.

In this regard, individuals simultaneously occupy two different types of generational positions, one defined by the rank order of the family lineage and the other defined by cohort membership and its corresponding age-based entitlements (Attias-Donfut & Arber, 2000). These generational positions are functionally interdependent, such that family transfers are sensitive to social policies that regulate the flow of resources across cohorts in the population. Current debate centers on whether generous state transfer programs disrupt or substitute for intra-family transfers. Evidence from European nations suggests that state and family contributions to older adults are best described as mutual and complementary, with a decided tilt toward public-mediated transfers in nations with the most elaborate welfare systems (Attias-Donfut & Wolff, 2000; Künemund & Rein, 1999).

Direct assessments of a compensatory linkage between social policy initiatives and intergenerational transfers point to just such a linkage. Comparative studies across European nations found that personal care and financial support were more commonly provided to parents in nations with weaker welfare provisions, though much of this effect was due to the higher rates of intergenerational co-residence found in those nations (Daatland & Herlofson, 2003; Glaser & Tomassini, 2000; Lowenstein, Katz, & Daatland, 2005). A study in Sweden found an increase in the proportion of elders served by families over the same historical period that public policies restricted eligibility for in-home services (Sundstrom, Johansson, & Hassing, 2002). In Germany, Kohli (2005) showed that an increase in transfers from older to younger generations was partially produced by the upgrading of state pensions among retirees in the former East Germany. The interdependence of personal and collective transfers can also be viewed in terms of the effects that public policy changes have on *anticipated* transfers from children. Yi (1994) found that fertility rates declined in an area of rural China where an experimental pension program was initiated. On further investigation, he found that pension availability weakened the belief that having children was necessary to ensure old age security.

Economists in particular have focused on transfer motivations, particularly altruism, as key to creating social policy that produces the most efficient balance between public and private support to older citizens. In this line of reasoning, public transfer programs partially neutralize the contributions of altruistically motivated children who would tend to increase their contributions were public transfers reduced. Thus, public transfer programs are viewed as compelling less-than-altruistic children to make transfers indirectly through payroll taxes, but such indirect transfers cease to be efficient when they are at a level that saves the altruistic child from contributing directly out-of-pocket. Minimalist transfer programs serving the elderly, however, may reinforce the exploitation of well-intentioned but self-sacrificing family members, especially daughters and daughters-in-law who bear the heaviest load of filial care. Attempts to advance the cause of generational equity by cutting benefits to the older generation may exacerbate gender inequity in the younger generation (Attias-Donfut & Arber, 2000).

In most modern, highly developed nations, economic transfers between generations are far more likely to flow downward from parents to children than in the reverse direction (Attias-Donfut & Wolf, 2000; Fritzell & Lennartsson, 2005; Künemund, Motel-Klingebiel, & Kohli, 2005; Lee, Parish, & Willis, 1994; Lowenstein et al., 2005; Spilerman, 2004). Further, the beneficiaries of downward transfers tend to be children with lower income and with social characteristics that suggest greater need. Künemund et al. (2005) found in Germany that children who were divorced or separated were more likely than married children to receive financial transfers from parents, supporting the premise that pensions are redistributive and reduce social class inequalities within families. There is evidence that the expectation for downward transfers has become institutionalized as a societal norm in modern societies, especially where the costs of household and family formation are prohibitively high for young adults (Spilerman & Elmelech, 2003).

That retirees have surplus wealth to transfer at all is sometimes taken as evidence that pensions in welfare states are too high. Some argue that an indirect circular flow of capital—from taxpayers to pensioners and back to taxpayers—only returns money to its source, and as such is an inefficient redistribution system. On the other hand, there may be advantages to be gained when transfers take a "detour" through the older generation. Parents are well positioned to evaluate the needs of their children and best able to make nuanced judgments about which of them deserve support. In addition, downward transfers may stimulate time transfers from children (visiting, social support) and serve to strengthen intergenerational solidarity (Attias-Donfut, 2000). Evidence also suggests that older people derive a greater sense of self-efficacy from being an altruistic provider to needy family members (Künemund & Rein, 1999).

The lifecycle transfer model advanced by R. D. Lee (2000, 2003) seeks to explain the intergenerational balance of made transfers by placing them in the context of how societies organize production and consumption schedules over the lifespan. In hunter and gatherer societies, the human life span is characterized by very low productivity in youth, surplus productivity in young adulthood that continues to middle-age, followed by an old age mostly devoted to

improving the production skills of children (Hill & Kaplan, 1999). Notably, the value of contributed labor exceeds consumption levels over almost the entire adult life span, such that net transfers are predominantly downward until a relatively short period of dependence before death.

By contrast, intergenerational reallocation in modern industrial societies operates through family transfers, as well as through market and public sector transfers. Sizable downward flows of resources to children in terms of cash, transfers, gifts, and bequests are balanced against upward flows to older adults through pension and other state-mediated programs (R. D. Lee, 2000). The high costs associated with raising children, especially education costs, "are more than offset by capital accumulation . . . and by strong upward transfers through the public sector" (R.D. Lee, 2000, p. 54). By comparing intergenerational flows across drastically different economic regimes, the lifecycle model challenges the orthodoxy of conventional demographic theory (Caldwell, 1976) by countering its assumption that modernization necessarily lowers the net value of children for old age security. Today, the value of children needs to be considered on a collective as well as a personal basis.

## III. Corporate and Mutual Aid Models

Older people in poorer nations of the world tend to rely predominantly or exclusively on family to satisfy their basic needs. For instance, many less developed Asian nations have few public provisions for their older populations and mandate that adult children provide eldercare as both a duty and a legal responsibility. In these contexts, cultural values of filial piety and the need to conserve scarce public resources are in alignment, with the burden put squarely on families. Viewed in this light, families serve a public function in that the state is saved the costs of supporting older adults.

Two related models of reciprocal exchange have been used to describe the interdependence of generations in less developed nations: the mutual aid model and the corporate-group model. The mutual aid model emphasizes the functional unity of the family and specifies that intergenerational transfers are isomorphic with the needs and resources of each generation. A "time-for-money" exchange between generations describes a common type of mutual aid in Asian families, where parents provide household labor and/or childcare services to the families of their adult children in exchange for money or food (Frankenberg, Lillard, & Willis, 2002; Lee et al., 1994; Lee & Xiao, 1998; Lillard & Willis, 1997; Sun, 2002).

A corporate model of transfers emphasizes the power of the household head to strategically allocate resources where they will produce the best benefit—much like Becker's altruistic dictator. Investing in the human capital of children exemplifies such a strategy. Funding higher education improves the quality of children and better ensures that they will have sufficient resources to provide for the old age security of their parents. Indeed, studies of intergenerational transfers in Malaysia, Taiwan, Indonesia, Korea, and China have demonstrated that older parents were more likely to receive financial support from their more highly educated children (Frankenberg et al., 2002; Y. J. Lee, 2000; Lee & Xiao, 1998; Lee et al., 1994; Lillard & Willis, 1997; Riley, 1994; Sun, 2002). Parents in these patrilineal societies found it particularly advantageous to invest in the education of sons over daughters (e.g., Lin et al., 2003), suggesting a cultural template that overlays power and exchange dynamics within families in the developing world.

Cultural values and economic conditions synergistically shape the nature of intergenerational transfers in less developed nations. Frankenberg and Kuhn (2005) compared patterns of transfers between older parents and their children in Bangladesh and Indonesia, two societies that are similar in many respects but differ in their levels of economic development and gender norms. They found that intergenerational transfer activity is higher overall, as well as more gender neutral, in Indonesia, where women have greater economic freedom, than in less affluent Bangladesh, where transfers are almost exclusively from son to parent. Research by Ofstedal, Reidy, and Knodel (2004) found similar patterns in a larger set of Asian nations, suggesting that greater prosperity and gender egalitarianism—both aspects of modernization—determine how resources are allocated within the family.

In Bangladesh, Kabir, Szebehely, and Tishelman (2002) also found a gendered division of labor, with sons predominating as financial providers to their parents, and daughters as providers of instrumental help. Older parents in rural areas also contributed substantial amounts of household labor to their children, enabled by high rates of intergenerational co-residence and neo-local living arrangements. The interdependence of generations in this poor region of Bangladesh is to a large degree the function of the strong need to pool resources across generations and the opportunity to do so. Thus, it is not surprising that high levels of international emigration from Bangladesh have imposed substantial economic burdens on sending households and communities. However, these costs appear to be at least somewhat offset by the return flow of capital from abroad, however; remittances appear to compensate for the travel and set-up costs of overseas migrants, as well as the opportunity costs of having children (mostly sons) who are absent from household production activities (Burholt & Wenger, 2005; Rahman, 1999). Research in Taiwan and the Philippines similarly found that remittances were greater from children who moved from rural to urban areas, confirming the remittance-as-reciprocity hypothesis (Domingo & Asis, 1995; Lee et al., 1994).

In summary, both mutual aid and corporate models are characterized by reciprocal exchanges between generations, the former a shorter-term strategy and the latter a longer-term strategy for reducing uncertainty in societies with weak public sectors. Each strategy enhances the ability of the recipient to reciprocate. Sun (2002) synthesized corporate and mutual aid frameworks into one systemic model "which treats family as a closely related network that cares for the well-being of all family members and seeks optimal distribution of resources within the family network" (p. 339). In developing nations where formal mechanisms of support are rare or nonexistent, exchanges do not necessarily take on the form of direct, dyadic reciprocity, but may be manifest as a complex diffusion of indirect and generalized flows of resources between and within generations (see Agree, Biddlecom, Valente, & Chang, 2001; Attias-Dunfut, 2003).

## IV. Normative-Moral Perspectives on Transfers

Exchange dynamics in families follow normative guidelines that are quite different from those found in market and other non-kin relationships. Particularly, with regard to parent-child relations, there is often an extended lag between the time that dependent children receive resources from parents and the time they are called on as adults to provide old age support to their parents. Long gaps between transfers may serve to depreciate the value of the parent's original investment and threaten confidence in the child's willingness to reciprocate. As a result, parents may come to count more on their children's internalized values than on their gratitude for contributions going back to childhood.

Given that intergenerational family relationships are without formal contracts, the possibility always remains that an opportunistic child may renege on the implicit expectation to reciprocate for earlier transfers. The potential for uncertainty in what is essentially a contractually unregulated transaction demands that motivations be reinforced by internalized commitments or a sense of moral duty on the part of the adult child. Becker formalized this notion in his Nobel lecture, suggesting that parents may attempt to instill "guilt, obligation, duty, and filial love that indirectly, but still very effectively, can 'commit' children to helping them out (in old age)" (1992, p. 50).

Social exchange theory provides a useful paradigm for understanding intergenerational transactions that goes beyond the rational self-interest model to include the nature of the role relationship between the exchange partners, as well as their mutual history of transactions and their degree of interdependence. Molm and Cook put it this way: "whereas classical microeconomic theory typically assumed the absence of long-term relations between exchange partners and the independence of sequential exchange transactions, social exchange theory took as its subject matter . . . the more or less enduring relations that form between specific partners (1995, p. 210)." This approach takes as its unit of analysis the relationship itself, and the social expectations for behavior that define the linked roles of "parent" and "child" in the family.

Yet family role expectations are not static. The moral hazard of having noncompliant children in modern societies such as the United States may be exacerbated by what some cultural critics have called the weakening fabric of social life over the last half-century (Bellah, Madsen, Sullivan, Swidler, & Tipton,

1985; Hareven, 1996; Putnam, 1995). Some scholars posit that radical changes in family structure resulting from historically unprecedented divorce and remarriage rates have weakened the capacity and willingness of adult children to provide support to their aging parents (Glenn, 1997; Popenoe, 1988). Others consider the family to be a resilient social institution and, even in its altered form, still capable of serving the needs of its vulnerable members (Bengtson, 2001; Kain, 1990). In fact, the obligation to provide care for older family members is a moral precept found in almost all social groupings (Stein et al., 1998). What then compels children to abide by cultural scripts associated with their position in the family? One line of thinking is that parents (as well as other family members, teachers, community institutions, and media) inculcate normative principles in their children that promote compassion and service to older parents (Silverstein & Conroy, in press). The intergenerational transmission of these values has implications for resource flows and the strength of the social contract between generations and may explain why intergenerational continuity and solidarity has endured in the face of disruptive social forces (Attias-Donfut, 2000).

## V. Conclusion

This review has touched on several themes in the family literature that place the motivations and conditions for intergenerational transfers within a larger social context. These contexts included the family as a social system of interacting individuals, the broader social-political-economic environments within which families function, and the cultural climate that sets parameters on expectations across generations. Although the principle of altruism appears to be the dominant motive behind intergenerational transfers, there are distinct variations on

this theme that bring into focus concepts of deference, power, competition, and reciprocity. These concepts advance our understanding of how families strategize to optimally satisfy individual and collective needs under resource constraints.

Among the most important and striking investigations of intergenerational transfers over the last decade are those that have taken historical-comparative or multinational approaches to the subject. Family members make choices within social structures, political economies, and cultural contexts that constrain or enhance opportunities and incentives to engage in transfer behavior across multiple generations. Social and economic changes currently under way in developing nations have altered family structures and household arrangements and, by some accounts, weakened traditional norms of filial piety. The consequences of these changes for family preferences and practices, and the well-being of older and younger generations, will be topics of research for many years to come.

Relatively recent changes in family size and structure have raised questions about the ability of the kinship unit to serve the needs of its members. Indeed, in some developed countries the very basis of intergenerational life—the availability of children—has been put in jeopardy by plummeting fertility rates, with possibly dire consequences for the vitality of intergenerational transfer programs. Current efforts to privatize Social Security in the United States and elsewhere threaten to disrupt the circular flow of resources across generations and abrogate the implicit intergenerational contract between the young and old in society, as well as in the family. Many of those in birth cohorts that experienced the brunt of the divorce revolution may in later life have doubtful prospects for upward and downward intergenerational transfers given the growth in step-relations and disrupted biological relations. Women in these cohorts, however, having benefited from the opening of education and labor market opportunities, may enter old age with enhanced personal resources to transfer to their children, if they have any.

Multigenerational families in developed and developing nations most likely will adapt to economic and cultural changes of the twenty-first century. Intergenerational transfers will undoubtedly remain an integral part of family life, even as the cross-generation calculus of resources and needs shifts in response to the pressures of globalization and the aging of populations. If Bengtson (2001) is correct about the positive influence of the longevity revolution on intergenerational solidarity, then the sheer increase in shared lifetimes between parents and children may give rise to new opportunities for resource-sharing across generations. Similarly, but more pragmatically, if public provisions to dependent populations have reached or surpassed their upper limit, then intergenerational transfers may become an ever more prominent survival strategy for families in the future.

## References

Aboderin, I. (2004). Decline in material family support for older people in urban Ghana, Africa: Understanding processes and causes of change. *Journals of Gerontology: Series B: Psychological Sciences and Social Sciences, 59B*(3), S128–S137.

Agree, E. M., Biddlecom, A. E., Chang, M., & Perez, A. E. (2002). Transfers from older parents to their adult children in Taiwan and the Philippines. *Journal of Cross-Cultural Gerontology, 17*, 269–294.

Agree, E. M., Biddlecom, A. E., Valente, T.W., & Chang, M. (2001). Social network measures of parent-child exchange: Applications in Taiwan & the Philippines. *Connections, 24*(2), 59–75.

Altonji, J. G., Hayashi, F., & Kotlikoff, L. J. (1992). Is the extended family altruistically linked? Direct tests using micro data. Panel Study of Income Dynamics. *The American Economic Review, 82*, 1177–1198.

Altonji, J., Hayashi, F., & Kotlikoff, L. (1997). Parental altruism and inter vivos transfers: Theory and evidence, *Journal of Political Economy, 105*(6), 1121–1166.

Altonji, J. G., Hayashi, F., & Kotlikoff, L. J. (2000). The effects of income and wealth on time and money transfers between parents and children. In A. Mason & G. Tapinos (Eds.), *Sharing the wealth: Demographic change and economic transfers between generations* (pp. 306–357). Oxford: Oxford University Press.

Amato, P. R., Rezac, S. J., & Booth, A. (1995). Helping between parents and young-adult offspring: The role of parental marital quality, divorce, and remarriage. *Journal of Marriage and the Family, 57*(2), 363–374.

Aquilino, W. S. (1994). Impact of childhood family disruption on young-adults' relationships with parents. *Journal of Marriage and the Family, 56*(2), 295–313.

Attias-Donfut, C. (2000). Cultural and economic transfers between generations: One aspect of age integration. *The Gerontologist, 40*, 270–272.

Attias-Donfut, C. (2003). Family transfers and cultural transmissions between three generations in France. In V. L. Bengtson & A. Lowenstein (Eds.), *Global aging and challenges to families* (pp. 214–252). Hawthorne, NY: Aldine de Gruyter.

Attias-Donfut, C., & Arber, S. (2000). Equity and solidarity across the generations. In S. Arber & C. Attias-Donfut (Eds.), *The myth of generational conflict: The family and state in ageing societies* (pp. 1–21). London: Routledge.

Attias-Donfut, C., & Wolff, F. (2000). Complementarity between private and public transfers. In S. Arber & C. Attias-Donfut (Eds.), *The myth of generational conflict: The family and state in ageing societies* (pp. 47–68). London: Routledge.

Bass, S. A., & Caro, F. G. (1996). The economic value of grandparent assistance. *Generations, 20*, 29–33.

Becker, G. S. (1974). A theory of social interactions. *Journal of Political Economy, 82*(6), 1063–1093.

Becker, G. S. (1991). *A treatise on the family.* (enlarged edition). Cambridge: Harvard University Press.

Becker, G. (1992). *The economic way of looking at life*, Nobel Lecture, December 9.

Bellah, R. N., Madsen, R., Sullivan, W. M., Swidler, A., & Tipton, S. M. (1985). *Habits of the heart: Individualism and commitment in American life*. Berkeley, CA: University of California Press.

Bengtson, V. L. (2001). Beyond the nuclear family: The increasing importance of multigenerational relationships in American society. The 1998 Burgess Award Lecture. *Journal of Marriage and Family, 63*, 1–16.

Bernheim, D., Shleifer, A., & Summers, L. (1985). The strategic bequest motive. *Journal of Political Economy, 33*, 1045–1076.

Burholt, V., & Wenger, G. C. (2005). Migration from South Asia to the United Kingdom and the maintenance of transnational intergenerational relationships. In M. Silverstein (Ed.), *Intergenerational relations across time and place. Annual Review of Gerontology and Geriatrics* (Vol. 24, pp. 153–176). New York: Springer.

Caffrey, R. A. (1992). Family care of the elderly in Northeast Thailand. *Journal of Cross Cultural Gerontology, 7*(2), 105–116.

Caldwell, J. C. (1976). Toward a restatement of demographic transition theory. *Population and Development Review, 2*(3–4), 321–66.

Caputo, R. K. (2002). Rational actors versus rational agents. *Journal of Family and Economic Issues, 23*(1), 27–50.

Cardia, E., & Ng, S. (2003). Intergenerational time transfers and childcare. *Review of Economic Dynamics, 6*(2), 431–454.

Chen, F., Short, S. E., & Entwisle, B. (2000). The impact of grandparental proximity on maternal childcare in China. *Population Research and Policy Review, 19*(6), 571–590.

Chow, N. (1993). Changing responsibilities of the state and family toward elders in Hong Kong. *Journal of Aging and Social Policy, 5*(1–2), 111–126.

Couch, K. A., Daly, M. C., & Wolf, D.A. (1999). Time? Money? Both? The allocation of resources to older parents. *Demography, 36*(2), 219–232.

Cox, D. (1987). Motives for private income transfers. *Journal of Political Economy, 95*, 508–546.

Cox, D., & Rank, M. R. (1992). Inter-vivos transfers and intergenerational exchange. *The Review of Economics and Statistics, 74*, 305–314.

Cox, D., & Stark, O. (1992). Intergenerational transfers and the demonstration effect (working paper). Unpublished.

Daatland, O. D., & Herlofson, K. (2003). 'Lost solidarity' or 'changed solidarity': A comparative European view of normative family solidarity. *Ageing and Society, 23*, 537–560.

Domingo, L. J., & Asis, M.M.B. (1995). Living arrangements and the flow of support between generations in the Philippines. *Journal of Cross-Cultural Gerontology, 10*, 21–51.

Estes, C. L. (2003). Theoretical perspectives on old age policy: A critique and a proposal. In S. Biggs, A. Lowenstein & J. Hendricks (Eds.), *The need for theory: Critical approaches to social gerontology* (pp. 219–243). Amityville, NY: Baywood.

Frankenberg, E., & Kuhn, R. (2005). The role of social context in shaping intergenerational relations in Indonesia and Bangladesh. In M. Silverstein (Ed.), *Intergenerational relations across time and place. Annual review of gerontology and geriatrics* (Vol. 24, pp. 177–199). New York: Springer.

Frankenberg, E., Lillard, L., & Willis, R. J. (2002). Patterns of intergenerational transfers in Southeast Asia. *Journal of Marriage and the Family, 64*, 627–641.

Fritzell, J., & Lennartsson, C. (2005). Financial transfers between generations in Sweden. *Ageing & Society 25*, 1–18.

Furstenberg, F. F., Hoffman, S.D., & Shrestha, L. (1995). The effect of divorce on intergenerational transfers: New evidence. *Demography, 32*, 319–333.

Ganong, L. H., & Coleman, M. (1998). Attitudes regarding filial responsibilities to help elderly divorced parents and stepparents. *Journal of Aging Studies, 12*(3), 271–290.

Gatti, R. (1999). *Family, altruism, and incentives*. Policy Research Working Paper Series, 2505. The World Bank.

Glaser, K., & Tomassini, C. (2000). Proximity of older women to their children: A comparison of Britain and Italy. *The Gerontologist, 40*(6), 7729–7737.

Glenn, N. D. (1997). A critique of twenty marriage and family textbooks. *Family Relations, 46*, 197–208.

Groger, L. (1992). Tied to each other through ties to the land: Informal support of Black elders in a southern U.S. community. *Journal of Cross-Cultural Gerontology, 7*(3), 205–220.

Gouldner, A. W. (1960). The norm of reciprocity: A preliminary statement. *American Sociological Review, 25,* 161–178.

Hareven, T. K. (1996). Historical perspectives on the family and aging. In R. Blieszner & V.H. Bedford (Eds.), *Aging and the family: Theory and research* (pp. 13–31). Westport, CT: Greenwood Press.

Hawkes, K., O'Connell, J. F., Jones, N. G. B., Alvarez, H., & Charnov, E. L. (1998). Grandmothering, menopause, and the evolution of human life histories. *Proceedings of the National Academy of Sciences, 95,* 1336–1339.

Henretta, J. C., Hill, M. S., Li, W., Soldo, B. J., & Wolf, D. A. (1997). Selection of children to provide care: The effect of earlier parental transfers. *Journal of Gerontology, Series B: Psychological Sciences and Social Sciences, 52,* 110–119.

Hermalin, A. I., Roan, C., & Perez, A.E. (1998). The emerging role of grandparents in Asia. *Elderly in Asia Research Report No. 98–52.* Ann Arbor, MI: University of Michigan.

Hill, K., & Kaplan, H. (1999). Life history traits in humans: Theory and empirical studies. *Annual Review of Anthropology 28,* 397–430.

Hogan, D. P., Eggebeen, D. J., & Clogg, C. C. (1993). The structure of intergenerational exchanges in American families. *American Journal of Sociology, 98*(6), 1428–1458.

Hollstein, B., & Bria, G. (1998). Reciprocity in parent-child relationships? Theoretical considerations and empirical evidence. *Berliner Journal fur Soziologie, 8,* 7–22.

Homans, G. C. (1950). *The human group.* New York: Harcourt, Brace and World.

Ikkink, K. K., Van Tilburg, T., & Knipscheer, K. (1999). Perceived instrumental support exchanges in relationships between elderly parents and their adult children: Normative and structural explanations. *Journal of Marriage and the Family, 61*(4), 831–844.

Kabir, Z. N., Szebehely, M., & Tishelman, C. (2002). Support in old age in the changing society of Bangladesh. *Ageing and Society, 22,* 615–636.

Kain, E. L. (1990). *The myth of family decline: Understanding families in a world of rapid social change.* Lexington, MA: Lexington Books.

King, V., Silverstein, M., Elder, G. H., Bengtson, V. L., & Conger, R. D. (2004). Relations with grandparents: Rural Midwest versus urban Southern California. *Journal of Family Issues, 24*(8), 1044–1069.

Klein, D. M., & White, J. M. (1996). *Family theories: An introduction.* Thousand Oaks, CA: Sage.

Kohli, M. (2005). Intergenerational transfers and inheritance: A comparative view. In M. Silverstein (Ed.), *Intergenerational relations across time and place. Annual review of gerontology and geriatrics* (Vol. 24, pp. 266–289). New York: Springer.

Kotlikoff, L. J., Razin, A., & Rosenthal, R. W. (1990). A strategic altruism model in which Ricardian equivalence does not hold. *Economic Journal, 100*(403), 1261–1268.

Künemund, H., Motel-Klingebiel, A., & Kohli, M. (2005). Do intergenerational transfers from elderly parents increase social inequality among their middle-aged children? Evidence from the German Aging Survey. *Journal of Gerontology: Social Sciences, 60B*(1), S30–S36.

Künemund, H., & Rein, M. (1999). There is more to receiving than needing: Theoretical arguments and empirical explorations of crowding in and crowding out. *Ageing and Society, 19*(1), 93–121.

Lee, R. D. (2000). Intergenerational transfers and the economic life cycle: A cross-cultural perspective. In A. Mason & G. Tapinos (Eds.), *Sharing the wealth: Demographic change and economic transfers between generations* (pp.17–56). Oxford: Oxford University Press.

Lee, R. D. (2003). Rethinking the evolutionary theory of aging: Transfers, not births, shape senescence in social species. *Proceedings of the National Academy of Sciences, 100*(16), 9637–9642.

Lee, Y. J. (2000). Support between rural parents and migrant children in a rapidly industrializing society: South Korea. In A. Mason & Liege (Eds.), *Sharing the wealth: Demographic change and economic transfers between generations* (pp. 282–305). Honolulu: IUSSP-East-West Center.

Lee, Y. J., Parish, W. L., & Willis, R. J. (1994). Sons, daughters, and intergenerational support in Taiwan. *American Journal of Sociology, 99*, 1010–1041.

Lee, Y. J., & Xiao, Z. (1998). Children's support for elderly parents in urban and rural China: Results from a national survey. *Journal of Cross-Cultural Gerontology, 13*, 39–62.

Lillard, L. A., & Willis, R. J. (1997). Motives for intergenerational transfers: Evidence from Malaysia. *Demography, 34*(1), 115–134.

Lin, I.-F., Goldman, N., Weinstein, M., Lin, Y.-H., Gorrindo, T., & Seeman, T. (2003). Gender differences in adult children's support of their parents. *Taiwan Journal of Marriage and the Family, 65*(1), 184–200.

Lowenstein, A., Katz, R., & Daatland, S. O. (2005). Filial norms and intergenerational support in Europe and Israel: A comparative perspective. In M. Silverstein (Ed.), *Intergenerational relations across time and place. Annual review of gerontology and geriatrics* (Vol. 24, pp. 200–223). New York: Springer.

Lundberg, S., & Pollak, R. A. (2001). Bargaining and distribution in families. In A. Thornton (Ed.), *The well-being of children and families: Research and data needs* (pp. 314–338). Ann Arbor: University of Michigan Press.

Mauss, M. (1967). *The gift: Forms and functions of exchange in archaic societies.* Translated by Ian Cunnison. New York: Norton (Original work published in 1923).

McGarry, K. (1999). Inter vivos transfers and intended bequests. *Journal of Public Economics, 73*, 321–351.

McGarry, K., & Schoeni, R. F. (1997). Transfer behavior within the family: Results from the Asset and Health Dynamics study. *Journal of Gerontology, Series B: Psychological Sciences and Social Sciences, 52*, 82–92.

Minkler, M., Fuller-Thomson, E., Miller, D., & Driver, D. (2000). Grandparent caregiving and depression. In B. Hayslip, Jr., & R. Goldberg-Glen, (Ed.), *Grandparents raising grandchildren: Theoretical, empirical, and clinical perspectives* (pp. 207–220). New York: Springer.

Minkler, M., & Roe, K. M. (1993). *Grandmothers as caregivers: Raising children of the crack cocaine epidemic.* Newbury Park. CA: Sage Publications.

Molm, L. D., & Cook, K. S. (1995). Social exchange and exchange networks. In K. S. Cook, G. A. Fine, & J. S. House (Eds.), *Sociological perspectives on social psychology* (pp. 209–235). Boston: Allyn and Bacon.

Ng, A. C., Phillips, D. R., & Lee, W.-K. (2002). Persistence and challenges to filial piety and informal support of older persons in a modern Chinese society: A case study in Tuen Mun, Hong Kong. *Journal of Aging Studies, 16*(2), 135–153.

Ofstedal, M., Reidy, E., & Knodel, J. (2004). Gender differences in economic support and well-being of older Asians. *Journal of Cross-Cultural Gerontology, 19*(3), 165–201.

O'Rand, A. M. (2003). The future of the life course: Late modernity and life course risks. In J. T. Mortimer & M. J. Shanahan (Eds.), *Handbook of the life course.* (pp. 693–702). New York: Kluwer Academic/Plenum.

Pezzin, L. E., Pollak, R. A., & Schone, B. (Revised, Jan. 2004). Long-term care and family decision making. Unpublished manuscript.

Pezzin, L. E., & Schone, B. S. (1999). Parental marital disruption and intergenerational transfers: An analysis of lone elderly parents and their children. *Demography, 36*(3), 287–297.

Phillipson, C. (2003). Globalization and the reconstruction of old age: New challenges for critical gerontology. In S. Biggs, A. Lowenstein, & J. Hendricks (Eds.), *The need for theory: Critical approaches to social gerontology* (pp. 163–179). New York: Baywood.

Pollak, R. A. (1988). Tied transfers and paternalistic preferences. *American Economic Review, 78*(2), 240–244.

Popenoe, D. (1988). *Disturbing the nest: Family change and decline in modern societies.* New York: Aldine De Gruyter.

Putnam, R. D. (1995). Bowling alone: America's declining social capital. *Journal of Democracy, 6*(1), 65–71.

Rahman, M. O. (1999). Family matters: The impact of kin on the mortality of the elderly in rural Bangladesh. *Population Studies, 53*(2), 227–235.

Riley, N. E. (1994). Interwoven lives: Parents, marriage, and Guanxi in China. *Journal of Marriage and the Family, 56*(4), 791–803.

Rossi, A. S., & Rossi, P. H. (1990). *Of human bonding: Parent-children relationship across the life course*. New York: Aldine de Gruyter.

Sando, R. (1986). Doing the work of two generations: The impact of out-migration on the elderly in rural Taiwan. *Journal of Cross-Cultural Gerontology, 1*(2), 163–175.

Silverstein, M., & Bengtson, V. L. (1997). Intergenerational solidarity and the structure of adult child-parent relationships in American families. *American Journal of Sociology, 103*, 429–460.

Silverstein, M., Burholt, V., Wenger, G. C., & Bengtson, V. L. (1998). Parent-child relations among very old parents in Wales and the United States: A test of modernization theory. *Journal of Aging Studies, 12*(4), 387–409.

Silverstein M., & Conroy S. (in press). Intergenerational transmission of moral capital across the family life course. In U. Schoenpflug (Ed.), *Cultural transmission*. Oxford: Oxford University Press.

Silverstein, M., Conroy, S., Wang H., Giarrusso, R., & Bengtson, V. L. (2002). Reciprocity in parent-child relations over the adult life course. *Journal of Gerontology: Social Sciences: 57*, S3–S13.

Silverstein, M., Parrott, T. M., & Bengtson, V. L. (1995). Factors that predispose middle-aged sons and daughters to provide social support to older parents. *Journal of Marriage and the Family, 57*, 465–475.

Sloan, F. A., Zhang, H. H., & Wang, J. (2002). Upstream intergenerational transfers. *Southern Economic Journal, 69*(2), 363–380.

Spilerman, S. (2004). The impact of parental wealth on early living standards in Israel. *American Journal of Sociology, 110*(1), 92–122.

Spilerman, S., & Elmelech, Y. (2003). Israeli attitudes about inter vivos transfers. In V. L. Bengtson & A. Lowenstein (Eds.), *Global aging and its challenge to families* (pp. 175–195). Hawthorne, NY: Aldine De Gruyter.

Spitze, G., & Logan, J. R. (1992). Helping as a component of parent-adult child relations. *Research on Aging, 14*(3), 291–312.

Stark, O. (1995). *Altruism and beyond: An economic analysis of transfers and exchanges within families and groups*. Cambridge, NY: Cambridge University Press.

Stark, O., & Falk, I. (1998). Transfers, empathy formation, and reverse transfers. *American Economic Review, 88*(2), 271–276.

Stein, C. H., Wemmerus, V. A., Ward, M., Gaines, M. E., Freeberg, A. L., & Jewell, T. (1998). "Because they're my parents": An intergenerational study of felt obligation and parental caregiving. *Journal of Marriage and the Family, 60*, 611–622.

Sun, R. (2002). Old age support in contemporary urban China from both parents' and children's perspectives. *Research on Aging, 24*(3), 337–359.

Sundstrom, G., Johansson, L., & Hassing, L. B. (2002). The shifting balance of long-term care in Sweden. *The Gerontologist, 42*, 350–355.

Tsuya, N. O., & Martin, L. G. (1992). Living arrangements of elderly Japanese and attitudes toward inheritance. *Journal of Gerontology: Social Sciences 47*(2), S45–S54.

Uhlenberg, P. (2005). Historical forces shaping grandparent-grandchild relationships: Demography and beyond. In M. Silverstein (Ed.), *Intergenerational relations across time and place. Annual review of gerontology and geriatrics* (Vol. 24, pp. 77–97). New York: Springer.

Whitbeck, L. B., Simons, R. L., & Conger, R. D. (1991). The effects of early family relationships on contemporary relationships and assistance patterns between adult children and their parents. *Journal of Gerontology: Social Sciences, 46*, S301–S337.

Wilhelm, M. O. (1996). Bequest behavior and the effect of heirs' earnings: Testing the altruistic model of bequests. *American Economic Review, 86*(4), 874–892.

The World Bank Group. Retrieved March 25, 2005 from the World Wide Web: http://web.worldbank.org/WBSITE/EXTERNAL/TOPICS/EXTCY/0,,contentMDK:20249126~menuPK:565284~pagePK:148956~piPK:216618~theSitePK:396445,00.html.

Yang, H. (1996). The distributive norm of monetary support to older parents: A look at a township in China. *Journal of Marriage and the Family, 58*, 404–415.

Yi, Z. (1994). China's agenda for an old-age insurance program in rural areas. *Journal of Aging and Social Policy, 6*(4), 101–114.

# Eleven

# Social Relationships in Late Life

Neal Krause

Social theorists have argued for decades that social relationships stand at the critical juncture between the individual and society. Individuals are shaped by society, and it is largely through interpersonal relationships that individuals change the social world in which they live (Berger & Luckman, 1966). Given the central role of interpersonal relationships in social life, it is not surprising that researchers have shown a good deal of interest in studying them across the life course. A large part of this work has focused on social relationships and health. Viewed broadly, this literature suggests that older people with strong social ties tend to enjoy better physical and mental health than older adults who do not maintain close relationships with others (Krause, 2001). These studies are important because they illustrate one way in which research in social gerontology can be used to improve the quality of life of our aging population.

The purpose of this chapter is to critically review the vast body of research on social relationships in late life. But this is a challenging task because there simply is

not enough space to adequately cover all the complex ways in which the lives of older people are joined with the lives of others. Therefore, the discussion that follows is, of necessity, selective. Given these constraints, it is important to identify the rationale that guided the selection of topics and structured the overall thrust of this review. Rather than merely presenting a catalog of what is known, the intent is to use current research as a point of departure for identifying promising new lines of inquiry that may help move the literature forward. Toward this end, the discussion that follows is divided into five main sections. First, an effort is made to define social relationships. The content domain of this broad construct is briefly sketched out at this juncture as well. Second, factors that influence the development and maintenance of social relationships are discussed. Third, a more detailed examination is made of various types of social relationships with an eye toward identifying how they may influence health and well-being in late life. Fourth, variations in social relationships by race are explored. Finally, the current state of theoretical perspectives on social relationships is examined.

# I. What Are Social Relationships?

Social relationships are recurrent patterns of interaction with other individuals. Some may equate social relationships with social support, but this is incorrect. Social relationships are broader, and serve a wider range of functions than crisis-oriented social support.

One way to get a better handle on the nature of social relationships is to stake out the content domain of this vast construct. At least four constructs are subsumed under the broad rubric of social relationships. The first is social support. Social support has to do with various types of assistance that are provided in an effort to help the recipient cope more effectively with stress. Included among the types of assistance that are typically provided for this purpose are emotional, tangible, and informational support (Barrera, 1986). Some researchers also include perceptual or evaluative measures of support (Barrera, 1986). These perceptual measures include satisfaction with assistance that has been exchanged as well as anticipated support. Anticipated support is defined as the belief that others stand ready to help in the future should the need arise.

Companionship represents a second type of social relationship that is quite different from social support. Rook (1987) defined companionship as social interaction that is engaged in primarily for the sake of enjoyment. Companionship involves shared leisure and recreational activities, as well as relationships that are based on the pursuit of common interests. When people interact with companions, they typically share fantasies and dreams, as well as expressions of affection and private jokes. As major stressful

events are relatively rare in late life, a good deal of the daily social interaction of older people takes place within the context of companionship.

The third type of social relationship is referred to as weak social ties. The term *weak social ties* was coined by Granovetter (1973) to capture relationships that lack the intimacy and frequency of interaction characteristic of family ties and relationships with close friends. Included among weak social ties are social encounters with bartenders, waitresses, as well as more distant neighbors and casual relationships with some co-workers. Formal social relationships represent another type of weak social tie. These are instrumental social relationships that take place within the context of formal organizations. Included among formal social ties are relationships with members of the clergy, mental health professionals, and medical professionals.

Negative interaction is the final type of social relationship examined in this chapter. Negative interaction involves unpleasant social encounters that are characterized by disagreements, criticism, rejection, and the invasion of privacy (Rook, 1984). Excessive helping as well as ineffective helping are sometimes included under the broad rubric of this construct.

# II. Exploring the Genesis of Social Relationships

Before discussing how social relationships influence health and well-being, it is important to first examine the factors that promote and maintain social relationships. Simply put, we need to approach the study of social relationships by thinking about them as dependent variables. Three issues are examined here that have not received considerable attention in the literature, but hold out the promise of deepening our understanding of social ties in late life. The first involves developmental differences in social relationships, the second has to do with cohort differences in social ties, and the third is concerned with social skills.

## A. Developmental Differences in Social Relationships

Any effort to understand the forces that shape social relationships in late life must ultimately come to grips with life course and developmental issues. We are a product of our own developmental histories, and any effort to assess current circumstances that is divorced from this personal past will invariably be incomplete. Cast within the context of this chapter, developmental differences in social relationships are concerned with how the ways people relate to others and the nature of the social ties they form change (or remain the same) over the life course.

Most theories of human development focus primarily on childhood, adolescence, and early adulthood. Even when theories extend into late life, researchers rarely focus on social relationships specifically. Carstensen's (1992) theory of socioemotional selectivity is a notable exception. According to this perspective, people tend to develop a greater preference for emotionally meaningful social relationships as they grow older. Consequently, social networks tend to become smaller as older adults disengage from more peripheral social ties and devote increasing attention to a smaller circle of relationships that are emotionally supportive. This work, however, is primarily concerned with change in the need for emotionally strong ties over the life course, and, as a result, it has little to say about other types of social relationships.

When taking a life course approach to the study of social relationships, it seems that researchers must inevitably confront the principle of primacy (Kermis, 1986). According to this view, experiences early in childhood play a critical role in shaping behavior across the remainder of the life course. A good deal of the impetus behind the principle of primacy comes from attachment theory (Bowlby, 1973). This perspective stipulates that human beings have a biologically based need to form long-lasting social bonds that provide a sense of security, safety, and comfort throughout life (see McCarthy & Davies, 2003, for a recent review of attachment theory and research). A central tenet in attachment theory is that relationships children form with their parents are prototypes for relationships in adult life. This suggests that the vestiges of early parent-child relationships should be evident across the life course. Unfortunately, as McCarthy and Davies point out, little research has been done in this area with older adults.

One of the few studies to examine the impact of early parent-child relationships on social ties in late life was conducted by Shaw and his colleagues (Shaw, Krause, Chatters, Connell, & Ingersoll-Dayton, 2004). The purpose of this study was to see whether the amount of emotional support from parents early in life shapes psychological resources (e.g., feelings of personal control), social relationships (emotional support and negative interaction), and health in adult life. Data provided by a nationwide sample of adults ages 25 to 74 revealed that more emotional support from parents early in life is associated with more emotional support from family members and friends, as well as less negative interaction with family members throughout adult life. Further unpublished analyses from this study indicate that the impact of early parent support on relationships with friends (both positive and negative interaction) did not change with advancing age; however, the relationship between early parental support and relationships with family members became weaker with age.

Thus it appears that early relationships with parents may have effects that last through late life; however, two factors must be taken into account when reviewing these findings. First, the magnitude of the effect is fairly modest. More specifically, the standardized regression coefficients associated with the relationships between early parental support and social relationships in adult life range from −.074 to .085. This suggests that a good deal of the variance in the quality of adult relationships is not explained by early ties with parents. Viewed in more general terms, this means that other factors arising later in life continue to shape the social bonds that people form with others. The second limitation in the work of Shaw et al. (2004) is that the age range of respondents in their study was truncated at 74, leaving the oldest-old outside the scope of inquiry.

If social relationships in adult life are shaped by more than just the quality of early ties with parents, then other factors arising later in life must come into play. This could involve other developmental changes, but change in social ties after childhood could also involve key life events and turning points. A turning point is defined simply as a time when a person's life takes a different direction (Clausen, 1993). Events involving career changes and marriage are among the most common turning points. The sheer number of potential life events and turning points that may arise after childhood seems almost limitless. Moreover, as little comprehensive work with large probability samples has been done in this area, there are significant blind spots in our understanding of the life course development of social relationships. This is especially true with respect to midlife. This is one reason why some refer to this period as the "last uncharted territory" of the life course (Brim, Ryff, & Kessler, 2004, p. 1). It is not possible to review all the potential life events, turning points, and developmental influences that shape social relationships after childhood. Speculating on some developmental influences that may arise in late life, however, should be useful for guiding research and shaping theory in the future.

In their insightful work on the oldest-old, Johnson and Barer (2003) reported that when people enter the final decades of life, they become increasingly introspective and evidence greater interiority, a concept that was discussed some time ago by Neugarten (1977). This is consistent with the observations of Aldwin and Gilmer (2004), who noted that advanced old age is often accompanied by a greater sense of wisdom and "gerotranscendence." As Tornstam (1997) pointed out, gerotranscendence involves a transition from a materialistic and pragmatic orientation to life to a more cosmic and transcendent one. It is not surprising to find that Tornstam traced the interpersonal implications of this shift in world view. In particular, he noted that as people enter late life, they become more selective in their relationships with others and prefer deep personal relationships with few individuals rather than more superficial ties with many people.

If the observations of Tornstam (1997) and Aldwin and Gilmer (2004) are correct, then we need to think more carefully about how to conceptualize and measure social relationships in late life. More specifically, steps must be taken to devise measures of the depth of interpersonal ties. Presently, most research involves assessing how many relationships an older person has, how often an older person comes into contact with others, and how much support is provided during these encounters, but variation in the depth of social ties is rarely evaluated empirically.

In the process of evaluating these developmental perspectives, it is important to keep another issue in mind. The work of Tornstam (1997) and others suggests that all older people follow the same path of development over time. But this may not be the case. As Goldhaber (2000) pointed out, this sort of developmental perspective is based on the assumption of essentialism. According to this view, there is a universal pattern of human development that is followed by all people. But researchers have begun to challenge this assumption (see Goldhaber, 2000, for a detailed discussion of this issue). Consistent with Dannefer and Sell's (1988) aged heterogeneity hypothesis, there may not be a single trajectory of change in social relationships across the life course. Instead, there may be multiple trajectories. Some people may never develop close ties with others over the life course, whereas others may have little difficulty doing so. And yet other individuals may go on to develop the kind of deep social ties that are described in Tornstam's (1997) notion of gerotranscendence. If this is true, then we must develop typologies of change in social relationships across the life course, and we need to determine the social forces that set some people on one path instead of another.

## B. Cohort Differences in Social Relationships

As Elder (1999) convincingly demonstrated, "Each generation is distinguished by the historical logic and shared experience of growing up in a different time period . . . individuals are thought to acquire a distinct outlook and philosophy from the historical world, defined by their birth date, an outlook that reflects lives lived interdependently in a particular historical context" (p. 15). This suggests that history has a profound effect on human life, and in the process, it is likely to shape the nature of the social bonds that are formed and maintained with others. With the exception of

Elder's work on the cohort growing up in the Great Depression, however, this issue is rarely discussed in the literature on social relationships. Even so, it is possible to piece together a few preliminary insights by pooling findings from current research.

Although there are no firm guidelines for determining the boundaries of different cohorts, Krause and his colleagues suggest that our older population is currently made up of three cohorts (Krause, Shaw, & Cairney, 2004). The first is the oldest-old (i.e., those individuals who are 85 years of age and over). Many entered adult life just as the Great Depression emerged. As a result, they are often referred to as the Depression Cohort (Meredith & Schewe, 2002). As research by Meredith and Schewe reveals, members of this cohort highly value independence and grittiness. These values may shape the way social support is exchanged. In particular, members of this cohort may be reluctant to accept tangible assistance from others. In addition, as Karner (2001) pointed out, members of the depression cohort disapprove of divorce and remarriage. This has implications for the kinds of social relationships that elders in this cohort are likely to have formed over the course of their lives.

For members of the second cohort, the old-old (ages 75–84), the big historical event was World War II. Consequently, Meredith and Schewe (2002) referred to people in this age group as the World War II cohort. Karner (2001) reported that this cohort is characterized by unprecedented patriotism and strong allegiance to country and community. But perhaps more important, she points out that members of this cohort place a premium on cooperation, mutual support, and teamwork. Clearly, these values may exert a positive influence on the nature and scope of social relationships formed by members of the World War II cohort.

Finally, Meredith and Schewe (2002) referred to members of the young-old cohort (ages 65–74) as the Postwar Cohort, but they are also known as the Eisenhower Cohort (Karner, 2001). This group was shaped by the good economic times and widespread political consensus after World War II. Members of this cohort tended to espouse an unquestioning belief in American social institutions and social conformity. They also place a high value on stability and living the American Dream (Karner, 2001). But perhaps more important, Karner (2001) pointed out that, "It was a profamily decade like no other" (p. 26). Although family ties are obviously important across all cohorts, this suggests that members of the Postwar Cohort may value them more highly than members of other cohorts.

The discussion of cohort differences provided here is sketchy and clearly in need of further development. In the process, care must be taken in investigating cohort-related issues. As Alwin, McCammon, and Hofer (2004) argued, cohort influences are neither uniform nor pervasive. Instead, as these investigators point out, different people may experience the same historical event in different ways. This suggests that cohort analysis may be far more challenging than we think because variations within and across cohorts must be considered. In addition, it is important to keep in mind that cohort and developmental influences on social relationships are not mutually exclusive. More specifically, there is no inherent reason why the developmental preference for emotionally close ties discussed by Carstensen (1992) cannot operate in conjunction with broad historical forces, such as the Great Depression, to shape the nature of social relationships in late life. This gives new meaning to the classic insights of C. Wright Mills (1959), who argued that the best way to study human behavior is to focus on the intersection between history (i.e., cohort influences) and biography (i.e., developmental influences).

## C. Social Skills

Social skills are interpersonal abilities that promote successful and beneficial relationships with others. Social skills are important for two reasons. First, they shape the development and maintenance of social relationships across the life course. Second, identification of key social skills represents an important point of departure for developing social support interventions. The meaning and nature of social skills is perhaps best clarified by focusing on specific types of skills. It would be impossible to discuss every social skill here. so reviewing a few should help highlight the need for further work in this area. Unfortunately, little research has been done on social skills in late life (for a notable exception, see the work of Hansson & Carpenter, 1990, as well as the Hogg & Heller, 1990). Consequently, a good deal of the discussion that follows is based on research in the general population.

A key social skill involves the ability to take the role of others. As Cooley (1902) put it, this involves the ability to enter the mind of another sympathetically. In fact, Schlenker (2003) argued that, "The ability to put oneself in the place of others and imagine how they are likely to interpret and respond to information is the basis for effective communication" (pp. 502–503). This means that to communicate effectively with others and build strong relationships with them, an individual must be able to put themselves in the place of others, carefully taking into account their knowledge and value systems, and packaging information using examples, ideas, and evidence that make sense to them (Schlenker, 2003). There is likely to be considerable variation in the ability to take the role of the other, but to verify this notion, good measures of this construct must first be devised.

As the previous discussion reveals, social relationships depend heavily on communication: The better the communication skills, the better the relationship. One key communication skill is expressiveness. This involves the verbal ability to properly convey thoughts, feelings, and needs to others (Schlenker, 2003).

As Aron (2003) noted, self-disclosure is one of the oldest topics in research on social relationships. Self-disclosure is a form of expressiveness, but the two differ in terms of focus. Expressiveness refers to the ability to convey a wide range of thoughts and feelings. In contrast, self-disclosure involves revealing information about the self to others, even when this information does not reflect positively on the self. The functions of self-disclosure are especially important when considering social support. Social network members are not typically together 24 hours a day. As a result, a potential support provider may not know that a close other is in need, and he or she may not have all the information necessary to deliver assistance effectively. Potential support recipients must, therefore, be willing to tell potential support providers what has happened, what they need, and when they need it.

When people help others, they sometimes do so at some expense to themselves. Although many do not look for compensation or reward, expressions of gratitude by the support recipient help ensure that support will be forthcoming in the future should the need arise. Gratitude is simply the expression of thankfulness for the supportive behavior and thoughtful acts of another. Looking at it the other way around, when help recipients fail to express gratitude, support providers may feel put upon, and they may believe they are being taken advantage of. The critical role of gratitude

in social interaction was highlighted in the classic sociological theory of Simmel (1950). He argued that gratitude is a key factor that sustains reciprocal relationships. The following quotation, taken from the work of Simmel, leaves little doubt about the importance he placed on this social skill: "... if every grateful action ... were suddenly eliminated, society (at least as we know it) would break apart" (Simmel, 1950, p. 388). Some investigators view gratitude as a psychological trait (e.g., McCullough, Tsang, & Emmons, 2004). However, as Simmel (1950) maintained, gratitude is an acquired social skill that is developed in the process of socialization and honed through continued interaction with others.

As discussed earlier, interpersonal difficulty and strife are sometimes encountered in social relationships. The skills that are brought to bear when negative interaction arises may determine the impact it has on health and well-being. To minimize the impact of negative interaction, people must be able to understand each other, see more than one side of an issue clearly, have good negotiation skills, and be able to arrange an outcome that is mutually satisfactory (Mirowsky & Ross, 2003). Unfortunately, the role of social skills in the process of responding to negative interaction has rarely been examined in the literature.

This brief overview of social skills hardly exhausts the list of those necessary to develop and maintain strong social relationships. At this point, we need good psychometric work aimed at staking out the content domain of this complex construct. Then, we must develop a comprehensive battery of measures that assess social skills that are especially relevant for older adults. Once this goal has been achieved, work can begin on identifying the factors that influence the adoption and utilization of social skills in late life. Although a number of factors are likely to come into play, the specific social skills that are cultivated by older people may be influenced by the developmental and cohort issues discussed previously. Viewed in this way, the study of social skills provides one-way bridging developmental and cohort issues with the study of social relationships in late life.

## III. Social Relationships and Health

Having examined how social relationships arise and are maintained, it is important to focus on how they function and the benefits they may provide. Social relationships may enhance the lives of older adults in a number of ways. Consistent with the overall theme of this chapter, the following discussion emphasizes how social relationships influence the health and psychological well-being of older people. This is accomplished by examining each of the facets of social relationships that were identified earlier.

### A. Social Support and Health

Undesirable stressful live events may affect health in a number of ways. Two are well documented in the literature. As research with older people reveals, stressful events tend to erode self-esteem and feelings of personal control (Krause & Borawski-Clark, 1994). But recent research by Krause (2004a) identified another pathway that has not been empirically evaluated by others. More specifically, his work suggests that stressors arising in highly valued roles exert an adverse effect on the physical health status of older adults primarily because they erode an older person's sense of meaning in life.

If stress compromises an older person's sense of self-esteem, feelings of control, and meaning in life, then perhaps social support operates by replenishing these important psychosocial resources. It is

important to reflect on how this takes place.

In his classic article on the stress process, Caplan (1981) argued that significant others help a person who has been exposed to a stressor define the problem situation and devise and implement a plan of action. Moreover, social network members provide advice, guidance, and feedback as the plan is being executed. Simply put, supportive others help older people confront the difficult events in their lives by helping them identify and adopt efficacious coping strategies. These insights are noteworthy because they suggest that instead of arising solely from within the individual, coping responses are the result of a social process in which older people and their significant others jointly negotiate the selection and implementation of the most effective coping strategies (see Lyons, Mickelson, Sullivan, & Coyne, 1998 for a detailed discussion of this issue).

Work by Krause (2004a) showed that when older people are confronted by undesirable life events, support from significant others also helps them maintain a sense of meaning in life. In his view, Krause (2004a) maintained that meaning in life arises from having a set of values, a purpose in life, and goals to work toward. He goes on to argue that meaning also arises from reflecting on the past. Here an older person finds meaning by reflecting on how his or her life has been lived, and making an effort to come to terms with, and reconcile, unpleasant things that have happened in the past. Findings from his nationwide survey reveal that social support helps replenish a sense of meaning in life. Moreover, this work suggests that others do so primarily by helping older people reconcile things that have happened in the past. In essence, this research shows that reminiscence is also the product of a social process. In addition, this work provides one way of integrating the vast literature on reminiscence into research on the stress process (Haight & Webster, 1995).

The discussion provided up to this point focuses solely on the ways in which social support helps offset the noxious effects of stressful life events on health and well-being. This focus may create the mistaken impression that social support is a universally effective coping resource; this may not always be so. Turning to a different kind of stressor, chronic strain, helps illustrate the ways in which the social support process may break down. Two factors differentiate chronic strains from stressful life events. First, as Pearlin and his colleagues pointed out, stressful life events are time-bound, and the effects of stressful life events tend to peak and dissipate in a relatively short period (e.g., one to two years) (Pearlin, Menaghan, Lieberman, & Mullan, 1981). In contrast, chronic strains are continuous and ongoing. Second, chronic strains are considered to have a more deleterious effect on health and well-being than stressful life events. Chronic strain associated with the caregiving process (Pearlin, Mullan, Semple, & Skaff, 1990) and strain associated with ongoing financial problems (Krause, 1987) are among the types of chronic strain that are encountered more frequently in late life. Chronic strains are important because there is some evidence they have a pernicious effect on social relationships in late life. More specifically, support providers may lack the resources needed to provide assistance over extended periods of time. This may eventually make support providers feel resentful and put upon (Coyne, Wortman, & Lehman, 1988). In addition, because of their continuous nature, chronic strains may erode an older person's resources, thereby making it difficult for them to reciprocate. And the inability to reciprocate may, in turn, create feelings of dependency (Gottlieb, 1997; Krause, 1987). Viewed more broadly, the literature that is reviewed here suggests that chronic strains may be especially noxious primarily because they tend to erode the very resources (i.e., social support) that older adults need to cope with them.

## B. Companionship and Health

As Rook (1987) insightfully pointed out, everyone wants to be understood. People also want to share their lives with others. In fact, the true value and meaning of many positive experiences in life are not fully understood or appreciated until they are shared with others. But perhaps even more important, people want to feel they are accepted; they want to feel as if they belong. Companionship performs all these functions. And as a result, older people are likely to experience a range of positive emotions. This is important because research reviewed by Ryff and Singer (1998) reveals that positive emotions may have beneficial physiological effects on the body (e.g., they may enhance immune functioning).

Research by Lee and Shehan (1989) highlights additional ways in which companions may enhance feelings of subjective well-being in late life. More specifically, their research indicates that interaction with friends tends to bolster feelings of self-worth, but interaction with family members fails to have a similar effect. These investigators argue that the beneficial effects of friendship ties arise because these relationships are entered into voluntarily, whereas relationships with family members are based on a sense of obligation. These findings are important because they suggest that companion relationships with age-peers have effects that are independent of relationships with family members and that companions may enhance the quality of life for older people in ways that are relatively unique.

But there are other health-related benefits of companionship that have not received sufficient attention in the literature. One of the main challenges facing older people arises from the need to feel they are useful and productive members of society. Lying behind this issue is another, more general, principle that was discussed some time ago by Cooley (1929). He argued that, "I can only say that I have found self-expression to be, in fact, as it is in principle, the heart of life" (Cooley, 1929, pp. 47–48). He went on to argue that, "The fuel that drives our engine is the self impulse, a certain ardor and craving to bring forth something of our own and make it work in general life" (Cooley, 1929, p. 192). The observations of Cooley (1929) fit well with more recent work on productive activities and aging (Rowe & Kahn, 1998). As Rook (1987) observed, one of the functions of companionship involves the pursuit of mutual interests and hobbies. Consistent with the views of Cooley (1929), this suggests that companions may facilitate and encourage self-expression, thereby helping people feel productive in late life. This is important because a number of investigators maintain that meaningful activity is a key to health and successful aging (Rowe & Kahn, 1998).

## C. Weak Social Ties and Health

Weak social ties may also have a beneficial effect on health and well-being in late life. However, as weak social ties are covered elsewhere in this volume (see Chapter 7), this facet of social relationships is examined only briefly here.

As noted earlier, weak ties are characterized by low levels of intimacy and relatively infrequent contact. As Adelman, Parks, and Albrecht (1987) pointed out, networks comprised of close ties tend to be relatively homogeneous, whereas weak ties are often formed with individuals who have different social characteristics. This ensures a greater diversity of views and opinions than may be found in close relationships. Simply put, weak

social ties may be an important source of informational support. Having a wider range of view may help older people select the best coping responses during difficult times. Moreover, as Adelman et al. argue, the social distance that is characteristic of weak ties may have important functions. When people seek out assistance from close others, they have to take into account how significant others will respond and how the request for help may affect the future of the relationship. These concerns are alleviated with weak ties. As a result, weak ties provide a context in which a person may experiment with new ideas and new behaviors with relatively low levels of accountability. This is especially evident in some types of formal social ties, such as relationships with physicians, members of the clergy, and mental health professionals.

The functions performed by weak social ties have important implications for the way older people cope with stress because the anonymity, low accountability, and diversity of views they provide typically cannot be found elsewhere. In this way, weak ties may have a unique influence on health and well-being in late life. Unfortunately, life course changes, such as retirement, may limit an older person's access to some types of weak social ties (e.g., co-workers).

In addition to the functions identified previously, formal social relationships may influence the health of older people in obvious ways. For example, good relationships with physicians are clearly associated with better health, and strong ties with mental health professionals can obviously enhance the psychological well-being of older people.

Unfortunately, researchers do not often acknowledge that interpersonal ties in formal settings may not always function smoothly, and at times they can have a detrimental effect on health and well-being. Evidence of this may be found in a study by Krause (2003) on interaction between older adults and members of the clergy. This work suggests that emotional support from the clergy may bolster feelings of self-worth in late life. This research further reveals, however, that relationships with the clergy may also become conflicted. And if they do, this study indicates that the self-esteem of older churchgoers is likely to suffer.

Social ties in formal settings may take a number of different forms. One that may be especially important for older people involves relationships that are associated with performing volunteer work. A recent report by the Department of Labor (2002) indicated that people age 65 and over spend more time performing volunteer work than individuals in any other age group. This is noteworthy because research reveals that volunteering may exert a positive influence on the health and well-being of older people (Musick & Wilson, 2003). Although there are a number of reasons why this may be so, there is some evidence that providing assistance to those in need benefits support providers as well as support recipients (Reissman, 1965). More specifically, helping others tends to bolster feelings of self-esteem as well as personal control among support providers. As the literature reviewed earlier reveals, these psychosocial resources are important determinants of health and well-being across the life course.

## D. Negative Interaction and Health

A fairly extensive body of research suggests that negative interaction exerts an adverse effect on the physical (Krause, 2005) and mental health (Rook, 1984) of older adults. In fact, some investigators maintain that the effects of negative interaction on health and well-being are larger in magnitude than the effects of positive support provided by significant others (Okun & Keith, 1998). But much less is known about how the pernicious effects of negative interaction arise.

Rook and Pietromonaco (1987) provided three reasons why negative interaction may have a greater impact on health and well-being than positive interaction with others. First, they point out that most people typically encounter a disproportionately greater amount of positive interaction in the course of daily life. This creates the impression that social relationships will continue on a positive course. But if negative interaction arises, it tends to violate these expectancies, often stunning the recipient. The second explanation has to do with the attributions that are typically made about social interaction. When people interact, they try to make inferences about the motives of others. But Rook and Pietromonaco maintain it is sometimes difficult to gauge the underlying motives behind supportive behavior because people may help out of genuine care and concern, or they may help purely out of a sense of duty. In contrast, there is no such ambiguity when negative interaction arises. This, coupled with the negative emotions it invokes, guarantees that the impact of negative interaction will be more forceful. Finally, because of inherited adaptive mechanisms, people are more vigilant to threats from the environment. As a result, they are more attuned to and more affected by negative encounters with others.

Although the work of Rook and Pietromonaco (1987) provided many valuable insights, there are at least two other ways in which the undesirable health-related effects of negative interaction may arise. First, as research reviewed by Ryff and Singer (1998) revealed, the negative emotions generated by interpersonal conflict can have direct, and undesirable, effects on physiological functioning. This is especially true with respect to immune functioning.

The second explanation of the deleterious effects of negative interaction may be found in Cooley's (1902) classic discussion of the looking-glass self. According to this view, a person's sense of self is shaped by the reflected appraisals and feedback from significant others. This suggests that negative self-images arising during unpleasant social encounters may become incorporated into the self, thereby lowering feelings of self-worth.

But the simple portrait provided by the looking-glass self may not correspond to what actually happens in daily life. Two factors mitigate against the direct incorporation of negative feedback from others into the self. First, the opinions and feedback of some individuals may carry greater weight than the opinions and feedback of others. Although many factors influence how important others are identified, there is some evidence that people seek out individuals who tend to view them in the same way they see themselves (Tice & Wallace, 2003). Second, research indicates that people distort the feedback provided by others, thereby protecting the self (Tice & Wallace, 2003).

Viewed broadly, the research discussed here suggests that negative feedback from others may have an adverse effect on health and well-being, but only under certain circumstances. We need to know more about the self-protective processes that are used so that older people who are at greatest risk can be more clearly identified.

Although negative interaction is typically viewed as having undesirable effects, this may not always be true. Consequently, to provide a more well-rounded discussion of this form of social interaction, it is important to consider the potentially positive outcomes of negative interaction as well. There are at least three ways in which negative interaction may have positive consequences for health and well-being.

First, as Rook, Thuras, and Lewis (1990) maintained, significant others may resort to the use of negative interaction to get a focal person to engage in positive health behaviors. So, for example, a wife may criticize her husband for drinking alcohol excessively. But if he takes this criticism to heart, and reduces his alcohol intake, then this form of negative interaction will have a positive influence on his health.

In addition, there may be times when negative interaction has positive long-term consequences for close relationships. Close relationships typically involve high levels of interaction, intimacy, and influence. Because these relationships are so intense, problems invariably arise in them. As a result, older adults need to ventilate, let off steam, and say potentially negative things to clear the air. Doing so allows them to get problematic aspects of the relationship into the open, thereby paving the way for smoother interpersonal functioning in the long run. Moreover, the process of airing grievances, coupled with reconciliation and renewed commitment to the relationship, may actually help older people develop social ties that are stronger than they were before negative interaction arose.

Finally, sometimes a focal person may actually have done something wrong, and as a result, the criticism received is justified. If the focal person takes this negative feedback to heart and changes his or her behavior for the better, then negative interaction may lead to personal growth even though it may be painful at the time it was first encountered.

Compared to the literature on positive interaction, research on negative interaction is vastly underdeveloped. Consequently, in an effort to encourage more work on negative interaction, five clusters of issues that have yet to be addressed are reviewed briefly next.

Most theoretical discussions of negative interaction focus solely on dyadic relationships. But more than one social network member may direct negative interaction at a focal elder for the same reason. We need to know how often this happens, and more research is needed to explore the effects of negative interaction arising from a group. It seems that a chorus of critical remarks from diverse sources should be especially destructive, but this issue has yet to be examined empirically.

When people encounter negative interaction, they are likely to ask whether it is justified. Sometimes, targets of negative interaction may believe they are indeed at fault and deserve the unpleasant feedback they are receiving. Other times, people may feel the negative interaction is not justified and they are being treated unfairly. We need to know which scenario has the greatest impact on physical and mental health. Does the guilt arising from knowing they are at fault have a greater effect, or does the anger and hurt associated with being unjustly attacked cause more damage?

We need to learn more about the potentially important role played by significant others who are not directly involved in a negative social encounter. On being told of a problem, they may fan the flames of righteous indignation by underscoring the unfounded nature of the injustice that has been perpetrated. Or they may contribute to the healing process by helping the focal person move toward a resolution and reconciliation. This raises the unexplored possibility that third parties not directly involved in negative interaction may help broker a solution. As these issues reveal, appraisals of negative interaction, and the way unpleasant interaction is handled, are often social products. We need to know more about this.

There is still little research on why a person decides to initiate a negative interaction. Sometimes, it is a cry for justice from an individual who believes he or she has been treated wrongly. But other times, darker motives are involved. In

particular, negative interaction may be an unhealthy and misguided effort to shore up the self. This is especially evident with gossip, which may be construed as a form of negative interaction, especially when it is vicious. Although few may realize it, Mead discussed this issue some time ago. He pointed out that, "There is a certain enjoyableness about the misfortunes of other people, especially those gathered about their personality. It finds its expression in what we term gossip" (Mead, 1934/1962, p. 206). These insights raise broader issues about the need to differentiate between the effects of negative interaction when one is the target, and negative interaction when one is the perpetrator. Moreover, it highlights the need to probe the underlying motives of the person initiating the unpleasant interaction.

In one sense, the dissolution of a relationship may be viewed as the ultimate expression of negative interaction and rejection. Divorce is an obvious example, but the complete rupture of ties with family members (e.g., siblings) or close friends should be included here as well. Does the sheer fact that a relationship has ended serve as an ever present reminder of failure, and is this realization capable of creating significant physical and mental health problems? Or is the dissolution of problematic social ties ultimately a relief? As the issues raised throughout this section reveal, the field of negative interaction is wide open.

## IV. Variations by Race

The study of social structural influences on social relationships represents one of the seminal contributions of social gerontology. Therefore, any review of social relationships in late life would be remiss if the important influence of social structure was ignored. The pillars of social structure are composed of socioeconomic status, race, gender, and age. Each has been shown to influence the relationships that older people develop and maintain with others. Unfortunately, it is not possible to review how each component of social structure may influence social ties in late life because such an undertaking would require a separate chapter. As a result, the discussion that follows focuses exclusively on the influence of race.

Different racial and ethnic groups have different cultural values that may influence the way they interact with others. For example, some researchers maintain that African Americans have a collectivist culture. More specifically, as Baldwin and Hopkins (1990) pointed out, African-American culture emphasizes inclusiveness, cooperation, interdependence, and collective responsibility. Given this collectivist worldview, one would expect to find that social relationships are more extensive, and more well-developed, among older African Americans than among older Caucasians.

Findings from the literature on race differences in social relationships, however, are by no means clear. A good deal of this work focuses on either social network composition or social support. With respect to social networks, Ajrouch, Antonucci, and Janevic (2001) reported that compared to Caucasians, African Americans tend to have smaller networks that contain disproportionately more family members. Even so, research on social network structure does not assess social relationships directly because this research is concerned with the form or structure of social ties rather than the content or function of the interaction that takes place within them. Instead, studies on factors such as social support are needed for this purpose. Silverstein and Waite (1993) conducted one of the better studies of race differences in social support. More specifically, they examined differences in instrumental and emotional support using data from the National Survey of Families and Households. Their complex series of analyses revealed that, overall, African Americans are no more likely than Caucasians to either give or receive instrumental and emotional support.

Even though there may not be differences in the amount of assistance exchanged by older Caucasians and older African Americans, it does not necessarily follow that social relationships are, therefore, comparable across racial groups in all respects. Instead, race differences may emerge in other ways. Four are examined briefly next.

First, elders in different racial groups may get assistance from different sources. This raises the possibility that the source of support may serve different functions and have differential effects on health across racial groups in late life. Some evidence of this may be found in the work of Krause (2002). He examined differences between older Caucasians and older African Americans with a comprehensive battery of measures assessing social support in the church. Substantial race differences emerged in the data. More specifically, the findings suggested that older African Americans give and receive more social support in church than their white counterparts. The fact that race differences emerge when the source of support is taken into consideration has important implications for the way we think about social relationships. Focusing on emotional support provides a good way to illustrate this point. People obviously receive and provide a good deal of emotional support outside, as well as inside, the church. That church-based support may be religiously motivated, however, suggests there may be subtle differences in the nature of emotional support that is exchanged in this setting. Compared to emotional support that is provided in secular settings, church-based emotional support may be driven by more altruistic motives, and the provider may be less likely to expect the recipient to reciprocate. If this difference exists, then we need to know if it has an especially beneficial effect on health. More fine-grained measures and more articulate theoretical frameworks are needed to evaluate this possibility.

Second, as discussed previously, certain social skills are needed to create and maintain social relationships. There do not appear to be any studies in the literature that examine race differences in social skills, but this is an important area to explore in the future. The skills needed to maintain relationships in collectivist cultures are likely to be quite different than the skills needed to function socially in more individualistically oriented cultures. In fact, given the unique historical experiences of African Americans, as well as the problems they face with racial injustice, there is a good chance that the social skills they need to function in society are unique and not likely to be found elsewhere. This possibility needs to be examined empirically.

Third, interpersonal assistance in different racial groups is likely to be put to different uses. In particular, research consistently shows that African Americans are exposed to disproportionately higher levels of prejudice and discrimination (Kessler, Mickelson, & Williams, 1999). Consequently, support from people of the same race may be critical in helping older African Americans cope effectively with the racial adversity they encounter. Evidence of this is provided in a study by Krause (2004b). This research revealed that older African Americans believe that religion has been an important source of strength in the face of racial difficulties. But more important, the data indicate that older African Americans who receive more emotional support from their fellow church members are especially likely to feel religion helps them in this way.

Fourth, most of the empirical research that has been done focuses on race differ-

ences in the amount or frequency of social support that has been exchanged. This is important information, but race differences can also arise in the impact of social support on health-related outcomes. This means that at the same level of assistance, the relationship between social support and health may be stronger for older African Americans than for older Caucasians. Differences in the impact of social support may arise because older African Americans are able to use support more effectively, or because there are subtle qualitative differences in the nature of the assistance that has been provided. Researchers rarely distinguish between differential levels of support and the differential impact of support on health, but they should.

These additional issues point to a new agenda in studying race differences in social relationships. More specifically, it is not sufficient to merely focus on how members of different racial groups respond to standard social support indicators. Instead, researchers need to throw a much wider net by studying race differences with a full complement of social relationship measures. For example, there do not appear to be any studies on race differences in companionship. Similarly, there is very little work on race differences in negative interaction. Okun and Keith (1998) provided simple bivariate correlations between race and negative interaction, but much more work needs to be done in this area. In addition, we need to know more about social relationships that involve people from different racial groups (e.g., support provided by older African Americans to older Caucasians). Cross-racial relationships obviously exist, but sufficient attention has not been given to them. This is especially true in social gerontology. What interpersonal adjustments are made when the parties in a biracial dyad come from cultural groups that rely on different social skills? A deeper understanding of how cross-racial relationships are formed and maintained is vitally important because it holds out the promise of helping to heal longstanding divisions in our society. Finally, we need more studies that look at cohort differences in social relationships among minority group members. For example, the oldest cohorts of African Americans grew up in a time when racism was prevalent and especially overt. We need to know more about how these historical experiences shape the way they relate to others, including those from different racial groups.

## V. The Current State of Theory on Social Relationships

As the discussion provided up to this point reveals, a good deal of empirical research has been done on social relationships in late life. Even so, the theoretical underpinnings of this work lag far behind. No one has provided a unified theoretical perspective that weaves the diverse empirical findings that have been generated into a more tightly integrated whole. Moreover, we have not fully exploited the broad-based and far-reaching insights provided by the grand theoretical masters in sociology.

As the literature currently stands, some investigators invoke social exchange theory to explain some facets of social relationships (e.g., Dowd, 1975), whereas others turn to the basic principles of symbolic interactionism to explain other dimensions (e.g., Krause & Borawski-Clark, 1994). More often than not, however, theoretical perspectives are not mentioned at all. Instead, focused hypotheses are tested that deal with circumscribed theoretical issues. For example, as discussed previously, some investigators report that social support offsets the deleterious effects of health because it bolsters self-esteem and feelings of personal control, or because

significant others help older people identify and implement new coping responses. But there are big gaps in this thinking. We do not have well-articulated theories that explain precisely how these support-based benefits arise. Viewed more broadly, we have assembled a disjointed list of empirical regularities in social interaction without a full understanding of what they reveal. Only by grounding this empirical work in more general principles of human nature and human behavior will we be able to tackle the deeper questions about who we become in old age and the forces that bring us to these points.

Researchers have bemoaned the state of theory in gerontology for decades (Birren & Bengtson, 1988), but relatively little progress has been made in many areas, including the study of social relationships. Part of the problem arises from the fact that many do not think well when faced with the task of sketching out the larger conceptual picture. One way to deal with this problem involves thinking inductively, looking across the collection of empirical findings for broader principles and regularities. An effort was made to lay the basic groundwork for doing this when the relationships between the various components of social interaction and health were discussed previously (see Section III). In particular, a deliberate attempt was made to examine these relationships from the symbolic interactionist perspective. The pieces are there; now someone needs to put them in place by filling in the gaps with classic insights of Cooley (1902) and Mead (1934/1962), as well as the more recent extensions of their work by Stryker (2001). Taking an inductive approach serves to highlight an essential point about grand theory and empirical research on social relationships: They form a two-way street. Although research on social relationships can benefit greatly from theory, theory may also benefit from research on social relationships.

# VI. Conclusions

Because the lives of older people are intimately connected with the lives of others, social relationships have far-reaching consequences for the health and well-being of our aging population. Social gerontologists have made great strides in illuminating the ways in which interpersonal ties affect health, but we need to think more about how the work we do can be used in intervention settings. The promise that the findings from our research will somehow improve the lives of older people is implicit in much of the work we do. It is time to make good on this promise. For example, there is a vast literature on interventions that attempt to enhance health and well-being by creating new social support systems or improving the quality of existing social ties (Hogan, Linden, & Najarian, 2002). But these support-based interventions have met with mixed success (Hogan et al., 2002). Although there are many reasons for this, at least part of the problem arises from the fact that our knowledge about social relationships, and the health-related benefits they provide, is still incomplete.

Many support-based interventions are designed to build new social relationships among people who have not known each other previously. Yet most of the research that has been done so far involves studying interpersonal relationships that have been in place for some time. So, for example, there is a good deal of work on intergenerational relationships. But if we want to design more effective interventions, then we need to know more about how new relationships are formed. The insights from research on weak social ties may be useful here because they represent the state of social relationships when support-based interventions are initiated. But this clearly is only a point of departure.

Presumably, many people are in support-based interventions because they have had difficulty forming strong social relationships on their own. They need to know precisely how to develop more effective ties with others. This is one reason why an emphasis was placed on social skills in the discussion provided previously. It seems that some people fail to develop close social relationships because they lack the necessary social skills to do so.

Other individuals are in support-based interventions because they are encountering significant negative interaction with the people they already know. Conducting research that shows that negative interaction has adverse effects on health is important, but it is of little help to these individuals. They need to find social skills that help resolve the interpersonal problems that confront them.

Thinking in terms of intervention design has an added benefit for social gerontologists. Virtually all the work that has been done so far relies on quasi-experimental designs, especially social surveys. This leads to nagging questions about the direction of causality between things like social relationships and mental health: Do people with strong ties have better mental health, or do people with initially good mental health subsequently develop better social ties? Moving into the intervention arena holds out the promise of resolving these thorny problems through the use of experimental designs. For example, older people who are depressed by the loss of a spouse can be assigned at random to treatment and control groups. Helping those in the treatment group to form new social relationships with others will make it possible to determine whether social relationships really do promote better mental health.

In many ways, the study of social relationships is as old as the discipline of sociology itself. As a result, from time to time, it is necessary to pause and reflect on the amount of progress that has been made. But progress is difficult to define.

Sometimes, we can judge our progress, not by the work that has been done, but by the questions that are raised and the new directions they propose. Using these criteria as a yardstick, it is hoped that the discussion provided in this chapter reveals that we have come a long way.

## Acknowledgment

Supported by the following grant from the National Institute on Aging: RO1 AG009221.

## References

Adelman, M. B., Parks, M. R., & Albrecht, T. L. (1987). Beyond close relationships: Support in weak ties. In T. L. Albrecht & M. B. Adelman (Eds.), *Communicating social support* (pp. 126–147). Newbury Park, CA: Sage.

Ajrouch, K. J., Antonucci, T. C., & Janevic, M. R. (2001). Social networks among blacks and whites: The interaction between race and age. *Journal of Gerontology: Social Sciences, 56B*, S112–S118.

Aldwin, C. M., & Gilmer, D. F. (2004). *Health, illness, and optimal aging*. Thousand Oaks, CA: Sage.

Alwin, D. F., McCammon, R.J., & Hofer, S. M. (2004). Studying baby boom cohorts with a demographic and developmental context: Conceptual and methodological issues. In S. K. Whitbourne & S. L. Willis (Eds.), *The baby boomers at midlife: Contemporary perspectives on midlife* (in press). Mahwah, NJ: Lawrence Erlbaum.

Aron, A. (2003). Self and close relationships. In M. R. Leary & J. P. Tangney (Eds.), *Handbook of self and identity* (pp. 442–461). New York: Guildford.

Baldwin, J. A., & Hopkins, R. (1990). African-American and European-American cultural differences as assessed by the Worldviews Paradigm: An empirical analysis. *Western Journal of Black Studies, 14*, 38–52.

Barrera, M. (1986). Distinctions between social support concepts, measures, and models. *American Journal of Community Psychology, 14*, 413–445.

Berger, P. L., & Luckman, T. (1966). *The social construction of reality: A treatise in the sociology of knowledge*. New York: Doubleday & Company.

Birren, J. E., & Bengtson, V. L. (1988). *Intergenerational perspectives on families, aging, and social support*. New York: Springer.

Bowlby, J. (1973). *Attachment and loss, Vol. 2: Separation*. New York: Basic Books.

Brim, O. G., Ryff, C. D., & Kessler, R. C. (2004). The MIDUS National Survey: An overview. In O. G. Brim, C. D. Ryff, & R. C. Kessler (Eds.), *How healthy are we? A national study of well-being in midlife* (pp. 1–34). Chicago: University of Chicago Press.

Caplan, G. (1981). Mastery of stress: Psychosocial aspects. *American Journal of Psychiatry, 138*, 413–420.

Carstensen, L. L. (1992). Social and emotional patterns in adulthood: Support for socioemotional selectivity theory. *Psychology and Aging, 7*, 331–338.

Clausen, J. A. (1993). *American lives: Looking back at the children of the Great Depression*. Berkeley, CA: University of California Press.

Cooley, C. H. (1902). *Human nature and the social order*. New York: Scribner's.

Cooley, C. H. (1929). *Life and the student: Roadside notes on human nature, society, and letters*. New York: Alfred A. Knopf.

Coyne, J. C., Wortman, C. B., & Lehman, D. R. (1988). The other side of support: Emotional overinvolvement and miscarried helping. In B. H. Gottlieb (Ed.), *Marshaling social support: Formats, processes, and effects* (pp. 305–330). Newbury Park, CA: Sage.

Dannefer, D., & Sell, R. (1988). Age structure, the life course, and "aged heterogeneity": Prospects for research and theory. *Comprehensive Gerontology, 2*, 1–10.

Department of Labor. (2002). *Volunteering in the United States*. From the following website: http://www.bls.gov.cps.

Dowd, J. J. (1975). Aging as exchange: A preface to a theory. *Journal of Gerontology, 30*, 584–594.

Elder, G. H. (1999). *Children of the Great Depression: Social change and life experience*. Boulder, CO: Westview.

Goldhaber, D. E. (2000). *Theories of human development: Integrative perspectives*. Mountain View, CA: Mayfield Publishing.

Gottlieb, B. H. (1997). Conceptual and measurement issues in the study of coping with chronic strain. In B. H. Gottlieb (Ed.),

*Coping with chronic stress* (pp. 3–40). New York: Plenum.

Granovetter, M. S. (1973). The strength of weak ties. *American Journal of Sociology, 78,* 1360–1380.

Haight, B. K., & Webster, J. D. (1995). *The art and science of reminiscing.* Washington, DC: Taylor & Francis.

Hansson, R. O., & Carpenter, B. N. (1990). Relational competence and adjustments in older adults: Implications for the demands of aging. In M. P. Stephens, J. H. Crowther, S. E. Hobfoll, & D. L. Tennenbaum (Eds.), *Stress and coping in later-life families* (pp. 131–151). New York: Hemisphere Publishing.

Hogan, B. E., Linden, W., & Najarian, B. (2002). Social support interventions: Do they work? *Clinical Psychology Review, 22,* 381–440.

Hogg, J. R., & Heller, K. (1990). A measure of relational competence for community-dwelling elderly. *Psychology and Aging, 5,* 580–588.

Johnson, C. L., & Barer, B. M. (2003). *Life beyond 85 years.* Amherst, NY: Prometheus Books.

Karner, T. X. (2001). Caring for an aging society: Cohort values and eldercare services. *Journal of Aging and Social Policy, 13,* 15–36.

Kermis, M. D. (1986). *Mental health in late life: Adaptive process.* Boston: Jones and Bartlett.

Kessler, R. C., Mickelson, K. D., & Williams, D. R. (1999). The prevalence, distribution, and mental health correlates of perceived discrimination in the United States. *Journal of Health and Social Behavior, 40,* 208–230.

Krause, N. (1987). Chronic financial strain, social support, and depressive symptoms among older adults. *Psychology and Aging, 2,* 185–192.

Krause, N. (2001). Social support. In R. H. Binstock & L. K. George (Eds.), *Handbook of aging and the social sciences* (5th ed., pp. 272–294). San Diego, CA: Academic Press.

Krause, N. (2002). Exploring race differences in a comprehensive battery of church-based social support measures. *Review of Religious Research, 44,* 126–149.

Krause, N. (2003). Exploring race differences in the relationship between social interac-tion with the clergy and feelings of self-worth in late life. *Sociology of Religion, 64,* 183–205.

Krause, N. (2004a). Stressors in highly valued roles, meaning in life, and the physical health status of older adults. *Journal of Gerontology: Social Sciences, 59,* S287– S297.

Krause, N. (2004b). Common facets of religion, unique facets of religion, and life satisfaction among older blacks. *Journal of Gerontology: Social Sciences, 59B,* S109– S117.

Krause, N. (2005). Negative interaction and heart disease in late life: Exploring varia-tions by socioeconomic status. *Journal of Aging and Health, 17,* 28–55.

Krause, N., & Borawski-Clark, E. (1994). Clarifying the functions of social support in later life. *Research on Aging, 16,* 251–279.

Krause, N., Shaw, B. A., & Cairney, J. (2004). A descriptive epidemiology of lifetime trauma and the physical health status of older adults. *Psychology and Aging, 19,* 637–648.

Lee, G. R., & Shehan, C. L. (1989). Social rela-tions and the self-esteem of older persons. *Research on Aging, 11,* 427–4442.

Lyons, R. F., Mickelson, K. D., Sullivan, M. J., & Coyne, J. C. (1998). Coping as a commu-nal process. *Journal of Social and Personal Relationships, 15,* 579–605.

McCarthy, G., & Davies, S. (2003). Some implications of attachment theory for understanding psychological functioning in old age. *Clinical Psychology and Psycho-therapy, 10,* 144–155.

McCullough, M. E., Tsang, J. A., & Emmons, R. A. (2004). Gratitude in intermediate affective terrain: Links of grateful moods to individual differences and daily emotional response. *Journal of Personality and Social Psychology, 86,* 295–309.

Mead, G. H. (1934/1962). *Mind, self, and soci-ety from the standpoint of a social behav-iorist.* Chicago: University of Chicago Press.

Meredith, G. E., & Schewe, C. D. (2002). *Defining markets, defining moments: America's 7 generational cohorts, their shared experiences, and why business should care.* New York: Hungry Minds, Inc.

Mills, C. W. (1959). *The sociological imagina-tion.* New York: Oxford.

Mirowsky, J., & Ross, C. E. (2003). *Education, social status, and health.* New York: Aldine De Gruyter.

Musick, M. A., & Wilson, J. (2003). Volunteering and depression: The role of psychological and social resources in different age groups. *Social Science and Medicine, 56,* 259–269.

Neugarten, B. L. (1977). Personality and aging. In J. E. Birren & K. W. Schaie (Eds.), *Handbook of the psychology of aging* (pp. 626–649). New York: Van Nostrand Reinhold.

Okun, M. A., & Keith, V. M. (1998). Effects of positive and negative social exchanges with various sources on depressive symptoms in younger and older adults. *Journal of Gerontology: Psychological Sciences, 53B,* P4–P20.

Pearlin, L. I., Menaghan, E. G., Lieberman, M. A., & Mullan, J. T. (1981). The stress process. *Journal of Health and Social Behavior, 22,* 337–356.

Pearlin, L. I., Mullan, J. T., Semple, S. J., & Skaff, M. M. (1990). Caregiving and the stress process: An overview of concepts and their measures. *The Gerontologist, 30,* 583–594.

Reissman, F. (1965). The helper therapy principle. *Social Work, 10,* 27–32.

Rook, K. S. (1984). The negative side of social interaction: Impact on psychological well-being. *Journal of Personality and Social Psychology, 46,* 1097–1108.

Rook, K. S. (1987). Social support versus companionship: Effects on life stress, loneliness, and evaluations of others. *Journal of Personality and Social Psychology, 52,* 1132–1147.

Rook, K. S., & Pietromonaco, P. (1987). Close relationships: Ties that heal or ties that bind? In W. H. Jones & D. Perlman (Eds.), *Advances in personal relationships* (Vol. 1, pp. 1–35). Greenwich, CT: JAI Press.

Rook, K. S., Thuras, P. D., & Lewis, M. A. (1990). Social control, health risk taking, and psychological distress among the elderly. *Psychology and Aging, 5,* 327–334.

Rowe, J. W., & Kahn, R. L. (1998). *Successful aging.* New York: Pantheon Books.

Ryff, C. D., & Singer, B. (1998). The contours of positive human health. *Psychological Inquiry, 9,* 1–28.

Schlenker, B. R. (2003). Self-presentation. In M. R. Leary & J. P. Tangney (Eds.), *Handbook of self and identity* (pp. 492–518). New York: Guilford.

Shaw, B. A., Krause, N., Chatters, L. M., Connell, C. M., & Ingersoll-Dayton, B. (2004). Emotional support from parents early in life, aging, and health. *Psychology and Aging, 19,* 4–12.

Silverstein, M., & Waite, L. J. (1993). Are blacks more likely than whites to receive and provide social support in middle and old age? Yes, no, and maybe. *Journal of Gerontology: Social Sciences, 48,* S212–S222.

Simmel, G. (1950). *The sociology of Georg Simmel.* Glencoe, IL: Free Press.

Stryker, S. (2001). Traditional symbolic interactionism, role theory, and structural symbolic interactionism: The road to identity theory. In J. H. Turner (Ed.), *Handbook of sociological theory* (pp. 211–231). New York: Plenum.

Tice, D. M., & Wallace, H. M. (2003). The reflected self: Creating yourself as (you think) others see you. In M. R. Leary & J. P. Tangney (Eds.), *Handbook of self and identity* (pp. 91–105). New York: Guilford.

Tornstam, L. (1997). Gerotranscendence: The contemplative dimensions of aging. *Journal of Aging Studies, 11,* 143–154.

Twelve

# Older Workers

Melissa Hardy

As the nations of the world address the challenges of population aging, two key issues of concern are whether a sufficient number of appropriately skilled workers will be available to maintain economic productivity and whether the existing retirement pension programs will be able to maintain the growing number of retirees. A multidisciplinary literature addresses various dimensions of these joined issues, including studies of the trends in employment rates among persons 55 years and older, the relationship between aging and changes in physical and mental capacity, the influence of current policies on the availability and utilization of older workers, and how new workplace programs and government policies may lead to improved opportunities for older workers. The policies proposed in response to these concerns differ in their targets for change and in their tone.

One set of strategies deals with the *supply* of older workers, their retirement decisions (and their preference for early retirement, in particular), and how changes in public policy could remove barriers to older workers' continuing attach-

ment to the labor force. This emphasis on increasing employment "opportunities" for older workers, however, has been coupled with new restrictions on pension entitlement, restructuring of retirement benefit programs, and attempts to make retirement less attractive or less affordable to older workers. Changing the terms of pension eligibility, reducing the level of income provided through pension benefits, and increasing taxation of Social Security benefits are examples of such policy changes that will likely increase the proportion of older workers who need to keep working and gradually increase the median age of retirement.

A second set of employment strategies focuses on the *demand* for the labor of older workers rather than on their supply decisions. Some of these strategies target employers' policies of hiring, retention, promotion, and retraining by challenging the negative and inaccurate stereotypes that continue to penalize older employees. Whereas some of the efforts involve redesigning human resource procedures within firms to encourage the retention and retraining of older workers, others target employers' actions by enforcing policies against age discrimination and strengthening the legal rights of older workers who have been the targets of discriminatory practices. Both of these policy streams occur against the larger backdrop of national economies, cultural views of distributional justice, and social constructions of intergenerational fairness.

The impact of population aging on the labor force is reflected in the attending changes in age structure. Among industrialized nations, declining fertility rates and slower population growth have been accompanied by a reduction in the proportion of economically active young adults (largely resulting from increases in educational attainment), a rising proportion of women in the labor force (including married women and mothers of young children), and a decreasing proportion of older men in the labor force. Although these correlated trends clearly have demographic roots, the organization of the life course around education, work, and family is also influenced by government and workplace policies that can either accommodate or inhibit an individual's attempts to engage these three domains in various combinations or sequences. But what may be desirable from the standpoint of individual development may not be feasible under prevailing institutional arrangements. As population processes have realigned, the industrial structure has also undergone some major transformations through downsizing, outsourcing, use of more sophisticated technology, and team-based approaches replacing the more traditional hierarchical organization of work activities. As employers search for ways to remain flexible and innovative and minimize fixed costs, their reliance on temporary workers, just-in-time inventories, and defined contribution pension plans has increased. Therefore, we examine issues related to older workers at a time when the composition of the labor force,

the nature of employment, and the labor market are all in flux.

## I. Who Are "Older" Workers in Today's Economy?

The lower age boundary defining "older worker" seems to depend on the context. Much of the retirement literature uses age 65 and older to define this category, a choice that reflects the salience of age 65 in previously enforced policies of mandatory retirement and entitlement for full Social Security benefits, as well as the general usage of the 18-to-64 age range in defining the "prime age" workforce. Within this context, "older worker" referred to someone whose continued attachment to the labor force ran counter to the normative pattern of retirement; by working beyond the "normal" retirement age of 65, these workers were considered categorically different from those who eschewed the option of "early" retirement.

The Age Discrimination in Employment Act (ADEA) of 1967 in the United States, however, uses age 40 and older to define the class of workers protected by the legislation. Although age 40 may seem too young to be an "older worker," the focus of the ADEA was not only on the perceived unfairness of forced terminations based on arbitrary age limits, but also on the problems being encountered by experienced workers who were not yet entitled to retirement benefits. Once out of a job, these workers found it difficult to secure comparable new jobs.

The wide range of ages used in these definitions of "older" or "aging" workers reflects the different policy questions underlying the classification. One fundamental question has been why workers 65 and older have not yet retired. At a time when retirement was an important management tool in maintaining a younger workforce and a major policy tool in minimizing unemployment, failure to retire was often viewed as problematic. In contrast, as average retirement ages steadily declined and the funding liabilities of defined benefit pension plans (including Social Security) grew, the underlying question in some quarters shifted to why so many people in their fifties were no longer working.

Recent government reports, including those issued by the U.S. Government Accounting Office, have used age 55 and older as their definition of "older workers." Here, the primary policy focus is on "early" retirement, with the underlying question being how the prevalence of early retirement can be reduced, the average age of retirement increased, and the typical working life span extended. Other questions addressed in the reports are: What types of employers hire, retain, and promote deserving older workers, and what types of employers would be willing to hire, retain, and promote deserving older workers if qualified workers in this range were available? Given the availability of suitable jobs, who in this age range wants to work, and how do they define "suitable" jobs?

## II. The Demographic Context of an Aging Labor Force

During the second half of the twentieth century, the rate of labor force participation (LFP) in the United States increased from 59% to 66%. A major component of that increase was due to a 14% climb in the LFP rate for women during the 20 years after 1970 (Fullerton, 1999). During the same period, LFP rates for men were gradually declining from 86% to 75%. The largest declines were associated with three age groups: 16- to 24-year-olds were down almost 9 points; rates for 55- to 64-year-olds dropped almost 19 points; and rates for those 65 and older were almost 30 points lower.

One consequence of these countervailing trends was a narrowing of the gender gap in LFP rates, especially among the youngest and oldest workers.

Increasing demographic diversity among U.S. workers has been a function of the changing race/ethnic composition of the population. Growth in the Hispanic, Asian, and Pacific Islander populations that began about 1970 has reintroduced a multicultural aspect to the labor force. As we begin the twenty-first century, the rate of labor force growth will slow, the gender composition will equalize (with about 48% of workers being women), the age structure will shift upward (with almost 1 in 5 workers being 55 and older by mid-century), and race/ethnic diversity will increase (with the proportion of white non-Hispanic workers dropping from 73% in 2000 to about 53% by 2050) (Toossi, 2002).

As the median age of the U.S. population increased, so did the median age of the workforce, although the trend has not been linear. In 1950, 17% of the labor force was 55 and older. Although this proportion dropped to 13% by the turn of the century, largely because of the distortion of the baby boom cohorts (born 1946–1964) having moved into early and then mid-career, workers 50 and older will become an increasingly large segment of the labor force (Toossi, 2002). As this unusually large cohort ages through its fifties and sixties, the median age of workers will increase.

This labor force aging will occur despite recent trends toward ever earlier retirement. Although lower than in 1950, the LFP rates of men 55 to 61 years old appear to have stabilized at about 72% (as of 2000); the LFP rates for women 55 to 61 years old have risen since 1950, reaching about 58% by 2000. Employment among men and women 62 to 64 years old actually increased between 1995 and 2001, from 42% to 46% for men and from 31% to almost 37% for women (Purcell, 2001).

## III. Age Discrimination in the Workplace

Beginning in the late 1800s, older workers faced increasing difficulties as the economy shifted from an agricultural to a manufacturing-based economy. Considered an obstacle to industrialization, older workers who resisted their loss of control over the labor process were viewed unfavorably by management. The "innovation" of the shorter workday also increased the pace of the production line, as employers attempted to recover the costs of the reduced schedule. In part, these changes involved a growing role for technology; however, it was not the technological change, per se, that made work more difficult for older workers. It was the speed at which the machines were operated. Within this context, employers seemed to find younger workers more pliable, less committed to union principles, and without the preindustrial work habits that management wanted to replace. As the twentieth century unfolded, older workers continued to have problems keeping their jobs. Census figures for 1930 reported an unemployment rate of 2.5% for 35- to 45-year-olds, 7% for persons 55 to 59 years old, and more than 13% for those 60 to 64 years old (Graebner, 1980). As the economy weakened, unemployment of older workers worsened. In response, a new federal policy enacted in 1935, Social Security, established wage replacement programs (unemployment insurance and retirement benefits). Entitled to an alternative source of income, older workers would not need to compete with younger workers for available jobs.

Providing older workers (and their families) with an adequate and dependable earnings replacement represented the primary method of addressing the difficulties older workers faced in keeping or finding jobs. Not only through Social Security, but also through post-World War II policies encouraging and regulating employer-sponsored pension plans, the federal government progressively strengthened older workers' claims to retirement benefits, thereby obviating the "need" for continued employment.

Although there had been several state laws prohibiting age discrimination before the mid-1950s (Neumark, 2003), the federal government did not prohibit age discrimination in the workplace until 1956 when the U.S. Civil Service banned maximum hiring ages in federal employment. Then in 1964, an Executive Order was issued by the President, disallowing age discrimination among federal contractors. The Older Americans Act of 1965, which encouraged research and assistance programs to help the elderly, also called for an end to age discrimination in the workplace. Unfortunately, none of these measures included any administrative procedures for implementation or enforcement. Therefore, the ADEA of 1967 was really the first federal policy that carried any significant weight. It prohibited mandatory retirement of federal and state employees before age 65, defining the protected group as those between 40 and 65 years old. A major impetus for legislating against age discrimination was the perception that older workers were being unfairly stereotyped. Although less likely to experience unemployment, if they did become unemployed, statistics showed that older workers had a more difficult time finding alternative employment and that their periods of unemployment were longer (Miller, 1966).

The Age Discrimination Act, passed in 1975, prohibited age discrimination in all programs receiving federal funds, including state or local government programs. In the years that followed, amendments progressively strengthened the ADEA. In 1978, protection was extended to nonfederal workers, and the protected group was expanded to age 70 (which thereby raised the minimum age of mandatory retirement to 70). Administrative responsibility for ADEA was shifted to the Equal Employment Opportunity Commission (EEOC) from the Department of Labor in 1979, and in 1986 the upper age limit was removed, thereby prohibiting mandatory retirement at any age except in jobs for which age is considered a bona fide criterion of ability (for the exceptions, see Chapter 23).

## A. Changing Retirement Transitions

Throughout most of the twentieth century, Americans viewed retirement as an event that occurred once in a lifetime and involved an immediate and complete withdrawal from full-time employment. Today, only about half of older workers experience retirement in this way. The other half passes through a period of partial retirement on the way to complete retirement or reverses the process by reentering the labor force (Hardy, 2002). Older workers are increasingly likely to follow an initial retirement with a period of part-time employment, spend some years between the end of their career job and retirement in "bridge" jobs, or interrupt their retirements with episodic spells of full-time employment. These new pathways into complete retirement have encouraged the view that "retirement" is now a somewhat individualized and evolving process that connects the end of "careers" with the end of "working life." If the time workers spend in specific jobs declines and job shifts increase, these pathways may grow longer and more diverse.

Reentry to the labor force (or "unretirement") is distinct from "partial" retirement (stepping down in hours worked per week or weeks worked per year) and from employment in "bridge" jobs. Displaced older workers must often move into lower-paying jobs to bridge the years to retirement. "Unretirement" is most common among retirees in their early to mid-fifties, and occurs within the first two years of retirement. It lasts an average of four years, and it involves jobs similar to bridge jobs, which pay lower wages, require fewer hours than the jobs previously held, and are more likely to involve self-employment (Hayward, Hardy, & Liu, 1994; Ruhm, 1990). At issue in this comparison, however, is not only what these jobs look like (as that depends on what jobs are available) but whether this transition appears to be planned or unanticipated.

# IV. Experiences of Older Workers in the Labor Market

As the financial circumstances of retirement improved, older workers began moving into retirement voluntarily at ever younger ages. A key element of the trend toward early retirement was a change in the structure of compensation. Whereas earnings from wages and salary had been the bases of negotiations between workers and employers, beginning in 1948, the National Labor Relations Board recognized fringe benefits, in general, and pensions, in particular, as a mandatory topic of contract negotiations between unions and management.

About half the U.S. labor force is covered by an employer-sponsored pension plan, either a defined benefit plan (DB) or a defined contribution plan (DC). DB plans were common among employers, particularly those in manufacturing, who wanted to encourage worker loyalty among young and middle-age workers, while managing the exit of older workers through mandatory retirement ages. But when these industries were being reorganized, moving older workers into retirement before the typical mandatory retirement age of 65 became more common, and DB plans provided a way to accomplish this goal. By structuring the accrual of pension wealth, firms could provide incentives for building seniority (30 years was a common career goal) and early retirement as well as disincentives for mid-career quits and delayed retirement.

In addition to their regular early retirement programs, beginning in the 1970s many firms used the DB plans to offer early retirement incentive packages (ERIPs) to encourage retirement at even earlier ages. Often coordinated with plant closings, ERIPs enabled firms to "shed" older workers and thereby minimize the number of layoffs among younger workers (Hardy, Hazelrigg, & Quadagno, 1996). The availability of employer-sponsored health insurance coverage for early retirees was an important component of the early retirement incentive package. Because retirees would not be eligible for Medicare coverage before age 65, potential early retirees were concerned not only about how much of their earnings would be replaced by pension benefits and ERIP buyouts, but also whether their health insurance coverage would continue. Firms that were straining under the long-term pension liabilities associated with DB plans were also looking for ways to cut back costs on health insurance. Promises of continued health coverage under regular retirement programs often included a clause that allowed employers to restructure coverage (e.g., increase retiree contributions), but because many of the incentive packages were considered separate retirement contracts, firms could not change the terms of the original offer. As health costs have increased, availability of employer-sponsored health insurance coverage for retirees under age 65 has declined (U.S. General Accounting Office, 2001).

Health insurance benefits for retirees are further jeopardized by company bankruptcies. Whereas DB pensions are insured by a federal agency, the Pension Benefit Guaranty Corporation (PBGC), health-care benefits are not. And although the Employee Retirement Income Security Act (which established the PBGC) regulates funding provisions for pension plans, companies are not required to put aside funds to cover promised retiree health care benefits. Under Chapter 11 of bankruptcy law, companies can file a plan for protection from their creditors, and workers' claims are often not a high priority in such plans. A company can "shed" its union contracts by arguing that the financial burden of those contracts makes it unattractive to prospective buyers. Once sold, the companies can be reopened as non-union operations.

Over time, increased federal regulation, ballooning pension liabilities, worker preference for portability, and employers' desire for flexibility in making labor force adjustments changed the mix of employer-sponsored pension plans. DB plan bankruptcies, conversions of DB to DC plans, and adoption of DC plans have made DC plans much more common. One consequence of this shift to DC plans is that DC plans influence retirement indirectly through their effect on individual wealth, thereby allowing the timing of retirement to be more individualized and less programmatically structured, and they include no penalties for delayed retirement. (See Chapter 20 for a fuller discussion of the trend to DC plans and the implications for retirement income.)

Although older workers have comparatively few spells of unemployment, the duration of these spells increases with age. Among those displaced, older workers have the lowest rates of reemployment. For those who find new jobs, older workers have high rates of reemployment in only part-time positions and the largest wage losses (Chan & Stevens, 1999). Recent studies indicate that there has been an increase in the relative rates of displacement among older workers

(Farber, 1997) and a deterioration of the circumstances of older workers in recent recessions. For example, between 1986 and 1991, involuntary job loss increased relative to quits, and this increase was particularly notable for older workers (Polsky, 1999). Further, the adverse consequences of these job losses became more severe as the century came to a close, especially for professionals, managers, and older workers (Polsky, 1999). The protection that seniority had once offered older workers has been eroding. Analysis of worker displacement and job loss during the recession of the early 1990s indicates that, with each successive recession, the risk to older workers has increased. Whereas evidence from earlier recessions indicated that older workers were less likely to be displaced than younger workers, during that particular recession this age difference disappeared, with younger and older workers being equally likely to have experienced job loss (Siegel, Muller, & Honig, 2000).

## V. Employment Opportunities for Older Workers

Nevertheless, the number of individuals 55 and older in the work force continues to grow (Hall & Mirvis, 1995). It is not unusual for workers to retire from one job and begin collecting pension benefits as they search for new jobs. Since the mid-1980s, full- and part-time work among "retirees" has increased significantly (Herz, 1995), but employers' views of older workers remain mixed. Positive traits associated with older workers include low absenteeism, low turnover, good work attitudes, strong motivation, good skills, and firm loyalty (Barth, McNaught, & Rizzi, 1993; Hassell & Perrewe, 1995). Unfortunately, studies indicate that many employers are influenced by the stereotypical view that older workers increase health costs, resist new

assignments, and are unsuited to retraining. Newly hired older workers are clustered in a smaller set of industries and occupations than newly hired younger workers or older workers in general (Hutchens, 1988). Occupations and industries in which older workers are employed tend not to hire older workers in entry-level positions (Garen, Berger, & Scott, 1996). Occupations with an older age profile are likely to be those with the fewest physical demands, flexible hours, flexible work schedules, and primarily low skill and training requirements. For example, older workers are generally not hired for jobs that require extensive use of computers (Hirsch, Macpherson, & Hardy, 2000).

Reeducating employers about the strengths and weaknesses of older workers might help to resolve this problem. Perhaps as a holdover from the production technologies of the earlier part of the twentieth century, older workers are thought to require more time than younger workers to complete their work—hence, the stereotype that they are less productive.

In fact, the research literature that deals with changes in productivity as workers age is spotty, and many of the studies refer to dated production technologies. The relationship between age and job performance is not well understood, nor is it empirically grounded in reliable data (Czaja, 1995). Much of the research on the relationship between aging and work performance fails to include contextual factors, such as job or occupational characteristics, specific mental and physical requirements of the job, organizational policies, the physical work environment, or the availability of necessary resources (Avolio, 1992; Waldman & Spangler, 1989). Age accounts for only a fraction of the between-individual variability in performance. In fact, experience appears to be a better predictor of job performance than age (Avolio, Waldman, & McDaniel, 1990).

## VI. Improving the Fit Between Human Resources and Jobs

Although the changing incentive structures of work and retirement embedded in public and workplace policy have also been studied in the context of European nations, a second important emphasis of European scholars has been the study of aging workers within the more general field of occupational health and the relationship of changes in human resources to work demands and the aging process. By demonstrating the effects of aging on work life, researchers hope to inform employment policies that will encourage increased LF participation of workers 55 and older.

A growing literature documents age-related changes in visual, auditory, and motor abilities that are relevant to work performance (Ketcham & Stelmach, 2004; Schieber, 2003). For example, rates of visual impairment increase with age, including a loss of static and dynamic visual acuity. Loss of contrast sensitivity, reduction in color sensitivity, greater sensitivity to problems of glare, and declines in dark adaptation are also age related (Fozard, 2000; Fozard & Gordon-Salant, 2001). Many older adults experience age-related hearing losses, including difficulty understanding speech and increased sensitivity to loudness (Irwin, 2000; Schieber, 2003). And, aging has been linked to slower response times, disruptions in coordination, loss of flexibility, and other declines in motor skills, such as reductions in strength, endurance, and dexterity (Fisk & Rogers, 2000; Walker, Philbin, & Fisk, 1997).

Changes in physical work capacity associated with aging include changes in the cardiovascular and musculoskeletal systems, body structure, and sensory systems. Although there are large individual differences, certain patterns of aggregate decline are apparent. For example, maximum oxygen consumption shows a clear, linear decline with age, although it is also responsive to regular exercise and can therefore be better maintained through adherence to a schedule of routine cardiorespiratory exercise. Even workers performing physically demanding work require positive physical exercise to maintain an average fitness level for their age. Regular physical exercise can keep physical capacity nearly unchanged between ages 45 and 65; however, failure to engage in regular exercise can make a 45-year-old worker less fit than an active 65-year-old (Ilmarinen, 2002; Nygard, Pohjonen, & Ilmarinen, 1999).

Cognitive declines with age have also been documented in experimental situations. Perception, memory, learning, thinking, and language use are cognitive functions that have received considerable attention from researchers (Kramer, Larish, Weber, & Bardell, 1999; Madden, 2001). The sensoriperceptive system that helps take in information, the cognitive system that processes information, and the motor systems that translate thoughts into actions slow with aging, although not uniformly. Working memory, problem solving and reasoning, inference formation, encoding and retrieval in memory, and information processing have all been shown to decline with age (Park, 1992; Salthouse, 1997). These changes in cognitive processing make it more difficult for older workers to shift their attention between displays, to multitask, and to maintain a rapid pace of information processing. But the evidence supporting these findings is largely experimental, produced in laboratory settings rather than in on-the-job situations.

In contrast, cognitive functions such as language use or processing complex problems in uncertain circumstances actually improve with age. Also, in many work situations, the motivation, experience, and wisdom of older workers can be effectively substituted for the speed and precision more characteristic of younger workers (Baltes & Staudinger, 2000; Czaja & Sharit, 1998). Further, the process of learning is not dependent on age, although the specific features of this process relative to brain structure may change with age, and the speed of learning may slow (Baltes & Smith, 1990; Salthouse, 1997; Schaie, 1994).

The complex connections among work experience, work performance, and aging require further study (McEvoy & Cascio, 1989; Salthouse & Maurer, 1996; Waldman & Avolio, 1986). Some research reports that older workers are as productive as younger workers in both skill-demanding and speed-demanding jobs (Spirduso, 1995). Ilmarinen (2002) argued that a large proportion of workers become physically weaker but mentally stronger as they age, and these changes should be reflected in work responsibilities that are less physically demanding but include more of the mental characteristics that improve with age. The concepts of *work ability* and *employability*, introduced by researchers at the Finnish Institute of Occupational Health (Ilmarinen, 1999a), address the connection between the capabilities of workers ("work ability"), the structure of job tasks, and the design of the work environment.

The changes in human resources discussed previously are one dimension of this concept, but the nature of work, including the structure of the work environment and the organization of the labor process, is another important aspect of work ability. As aging workers experience changes in their own levels of physical and mental functioning, or changes in their "work ability" (Ilmarinen, 1999b), they also encounter changes in work techniques and the tools of the trade, work expectations and work loads, the introduction of new technologies, and different methods of organizing the labor process (e.g., team approaches versus sequential individually performed operations). In past decades, such changes have

been used to justify the displacement of older workers under the assumption that older workers are unable to learn new techniques or adjust to new approaches. But researchers argue that instead, measuring "work ability" can become a tool for human resource managers and serve as a guide for how employers can build in adjustment periods for older workers that permit the identification of sources of friction in new labor regimens. Then they can develop appropriate training and design ergonomically superior work settings that allow work to flow smoothly. The complement to the work ability concept, *employability*, refers to the policies needed to increase the rate of labor force participation among older workers, including employment, education, and retirement policies; access to social and health services; programs to combat negative stereotypes; and legislation against age discrimination.

Neither *work ability* nor *employability* is limited in application to older workers; rather, both aim at the kind of social change needed to achieve better employment for workers of all ages. Although employers generally voice attitudes accepting of older workers, corporate policies and the actions of human resource officers may not be actively supportive of this rhetoric. Human resource managers also offer older workers little support for career development or career counseling (Hassell & Perrewe, 1995). As industries become more knowledge-based, employers need to reassess the value of older workers, the organizational roles they play, the institutional memory they represent, and the array of experiences they have accrued (DeLong, 2004).

## VII. Older Worker Policies in Comparative Perspective

Population aging is an issue for both developed and developing nations of the world. Whereas developing nations are often experiencing fundamental changes in industrial structure while at the same time trying to develop mechanisms to support elders in poverty, developed countries face problems ranging from severe strain on national pension systems to labor shortages. In spite of the rhetoric of "crisis" that often accompanies discussions of population aging in the United States, most other high-income nations will face circumstances more severe. The United States, Japan, Sweden, and the United Kingdom are high-income nations with relatively high rates of labor force participation among people 55 years and older. The United States has a higher total fertility rate (2.11 compared to 1.32 in Japan, 1.77 in Sweden, and 1.58 in the United Kingdom) and a higher net migration rate (3.7 compared to 0.4 in Japan, 1.1 in Sweden, and 2.3 in the United Kingdom), which slow the rate of population aging. Japan is experiencing much more rapid aging compared to the United States. Projections indicate that by 2050 the median age in Japan will be 53.2, or almost 12 years older than the expected median age of 41.4 in the United States (United Nations Population Division, 2005).

Not only is the rate of U.S. population aging lower than in many other nations, but its LFP rates for older workers are expected to remain higher than in most other high-income nations as we move through the years ahead. In France, Germany, and Italy, for example, only 2% to 4% of people 65 and older were in the labor force in 2000 compared to 10% in the United States. LFP rates for those 55 to 64 years old were less than 50% for men and women in Finland, France, and the Netherlands (International Labor Organization, 2002). The LFP rate for U.S. workers 50 to 64 years old was 66%, which ranked third behind Sweden (79%) and Japan (73%), and roughly the same as the United Kingdom (International Labor Organization, 2002). These relatively high rates of LFP are due to an increase in

employment among older women at the same time that the participation of older men has declined. The proportion of women among older workers has been increasing in most high-income nations since 1970 (although Japan is a notable exception), and many developing countries are now experiencing a similar trend. For example, for the period 1950 to 2010, Sweden will experience a tripling of LFP rates among women 50 to 64 years old (from 25% to 76%), and in the United States there will be a near doubling of the rate (from 31% to 58%) (U.S. General Accounting Office, 2003). However, the pattern is not uniform. Hungary has experienced declining LFP rates for older women since 1970 (International Labor Organization, 2002).

The countries with the highest LFP rates among older workers—Japan, Sweden, the United Kingdom, and the United States—have been modifying policies in an attempt to encourage employment of older workers and reduce pension costs. The United States began changing the structure of Social Security in 1983 by legislation that gradually increased the "normal" age for retirement benefit eligibility from 65 to 67 over a 25-year period from 2003 through 2027; the actuarial reduction in benefits for retiring early at age 62 is being increased from 20% to 30% during the same period. In addition, the Senior Citizens Freedom to Work Act of 2000 abolished the Social Security earnings test for persons 65 and older; they can work full-time and still receive full Social Security benefits.

Japan has substantially cut national pension benefits by raising the earliest eligibility age to 65 (from age 60) and reducing benefit levels. Sweden allows older workers to take full or partial national pensions benefits at age 61. Workers who take a one-quarter, one-half, or three-quarter pension are able to add to the value of their pension accounts while they continue to earn. When they finally move into full retirement, their benefits will be recalculated to reflect the additional earnings. The United Kingdom is gradually raising the national pension eligibility age for women to age 65, the age currently set for men, and they have introduced financial incentives for delaying retirement.

In addition to revising their national pension systems, some countries have also tightened eligibility for their disability programs, making it more difficult for older workers to replace earnings with disability benefits. Sweden previously allowed older workers to qualify for disability benefits on the basis of longterm unemployment or a combination of unemployment and medical conditions. Recent reforms now limit disability benefits to those who qualify on the basis of physical or mental impairments. The United Kingdom, which also requires a medical determination of eligibility for disability benefits, has initiated routine 3-year reviews of all disability claims. The United States tightened eligibility rules of disability benefits in the 1980s.

As indicated previously, employersponsored plans in the United States have been shifting from DB to DC plans, which are more portable than DB plans, but require individual workers to manage the investment risks. In Sweden, where employer-sponsored pensions cover 90% of workers, the same type of conversion of DB to a pure DC plan or a plan that combines DB with DC features has occurred. In the United Kingdom, many employers closed their DB plans to new workers, although workers already covered by a DB plan continue to be covered by them. New workers, however, are channeled into DC plans.

## A. Addressing the Structure of the Labor Market

Whereas modifying the structure of pension plans is likely to make early retirement more difficult to afford, making retirement less attractive can only increase the need or the desire of older workers to remain active in the labor force. The other half of the policy picture involves the behavior of employers and the opportunity structure that older workers encounter in the labor market. For this reason, a broad range of policy reforms that also address the labor market are required.

The United States was a world leader in passing legislation against age discrimination in the 1960s, 1970s, and 1980s, in an attempt to remove some of the barriers to the hiring and retention of older workers. In 2000, the European Union adopted a Council Directive that requires all member countries to introduce legislation prohibiting age discrimination in the workplace by the end of 2006; however, the directive allows countries considerable latitude in developing these policies (e.g., whether to eliminate mandatory retirement).

In 1997, Sweden raised the minimum mandatory retirement age from 65 to 67, and in 2001, the Swedish Parliament passed the Employment Protection Act, which requires firms attempting to downsize to follow the "first-in-last-out rule" (U.S. General Accounting Office, 2003). The United Kingdom and Japan have been relying on employers to voluntarily change policies that hinder older workers. For example, in 1999 the United Kingdom adopted a voluntary Code of Practice on Age Diversity, which set forth good practice standards for employers.

Although other countries are contemplating age discrimination legislation, the implementation of the ADEA in the United States has been significantly narrowed by Supreme Court rulings. For example, in 1993, the Supreme Court ruled that an adverse employment decision based on a factor highly correlated with age (e.g., service or salary) did not violate the ADEA (Hazen Paper Co.

v. Biggins, 91–1600 Supreme Court of the US, 507 U.S. 604, 1993). In 2000, the Supreme Court ruled that the Eleventh Amendment bars state employees from suing their employers in federal court for money damages under the ADEA (Kimel v. Florida Board of Regents, 98–791 Supreme Court of US, 527 U.S. 1067, 2000). Further, in writing their opinions, justices argued that for a state to discriminate on the basis of age was not necessarily an "irrational" employment policy. The most recent case involved the fundamental question of evidence. Claims of discrimination have been made on the basis of disparate treatment, as well as disparate impact. Disparate treatment requires the demonstration of intent to discriminate; however, disparate impact theory holds that practices that adversely affect older workers or other protected groups, such as those defined by race, color, religion, gender, or national origin, regardless of whether such practices were intentional, could be viewed as discrimination. Although a Supreme Court ruling issued in 1971 stated that Title VII of the Civil Rights Act of 1964 supports disparate impact as a cause of action, in 2002 the Supreme Court refused to review a lower court ruling that disparate impact was not available under ADEA (Adams v. Florida Power, 01–584 Supreme Court of the US, 535 U.S. 228, 2002).

The disallowance of disparate impact has important implications for the future of age discrimination claims. Proving intent to discriminate has always been difficult. Disparate impact allowed plaintiffs to demonstrate that a policy had a disproportionately negative impact on members of the protected group—in this case, older workers. Statistical evidence of this disproportionate effect was useful as evidence of discrimination. The elimination of disparate impact as the basis for a claim mandates proof of intent, but the proof does not necessarily have to be direct. In Reeves v. Sanderson Plumbing

(120 S. Ct. 2097 [2000]), the Supreme Court approved the framework necessary for establishing intentional discrimination. After Reeves established a prima facie case (Reeves was 57—a member of the protected group—when he was fired, qualified, and replaced by a younger worker), the burden of proof shifted to the employer, who claimed Reeves failed to maintain adequate employee records. Reeves then refuted this claim with witnesses who challenged the employer's testimony, reported that the employer had made negative age-based comments about Reeves, and treated Reeves especially harshly compared to younger workers. The jury found for Reeves, but the Fifth Circuit Court of Appeals overturned because Reeves had not convincingly established that the firing was motivated by age. The Supreme Court, however, unanimously found that "sufficient evidence to find the employer's asserted justification is false may permit the [conclusion] that the employer unlawfully discriminated" (Reeves v. Sanderson, 197 F. 3d 688, 693–694 [5th Cir. 1999]). In other words, plaintiffs do not need to directly demonstrate that the action was because of their age; discrediting the grounds claimed by the employer or showing the employer's justification to be a pretext provides circumstantial evidence consistent with a conclusion of intentional discrimination.

Japan, Sweden, and the United Kingdom have taken positive steps to help older workers remain competitive and to assist them in finding employment. For example, Japan has established wage subsidies to encourage the retention of older workers, and both Japan and the United Kingdom have allocated resources to organizations and services that help older workers find new jobs. Japanese job assistance centers provide older workers with temporary jobs or with volunteer opportunities, and they have also developed a program to match older workers with suitable employers. Recognizing that more flexibility in work arrangements may be attractive to older workers, Sweden is exploring policies to promote greater access to part-time work. In addition, in an effort to ensure that older workers have the necessary skills to make them employable, Sweden has begun promoting skill enhancement for them as part of the public education system (U.S. General Accounting Office, 2003).

In some high-income countries, part-time work is especially common for older workers. Older men and women in Japan frequently work part-time as a way of transitioning from full employment to complete retirement (International Labor Organization, 2002). Three-quarters of older workers (age 55 and over) in the Netherlands are in part-time positions, as well as more than half of older workers in the United Kingdom and Denmark (International Labor Organization, 2002). In the Netherlands, the aging of the labor force has been offset, in part, by a significant upsurge in early retirement and its large number of disability beneficiaries. In terms of industries, education and agriculture employ the highest proportion of older workers, with 10% to 15% of their workers age 55 or older. Some Dutch employers have adopted supportive "age-conscious" personnel policies, including ergonomic adjustments, additional leave or increased holiday time, flexible working hours, and age limits for irregular work or overtime hours. The 60% of all Dutch companies that have been formed during the last 10 years, however, tend to employ younger workers, and, when faced with a need for additional workers, employers tend not to look to older workers to fill that need (Remery, Hekens, Schippers, & Ekamper, 2003).

In sum, countries differ in their approaches to older workers. In many cases, policy changes shift to individuals some of the risks associated with retirement financing. Whereas many high-income countries cite a need for workers to remain in the labor force at older ages, they differ in what steps they take to create employment opportunities for older workers. Although many are eliminating or relaxing mandatory retirement policies, legislating or encouraging the elimination of age discrimination in the workplace, and putting in place incentives for continued earnings, fewer countries are improving and subsidizing the training of older workers, assisting older workers in job searches, and exploring ways to increase the flexibility of work schedules, the quality of work conditions, and the desirability of continued employment.

## B. Macro Influences

In surveying the changes in LFP rates for older men and women, we cannot ignore the social, economic, and political conditions that provide the broader context for individual actions. Although much has been written about retirement planning and decision making, workers attempting to engage these issues must proceed under conditions of considerable uncertainty, not only with regard to life events that are difficult to predict, but also with regard to larger-scale conditions that are beyond their control. Retirement planning requires certain assumptions about longevity (for self and spouse), health trajectories, labor markets, financial markets, and political sentiments that shape employment policies, retirement programs, and tax structures

The observed increase in LFP rates for men and women 55 and older that was observed at the end of the twentieth century occurred when the economy was strong and the unemployment rate was falling. The process of globalization will have a profound impact on the nature and intensity of competition among workers, firms, and national economies. Increased productivity occurs when firms compete more aggressively for shrinking orders;

workers compete more aggressively for limited job openings; firms are forced to improve efficiencies to protect profits (e.g., cost cutting measures and restructuring). But increased efficiencies can be due to improved management of organizational productivity, as well as to innovative technologies.

Maintaining a low rate of unemployment and industrial "restructuring" have often included the early retirement of older workers as a major strategy for achieving these goals. As noted previously, downsizing, especially in unionized firms, has been primarily accomplished by enticing older workers to accept early retirement incentive programs. Although these changes have often been legitimized as an attempt to reduce the size of the internal labor force, it has often been primarily a reconfiguration of the labor force—closing plants in one state only to open a new plant elsewhere, moving older workers into early retirement only to hire younger workers for the new plant.

In the Netherlands, for example, restricting early retirement was a high priority because the attractiveness of retirement was seen as a deterrent to continued employment among older workers. And there has been an increase in LFP rates among older Dutch workers; however, this shift preceded the early retirement reforms. It was coupled with a significant shift in public sentiment with regard to employment. Whereas sentiment in the 1970s and 1980s favored early retirement for older workers as a way to make room for younger workers, Dutch citizens currently favor "age-equality" in job opportunities (Van Dalen & Henkens, 2002).

One dilemma is how to manage the transition of more highly paid, older workers (for whom speed in the use of modern technologies as currently configured is an issue) into either self-financed early retirement or lower-paid, less attractive jobs. Technological change—

particularly the increased use of information technology equipment and software—has been a major reason for the recent acceleration of productivity growth, accounting for between a third and a half of the greater productivity growth in the late 1990s, relative to that of the 1974–1990 period.

Because age-related changes could pose difficulties for older workers in jobs that require an increasing amount of technological proficiency, training opportunities and appropriate training strategies are a particularly important component of an overall effort to address the fit between workers and jobs. As the skills that are linked to earlier technologies are rendered obsolete, workers must learn new skills and maintain their currency in a rapidly changing environment.

## VIII. Conclusions

Older workers of today are healthier, better educated, more highly skilled, and a larger proportion of the labor market than in any previous era. Yet, many employers continue to view older workers through a lens distorted by negative stereotypes that developed during the early days of the industrialization process. High rates of unemployment and a sense that human capital, developed in early adulthood, should be sufficient to see workers through their careers made "shedding" older workers a seemingly affordable solution. The long-term costs of that "solution" are now being realized, not only in terms of the pension liabilities that encumber the finances of firms, but also in terms of the organizational loss that occurs when senior workers disappear (DeLong, 2004).

On the surface, it appears that the initial "solution" for managing unemployment through early retirement will now be restructured to find a new "solution" to the growing cost of retirement. Early retirement will increasingly need to be self-financed, through personal savings, in general, and the accumulation of pension wealth through DC plans, in particular. But it is unlikely that the DC accounts currently being nurtured by younger workers will allow them to afford the early retirement of their parents' generation. The restructuring of retirement plans—both national pensions and employer-sponsored pensions—will encourage (or require) later exits. To varying degrees, nations are trying to coordinate pension reorganization with policies that improve work conditions and job opportunities for older workers.

But before we can intelligently design policy, we must build a better understanding of how workers age, how aging workers function, and how jobs, training strategies, workplace design, employment law, and workplace regulations influence these dynamic processes. We know too little about the diversity of work patterns in later life or how aging affects work performance. We have identified a variety of age-related changes in functioning, but we need more research on how these changes connect to job requirements in different types of employment. Although researchers have paid considerable attention to the role of pensions in retirement behavior, work satisfaction, schedule flexibility, phased retirement options, and supportive work environments have received much less attention. Whereas some jobs provide opportunities for personal growth and creative expression, other jobs subject workers to physical strain, emotional stress, and hazardous conditions. Careful study of workplace interventions may provide evidence of how to make work less stressful, how to increase worker satisfaction, how to reconfigure jobs or better train workers, and how technology is changing the workplace. Research that addresses these fundamental questions may be tackled productively within a variety of disciplines, as well as through

interdisciplinary teams, but it needs to go beyond comparisons of averages and address other distributional features. Once we have developed these areas through basic science, we can translate what we have learned into the design of tools and work environments that optimize performance while keeping injuries to a minimum.

Increasing the average age of retirement may be a legitimate goal for many nations of the world, but doing so in a responsible way requires doing more than rescinding the individual-level incentives that have made early retirement so attractive. By addressing aging as a developmental process—a process that is responsive to the opportunities and the constraints encountered in the environment—we can develop employment policies to manage the fit between worker skills and capabilities and the way work is organized. Crafting creative responses to these issues may make it possible to structure jobs, job tasks, and work environments for a diverse work force that will benefit workers of all ages.

## References

Avolio, B. J. (1992). A levels of analysis perspective of aging and work research. In K.W. Schaie & M. P. Lawton (Eds.), *Annual review of gerontology and geriatrics* (pp. 239–260). New York: Springer.

Avolio, B. J., Waldman, D. A., & McDaniel, M. A. (1990). Age and work performance in nonmanagerial jobs: The effects of experience and occupational type. *Academy of Management Journal, 33,* 407–422.

Baltes, P., & Smith J. (1990). Toward a psychology of wisdom. In R. J. Stenberg (Ed.), *Wisdom: Its nature, origin and development* (pp. 87–120). New York: Cambridge University Press.

Baltes, P. B., & Staudinger, U. M. (2000). Wisdom: A metaheuristic (pragmatic) to orchestrate mind and virtue toward excellence. *American Psychologist, 55*(1), 122–136.

Barth, M. C., McNaught, W., and Rizzi, P. (1993). Corporations and the aging workforce. In P. H. Mirvis (Ed.), *Building the competitive workforce: Investing in human capital for corporate success*. New York: Wiley, 1993.

Chan, S., & Stevens, A. H. (1999). Employment and retirement following a late-career job loss. *American Economic Review, 70*(3), 355–371.

Czaja, S. J. (1995). Aging and work performance. *Review of Public Personnel Administration, 15*(2), 46–61.

Czaja, S. J., & Sharit, J. (1998). Ability-performance relationships as a function of age and task experience for a data entry task. *Journal of Experimental Psychology: Applied, 4*(4), 332–351.

DeLong, D. W. (2004). *Lost knowledge: Confronting the threat of an aging workforce*. New York: Oxford University Press.

Farber, H. S. (1997). The changing face of job loss in the United States, 1981–1995. *Brookings Papers on Microeconomic Activity: Microeconomics*, 55–128. Washington, DC: The Brookings Institution.

Fisk, A. D., & Rogers, W. A. (2000). Influence of training and experience on skill acquisition and maintenance in older adults. *Journal of Aging and Physical Activity, 8*, 373–378.

Fozard, J. L. (2000). Sensory and cognitive changes with age. In K. W. Schaie & M. Pietrucha (Eds.), *Mobility and transportation in the elderly* (pp. 1–44). New York: Springer.

Fozard, J. L., & Gordon-Salant, S. (2001). Changes in vision and hearing with aging. In J. E. Birren & K. W. Schaie (Eds.), *Handbook of psychology of aging* (pp. 241–266). San Diego, CA: Academic Press.

Fullerton, H. (1999). Labor force participation: 75 years of change, 1950–98 and 1998–2025. *Monthly Labor Review, 122*(12), 3–12.

Garen, J., Berger, M., & Scott, F. (1996). Pensions, non-discrimination policies, and the employment of older workers. *Quarterly Review of Economics and Finance, 36*(4), 417–429.

Graebner, W. (1980). *A history of retirement: The meaning and function of the American institution, 1885–1978*. New Haven, CT: Yale University Press.

Hall, D. T., & Mirvis, P. H. (1995). The new workplace and older workers. In J. A. Auerbach & J. C. Welsh (Eds.), *Aging and competition: Rebuilding the U.S. workforce* (pp. 58–63). Washington, DC: National Council on the Aging and National Planning Associates.

Hardy, M. A. (2002). The transformation of retirement in 20th century America. *Generations, 26*(2), 9–16.

Hardy, M. A., Hazelrigg, L. E., and Quadagno, J. (1996). *Ending a career in the auto industry: Thirty and out*. New York: Plenum Publishing.

Hassell, B. L., & Perrewe, P. L. (1995). An examination of beliefs about older workers: Do stereotypes still exist? *Journal of Organizational Behavior, 16*(5), 457–468.

Hayward, M. D., Hardy, M. A., & Liu, M. C. (1994). Work after retirement: The experience of older men in the U.S. *Social Science Research, 23*, 82–107.

Herz, D. (1995). Work after early retirement: An increasing trend among men. *Monthly Labor Review, 118*(4), 13–20.

Hirsch, B., Macpherson, D., & Hardy, M. (2000). Occupational age structure and access for older workers. *Industrial and Labor Relations Review, 53*, 401–418.

Hutchens, R. M. (1988). Do job opportunities decline with age? *Industrial and Labor Relations Review, 42*, 89–99.

Ilmarinen, J. E. (1999a). *Ageing workers in the European Union—status and promotion of work ability, employability and employment*. Helsinki: Finnish Institute of Occupational Health, Ministry of Social Affairs and Health, Ministry of Labour.

Ilmarinen, J. E. (1999b). Promotion of work ability during ageing. *American Journal of Industrial Medicine Supplement, 1*, 21–23.

Ilmarinen, J. E. (2002). Physical requirements associated with the work of aging workers in the European Union. *Experimental Aging Research, 28*(1), 7–23.

International Labour Organization (2002). *Estimates and projections of the economically active population, 1950–2010*, 4th ed., rev. 2. Geneva.

Irwin, J. (2000). What are the causes, prevention and treatment of hearing loss in the ageing worker? *Occupational Medicine, 50*, 492–495.

Ketcham, C. J., & Stelmach, G. E. (2004). Movement control in the older adult. In R. W. Pew & S. B. Van Hemel (Eds.), *Technology for adaptive aging* (pp. 64–92). Washington, DC: The National Academies Press.

Kramer, A. F., Larish, J. L., Weber, T. A., & Bardell, L. (1999). Training for executive control: Task coordination strategies and aging. In D. Gopher & A. Koriat (Eds.), *Attention and performance XVII: Cognitive regulation of performance: Interaction of theory and application* (pp. 617–652). Cambridge, MA: MIT Press.

Madden, D. J. (2001). Speed and timing of behavioral processes. In J. E. Birren & K. W. Schaie (Eds.), *Handbook of the psychology of aging* (5th ed., pp. 288–312). San Diego, CA: Academic Press.

McEvoy, G. M., & Cascio, W. F. (1989). Cumulative evidence of the relationship between employee age and job performance. *Journal of Applied Psychology, 74*(1), 11–17.

Miller, D. G. (1966). Age discrimination in employment: The problem of the older worker. *New York University Law Review, 41*(2), 383–424.

Neumark, D. (2003). Age discrimination legislation in the United States. *Contemporary Economic Policy, 21*(3), 297–317.

Nygard, C. H., Pohjonen, T., & Ilmarinen, J. (1999). Muscular strength of ageing employees over an 11-year period. In J. Ilmarinen & V. Louhevaara (Eds.), *FinnAge—Respect for the ageing. People and work, Research reports 26* (pp. 240–249.). Helsinki: Finnish Institute of Occupational Health.

Park, D. C. (1992). Applied cognitive aging research. In F. I. M. Crail & T. A. Salthouse (Eds.), *The handbook of aging and cognition* (pp. 449–494). Mahwah, NJ: Laurence Erlbaum Associates.

Polsky, D. (1999). Changing consequences of job separation in the United States. *Industrial and Labor Relations Review, 52*, 565–580.

Purcell, P. J. (2001). Older workers: Employment and retirement trends. *Congressional Research Service Report RL30629.* Washington, D.C.: U.S. Library of Congress.

Remery, C., Henkens, K., Schippers, J., & Ekamper, P. (2003). Managing an aging workforce and a tight labor market: Views held by Dutch employers. *Population Research and Policy Review, 22*, 21–40.

Ruhm, C. (1990). Bridge jobs and partial retirement. *Journal of Labor Economics, 8*(4), 482–501.

Salthouse, T. A. (1997). Implications of adult age differences in cognition for work performance. In A. Kilborn, P. Westerholm, & L. Hallsten (Eds.), *Work after 45!* (Vol. 1, pp. 15–28). Arbete och Halsa. Arbetslivsinstitutet. Solna.

Salthouse, T. A., & Maurer, T. J. (1996). Aging, job performance, and career development. In J. E. Birren & K. W. Schaie (Eds.), *Handbook of the psychology of aging* (4th ed., pp. 353–364). San Diego, CA: Academic Press.

Schaie, K. W. (1994). The course of adult intellectual development. *American Psychologist, 38*, 239–313.

Schieber, F. (2003). Human factors and aging: Identifying and compensating for age-related deficits in sensory and cognitive function. In N. Charness & K. W. Schaie (Eds.), *Impact of technology on successful aging* (pp. 42–84). New York: Springer.

Siegel, M., Muller, C., & Honig, M. (2000). The incidence of job loss: The shift from younger to older workers, 1981–1996. (December 2000). New York: International Longevity Center, Working Paper No. 2000–03.

Spirduso, W. W. (1995). Job performance of the older worker. In W. W. Spirduso (Ed.), *Physical dimensions of aging* (pp. 367–387). Champaign, IL: Human Kinetics.

Toossi, M. (2002). A century of change: The U.S. labor force, 1950–2050. *Monthly Labor Review, 125*(5), 15–28.

United Nations Population Division. (2005). World Populations Prospects, The 2004 Revision. New York: United Nations.

U.S. General Accounting Office. (2001). *Retiree health insurance: Gaps in coverage and availability.* GAO-02-178T. Washington, DC: Government Printing Office.

U.S. General Accounting Office. (2003). *Older workers: Policies of other nations to increase labor force participation.* Report GAO-03-307. Washington, DC: Government Printing Office.

Van Dalen, H. P., & Henkens, K. (2002). Early-retirement reform: Can it and will it work? *Ageing and Society, 22,* 209–231.

Waldman, D. A., & Avolio, B. J. (1986). A meta-analysis of age differences in job performance. *Journal of Applied Psychology, 71*(1), 33–38.

Waldman, D. A., & Spangler, W. D. (1989). Putting together the pieces: A closer look at the determinants of job performance. *Human Performance, 2,* 29–59.

Walker, N., Philbin, D. A., & Fisk, A. D. (1997). Age-related differences in movement control: Adjusting submovement structure to optimize performance. *Journals of Gerontology, Series B: Psychological Sciences and Social Sciences, 52*(1), P40–P52.

Thirteen

# Economic Status of the Aged

Karen Holden and Charles Hatcher

The ability of individuals to maintain some expected standard of living after labor market work ceases at retirement is an issue confronting all societies at all levels of economic development. It has moved to the forefront of the public discussion in the United States as the population ages, a consequence of declining fertility and increases in life expectancy. This aging of the population has called into question the adequacy of individuals' retirement savings behavior and the appropriateness of current retirement-income policies. Economic support subsequent to labor force withdrawal can come from one's own retirement savings, employer-provided pension plans, social insurance payments, or transfers from family and friends. Longer lives present challenges to all these sources. One's own savings must be drawn down over an ever-increasing retired lifetime, and employers, governments, and families must expect to have sufficient foresight to fund the current and future retiree population for lives that continue to increase with imprecise predictability. Thus, the well-being of the older population is a key part of policy discussion about the

adequacy of savings for retirement among younger birth cohorts and the appropriate role of government as a direct provider, subsidizer, or regulator of retirement pension and savings programs.

Central to the discussion of individuals' level of economic well-being and the role of government in income provision to older adults is agreement on a conceptual definition of economic well-being, of the measure that is used to quantify and assess levels and changes in well-being over time and across population groups. In this chapter, we first present statistical data on money income levels and the distribution of income among individuals and households in the United States. This is the most frequently reported measure of well-being, largely because of its ease, and therefore frequency, of collection. To provide a more complete picture of resources available to older households, we describe levels and distributions of wealth holdings across households. We follow these descriptions with a discussion of a variety of approaches to measuring economic well-being that go beyond measures of income and wealth. We end with a consideration of future research

*Handbook of Aging and the Social Sciences, Sixth Edition*

issues concerning the economic status of older individuals, including future cohorts of older persons.

# I. Income and Asset Status of Older Adults

Table 13.1 shows the mean and median incomes of U.S. households in 2001, classified by the age of the head of the household. Both measures are presented since the mean (the total of the income of all households in the group divided by the number of households in the group) is more sensitive than the median (the income level where 50% of households are below the level) to the presence of unusually high- or low-income households. The numbers in Table 13.1 indicate that as the age of the head of the household rises, income increases until it peaks in the 45- to 54-year age range, declining thereafter.

Differences between means and medians for a group of households imply an income distribution that is distributed unevenly in that group. A higher mean than median implies an income distribution skewed toward higher incomes. The ratio of the mean to the median suggests relative stability in income distribution during the prime working years, with income becoming more skewed toward higher incomes during the early retirement years. A more direct measure commonly used to measure inequality is the Gini coefficient, which measures how concentrated income is within a group. The Gini coefficient ranges between 0 and 1, zero being a perfectly even distribution of income (all households have the same income) and 1 being a perfectly uneven distribution (1 household has all the income). With the exception at the youngest age (of household heads), the distribution of wealth first equalizes with increasing age and then, as shown by the increasing Gini, becomes more unequal for households headed by older persons. Among younger households differences in levels and the distribution of income are largely driven by differences across households in labor force participation and labor market earnings, whereas at older ages differences among households in retirement timing and access to and benefits received from pensions and Social Security are major influences on income inequality.

Figure 13.1 shows median household income (in price-adjusted dollars) by age at several points in time. As a group, older households have made progress in income relative to other groups, although incomes remain absolutely lower com-

### Table 13.1
Income of U.S. Households by Age of Head of Household, 2001

| Age | Mean | Median | Mean/Median | Gini |
|---|---|---|---|---|
| 15–24 | $35,340 | $26,900 | 1.31 | 0.449 |
| 25–34 | 56,202 | 46,272 | 1.21 | 0.405 |
| 35–44 | 71,704 | 57,492 | 1.25 | 0.391 |
| 45–54 | 83,923 | 68,114 | 1.23 | 0.366 |
| 55–64 | 76,157 | 54,457 | 1.40 | 0.409 |
| 65–74 | 53,279 | 36,985 | 1.44 | 0.428 |
| Over 75 | 40,976 | 30,126 | 1.36 | 0.396 |
| All Households | $66,863 | 51,407 | 1.30 | 0.414 |
| Under 65 | $70,306 | 55,645 | 1.26 | 0.405 |
| Over 65 | $48,318 | 33,816 | 1.43 | 0.423 |

Source: U.S. Census Bureau, 2002.

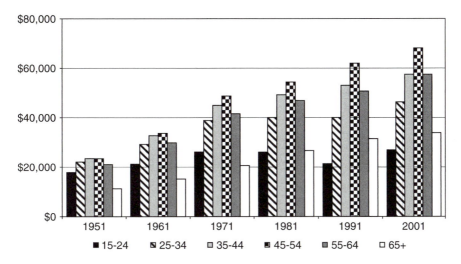

**Figure 1**   Median Income by Age of U.S. Household Head and Survey Year (in 2001 dollars)
**Source**: U.S. Bureau of the Census (various years).

pared to younger age groups. The median income level of older households (age 65 and over) has tripled in the last 50 years, compared to only a doubling for the median of age 25–34 households. The median household income for the over-65 population was only about half that of households 25 to 34 years old in 1951, but that ratio was nearly three-quarters in 2001. The story is the same, whether growth in median income is calculated with 1951, 1961, or 1971 as the base year.

Data in Figure 13.1 compare age groups at a point in time and exhibit an age-related pattern that may not conform to how incomes actually change as individuals (or household heads) age over time. One must follow the same group of individuals over time as they age, for example those 15 to 24 years old in 1951, 25 to 34 years old in 1961, 35 to 44 years old in 1971, 45 to 54 years old in 1981, and 55 to 64 years old in 1991, to observe "cohort" patterns of income growth and decline. For this cohort (15–24 years old in 1951), increases in median income were greater over the preretirement years, and declines

were smaller than would have been predicted based on 1951 or 1961 cross-sectional age patterns. For this reason it is difficult to predict with any degree of certainty what might be the income experiences of more recent cohorts (e.g., 15 to 24 years old in 1991 or 2001), although median income increases appear to promise continuing gains in average economic well-being.

## A. Poverty

Another way to look at differences in income among the aged and between the aged and other groups is to observe the percentage that falls below some measure of income adequacy and to see how that has changed absolutely for older adults and relative to the risk of poverty facing younger families. The poverty threshold is specific to household size and thus takes account of lower consumption requirements of smaller households. In 2004, the official government poverty threshold was $9,060 for an individual 65 and older and $11,418 for a two-older-adult household, a threshold that is adjusted each year with price changes. These thresholds are 8% and 10%, respectively, below the equivalent thresholds for households of similar size headed by persons of younger ages. These differences are controversial and are often rationalized by the supposed lower work-related expenses and taxes imposed on older individuals.

Table 13.2 shows the percentage of the aged and non-aged who lived in households with incomes below the official government poverty threshold. Older individuals are now less likely to be in poverty than are younger individuals. The difference is striking when comparing the older population to children, who are more than 70 percent more likely to live in poverty. This gap is quite different from 30 years ago, when the poverty rates for older and younger Americans were quite close. Since 1973, we have seen a significant decline in poverty rates among the old (by about 40%), while the period 1973–1983 saw poverty rates among children nearly double, and then decline over the last 10 years. Earnings gains by each new cohort entering the labor market (as seen in Figure 13.1), and the consequent higher benefits from employer-provided pensions and Social Security, are generally credited with bringing poverty rates down among the older population. The higher poverty among younger families is attributed to a slowing of income growth

among younger cohorts (as seen in Figure 13.1) and rising percentages of single parent families.

Table 13.3 compares poverty rates by age groups in 2001 for African Americans, Hispanic Americans, and the total U.S. population. In each age group, African-American and Hispanic households have higher poverty rates than does the total population of the same age. Compared to a poverty rate of 10.1% for all individuals 65 and older, 21.9% of older African Americans and 21.8% of older Hispanics are poor. As is the case for the total population, among African Americans and Hispanics older individuals are less likely to be poor than are children in their racial categories. African-American children are about 38% more likely to be poor (30.2% are poor) and Hispanic children about 28% more (28.0% are poor) likely to be poor than are those 65 and older. This is a smaller difference than between children and older adults in the total population (all children are 61% more likely to be

**Table 13.2**
Percent of Individuals Living in U.S. Households with Income Below Poverty Threshold by Age, 1973–2003

|  | 1973 | 1983 | 1993 | 2003 |
|---|---|---|---|---|
| **All Americans** |  |  |  |  |
| Under 18 | 14.4% | 22.3% | 22.7% | 17.6% |
| 18–64 | 8.3 | 12.4 | 12.4 | 10.8 |
| 65 and older | 14.6 | 10.3 | 9.6 | 10.2 |

Source: U.S. Census Bureau, 2002.

**Table 13.3**
Percent of U.S. Age Groups Living in Households with Income Below Poverty and Near-Poverty Thresholds, by Race, 2001

|  | Household with Income Below | |
|---|---|---|
|  | Poverty Threshold | 150% of Poverty Threshold |
| **All Individuals** |  |  |
| Under 18 | 16.3% | 27.5% |
| 18–64 | 10.1 | 17.4 |
| 65 and older | 10.1 | 24.2 |
| **African Americans** |  |  |
| Under 18 | 30.2 | 45.8 |
| 18–64 | 16.9 | 27.6 |
| 65 and older | 21.9 | 41.3 |
| **Hispanic Americans** |  |  |
| Under 18 | 28.0 | 46.6 |
| 18–64 | 17.7 | 32.1 |
| 65 and older | 21.8 | 42.1 |

Source: U.S. Census Bureau, 2002.

poor), but it does not necessarily reflect greater success in securing incomes for African-American and Hispanic children. Rather, it is more likely that it is the legacy of labor market discrimination that limited for minority workers and retirees the increases in wages and pension coverage to which the gains for older Americans in general have been attributed.

The relative economic status of older adults looks somewhat different if one considers the percentage of households that are below 150% of the poverty threshold. Although older Americans were no more likely to be poor in 2001 than individuals 18 to 64 years old, and far less likely to be poor than children, they are much more likely to have incomes that fall below this higher, but still low, threshold than were nonolder adults, and only slightly less likely than were children. The relatively low poverty rates can be attributed in part to the Social Security program. An average wage earner (earning at the mean of the

national wage index throughout his or her working life) would receive Social Security benefits at age 62 equal to approximately 150% of the poverty threshold if married and about 125% of the threshold as a single individual (Social Security Administration, 2004). As is suggested in Table 13.3, Social Security benefits appear to substantially reduce the risk of poverty for older Americans, but if they are the sole source of income, beneficiaries are at relatively high risk of clustering just above that threshold. Moving beyond "near poverty" requires access to other sources of retirement income.

Figure 13.2 compares median money income of married and unmarried units by age. With the exception of the oldest age group, the median couple has more than twice the income of unmarried men or women. This means that even taking account of the differing consumption needs of two- and one-person households, women and men living alone have, on average, fewer income resources per

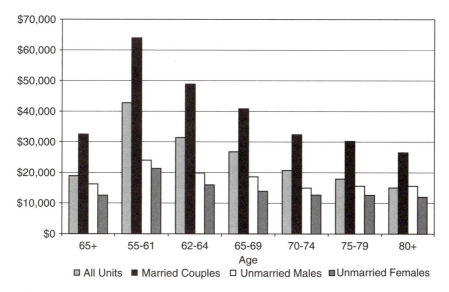

**Figure 2**   Median Income by Age and Marital Status; Aged Units, 2001
**Source**: U.S. Census Bureau (various years).

person than do married older persons. This translates into higher individual poverty rates for unmarried women and men than for couples (Table 13.4). The disadvantaged position of unmarried older individuals, particularly women, is unrelated to how "poverty" is defined; if the threshold is raised by half again, single men and women are still far more likely to be poor than are married men and women.

## B. Sources of Income

Table 13.5 demonstrates the importance of Social Security for individuals over age 65; 90% of all persons 65 and over receive some benefits from this program, which accounts for more than one-third of the aggregate income of older adults. A much smaller percentage receives income from the other three main sources of income: earnings, retirement benefits (employment-related pensions, private annuities, government employee pensions, and Railroad Retirement), and assets (interest, dividends, and rents). (Excluded from the table is the 2% to 4% of income from

aggregated "other sources," such as cash gifts and gambling winnings.) The U.S. retirement system is sometimes described as a "three-legged stool," composed of income from Social Security, employer-provided pensions, and private savings. However, not all older Americans are fully retired. Earnings by older persons remain an additional important "leg" as older Americans continue to work (mainly part-time) while either receiving Social Security benefits or by postponing receipt of benefits. Nevertheless, for older Americans generally, asset and pension incomes are shorter legs than is Social Security. One reason for the relatively low share of income from assets is that "pension" income includes annuities from tax-advantaged individual savings vehicles such as Individual Retirement Accounts and 401(k) accounts; these are classified as "pensions" even though, strictly speaking, they are not deferred compensation accounts provided by an employer.

Table 13.5 also shows the difference between the incomes of married couples and unmarried older women and men. That women have even lower income, and far lower pension income when received, is consistent with lower earnings of working women being translated into lower Social Security benefits and private pension coverage and income. Single women, the majority of whom are widows, are more dependent than are married couples and unmarried men on Social Security benefits. The greater dependence by certain groups on Social Security implies the importance of that program to the economic status of older households, particularly for unmarried women.

## C. Wealth

While older households tend to have less income than younger adults, the situation is the reverse when considering the

**Table 13.4**
Percent of U.S. Older Individuals Living in Households with Income Below Poverty and Near-Poverty Thresholds, by Gender and Marital Status, 2001

|  | Percent Below Poverty Threshold | Percent Below 150% of Poverty Threshold |
|---|---|---|
| All individuals 65+ | 10.1% | 24.2% |
| Men 65+ | 7.0 | 17.9 |
| Women 65+ | 12.4 | 25.7 |
| In married couple households |  |  |
| Men 65+ | 4.4 | 12.8 |
| Women 65+ | 4.9 | 10.7 |
| Unrelated individuals, living alone |  |  |
| Women 65 + | 21.2 | 47.0 |
| Men 65+ | 15.1 | 34.8 |

**Source**: U.S. Census Bureau, 2002.

**Table 13.5**

Median Income of U.S. Household Units, Household Heads Aged 65+, by Source of Income and Marital Status, 2002

|  | All Older Units | Married Couples | Single Women | Single Men |
|---|---|---|---|---|
| **Social Security (SS)** |  |  |  |  |
| % Collecting | 90% | 91% | 89% | 87% |
| Share of total income | 39% | 35% | 52% | 38% |
| Median amount | $12,000 | $17,136 | $9,900 | $11,400 |
| **Earnings (incl. self-employment)** |  |  |  |  |
| % Collecting | 22% | 35% | 12% | 18% |
| Share of total income | 25% | 30% | 13% | 23% |
| Median amount | $20,000 | $24,000 | $11,700 | $18,000 |
| **Retirement Benefits Other than SS** |  |  |  |  |
| % Collecting | 41% | 51% | 32% | 39% |
| Share of total income | 19% | 20% | 17% | 20% |
| Median amount | $6,588 | $8,460 | $3,600 | $7,200 |
| **Asset Income (interest, dividend, rents)** |  |  |  |  |
| % Collecting | 55% | 67% | 48% | 47% |
| Share of total income | 14% | 13% | 14% | 15% |
| Median amount | $1,531 | $2,118 | $1,028 | $1,461 |
| **Median Total Income** | $18,938 | $32,460 | $12,548 | $16,248 |

**Source**: Social Security Administration, 2005.
**Note**: Aged units are married couples living together—at least one of whom is 65 or older—and nonmarried persons 65 or older.
Not included is "other sources" of income (e.g., income from family, other gifts, gambling/lottery winnings) that account for 2% to 4% of income.
Median income for recipients only.

net worth of households. Table 13.6 shows the net worth (assets minus liabilities) by age of household heads in 2001. These assets do not include the wealth value that is represented by life-contingent claims such as the present value of promised defined benefit pension plans or Social Security. Net worth is distributed more unequally than is income, as indicated by the differences between mean and median net worth (and their ratio); relatively few households hold a high proportion of assets, which skews the mean upward. By this measure of inequality, with the exception of the youngest households among which a high proportion have not begun any wealth accumulation, wealth is most unequally distributed among households of retirement age, the age at which both median and mean wealth declines.

Figure 13.3 presents the two components of median net worth, total assets and liabilities (or debt), showing the relative role of debt in modifying or exacerbating differences in wealth accumulation

**Table 13.6**

Median and Mean Net Worth of U.S. Households by Age of Household Head, 2001

|  | Mean | Median | Mean/ Median |
|---|---|---|---|
| 34 and younger | $ 85,025 | $ 11,600 | 7.33 |
| 35–44 | $259,199 | $ 77,600 | 3.34 |
| 45–54 | $491,580 | $132,000 | 3.72 |
| 55–64 | $730,729 | $281,500 | 2.60 |
| 65–74 | $671,649 | $176,300 | 3.81 |
| 75 and older | $464,989 | $151,400 | 3.07 |

**Source**: Authors' calculations from Survey of Consumer Finances. Board of Governors of the Federal Reserve System, 2001.

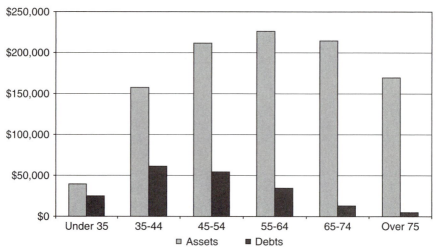

**Figure 13.3** Median Assets and Debts by Age, 2001
**Source**: Aizcorbe, Kennickell, and Moore (2003).

across households by age. Although liability variation certainly exists across
ages, differences in total assets most contribute to net worth differences by age.
On the other hand, it is not apparent from
these cross-sectional data whether the
higher debt at younger ages is merely

wise financing of human (e.g., education)
and physical (e.g., housing) capital investments or the consequence of higher consumer debt that may jeopardize future
financial security. Therefore, in Figure
13.4, we disaggregate total debt into
secured debt (such as mortgages) and

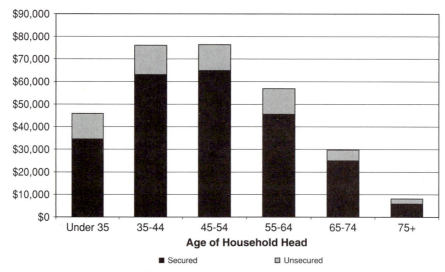

**Figure 13.4** Median Assets and Secured vs. Unsecured Debts by Age, 2001
**Source:** Authors's calculations from Survey of Consumer Finances Board of Governors of the Federal Reserve System, 2001

unsecured debt (consumer loans including credit card debt). Although there is a relationship between debt levels and age, with households headed by older individuals holding less debt, there does not seem to be a strong relationship between age and debt type as a proportion of total debt. Neither level nor type of debt plays a major role in net wealth differences across age groups.

Although the age differences in wealth in 2001 are consistent with the notion that one accumulates savings during the working years and spends down assets in later life, we must remember that these differences are not just a consequence of individuals spending and saving assets over time, but also of different savings behavior across birth cohorts. The data in Table 13.7 show persistence in the cross-sectional, age-related accumulation and spending pattern over time, implying wealth accumulation during the working-age years followed by conversion of wealth into income during retirement. It also shows that the difference between the wealth holdings of younger and older households (measured in the bottom row of the table as the ratio of median net worth of the 75 and older group divided by the median for the under 35 group) first decreased between 1992 and 1995 and then increased dramatically, a change that reflects the importance in wealth

accumulation of capital markets. It would appear that in periods when asset returns were modest (1992–1995), older groups lost ground to younger groups who were building net worth mainly through saving of income and housing purchases as opposed to capital gains. When asset returns are larger (1995–1998), higher-asset groups (i.e., the older groups) gained more relative ground.

Comparing cohorts across time, however, shows that on average wealth grew for all cohorts. Comparing 1992 data with the 10-year older age group in 2001, the youngest households, who were both saving and advantaged by capital and housing value growth in the latter part of the decade, experienced higher growth in net wealth than did the oldest cohorts whose assets grew nevertheless.

Older households tend to have more assets than younger ones, but that wealth growth may slow as retirement age approaches. This is not surprising, as one would expect asset spend-down because of retirement and long-term care costs. What is somewhat surprising is that the differences between the net worth of the old and young seem to be increasing over time. For example, the median household net worth of the 75 and over subgroup was roughly 9.4 times that of the 34 and under median in 1992; that multiplier was more than 13.0 nine years later. The

**Table 13.7**
Median Net U.S. Household Worth, by Age of Household Head, 1992–2001 (in 2001 Dollars)

|                | 1992 | 1995 | 1998 | 2001 |
|----------------|------|------|------|------|
| 34 and Younger | $11,400 | $13,900 | $9,900 | $11,600 |
| 35–44 | **55,100** | 60,300 | 69,000 | 77,600 |
| 45–54 | *96,800* | 107,500 | 114,800 | **132,000** |
| 55–64 | **141,100** | 133,200 | 139,200 | *281,500* |
| 65–74 | 121,700 | 128,000 | 159,500 | **176,300** |
| 75 and Older | 107,500 | 107,500 | 136,700 | 151,400 |
| (75+)/(34u) | 9.4 | 7.7 | 13.8 | 13.1 |

**Source**: Authors' calculation from the Survey of Consumer Finances, 1992, 1995, 1998, 2001. Board of Governors of the Federal Reserve System, 2001.
**Note**: Bolded and italicized figures show cohort values (see text).

median for households under age 35 barely changed from 1992 to 2001; it increased by almost 50% in that time period for households over age 75, and nearly doubled for the 55- to 64-year age group. Part of these changes must be examined within the context of a pronounced bull market over this time period, but one must also keep in mind, when examining this phenomenon, that it is younger households that would be expected to benefit from a bull market.

Prudent financial planning would dictate a more aggressive investment style among younger cohorts who are in a better position to take advantage of the higher long-run average returns to risky investments, followed by a switch to more secure investments as retirement approaches. This may be countered by younger cohorts' heavier investments (and debt) in housing (as measured by the ratio of housing to total wealth) that may lead to more conservative choices in the rest of the portfolio (Flavin & Yamashita, 2002). Thus some of the differences in asset growth between younger and older cohorts may be attributed to changes in

investment strategy as housing and stock returns grew, rather than only to lower net additional savings.

Figure 13.5 breaks down asset composition by age, separating total assets into monetary assets (i.e., bank and money market accounts), investment assets (i.e., stocks, bonds, mutual funds, retirement accounts), real assets (i.e., housing, vehicles), and other assets. One would expect younger households to have relatively more of their savings invested in higher risk investment and real estate assets, and older households to have savings in more secure monetary assets. Figure 13.5 does not confirm this, which means, perhaps, that risk preference differences by age are not a major factor in differential wealth growth.

Indeed, as shown in Table 13.8, in 1992 older households were about as likely to own stocks or mutual funds as younger households (except the under-35 age group) and much less likely to participate in saving money in retirement accounts, which in these data from the Survey of Consumer Finance include defined-contribution pension balances ("account type

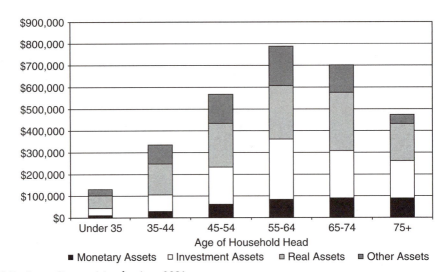

**Figure 13.5** Asset Composition by Age, 2001

**Source:** Authors' calculations from Survey of Consumer Finances Board of Goveemors of the Federal Reserve System, 2001

Table 13.8

Percent of U.S. Households Owning Stocks, Mutual Funds, and Retirement Accounts: By Age of Household Head and Year

| | 1992 | | | 2001 | | |
|---|---|---|---|---|---|---|
| | Stocks | Mutual Funds | Retirement Accounts* | Stocks | Mutual Funds | Retirement Accounts* |
| 34 and Younger | 10.9 | 2.2 | 26.6 | 17.4 | 11.5 | 45.1 |
| 35–44 | **16.9** | **7.9** | **47.8** | 21.6 | 17.5 | 61.4 |
| 45–54 | 20.7 | 9.2 | 49.8 | **22.0** | **20.2** | **63.4** |
| 55–64 | **18.6** | **9.7** | **42.4** | 26.7 | 21.3 | 59.1 |
| 65–74 | 17.1 | 9.3 | 27.6 | **20.5** | **19.9** | **44.0** |
| 75 and Older | 18.5 | 9.8 | 6.0 | 21.8 | 19.5 | 25.7 |

Source: Authors' calculation from the Survey of Consumer Finances, 1992, 2001. Board of Governors of the Federal Reserve System, 2001.
Note: Bolded figures show approximate cohort values (see text).
*Any defined contribution pension balance

pension plans"). In 2001, there is little difference between old and young in holdings of mutual funds, though there appears to be a secular trend upward among all age groups. The bolded figures correspond to approximate cohorts and show growth in percentages holding stocks and mutual funds for all cohorts. The stability in retirement accounts for older age cohorts in contrast to growth for younger age cohorts could be due to life cycle patterns of retirement savings (i.e., retirement accounts are initiated primarily during the prime working years) or because during the older cohorts' working years, legislation and savings through 401(k) and 403(b) accounts were still new savings options. These accounts were first introduced in 1978 federal legislation, effective January 1, 1980, with IRS regulations following in January 1981 (see Chapter 20).

Table 13.9 shows the effective equity participation of households in various years by age. By "effective," we mean direct stock investments, plus stock mutual funds or stock holdings in retirement savings accounts. Here, it appears that the net rate of growth in equity participation for older households has been

less than that of other age groups, a conclusion that differs slightly from the one drawn from the separate types of investments, where for each the increased participation of older Americans seemed to go in step with younger cohorts. Indeed, examining the bolded cohort rates shows that the percentage of households holding any stock slowed considerably over the decade among the older cohorts, suggesting overall modification of risk preferences at older ages, which is consistent

Table 13.9

Effective Percent of U.S. Households Owning Stock* by Age of Household Head, 1992–2001

| | 1992 | 1995 | 1998 | 2001 |
|---|---|---|---|---|
| 34 and Younger | 28.4 | 36.6 | 40.8 | 48.9 |
| 35–44 | **42.4** | 46.4 | 56.7 | 59.5 |
| 45–54 | **46.4** | 48.9 | 58.6 | **59.2** |
| 55–64 | **45.3** | 40.0 | 55.9 | **57.1** |
| 65–74 | 30.2 | 34.4 | 42.7 | **39.2** |
| 75 and Older | 25.7 | 27.9 | 29.4 | 34.2 |

Source: Authors' calculation from the Survey of Consumer Finances, 1992, 1995, 1998, 2001. Board of Governors of the Federal Reserve System, 2001.
Note: Bolded figures show cohort values (see text).
*Includes households that own stock through mutual funds or retirement accounts.

with standard financial advice. That younger cohorts have higher effective equity participation at each age than did older cohorts, suggests differences in risk preferences among these cohorts which could portend quite different investment behavior and asset growth among future older cohorts.

## II. Measures of Economic Well-Being

The increasing availability of data on wealth holdings that document the different distribution of wealth and income across and within age groups has led to calls to incorporate wealth into measures of economic well-being. That wealth is distributed more unequally than income (described previously) suggests that economic security measures that include wealth accumulation would be more skewed toward households with higher income and wealth. Caner and Wolff (2004) have shown that this greater concentration of wealth than income means that incorporating wealth into an "asset poor" measure reduces poverty for some older groups, particularly married couples, but increases poverty among unmarried women. They define "asset poor" as households who do not have sufficient wealth to sustain poverty level consumption for three months or more. Including housing in net wealth measures, asset poverty among older adults was about comparable to income poverty, but when housing was excluded, asset poverty rate was more than twice as high as income poverty, particularly for older unmarried women. Haveman, Holden, Wolfe and Sherlund (2005) estimated the percent of older adults who could not sustain a poverty level of consumption throughout their remaining lifetime even if all wealth, including expected Social Security and pension benefits, were annuitized and added to retirement income

flows. Although poverty rates fall substantially for their sample because of inclusion of wealth, poverty rates among unmarried women and men are about five times higher than that of married couples.

Incorporating wealth in measures of well-being is only one way of improving how economic well-being is measured. Although income and wealth are arguably among the most important determinants of the quality of life for a family or individual, they are not the only factors involved. Indeed, some would argue, the term *economic well-being* implies that it is not just the receipt of income and wealth that matters to quality of economic life, but individuals' command over resources that enable the consumption of goods and services. These broader measures of economic well-being include measures of subjective well-being and its relationship to income (Easterlin, 2001), consumption of goods and services (U.S. Census Bureau, 2003), and the "full resources" that are available to fund consumption and, consequently, consumer satisfaction.

### A. Subjective Well-Being

In general, studies of subjective well-being find that although individuals with more goods (or potential command over goods) are somewhat happier than others in the cross section, the correlation is small, and over time income gains are not associated with an increase in subjective well-being (Blanchflower & Oswald, 2004; Diener & Biswas-Diener, 2002). Two possible explanations are given for this contrast between cross-sectional and time-series findings: (1) individuals' happiness depends not on their absolute income or consumption but on their position relative to others with whom they compare themselves, and (2) individuals adapt over time to changes in their fortune. The first implies that if one's income rises but one's relative income position remains the same, there will be no long-run gain in individual subjective well-being. The second implies that though individuals may at first rejoice at their good fortune, the euphoria from the gain diminishes as the person adapts to the new lifestyle or circumstances. Studies that examined predictors of subjective well-being among older adults do not contradict general conclusions drawn from income-based measures. They found that older age alone is associated with higher subjective well-being (Clark & Oswald, 1996) but also that poorer health, widowhood, and divorce appear to be associated with lower subjective well-being (Diener, Suh, Lucus, & Smith, 1999; Shields & Wooden, 2003). In addition, Clark and Oswald (1966) and others have documented the association between satisfaction and voluntary versus involuntary withdrawals from work. Bender (2004), using data from the Health and Retirement Survey, found that income and wealth have only marginal effects on satisfaction, but higher levels of satisfaction were reported by those who retired voluntarily, were older, were in good health, were married, or were covered by both an employer-provided pension and Social Security.

Despite the overall weak association between income and satisfaction, findings suggest important differences in subjective economic well-being among older adults, as well as the importance of studying these. First, the relative position of groups and individuals in the income and wealth distribution matters. Subjective well-being is linked to the income position of older Americans relative to other age groups, of other older subgroups, and of older individuals relative to their preretirement experiences. Thus, lower incomes may indeed reflect lower subjective well-being. Second, that older age (controlling for other factors) is associated with greater life satisfaction is consistent with hypotheses about long-run adaptation to social, health, and economic circumstances, as well as the role of aspirations and expectations in shaping satisfaction (Easterlin, 2001). Third, declines in health status appear to have long-run consequences for subjective well-being. Consequently resources matter to the extent they affect access to health care and the ability to pay for appropriate care. Fourth, changes in marital status appear to have long-run consequences for subjective well-being. It may be that the declines in income that accompany widowhood compound the effect of the spousal loss on subjective well-being (Holden & Smock, 1991; Zick & Holden, 2000). This implies a greater difference in subjective well-being between older married couples and unmarried women than is implied by simple resources differences described earlier. Fifth, Bender's findings on the positive effect on happiness for those receiving secure pension and Social Security, compared to those with no secure pension coverage, controlling for current income, suggests that the long-run security of income sources matters. This would imply that dependence on Social Security income among the low-income older population comes with a security that enhances well-being even at low-income levels. Finally, even short-run changes in satisfaction and the causes of those changes have consequences for individuals and families. Adaptation of individuals in the long run to change does not negate the consequences for families and individuals (and public policy) of sharp changes in income.

B. Consumption Measures of Well-Being

Another approach to assessing well-being is to measure the consumption of good and services. The argument is that individuals derive satisfaction from consumption itself, and thus directly measuring consumption provides a better indicator of absolute and relative well-being than does a resource measure (or income-based measure). Income-based and consumption measures of well-being will not produce identical levels of well-being and may place individuals in different positions in the "well-being" distribution, in part because income (even if expanded to include wealth) is an imperfect representation of the ability to consume. Individuals may have access to services and goods for which they do not pay the full market price or do not pay at all. Durables purchased many years earlier may continue to provide services, allowing individuals to consume those services even when income is diminished. Home owners do not pay the rent for housing that nonowners must pay. Government expenditures raise consumption of individuals and families without direct expenditures by them, for example, for highway services and fire and police protections (Musgrave, Case & Leonard 1974; Wolff, Zacharias, & Caner, 2003). Finally, higher income may enable the purchase of additional leisure hours, a consumption item that is entirely neglected in pure resource measures. Osberg and Sharp (2002) argue, however, that leisure is an important component of differential economic well-being across countries and individuals.

An additional argument for the preference of consumption over income measures of well-being is the diminished volatility from year-to-year that is exhibited by consumption (Slesnick, 2001). Individuals experience fluctuations in income over time that do not cause comparable year-to-year fluctuations in consumption (and well-being). They may have saved against such dips in income or have access to credit markets that allow them to borrow and pay back when income rises. This is not captured in resource measures of well-being, affected by short-term fluctuations that are not fully translated into consumption changes.

Defining "consumption" is difficult, and there is little consensus on methodological issues, including data collection and comparability of its measurement over time (U.S. Census Bureau, 2003). Few surveys gather full consumption measures. They generally exclude, for example, the consumption of goods not directly purchased by individuals, such as health care and government-provided services. The alleged advantages of consumption measures, however, have led to improved resource measures of well-being. These include adjustments to traditional income measures to take account of:

- The value of nonmonetary benefits such as the value of health insurance provided through employers or government.
- Adjustments to income for the consumption requirements of households of different sizes.
- Multiyear measures of resources to smooth out year-to-year changes.
- Annuitizing assets to estimate consumption potential from household savings and assets.

## C. Resource Measures of Well-Being

The most common approach to measuring economic well-being, and the one taken earlier in this chapter, is the use of "resource-based" measures or those that look at income, assets, and in-kind resources that enable financing the consumption of goods and services. This approach always includes income receipt and, to the extent possible, assets that could be accessed for consumption purposes (i.e., for smoothing consumption when income fluctuates). Also included are the value of nonmonetary economic resources, in-kind benefits that enable individuals to consume goods and services without direct income outlays (e.g., the face value of food stamps, the insurance premium equivalence of Medicare and Medicaid coverage), and the value of employer-provided fringe benefits that noncovered individuals must pay out of pocket (e.g., the premium for health insurance) (U.S. Bureau of the Census, 1996).

Resource measures have the advantage of sharing a common metric (the monetary unit), are easily and therefore most frequently gathered, and can be compared across units, time, and space with appropriate adjustments for differences in prices. Although such measures provide a more comprehensive view of economic resources, it is not necessarily the case that these broader measures of resources change the conclusions drawn from income alone.

## D. Equivalence Scales

Consumption measures of well-being directly argue the necessity of adjusting resource measures for differences across households in consumption requirements. A married couple and a single person receiving identical incomes would not be equally well-off in terms of consumption potential. For some consumption items, two individuals require twice as much. Clothing is unlikely to be shared between spouses; a couple would require twice as much income for these expenditures. On the other hand, two individuals sharing housing space would not consume twice as much space or heat, twice as many automobile trips and home appliances; there are large economies of scale in the consumption of these services. For other items such as food cooked at home, the economies of scale are smaller.

The appropriate adjustment for the consumption needs of different size households remains an unsettled issue. Alternative scales can make a difference

to levels and changes in well-being and to relative position where family size is different across resource levels (OECD, 1982). Buhmann, Rainwater, Schmaus, and Smeeding (1988) compared equivalence scales, their use, and the comparative results when used to study economic well-being and inequality. The official U.S. poverty thresholds, developed in 1963–1964 represent one implied and widely used set of equivalence scales (Fisher, 1992). More recently, the National Research Council recommended a comprehensive change in the poverty threshold (Citro & Michael, 1995). Their recommendations included the adoption of equivalence scales that have explicit weights that represent the additional (but different) consumption requirements of children and of additional adults beyond the first in the household, and an explicit economy of scale factor not found in most other measures.

It is worth noting briefly a debate over the interpretation of equivalence scales because it is akin to the debate over subjective versus resource measures of well-being and the interpretation of each in public policy discussions. Adjusting for consumption needs of larger households results in a single-earner couple being less well-off than a single person with identical total income. The implication is that the married earner would have been better off if she or he had not married. Yet, it is argued, and probably correctly so, that the married earner prefers the married state over the single status (for a variety of reasons). Thus, a single earner may be subjectively better off when married even though the objective equivalence scale would show otherwise. Thus it is argued that these objective equivalence scales are what might be called "conditional equivalence" scales reflecting the consumption costs of larger families but not the subjective benefits (Pollack & Wales, 1979). Conversely, the death of a nonearning spouse, which would raise the objective well-being of the surviving and primary earner, reflects the economic gains from spousal loss but not the subjective costs. By this implication, widowed women and men may be even worse off than their objective equivalence would suggest.

### E. The Income Reference Period

Well-being measures take account of resources received over a specific time period (or "reference period") and count assets held at a moment in time. Because access to in-kind benefits, income flows, and household composition fluctuates over time, the length of the reference period over which these resources are counted will affect observed economic characteristics. Longer reference periods may smooth out short-period income variations. Yet changes in household composition during that time period may make it difficult to obtain an accurate accounting of any single individual's access to income and consumption. For example, standard interviewing practice asks current household members about income received during some previous months. A recent spousal death will cause that spouse's income not to be accounted for, underestimating the resources that were available to the surviving spouse (Burkhauser, Holden, & Myers, 1986; Holden, 1992). Well-being measures estimated over longer reference periods are also subject to error because of moves out of the unit by individuals who had provided income to that household during the reference period. Shorter reference periods, however, are subject to short-term changes in income, which while accurately identified, are not representative of a household's longer term economic status. Poverty measures find more individuals ever poor when income reference periods are shorter than over longer reference periods (Bane & Ellwood, 1986).

## III. Conclusions and Directions for Future Research

Measures of satisfaction, consumption, and resources capture different aspects of economic well-being. Income remains the most frequently reported measure of economic status, primarily because it is most easily, and therefore most frequently and uniformly, gathered in national surveys. Income measures of well-being, however, are increasingly expanded to include assets and in-kind benefits. For this reason the relative economic status of older adults remains an empirical question that promises to provide new dimensions of understanding.

Income measures were described in this chapter because these are available over time and over population groups. They show a diminishing rate of poverty among the older population. Many older Americans with incomes above the U.S. poverty threshold, however, have incomes that are extremely modest—just over the threshold.

Asset data are less consistently available but also show gains in older American economic status over time, both comparing across age groups and over time for individual cohorts. On the other hand, assets are highly skewed toward higher income households, and their inclusion does not much alter conclusions about relative poverty risk. In part it appears the income in assets is due to both older and younger populations taking advantage of opportunities for asset growth through equity investments. Assets ownership and value have grown among the young and old, though at a somewhat slower pace at older ages. Although this is consistent with life-cycle asset accumulation/decumulation patterns and with advice to reduce holdings of risky assets at older ages, the slower growth among older cohorts may also be due to the fact that tax deferred retirement accounts were introduced fairly late in their working lives.

What may the future hold for current younger cohorts as they age? The data show more modest income increases for younger cohorts, though this does not appear to have occurred in median asset holdings. Debt is higher among younger cohorts but does not appear to be a source of diminished asset growth, though to the extent that mean asset and debt holdings reflect different owners of debt and assets, debt may be a source of economic insecurity for some individuals.

If the lower incomes of younger cohorts are offset over time by the apparent growing aggressiveness of their asset holdings and investments, then one can anticipate increased well-being over time of future cohorts of older Americans. To the extent that slower income growth reduces savings and thus asset holding, however, the older population in the future may be characterized by greater economic insecurity. Data on women and minorities show the persistence of disparities in economic well-being by gender and ethnicity/race, despite absolute gains across all groups. Policies aimed at reducing income tax rates and increasing tax-advantaged savings are not likely to alter the economic well-being of these most vulnerable groups. In addition, studies of subjective well-being suggest that policies that reduce the security of retirement income by placing greater risk of market shifts on retirees and away from employers and government, such as partial privatization of Social Security, would reduce economic well-being.

There is still much to be learned about how to measure economic well-being and consequently how well-being has changed over time, among age groups, and between cohorts. The gathering of richer demographic and economic data promises to expand our knowledge of economic well-being of all Americans. Each new cohort entering the work force brings with it a combination of educational preparation, family responsibili-

ties, and aspirations and makes decisions within the context of changing job opportunities, taxation policies, and savings and consumption options.

Economic well-being of older people, although exhibiting some persistence in patterns over groups and age, is an ever evolving phenomenon. Ongoing national surveys that gather data on individuals over time are providing the means to understand how economic status changes over time, age, and with the events that are increasingly likely as one grows older (e.g., the death of a spouse, the onset of chronic diseases and disabilities, and retirement). The Health and Retirement Study (University of Michigan, 2005), the Wisconsin Longitudinal Study (1957–2003), and the National Survey of Families and Households (Sweet and Bumpass, 2003) have been developed explicitly to provide richer, longer run, more accurate information, and more useful views for policy purposes of economic well-being of older Americans.

## References

Aizcorbe, A. N., Kennickell, A. B., & Moore, K. B. (2003). Recent changes in U.S. family finances: Evidence from the 1998 and 2001 Survey of Consumer Finances. *Federal Reserve Bulletin, 89* (January), 1–32.

Bane, M. J., & Ellwood, D. (1986). Slipping into and out of poverty: The dynamics of spells. *Journal of Human Resources, 21*(1), 1–23.

Bender, K. (2004). The well-being of retirees: Evidence using subjective data, Newton, MA. Center for Retirement Research, Boston College, WP (2004–24). Retrieved March 15, 2005, from http://www.bc.edu/centers/crr/papers/wp_2004–24.pdf

Blanchflower, D. G., & Oswald, A. J. (2004). Well-being over time in Britain and the USA. *Journal of Public Economics, 88,* 1359–1386.

Board of Governors of the Federal Reserve System. (2001). *Codebook for the 2001 Survey of Consumer Finance.* Washington, D.C.: Retrieved March 15, 2005 from http://www.federalreserve.gov/pubs/oss/oss2/2001/codebk2001.txt

Buhmann, B., Rainwater, L., Schmaus, G., & Smeeding, T. N. (1988), Equivalence scales, well-being, inequality and poverty: Sensitivity estimates across ten countries, using the Luxembourg Income Study (LIS) database. *The Review of Income and Wealth, 34*, 115–142.

Burkhauser, R. V., Holden, K. C., & Myers, D. A. (1986). Marital disruption and poverty: The role of survey procedures in artificially creating poverty. *Demography, 23*, 621–631.

Caner, A. & Wolff, E. (2004). *Asset poverty in the United States: Its persistence in an expansionary economy.* Annandale-on-Hudson, NY: The Levy Institute at Bard College, Public Policy Brief No. 76A.

Clark, A. E., & Oswald, A. J. (1996). Satisfaction and comparison income. *Journal of Public Economics, 61*, 359–381.

Citro, C. F., & Michael, R. T. (Eds). (1995). *Measuring poverty: A new approach.* Washington, D.C.: National Academy Press.

Diener, E., & Biswas-Diener, R. (2002). Will money increase subjective well-being? A literature review and guide to needed research. *Social Indicators Research, 57*, 119–169.

Diener, E., Suh, E. M., Lucus, R. E., & Smith, H. L. (1999), Subjective well-being: Three decades of progress. *Psychological Bulletin, 125*, 276–302.

Easterlin, R. A. (2001). Income and happiness: Towards a unified theory. *Economic Journal, 111*, 465–484.

Fisher, G., (1992). The development and history of the poverty thresholds. *Social Security Bulletin, 55*(4), 3–14.

Flavin, M. & Yamashita, T. (2002). Owner-occupied housing and the composition of the household portfolio, *American Economic Review, 92*, 345–362.

Haveman, R., Holden, K., Wolfe, B., & Sherlund, S. (2005) Do newly retired workers in the U.S. have sufficient resources to maintain well-being? La Follette School of Public Affairs Working Paper No. 2005–0012. Retrieved on May 1 from: http://www.lafollette.wisc.edu/publications/workingpapers

Holden, K. C. (1992) SIPP and the measurement of income transitions among the elderly: Limitations and suggestions for modification. *Journal of Economic and Social Measurement, 18*(1–4),193–212.

Holden, K. C., & Smock, P. J. (1991). The economic costs of marital dissolution: Why do women bear a disproportionate cost? *Annual Review of Sociology, 17*, 51–78.

Musgrave, R. A., Case, K. S., & Leonard, H. (1974). The distribution of fiscal burdens. *Public Finance Quarterly, 2*, 259–311.

Organization for Economic Cooperation and Development. (1982). *The OECD list of social indicators.* Paris: Organization for Economic Cooperation and Development.

Osberg, L., & Sharpe, A. (2002). An index of economic well-being for selected OECD countries. *Review of Income and Wealth, 48*, 291–316.

Pollack, R. A., & Wales, T. J. (1979). Welfare comparisons and equivalence scales. *The American Economic Review, 69*, 216–221.

Shields, M., & Wooden, M. (2003). Marriage, children and subjective well-being. Paper presented at the Eighth Australian Institute of Family Studies Conference. Retrieved March 15, 2005 from http://www.melbourneinstitute.com/hilda/Biblio/hbibliocp.html

Slesnick, D. T. (2001). *Consumption and social welfare: Living standards and their distribution in the United States.* New York: Cambridge University Press,

Social Security Administration. (2004). *Fast facts and figures about Social Security, 2004.* Washington, D.C.: Office of Policy and Research, Social Security Administration.

Social Security Administration (2005). *Income of the population 55 or older, 2002*, SSA Publication No. 13–11871 Washington, D.C.: Office of Research and Statistics. Retrieved March 15, 2005, from http://www.ssa.gov/policy/docs/statcomps/income_pop55/

Sweet, J. A., & Bumpass, L. (2003). The national survey of families and households: Data description and documentation. Retrieved April 1, 2005, from http://www.ssc.wisc.edu/nsfh/

University of Michigan. (2005) *Health and Retirement Study: An overview of Health and Retirement Study components.* Retrieved April 1, 2005, from http://hrsonline.isr.umich.edu/intro/sho_uinfo.php?hfyle=overview&xtyp=2

U.S. Bureau of the Census (1996). *Income, poverty and the valuation of noncash benefits: 1994*, Current Population Reports. Consumer Income P60–18. Washington D.C.: U.S. Department of Commerce, Economics and Statistics Administration. Retrieved March 1, 2005, from www.census.gov/prod/1/pop/p60–189.pdf

U.S. Census Bureau (various years). *Annual Demographic Survey*, various years. Retrieved March 1, 2005, from http://www.bls.census.gov/cps/ads/sdata.htm

U.S. Census Bureau, (2002). *Annual demographic survey: March supplement: 2002 data*. Retrieved March 1, 2005, from http://www.bls.census.gov/cps/ads/sdata.htm

U.S. Census Bureau. (2003). *Supplemental measures of material well-being: Expenditures, consumption, and poverty 1998 and 2001*. Current Population Reports. Retrieved March 1, 2005 from www.census.gov/prod/2003pubs/p23–201.pdf

Wisconsin Longitudinal Study (WLS). (1957–2003). [machine-readable data file] / Hauser, Robert M. [principal investigator(s)]. Madison, WI: University of Wisconsin-Madison, WLS. [distributor]; <http://www.ssc.wisc.edu/~wls/

Wolff, E.N., Zacharias, A., & Caner, A. (2003). *Household wealth, public consumption, and economic well-being in the United States.* Annandale-on-Hudson, NY: Levy Economics Institute Working Paper No. 386.

Zick, C., & Holden, K. C. (2000). An assessment of the wealth holdings of recent widows. *Journal of Gerontology: Social Sciences, 55*, S90–S97.

# Fourteen

# Health and Aging

Kenneth F. Ferraro

The study of health has been *the* issue that has generated the most social science research on aging during the last 50 years. Health is so pivotal to the aging experience that even in research on other topics, such as retirement, relocation, and religion, health often emerges as an independent variable. Health is a critical part of the aging process, and an enormous research infrastructure is focused on understanding the relationship between health and aging. The ultimate goal is that discoveries related to health and aging will enhance quality of life over the life course, thereby reducing the likelihood of premature morbidity, disability, and death.

Although other chapters in this volume give explicit attention to the topics of morbidity and mortality (see Chapter 3) and quality of life (see Chapter 18), the focus of the present chapter is the relationship between health and aging. The aim is to systematically examine the way in which research on health and aging has changed over the last 50 years and identify points of emphasis in current and future studies. In the process, this review considers theoretical and methodological innovations that are helping to guide research on health and aging.

## I. Fifty Years of Research on Health and Aging

Social scientific approaches to the study of health have changed considerably over time. Thus, it may be useful to briefly consider some of the major changes in the theories and methods used to study health and aging. Scientific knowledge is socially constructed, and briefly reviewing the paradigmatic approaches to the study of health and aging may help us understand why the literature emphasizes certain findings and topical issues.

### A. The Health of Older People

It is probably not an oversimplification to assert that the earliest studies of health and aging were focused on the health problems of later life. Charcot's (1881) *Clinical lectures on the diseases of old age* emphasized the problems of aging, the predominant view at the time. The term *geriatrics* was coined in the second decade of the twentieth century, and the focus of Nascher (1909, 1914) and other early geriatricians was disease in later life. This problem orientation pervaded many of the early social science studies that sought to describe the diseases common among older people (Achenbaum, 1995).

It should be noted that studies of the prevalence of various diseases and their correlation with age were helpful for describing the population of older people and identifying risk factors. Human history was replete with deaths resulting from acute disease, so the shift to chronic disease and a different type of mortality merited study (Rogers, Hummer, & Nam, 2000). Chronic diseases such as heart disease, stroke, cancer, and diabetes became more prevalent, and there was great concern about how these chronic diseases would impact the older population and society as a whole.

Nevertheless, research on health and aging during the mid-twentieth century implied an analytical focus on the diseases common to older people. Most early studies were cohort-centric; that is, older people were the object of study, and there was relatively little research comparing the prevalence of such diseases with persons in the earlier periods of life. Five decades ago, the focus was more on describing the older population, usually defined as 65 years and older, and the health problems common to this stage of life.

One of the major problems with descriptions of the older adult population is the tremendous heterogeneity within it. As Quinn (1987) aptly stated, "The most important characteristic of the aged is their diversity. The average can be very deceptive, because it ignores the tremendous dispersion around it. Beware of the mean" (p. 64). In addition, on the health front, age may not be a meaningful predictor variable. Age is correlated with many health conditions, but at any given age, there are tremendous differences in health and functional ability. Thus, descriptive studies of age differences in health could take the field only so far.

## B. The Health of People Who Are Aging

Instead of an emphasis on studying the health problems of older people, the field shifted to an emphasis on understanding change in health status. This shift was probably due to many factors, both methodological and theoretical. On the methodological front, longitudinal studies of aging provided unique insights into how health status changes over the life course. Although this type of study started in the 1950s, the influence of the Duke Longitudinal Studies of Normal Aging (Busse & Maddox, 1985) and the Baltimore Longitudinal Study of Aging (Shock et al., 1984) grew substantially in the late 1960s and early 1970s. Those and other studies began to reshape the way social scientists thought about studying health. The emphasis shifted from the diseases of older people to the *process of aging*, with special attention on "normal aging." The idea was to separate pathology from overall health and functioning, noting that people could live many years with chronic diseases.

Although the methodological innovations, especially the emphasis on longitudinal studies, were central to reshaping the field, there were also important theoretical and conceptual developments that helped move the study of health and aging to more dynamic analyses. The 1970s was a period of considerable change in the way social scientists theorized about aging. On the conceptual and theoretical front, Volumes 1 and 3 of *Aging and Society* by Riley and colleagues (1968, 1972, see also Riley, 1987) helped sociologists see more clearly the processes of aging over the life course and cohort flow, as well as the interplay between aging and social change. Various theories, from modernization to activity theory, were anchored in the study of social change, and this conceptual focus on changing lives (and societies) helped social gerontologists give greater attention to *change* in health status, not simply cross-sectional descriptions of age differences in health.

Research on adjustment in later life was also increasingly based on longitudinal studies and spurred interest in aging and the life course, as opposed to just studying older people. Whether it was life events such as retirement (e.g., Ekerdt, Baden, Bosse, & Dibbs, 1983) or widowhood (e.g., Ferraro, Mutran, & Barresi, 1984), biography and history were important for understanding physical or mental health outcomes (Elder, 1974, 1994; George, 1980; Wheaton, 1990). The value of taking the "long view of aging" had been established, and longitudinal studies have become the norm rather than the exception in research on health and aging.

One of the major theses regarding health and aging in the past three decades was that the rectangularization of the survival curve is leading to a compression of morbidity (Fries, 1980). Fries predicted a future compression where the span of life that is free of chronic disease will increase, and the time between disease onset and death will decrease. If it transpires, it would be a major public health achievement and provide good news for the image of aging in modern societies. The meaning of age 65 would likely change as society becomes more accustomed to seeing senior athletes and a more active senior population. Despite enthusiasm for the thesis, however, others have argued that the prediction may be overstated.

Guralnik (1991) noted that the idea of a compression of morbidity was premised on the fact that life expectancy has stopped increasing. Data over the last 20 years and most projections for the next 30 years, however, show that life

expectancy will continue to increase, albeit at a modest pace (Kaplan, 1991). Hubert, Bloch, Oehlert, and Fries (2002) countered that compression of morbidity remains likely, even if life expectancy rises, largely because of the continuing decline in health destructive behaviors such as smoking.

The debate ensues, but there appears to be agreement that the period of coping with functional limitations is being pushed back to advanced ages (Guralnik, 1991; Verbrugge, 1991; Wolinsky, Armbrecht, & Wyrwich, 2000). This means that research increasingly emphasizes studying the processes of disablement and health decline (Glass, 1998; Lawrence, & Jette, 1996; Taylor, & Lynch, 2004; Verbrugge, & Jette, 1994).

Disability has been one topic where this shift is seen most clearly. Early studies focused on the development of sound measures of disability (Nagi, 1965), followed by efforts to enhance the epidemiology of disability in adulthood (Nagi, 1976). Nearly three decades later, it is clear that Nagi's call has been heard. More dynamic studies of disability have become the norm and stimulated by findings from Manton, Corder, and Stallard (1993) that disability has *declined* among older people. Using data from the National Long-Term Care Survey (NLTCS), they showed that the prevalence of disability declined among "chronically disabled community-dwelling and institutionalized elderly populations" (Manton, Corder, & Stallard, 1993, p. S194). Others have questioned these findings on several fronts, especially because the NLTCS uses a screener question so that some disability is required for sample inclusion. Thus, the people who made the transition from no disability to some disability were excluded in their longitudinal analyses. Crimmins, Saito, and Reynolds (1997) reported fluctuation rather than a clear trend in the prevalence of disability in two other national surveys. Still, investigators of other studies such as the Framingham Heart Study have reported declines in disability (Allaire et al., 1999). Whether the disability decline occurs will continue to be debated, but the finding spurred many longitudinal investigations on disability transitions (Anderson, James, Miller, Worley, & Longino, 1998; Kelley-Moore & Ferraro, 2004).

## II. Life Course Epidemiology

As research on health and aging shifted from studying older people to the aging process, studies using the long view of aging generated important insights regarding how health and social status in early life influence health in later life. Applying the life course perspective to the study of health yields what may be referred to as life course epidemiology (Kuh & Ben-Shlomo, 1997; Wadsworth, 1991). For health gerontology, the idea is that the best models of health in later life will incorporate elements of early life—from birth and middle-age to the early periods of later life. According to Wadsworth (1997), there is growing interest in taking a "lifetime view of the natural history of some common serious illnesses which usually begin in middle or later life" (p. 860).

### A. Early Origins of Adult Health

Some of the most compelling research for establishing the value of a life course approach to epidemiology was completed in Europe, especially the British studies of the fetal origins of adult health. The work of David Barker and colleagues (1991, 1997, 1998) has been both enlightening and controversial. Their research program on *fetal* origins of adult health shows persuasively that gestation and birth weight are correlated with a host of health outcomes in childhood and adulthood. For

instance, can a pregnant mother's exposure to famine influence the health of her progeny 50 years after the child's birth? The answer is *yes*. Dutch adults "who had been exposed to famine in early gestation" were more likely than those exposed to the famine in mid- or late gestation to report poor health in adulthood—at about age 50 (Roseboom, Van Der Meulen, Ravelli, Osmond, Barker, & Bleker, 2003, p. 391). This is just one study that shows clearly how research on the early origins of adult health is worth the effort. Beyond such historical effects, the fetal-origins research has also elucidated the long-term consequences of health-destructive behaviors during pregnancy (Cheung, 2002). The scientific innovation in this genre of research is to track the subjects from birth to later life and systematically document the associations (Sayer, Syddall, Gilbody, Dennison, & Cooper, 2004). This is the long view of aging par excellence, an important contribution for both maternal and gerontological health.

At the same time, criticism has been leveled at what some consider an oversimplified view of the link between fetal origins and health in later life. To begin, it is possible that some of the link can be explained by genetics. This is a valid criticism, and one that merits evaluation in future research, especially with twin studies. Second, there is concern about the etiological links between early and later life. Admittedly, the links are complex. For example, can low birth weight increase the risk of diabetes? Research has shown that low birth weight raises the risk of obesity in modern and developing countries (Schroeder, Martorell, & Flores, 1999). Obesity, in turn, is highly correlated with diabetes. Thus, low birth weight does not directly cause diabetes mellitus, but the mechanism may be through greater risk of obesity and compromised insulin metabolism (Eriksson, Forsen, Osmond, & Barker, 2003). Granted, the links over the life course are complex, but this is the work of life course epidemiology.

Third, some researchers contend that the relationship between early origins and adult health reported in some studies may be misleading because of "inappropriate statistical adjustment for variables on the causal pathway" (Tu, West, Ellison, & Gilthorpe, 2005, p. 27). This can lead to a statistical effect known as the "reversal paradox," whereby the relationship between the early-origin risk factor and adult health is highly dependent on the relationship between the early and adult risk factors.

Fourth, there remains concern about the purported inexorability of effects by some who study the early origins of adult health. For instance, does low birth weight establish a health trajectory that is insurmountable? Risk is higher, but can it be reversed? The concern is that positing an inexorable effect because of early life risks may lead to a sense of fatalism among both the public and those in the public health arena. Such beliefs can be dangerous in their effects, so it is important to learn about heightened risk resulting from early disadvantages without succumbing to a deterministic model of health. Is health in later life scripted through earlier disadvantage, or is it more likely due to the accumulated risks?

The work of Felitti and colleagues is another example of the early origins research, albeit focused on the effect of adverse *childhood* experiences. Using data from 17,421 adults enrolled in the Kaiser Permanente health maintenance organization in San Diego, Felitti and colleagues have been collecting retrospective data linking adverse childhood experiences with both physical and mental health in adulthood. They found that adverse childhood experiences (ranging from parental divorce to sexual abuse) are much more common than widely acknowledged and consequential in their effects on adult health 50 years later (Felitti, 2002; Felitti et al., 1998). On a host of outcomes, adults who reported abuse as a child or living in a dysfunctional family were more likely to fare worse than those who did not have such adverse experiences.

### B. Cumulative Disadvantage and Health

Research on how health risks accumulate over the life course has also benefited from the development of cumulative disadvantage theory. The idea behind the early-origins research is that disadvantages in early life, even at gestation and birth, lead to additional disadvantages. In a sense, "the deck is stacked" against those who start out disadvantaged (Blackwell, Hayward, & Crimmins, 2001).

Cumulative disadvantage theory addresses such *life course inequalities*, but gives explicit attention to how this also involves a process of cohort differentiation (Dannefer, 1987, 2003). Certain cohorts are more advantaged than others from the start, but each cohort also becomes more heterogeneous because of social stratification and accumulated experiences. For health, one sees the substantial variation in functional ability and health behavior in later life and looks backward over cohort history and personal biography to the events, experiences, and inequalities that raise the risk of adverse health outcomes.

This view over the life course typically shows that some persons are advantaged in their early years, and this advantage compounds over time. Others are disadvantaged because of genetic or environmental factors, and these disadvantages also accumulate. In a sense, disadvantages may "scar" the person's life chances (Preston, Hill, & Drevenstedt, 1998), and many of the inequalities that we observe in later life were established earlier. For instance, racial inequalities in health do not emerge during later life. There are well-documented racial differences in health at birth, in infancy and childhood, and throughout most of adulthood (Ahmed, 1994; Ferraro & Farmer, 1996; Mangold & Powell-Griner, 1991; Manton, 1980). Though racial differences in health in later life have generated considerable interest among gerontologists, most of the longitudinal research on the subject shows that the inequalities are present early and remain fairly stable over the life course. Indeed, once one accounts for the adverse mortality processes among African Americans, there may actually be a leveling or reversal of differences, as posited in the racial mortality crossover thesis (Manton & Stallard, 1981).

Parallel to research on race and health, considerable interest has been shown in testing cumulative disadvantage theory by examining the relationship between socioeconomic status (SES) and health. There is little debate that SES is related to health, but the results have been inconsistent with regard to when the relationship is strongest across the life course. Some studies have shown that health disparities resulting from education increase over the life course (Ross & Wu, 1995, 1996), but other studies show that health disparities resulting from education and income are greatest in middle age—advanced age levels the salubrious effects of SES on health (House, Kessler, Herzog, Mero, Kinney, & Breslow, 1990; House, Lepkowski, Kinney, Mero, Kessler, & Herzog, 1994). The inconsistency in findings may be due to many reasons, but a growing body of research suggests the importance of identifying the mechanisms by which SES links early-life risk factors to later-life health. For instance, Pampel and Rogers (2004) not only reported an inverse relationship between SES and smoking, but that the effects of smoking on health were exacerbated for the SES disadvantaged groups. In other words, low SES is associated with both risk exposure and risk amplification.

A related body of research has shown that the effects of SES on health are contingent on residential history (Angel, Buckley, & Sakamoto, 2001), especially because early disadvantage increases the risk of living in a health-damaging environment (Holland, Berney, Blane, Smith, Gunnell, & Montgomery, 2000).

Beyond racial and SES differences in health, research applying cumulative disadvantage theory has examined other risk factors associated with poor health in later life. For example, Ferraro and Kelley-Moore (2003b) found that obesity was a turning point in the health of adults. Using data from a 20-year follow-up of a national sample, they found that obesity had long-term effects on disability: exceeding the body mass index threshold of 30 was associated with premature disability for both men and women. They also found, however, that those subjects who exercised regularly were able to compensate somewhat for the effects of obesity. In this and other cases, there was evidence that there are ways to overcome health risks from earlier life—early risks are not necessarily inexorable in their effects (U.S. Department of Health and Human Services, 1990).

It is not surprising that the study of cumulative disadvantage has spurred interest in health trajectories over the life course. "Life-course trajectories are simply long-term patterns of change and stability" (George, 2003, p. 162). Health trajectories incorporate multiple indicators of health over several measurement occasions, perhaps over decades of a person's life. For instance, Elder, Shanahan, and Clipp (1994) used data from the Stanford Terman study panel study to examine the effects of military service on health trajectories over several decades of adult life—a wide angle view. Considerable criticism has been leveled at the early-origins research for the lack of information on intervening events and changes (i.e., mechanisms of change). Research on health trajectories, however, makes use of multiple measurement occasions to track the changes, thereby permitting more rigorous tests of competing mechanisms such as life events and health behavior.

## C. Health-Protective and Health-Destructive Behavior

Ways in which to reduce or reverse health decline have long been of interest to scientists, clinicians, and public health officials. Without unduly privileging human agency and individual responsibility, there are important differences in health over the life course that may be shaped by behaviors over which humans have some degree of control. This is not to backtrack on the importance of early disadvantage in shaping health over the life course. It is, however, a recognition that even among those exposed to the same levels of risk, there are behaviors that can make a difference. As we shall make clearer at the conclusion of the chapter, we need public health initiatives that address *both* structural arrangements and individual choice.

Research on health-protective and health-destructive behavior generally falls into two types. There are the behavior-specific studies such as smoking (Barbeau, Krieger, & Soobader, 2004), substance abuse (Oman, Vesely, Aspy, McLeroy, Rodine, & Marshall, 2004), and eating disorders/nutrition (Flegal, Williamson, Pamuk, & Rosenberg, 2004), and there are studies that aim to consider the complex of these behaviors (Bryant, Shetterly, Baxter, & Hamman, 2002; Merzel & D'Afflitti, 2003; Newsom, Kaplan, Huguet, & McFarland, 2004; Nigg et al., 1999). As one surveys both literatures, three conclusions related to health and aging are quite clear.

First, the effect of accumulated life experiences is substantial. Not only did

Felitti and colleagues find that adverse childhood experiences influence health, but they also found that childhood adversity raised the risk of participating in risky or health-destructive acts. Evidence is accumulating that child abuse or other adversities increase the likelihood of risky sex (Hillis, Anda, Felitti, & Marchbanks, 2001), having an unintended pregnancy (Dietz et al., 1999), smoking (Anda et al., 1999), adult obesity (Williamson, Thompson, Anda, Dietz, & Felitti, 2002), and attempted suicide (Dube, Anda, Felitti, Chapman, Williamson, & Giles, 2001). There is ample evidence that adverse childhood experiences are related to adult health, but an emerging body of research now identifies some of the mechanisms by which adversity in childhood leads to poor health in later life. The emotional scars of childhood abuse and adversity are associated with a host of health-destructive behaviors that compromise health over the long term.

Second, evidence has emerged over the past three decades that health behavior is intricately related to social stratification. Most of the health-destructive behaviors are much more likely among persons of lower social class. Persons of lower SES are far more likely to smoke (Barbeau et al., 2004; Jefferis, Power, Graham, & Manor, 2004), be physically inactive (Crespo, Smit, Andersen, Carter-Pokras, & Ainsworth, 2000), be obese (Sobal, 1991) or severely obese (Ferraro, Thorpe, & Wilkinson, 2003), and engage in other risky behaviors such as alcohol and drug abuse (Oman et al., 2004).

It should also be recognized that poverty exposes children to greater risk of adversity in the early years. If children grow up in a poor neighborhood, they are more likely to be exposed to environmental risks and a social order in which there are more risky behaviors (e.g., smoking, substance abuse). In other words, poverty and childhood adversity often overlap, thereby increasing the likelihood that children born in poor neighborhoods will begin life health disadvantaged. For instance, smoking is more prevalent in poor neighborhoods, and pregnant women who smoke are more likely to have babies of low birth weight. Low birth weight, in turn, may lead to early health disadvantages, thereby setting a trajectory that is less than desirable. The relationship between social class and health-destructive behaviors may create a cascade of risks to those of lower SES.

It should be noted that even though the SES/health relationship is strong, there are exceptions. Noting that Mexican Americans have better health and longevity than what one would predict based on their comparatively lower SES, Markides and Coreil (1986) described the situation as an epidemiological paradox. Indeed, on a number of health indicators, Mexican Americans fare better than Caucasian Americans given their generally poorer SES (see, for example, Gillum, 1997).

Third, despite what may appear to be strong patterns of social influence, health behaviors are modifiable. Even in poor neighborhoods, there is evidence that health promotion interventions can be effective in increasing participation in a regular exercise program, weight reduction (Clark, Stump, & Damush, 2003), and medication compliance (Murray et al., 2004). In addition, the evidence is clear that such behavioral change is consequential. It cannot undo a lifetime of destructive behavior, but eliminating a risky behavior or initiating a health-protective behavior, even in later life, is in most cases consequential to longevity, functional ability, and quality of life.

## III. Health and Illness Behavior

Health behavior involves more than simply deciding to avoid practices that are widely known to harm health. Health and illness behavior also includes the early stages of reacting to the threat of compromised health (health awareness and symptom interpretation) and the later stages of dealing with health problems (help seeking and medical care use). Through it all, there are important differences in the way in which aging influences responses to health problems.

### A. Symptom Interpretation and Health Assessment

It is well established that most people experience a host of bodily sensations that may be indicative of a chronic health problem long before they seek help for it. Early on in the development of a chronic disease, people may experience symptoms that merit attention, but they may not be sufficiently definitive to initiate a plan of action or watchful waiting. For some conditions, there may be no symptoms that offer clues as to a bodily abnormality. In those cases in which the person is cognizant of a potential health problem, however, he or she may ignore the symptoms or seek lay and/or professional information to determine how to respond (Haug, Musil, Warner, & Morris, 1998).

Whereas younger people are much less likely to experience chronic health problems, there is less discussion among age peers regarding such matters. Aging, however, often erodes the feelings of health invincibility as functional ability is compromised. Aging also introduces age peers to more conversations about bodily changes and symptoms with which the person may not be familiar. This period of symptom interpretation and information seeking involves assessment of preclinical morbidity because there is no diagnosis. Rather, the person senses a configuration of symptoms and gathers information regarding the seriousness of and susceptibility to a disease (Becker, 1974; Haug et al., 1998).

One of the health topics garnering the most research attention over the last three decades is health assessment. The single-item indicator known as self-rated health has been widely studied. Interest in this item is due to a variety of reasons, not the least of which is how useful it is as an overall assessment of health status (Deeg, van Zonneveld, van der Maas, & Habbema, 1989; Idler & Kasl, 1991). Interest was also stimulated by the paradox that despite the fact that older people are more likely to have chronic diseases and higher disability, they may actually be somewhat more optimistic in rating their health (Ferraro, 1980; Maddox, 1962). Moreover, research has repeatedly shown that self-rated health has prognostic validity in predicting both health service use (Angel & Gronfein, 1988) and mortality (Idler & Benyamini, 1997).

The link between self-rated health and mortality—above and beyond indicators of morbidity and disability—raises the question: What are people communicating in this rating of their health that is so predictive of important health outcomes? The answer appears to include both the preclinical symptoms (Krause & Jay, 1994) and a sense of how one's health is changing (Strawbridge & Wallhagen, 1999; Wolinsky & Tierney, 1998). We now know that health ratings are quite responsive to changes in morbidity and disability and that changes in health ratings are robust predictors of mortality (Ferraro & Kelley-Moore, 2001; Svärdsudd & Tibblin, 1990). Adults, especially older adults, have much biographical and symptomatic information that is expressed in self-rated health. As such, it is a useful predictor of health trajectories and may be why self-rated health is typically a better predictor of mortality than is physician-rated health (Markides, Lee, Ray, & Black, 1993).

## B. Help Seeking

Once a decision is made to seek help for a health problem, early efforts are often ori-ented toward lay referral networks. The Internet has opened up the lay referral and public information system in ways that were not imagined just a decade ago. Beyond conversing with family and friends, people have electronic access to thousands of sites with information related to diseases, medications, and the use of health services. Of course, there is little, if any, quality control over Internet content, so it is rarely a replacement for discussing health issues with significant others in the lay referral network. With chronic illness, the period of coping may be long. Thus, there are repeated efforts to get information to manage the intrusiveness of the condition (Charmaz, 1991).

Early stages of information gathering often lead to a period of self-care. Self-care may involve changes in the health-related behaviors noted earlier, such as increased physical activity, smoking cessation, and/or weight management. The historical move toward more health-protective behavior has been encouraging in many respects, especially with regard to smoking cessation. On the other hand, the rise in obesity during this time is a major public health concern (Flegal, Carroll, Kuczmarski, & Johnson, 1998). Social change and cohort flow shape the adoption of health behaviors and self-care, but individual aging also alters interest in and adoption of such activities.

The literature shows that a wide array of complementary and alternative therapies is incorporated into self-care across the life course. Ranging from acupuncture to yoga, use of such therapies appears to be growing in the United States. Aging, however, does not necessarily mean greater use of such therapies. Self-care that involves prayer and either megavitamin or mind/body therapies are common among older people in the United States, but other therapies such as chiropractic and massage are more common in middle age than in later life (Barnes,

Powell-Griner, McFann, & Nahin, 2004). Despite the growing prevalence of such therapies in the United States, American elders appear to be less likely than Japanese elders to stay with self-care in the face of more serious conditions (Haug, Akiyama, Tryban, Sonoda, & Wykle, 1991). Americans rely on the benefits of scientific medicine, even to the point of expecting surgical procedures to solve preventable health problems (e.g., gastric-bypass surgery).

In response to limitations in functional status, there is evidence that the use of equipment and environmental modifications is prevalent and growing in modern societies. The likelihood of engaging in such practices generally increases with the severity of the functional limitations, but there appears to be a threshold: use of such self-care measures is somewhat less frequent among persons with the most substantial limitations in physical functioning (Norburn et al., 1995). Self-care is preferred, but as conditions disrupt daily life, self-care seems to be a less suitable approach.

## C. Medical Care Use

People use medical care services over the life course, but aging increases the frequency of interactions with health care personnel. Self-care may continue to play a significant role in the management of chronic disease, but older adults in most modern societies rely heavily on the medical care system for handling morbidity. Other chapters in this volume focus on more structural topics such as the organization and financing of health care (see Chapter 21) and emerging issues in long-term care (see Chapter 22). In this section, however, the focus is on what we know about who uses medical care and the health consequences of it.

During the last three decades, scores of researchers have applied the behavioral model of health service use to the study of many forms of care—from physician visits to dementia care. Andersen (1968) first articulated the model with an interest in why families use health care. He developed the model with three sets of influences on health service use: predisposing characteristics, enabling resources, and need. The model has undergone repeated revisions and remains both widely applied and critiqued (Andersen, 1995).

Among the most important contributions from scholars applying the model has been the finding that *need* remains a strong predictor of use. Of course, there are variations in the degree to which this occurs, but the greatest contribution to the explained variance in multivariate models remains the need variables (Wolinsky, Stump, & Johnson, 1995). The relative influence of need on medical care use also varies across types of care. Need is a strong predictor of hospitalization, but less so for physician or dentist visits, which are more discretionary in nature.

A second major contribution of the model is the identification of inequalities in care (Aday & Andersen, 1981; Aday, Andersen, & Fleming, 1980). There are substantial inequalities in medical care in the United States. For example, African-American and Caucasian patients are, by and large, treated by different physicians. Recent research shows that African-American patients are more likely than Caucasian patients to obtain their medical care from physicians who have less access to high-quality clinical resources (Bach, Pham, Schrag, Tage, & Hargrace, 2004). Thus, it should not be altogether surprising that there are African-American/Caucasian differences in medical care use. African-American heart patients are less likely than their Caucasian counterparts to receive cardiac revascularization (Ibrahim, Whittle, Bean-Mayberry, Kelley, Good, & Conigliaro, 2003). Consequently, African Americans are more likely to experience sudden coronary death (either outside of the hospital or in an emergency room) than Caucasian Americans (Gillum, 1997).

Research on medical care use also reflects some of the design changes noted earlier with regard to health research. Most health services research in the 1970s and early 1980s was based on cross-sectional analyses, but longitudinal investigations are becoming more common (e.g., Wolinsky, Krygiel, & Wyrwich, 2002). There is also a critical distinction regarding analyses of "first" visits versus repeated events. When modeling a single hospitalization event, it is most unlikely that it is the first time such an event has occurred. For practicality, however, it is customary to recognize that such events may have occurred before the study observation period. Although this problem pervades virtually every study, the analysis of repeated events moves the inquiry to a higher level. Especially with regard to growing older, the analysis of repeated events is critical. For instance, one of the concerns about the implementation of the Prospective Payment System, based on diagnostic-related groups, is that older people may be discharged "quicker and sicker." Thus, it was essential that studies of hospitalization incorporate temporal dimensions and analyze repeated events to detect the possibility of adverse outcomes such as discharge instability (Weissman & Epstein, 1994) and early readmission (Ashton, Kuykendall, Johnson, Wray, & Wu, 1995). These studies have helped to clarify the enduring inequalities over the life course, as well as the precarious position in which many frail older people find themselves.

## IV. Future Research Directions

Although several specific research directions have been noted throughout the chapter, it might be valuable to highlight a few ideas that could substantially aid research on aging and health.

### A. Social Structure and Human Agency in the Development of Health Disparities

For many of the research topics discussed, there is the question of inequality—its genesis and consequences. As reviewed herein, there are strong social and environmental influences on health. Inequality is present in all societies, but the health consequences of inequality are of immense public health import; hence, there is much interest in both studying and eliminating *health disparities* (U.S. Department of Health and Human Services, 2000).

To better explicate these disparities, the field has shifted to studying the cumulative effects of disadvantage on health and well-being. This research shows clearly how disadvantaged are those who have a poor start. In this sense, gerontologists should see and appreciate the long-term health consequences of maternal and child health. A good start in life aids the chances for a good finish.

It is hard to overstate the influence of early disadvantages. When disadvantaged early in life, the likely outcome is additional risk exposure, which most often leads to further disadvantage. At the same time, one cannot neglect human agency. Despite the toughest of circumstances, some people not only survive, but they thrive. This is, to some degree, still a mystery. At a minimum, it would be useful to ask people about what led and enabled them to stave off the disadvantage. How can one steer clear of the harmful effects of social disorganization? What resources helped these "success stories" to persevere or overcome the odds? Identifying these resources may help others. If "the race is to the swift," what enabled those who started out poorly to catch up? At a minimum, studies of the compensatory mechanisms will help keep hope alive that one can overcome earlier disadvantages. It also validates the value of health-protective behavior.

Research on health disparities needs to explicate the ways in which social structures generate health risks, as well as the ways in which people can compensate for cumulative adversity. At the same time, we need evidence-based interventions to address both the social structures that generate health inequality and the mechanisms to promote health behaviors.

## B. Enhancing the Long View of Aging and Health

Several tangible steps on the research front should be clearly understood as enabling major contributions to our understanding of aging and health. To begin, the valuable role of panel studies is profound. There has been a demonstrable increase during the last 50 years in the use of longitudinal panel designs in articles published in the flagship journal devoted to social scientific research on aging (Ferraro & Kelley-Moore, 2003a). The greater use of longitudinal data has helped to illuminate the dynamic nature of the aging process.

Not only have we witnessed greater use of longitudinal data to study health, but we are seeing more studies with more waves of data. The two-wave study helps one to see so much more than a cross-sectional study, but when studying something as complex and dynamic as health, the advantage of having three or more waves of data is clear. Fortunately, there are many excellent multi-wave panel studies that are very resourceful for studying health and aging. And excellent methods for handling these rich data sets are increasingly being applied. For example, in a relatively short period of time, we have moved from predominance on cross-sectional studies of health to multi-wave studies that apply growth curves and/or time-dependent covariates to better understand health transitions.

Moreover, with changes observed in both health behaviors and health status during these panel studies, we can take advantage of such sequencing to map out the contribution of behavior on health.

Beyond the increasing use of longitudinal data, more studies are incorporating biomarkers into epidemiological and social science studies of health. Whether the measures cover blood pressure or cholesterol, allostatic load, or genetics, there is a movement to more interdisciplinary teams investigating how biological factors can be incorporated into social science research (Conley, & Bennett, 2000; Seeman, McEwen, Rowe, & Singer, 2001). This is a welcome development but investigators must be vigilant with regard to the protection of human subjects while incorporating biomarker data (National Research Council, 2001).

Data on childhood experiences, even if retrospective, are another way to enhance research on the "long view" of aging. There is now sufficient evidence to demonstrate the utility of gathering information on childhood experiences in studying adult health. Merging social and biomarker data from childhood to later life would be a special resource for identifying the etiologic mechanisms by which adverse childhood experiences influence adult health.

Finally, a promising development is linking social and health surveys with medical record or health service use data. These studies allow one to compare and contrast what the person reports versus what he or she was treated for by a health care provider. In addition, studies that link community-based surveys to health service records offer a special opportunity in studying health disparities in accessing care, as well as differences in the sequelae of using services. Movement toward more dynamic models of health and health service use is clear, and understanding each step in the process of health decline should open up avenues for effective public health intervention.

# V. Social Forces and Health Across the Life Course

The last 50 years have ushered in robust research activity on the health of older people and, more recently, the systematic study of the aging process per se. Social and behavioral research has done much to advance our understanding of health across the life course, explicating the diversity within the older adult population and the antecedents of more rapid health decline. We now know that many health problems are preventable and that social forces are critical to risk exposure across the life course. Although there are biological and genetic limits to extending and improving health, our aim should be to harness the available knowledge to optimize health for a diverse society.

In his pioneering efforts to draw medical attention to the study of later life, Jean Martin Charcot (1881) noted that there is a "particular stamp which old age imprints on all morbid manifestations" (p. 26). His insight was profound at the time and spurred the systematic study of aging and disease. Much has transpired in the 125 years since his clinical lectures were collected, and contemporary scientists are still studying imprints. The imprints that fuel the interests of today's social and behavioral epidemiologists, however, are those not stamped by "old age" but by the life course itself. In a sense, the study of aging and health begins with maternal and child health, noting how many of the diseases and disabilities of later life have early origins that are socially patterned. It could be argued that the early and social origins of disease and disability are largely irrelevant once the person enters the medical care system as a patient. The social origins perspective, however, notes that even the time and portal of entry into the medical care system is conditioned by events and inequalities manifest over the life course (Kaplan, 2004). We need social science research that uses various lenses to understand aging and health, from studies examining processes within a short span of time to those considering the entire life course. Together, they enable us to identify the stamps that imprint health across the life course.

## References

Achenbaum, W. A. (1995). *Crossing frontiers: Gerontology emerges as a science.* Cambridge: Cambridge University Press.

Aday, L. A., & Andersen, R. M. (1981). Equity of access to medical care—A conceptual and empirical overview. *Medical Care, 19 (12),* 4–27.

Aday, L. A., Andersen, R. M., & Fleming, G. V. (1980). *Health care in the US: Equitable for whom?* Beverly Hills, CA: Sage.

Ahmed, F. (1994). Infant mortality and related issues. In I. L. Livingston (Ed.), *Handbook of Black American health: The mosaic of conditions, issues, policies, and prospects* (pp. 216–235). Westport, CT: Greenwood Press.

Allaire, S. H., LaValley, M. P., Evans, S. R., O'Connor, G. T., Kelly-Hayes, M., Meenan, R. F., Levy, D., & Felson, D. T. (1999). Evidence for decline in disability and improved health among persons aged 55 to 70 Years: The Framingham Heart Study. *American Journal of Public Health, 89,* 1678–1683.

Anda, R. F., Croft, J. B., Felitti, V. J., Nordenberg, D., Giles, W. H., Williamson, D. F., & Giovino, G. A. (1999). Adverse childhood experiences and smoking during adolescence and adulthood. *Journal of the American Medical Association, 282,* 1652–1658.

Andersen, R. M. (1968). *Behavioral model of families' use of health services.* Research series No. 25. Chicago, IL: Center for the Study of Health Administration Studies, University of Chicago.

Andersen, R. M. (1995). Revisiting the behavioral model and access to medical care: Does it matter? *Journal of Health and Social Behavior, 36,* 1–10.

Anderson, R. T., James, M. K., Miller, M. E., Worley, A. S., & Longino, C. F., Jr. (1998). The timing of change: Patterns in transitions in functional status among elderly persons. *Journal of Gerontology: Social Sciences, 53B*, S17–S27.

Angel, J. L., Buckley, C. J., & Sakamoto, A. (2001). Duration or disadvantage? Exploring nativity, ethnicity, and health in midlife. *Journal of Gerontology: Social Sciences, 56(5)*, S275–S284.

Angel, R., & Gronfein, W. (1988). The use of subjective information in statistical models. *American Sociological Review, 53*, 464–73.

Ashton, C., Kuykendall, D. H., Johnson, M. L., Wray, N. P., & Wu, L. (1995). The association between the quality of inpatient care and early readmission. *Annals of Internal Medicine, 122(6)*, 415–421.

Bach, P. B., Pham, H. H., Schrag, D., Tate, R. C., & Hargraves, J. L. (2004). Primary care physicians who treat blacks and whites. *New England Journal of Medicine, 351(6)*, 575–584.

Barbeau, E. M., Krieger, N., & Soobader, M. J. (2004). Working class matters: Socioeconomic disadvantage, race/ethnicity, gender, and smoking in NHIS 2000. *American Journal of Public Health, 94(2)*, 269–278.

Barker, D. J. P. (1991). *Fetal and infant origins of adult disease*. London: British Medical Journal.

Barker, D. J. (1997). Maternal nutrition, fetal nutrition, and disease in later life. *Nutrition, 13*, 807–813.

Barker, D. J. P. (1998). *Mothers, babies and health in later life*. Edinburgh: Churchill Livingstone.

Barnes, P. M., Powell-Griner, E., McFann, K., & Nahin, R. L. (2004). Complementary and alternative medicine use among adults: United States, 2002. *Advance Data from Vital and Health Statistics, 343*, 1–19.

Becker, M. H. (Ed.) (1974). *The health belief model and personal health behavior*. San Francisco: Society for Public Health Education.

Blackwell, D. L., Hayward, M. D., & Crimmins, E. M. (2001). Does childhood health affect chronic morbidity in later life? *Social Science and Medicine, 52*, 1269–1284.

Bryant, L. L., Shetterly, S. M., Baxter, J., & Hamman, R. F. (2002). Modifiable risks of incident functional dependence in Hispanic and non-Hispanic White elders: The San

Luis Valley Health and Aging Study. *The Gerontologist, 42*, 690–697.

Busse, E. W., & Maddox, G. L. (1985). *The Duke longitudinal studies of normal aging: 1955–1980*. New York: Springer Publishing Co.

Charcot, J. M. (1881). *Clinical lectures on the diseases of old age* (Trans. by Leigh H. Hunt, with additional lectures by Alfred L. Loomis). New York, William Wood & Co.

Charmaz, K. (1991). *Good days, bad days: The self in chronic illness and time*. New Brunswick, NJ: Rutgers University Press.

Cheung, Y. B. (2002). Early origins and adult correlates of psychosomatic distress. *Social Science and Medicine, 55(6)*, 937–948.

Clark, D. O., Stump, T. E., & Damush, T. M. (2003). Outcomes of an exercise program for older women recruited through primary care. *Journal of Aging and Health, 15(3)*, 567–585.

Conley, D., & Bennett, N. G. (2000). Is biology destiny? Birth weight and life chances. *American Sociological Review, 65*, 458–467.

Crespo, C. J., Smit, E., Andersen, R. E., Carter-Pokras, O., & Ainsworth, B. E. (2000). Race/ethnicity, social class and their relation to physical inactivity during leisure time: Results from the Third National Health and Nutrition Examination Survey 1988–1994. *American Journal of Preventive Medicine, 18(1)*, 46–53.

Crimmins, E. M., Saito, H., & Reynolds, S. L. (1997). Further evidence on recent trends in the prevalence and incidence of disability among older Americans from two sources: The LSOA and the NHIS. *Journal of Gerontology: Social Sciences, 52B*, S59–S71.

Dannefer, D. (1987). Aging as intracohort differentiation: Accentuation, the Matthew effect, and the life course. *Sociological Forum, 2*, 211–236.

Dannefer, D. (2003). Cumulative advantage/disadvantage and the life course: Cross-fertilizing age and social science theory. *Journal of Gerontology: Social Sciences, 58B(6)*, S327–S337.

Deeg, D. J. H., van Zonneveld, R. J., van der Maas, P. J., & Habbema, J. D. F. (1989). Medical and social predictors of longevity in the elderly: Total predictive value and interdependence. *Social Science and Medicine, 29*, 1271–1280.

Dietz, P. M, Spitz, A. M., Anda, R. F., William-son, D. F., McMahon, P. M., Santelli, J. S., Nordenberg, D. F., Felitti, V. J., & Kendrick, J. S. (1999). Unintended pregnancy among adult women exposed to abuse or household dysfunction during their childhood. *Journal of the American Medical Association, 282,* 1359–1364.

Dube, S. R., Anda, R. F., Felitti, V. J., Chapman, D., Williamson, D. F., & Giles, W. H. (2001). Childhood abuse, household dysfunction and the risk of attempted suicide throughout the life span: Findings from the Adverse Childhood Experiences Study. *Journal of the American Medical Association, 286,* 3089–3096.

Ekerdt, D. J., Baden, L., Bosse, R., & Dibbs, E. (1983). The effect of retirement on physical health. *American Journal of Public Health, 73,* 779–783.

Elder, G. H., Jr. (1974). *Children of the Great Depression: Social change in life experience.* Chicago: University of Chicago Press.

Elder, G. H., Jr. (1994). Time, human agency, and social change: Perspectives on the life course. *Social Psychology Quarterly, 57,* 4–15.

Elder, G. H., Jr., Shanahan, M. J., & Clipp, E. C. (1994). When war comes to men's lives: Life-course patterns in family, work, and health. *Psychology and Aging, 9*(1), 5–16.

Eriksson, J. G., Forsen, T. J, Osmond, C., & Barker, D. J. P. (2003). Pathways of infant and childhood growth that lead to type 2 diabetes. *Diabetes Care, 26 (11),* 3006–3010.

Felitti, V. J. (2002). The relationship between adverse childhood experiences and adult health: Turning gold into lead. *The Permanente Journal, 6,* 44–47.

Felitti, V. J., Anda, R. F., Nordenberg, D., Williamson, D. F., Spitz, A. M., Edwards, V., Koss, M. P., & Marks J. S. (1998). The relationship of adult health status to childhood abuse and household dysfunction. *American Journal of Preventive Medicine, 14,* 245–258.

Ferraro, K. F. (1980). Self-ratings of health among the old and the old-old. *Journal of Health and Social Behavior, 21,* 377–383.

Ferraro, K. F., & Farmer, M. M. (1996). Double jeopardy to health hypothesis for African Americans: Analysis and critique. *Journal of Health and Social Behavior, 37,* 27–43.

Ferraro, K. F., & Kelley-Moore, J. A. (2001). Self-rated health and mortality among Black and White adults: Examining the dynamic evaluation thesis. *Journal of Gerontology: Social Sciences, 56B,* S195–S205.

Ferraro, K. F., & Kelley-Moore, J. A. (2003a). A half-century of longitudinal methods in social gerontology: Evidence of change in the *Journal. Journal of Gerontology: Social Sciences, 58B,* S264–S270.

Ferraro, K. F., & Kelley-Moore, J. A. (2003b). Cumulative disadvantage and health: Long-term consequences of obesity?" *American Sociological Review, 68,* 707–729.

Ferraro, K. F., Mutran, E., & Barresi, C. M. (1984). Widowhood, health, and friendship support in later life. *Journal of Health and Social Behavior, 25,* 245–259.

Ferraro, K. F., Thorpe, R. J., Jr., & Wilkinson, J. A. (2003). The life course of severe obesity: Does childhood overweight matter?" *Journal of Gerontology: Social Sciences, 58B,* S110–S119.

Flegal, K. M., Carroll, M. D., Kuczmarski, R. J., & Johnson, C. L. (1998). Overweight and obesity in the United States: Prevalence and trends, 1960–1994. *International Journal of Obesity and Related Metabolic Disorders, 22*(1), 39–47.

Flegal, K. M., Williamson, D. F., Pamuk, E. R., & Rosenberg, H. M. (2004). Estimating deaths attributable to obesity in the United States. *American Journal of Public Health, 94*(9), 1486–1489.

Fries, J. F. (1980). Aging, natural death and the compression of morbidity. *New England Journal of Medicine, 303,* 130–135.

George, L. K. (1980). *Role transitions in later life.* Monterey, CA: Brooks/Cole.

George, L. K. (2003). What life-course perspectives offer the study of aging and health. In R. A. Settersten Jr. (Ed.), *Invitation to the life course: Toward new understandings of later life* (pp. 161–188). Amityville, NY: Baywood Publishing.

Gillum, R. F. (1997). Sudden cardiac death in Hispanic American and African Americans. *American Journal of Public Health, 87,* 1461–1466.

Glass, T. (1998). Conjugating the "tenses" of function: Discordance among hypothetical, experimental, and enacted function in older adults. *The Gerontologist, 38,* 101–112.

Guralnik, J. M. (1991). Prospects for the compression of morbidity: The challenge posed by increasing disability in the years prior to death. *Journal of Aging and Health*, 3, 138–154.

Haug, M. R., Akiyama, H., Tryban, G., Sonoda, K., & Wykle, M. (1991). Self care: Japan and the U.S. compared. *Social Science and Medicine*, 33(9), 1011–1022.

Haug, M. R., Musil, C. M., Warner, C. D., & Morris, D. L. (1998). Interpreting bodily changes as illness: a longitudinal study of older adults. *Social Science and Medicine*, 46(12), 1553–1567.

Hillis, S. D., Anda, R. F., Felitti, V. J., & Marchbanks, P. A. (2001). Adverse childhood experiences and sexual risk behaviors in women: A retrospective cohort study. *Family Planning Perspectives*, 33, 206–211.

Holland, P., Berney, L., Blane, D., Smith, G. D., Gunnell, D. J., & Montgomery, S. M. (2000). Life course accumulation of disadvantage: Childhood health and hazard exposure during adulthood. *Social Science and Medicine*, 50(9), 1285–1295.

House, J. S., Kessler, R. C., Herzog, A. R., Mero, R. P., Kinney, A. M., & Breslow, M. J. (1990). Age, socioeconomic status, and health. *Milbank Quarterly*, 68, 383–411.

House, J. S., Lepkowski, J. M., Kinney, A. M., Mero, R. P., Kessler, R. C., & Herzog, A. R. (1994). The social stratification of aging and health. *Journal of Health and Social Behavior*, 35, 213–234.

Hubert, H. B., Bloch, D. A., Oehlert, J. W., & Fries, J. F. (2002). Lifestyle habits and compression of morbidity. *Journal of Gerontology: Medical Sciences*, 57(6), M347–M51.

Ibrahim, S. A., Whittle, J., Bean-Mayberry, B., Kelley, M. E., Good, C., & Conigliaro, J. (2003). Racial/ethnic variations in physician recommendations for cardiac revascularization. *American Journal of Public Health*, 93(10), 1689–1693.

Idler, E. L., & Benyamini, Y. (1997). Self-rated health and mortality: A review of twenty-seven community studies. *Journal of Health and Social Behavior*, 38, 21–37.

Idler, E. L., & Kasl, S. (1991). Health perceptions and survival: Do global evaluations of health status really predict mortality? *Journal of Gerontology: Social Sciences*, 46, S55–S65.

Jefferis, B. J., Power, C., Graham, H., & Manor, O. (2004). Effects of childhood socioeconomic circumstances on persistent smoking. *American Journal of Public Health*, 94(2), 279–285.

Kaplan, G. A. (1991). Epidemiologic observations on the compression of morbidity: Evidence from the Alameda County Study. *Journal of Aging and Health*, 3, 155–171.

Kaplan, G. A. (2004). What's wrong with social epidemiology, and how can we make it better? *Epidemiologic Reviews*, 26, 124–135.

Kelley-Moore, J. A., & Ferraro, K. F. (2004). The Black/White disability gap: Persistent inequality in later life? *Journal of Gerontology: Social Sciences*, 59B, S34–S43.

Krause, N. M., & Jay, G. M. (1994). What do global self-rated health items measure? *Medical Care*, 32, 930–942.

Kuh, D., & Ben-Shlomo, Y. (1997). Introduction: A life course approach to the aetiology of adult chronic disease. In D. Kuh & Y. Ben-Shlomo (Eds.), *A life course approach to chronic disease epidemiology* (pp. 3–14). New York: Oxford University Press.

Lawrence, R., & Jette, A. (1996). Disentangling the disablement process. *Journal of Gerontology: Social Sciences*, 51B, S173–S182.

Maddox, G. L. (1962). Some correlates of differences in self-assessment of health status among the elderly. *Journal of Gerontology*, 17, 180–185.

Mangold, W. D., & Powell-Griner, E. (1991). Race of parents and infant birthweight in the United States. *Social Biology*, 38, 13–27.

Manton, K. G. (1980). Sex and race specific mortality differentials in multi-cause of death data. *The Gerontologist*, 20, 480–493.

Manton, K. G., Corder, L. S., & Stallard, E. (1993). Estimates of change in chronic disability and institutional incidence and prevalence rates in the U.S. elderly population from 1982, 1984, and 1989 National Long Term Care Survey. *Journal of Gerontology: Social Sciences*, 48, S153–S166.

Manton, K. G., & Stallard, E. (1981). Methods for evaluating the heterogeneity of aging processes in human populations using vital statistics data: Explaining the black/white mortality crossover by a model of mortality selection. *Human Biology*, 53(1), 47–67.

Markides, K., & Coreil, J. (1986). The health of Hispanics in the southwestern United

States: An epidemiological paradox. *Public Health Reports, 101,* 253–265.

Markides, K. S., Lee, D. J., Ray, L. A., & Black, S. M. (1993). Physicians' ratings of health in middle and old age: A cautionary note. *Journal of Gerontology: Social Sciences, 48,* S24–S27.

Merzel, C., & D'Afflitti, J. (2003). Reconsidering community-based health promotion: Promise, performance, and potential. *American Journal of Public Health, 93*(4), 557–574.

Murray, M. D., Young, J. M., Morrow, D. G., Weiner, M., Tu, W., Hoke, S.C., Clark, D. O., Stroupe, K. T, Wu, J., Deer, M. M., Bruner-England, T. E., Sowinski, K. M., Smith, F. E., Oldridge, N. B., Gradus-Pizlo, I., Murray, L. L., Brater, D. C., & Weinberger, M. (2004). Methodology of an ongoing, randomized, controlled trial to improve drug use for elderly patients with chronic heart failure. *American Journal of Geriatric Pharmacotherapy, 2*(1), 53–65.

Nagi, S. Z. (1965). Some conceptual issues in disability and rehabilitation. In Sussman M. B. (Ed.), *Sociology and rehabilitation* (pp. 100–113). Washington, DC: American Sociological Association.

Nagi, S. Z. (1976). An epidemiology of disability among adults in the United States. *Milbank Memorial Fund Quarterly/Health and Society, 54,* 439–467.

Nascher, I. L. (1909). Geriatrics. *New York Medical Journal, 90,* 358.

Nascher, I. L. (1914). *Geriatrics.* Philadelphia: P. Blakiston's Son & Co.

National Research Council. (2000). *Cells and surveys: Should biological measures be included in social science research?* Committee on Population. In C. E. Finch, J. W. Vaupel, & K. Kinsella (Eds.), Commission on Behavioral and Social Sciences and Education. Washington, DC: National Academy Press.

Newsom, J. T., Kaplan, M. S., Huguet, N., & McFarland, B. H. (2004). Health behaviors in a representative sample of older Canadians: Prevalences, reported change, motivation to change, and perceived barriers. *The Gerontologist, 44,* 193–205.

Nigg, C. R., Burbank, P. M., Padula, C., Dufresne, R., Rossi, J. S., Velicer, W. F. Laforge, R. G., & Prochaska, J. O. (1999).

Stages of change across ten health risk behaviors for older adults. *The Gerontologist, 39,* 473–482.

Norburn, J. E., Bernard, S. L., Konrad, T. R., Woomert, A., DeFriese, G. H., Kalsbeek, W. D., Koch, G. G., & Ory, M. G. (1995). Self-care and assistance from others in coping with functional status limitations among a national sample of older adults. *Journal of Gerontology: Social Sciences, 50*(2), S101–S109.

Oman, R. F., Vesely, S., Aspy, C. B., McLeroy, K. R., Rodine, S., & Marshall, L. (2004). The potential protective effect of youth assets on adolescent alcohol and drug use. *American Journal of Public Health, 94*(8), 1425–1430.

Pampel, F. C., & Rogers, R. G. (2004). Socioeconomic status, smoking, and health: A test of competing theories of cumulative advantage. *Journal of Health and Social Behavior, 45*(3), 306–321.

Preston, S. H., Hill, M. E., & Drevenstedt, G. L. (1998). Childhood conditions that predict survival to advanced ages among African-Americans. *Social Science Medicine, 47,* 1231–1246.

Quinn, J. F. (1987). The economic status of the elderly: Beware of the mean. *Review of Income and Wealth, 33,* 63–82.

Riley, M. W. (1987). On the significance of age in sociology. *American Sociological Review, 52,* 1–14.

Riley, M. W., Foner, A., Moore, M. E., Hess, B. B., & Roth, B. K. (1968). *Aging and society: Vol. 1. A sociology of age stratification.* New York: Russell Sage Foundation.

Riley, M. W., Johnson, M., & Foner, A. (1972). *Aging and society: Vol. 3. An inventory of research findings.* New York: Russell Sage Foundation.

Rogers, R. G., Hummer, R. A., & Nam, C. B. (2000). *Living and dying in the USA: Behavioral, health and social differentials of adult mortality.* San Diego: Academic Press.

Roseboom, T. J., Van Der Meulen, J. H., Ravelli, A. C., Osmond, C., Barker, D. J., & Bleker, O. P. (2003). Perceived health of adults after prenatal exposure to the Dutch famine. *Paediatrics and Perinatal Epidemiology, 17*(4), 391–397.

Ross, C. E., & Wu, C. L. (1995). The links between education and health. *American Sociological Review, 60,* 719–745.

Ross, C. E., & Wu, C. L. (1996). Education, age, and the cumulative advantage in health. *Journal of Health and Social Behavior, 37,* 104–120.

Sayer, A. A., Syddall, H. E., Gilbody, H. J., Dennison, E. M., & Cooper, C. (2004). Does sarcopenia originate in early life? Findings from the Hertfordshire cohort study. *Journal of Gerontology: Medical Sciences, 59*(9), M930–M934.

Schroeder, D. G., Martorell, R., & Flores, R. (1999). Infant and child growth and fatness and fat distribution in Guatemalan adults. *American Journal of Epidemiology, 149,* 177–185.

Seeman, T. E., McEwen, B. S., Rowe, J. W., & Singer, B. H. (2001). Allostatic load as a marker of cumulative biological risk: MacArthur Studies of Successful Aging. *Proceedings of the National Academy of Sciences of the United States of America, 98,* 4770–4775.

Shock, N. W., Gruelich, R. C., Costa, P. T., Jr., Andres, R., Lakatta, E. G., Arenberg, D., & Tobin, J. D. (1984). *Normal human aging: The Baltimore Longitudinal Study of Aging,* NIH publication No. 84–2450. Washington, DC: U.S. Department of Health and Human Services.

Sobal, J. (1991). Obesity and socioeconomic status: A framework for examining relationships between physical and social variables. *Medical Anthropology, 13,* 231–247.

Strawbridge, W. J., & Wallhagen, M. I. (1999). Self-rated health and mortality over three decades: Results from a time-dependent covariate analysis. *Research on Aging, 21,* 402–416.

Svärdsudd, K., & Tibblin, G. (1990). Is quality of life affecting survival? The study of men born in 1913. *Scandinavian Journal of Primary Health Care, 1* (Supplement), 55–60.

Taylor, M. G., & Lynch, S. M. (2004). Trajectories of impairment, social support, and depressive symptoms in later life. *Journal of Gerontology: Social Sciences, 59*(4), S238–S246.

Tu, Y. K., West, R., Ellison, G. T., & Gilthorpe, M. S. (2005). Why evidence for the fetal origins of adult disease might be a statistical artifact: The "reversal paradox" for the relation between birth weight and blood pressure in later life. *American Journal of Epidemiology, 161*(1), 27–32.

U.S. Department of Health and Human Services. (1990). *The health benefits of smoking cessation: A report of the surgeon general.* Rockville, MD: Centers for Disease Control, Center for Chronic Disease Prevention and Health Promotion, Office on Smoking and Health.

U.S. Department of Health and Human Services. (2000). *Healthy people 2010: Understanding and improving health,* 2nd ed. Washington, DC: U.S. Government Printing Office.

Verbrugge, L. M. (1991). Survival curves, prevalence rates, and dark matters therein. *Journal of Aging and Health, 3,* 217–236.

Verbrugge, L. M., & Jette, A. M. (1994). The disablement process. *Social Science and Medicine, 38,* 1–14.

Wadsworth, M. E. J. (1991). *The imprint of time: Childhood, history, and adult life.* Oxford: Clarendon Press.

Wadsworth, M. E. J. (1997). Health inequalities in the life course perspective. *Social Science and Medicine, 44,* 859–869.

Weissman, J. S., & Epstein, A. M. (1994). *Falling through the safety net: Insurance status and access to health care.* Baltimore, MD: Johns Hopkins University Press.

Wheaton, B. (1990). Life transitions, role histories, and mental health. *American Sociological Review, 55*(2), 209–223.

Williamson, D. F., Thompson, T. J., Anda, R. F., Dietz, W. H., & Felitti, V. J. (2002). Adult body weight, obesity, and self-reported abuse in childhood. *International Journal of Obesity, 26,* 1075–1082.

Wolinsky, F. D., Armbrecht, E. S., & Wyrwich, K. W. (2000). Rethinking functional limitation pathways. *The Gerontologist, 40,* 137–146.

Wolinsky, F. D., Krygiel, J., & Wyrwich, K. W. (2002). Hospitalization for prostate cancer among the older men in the Longitudinal Study on Aging, 1984–1991. *Journal of Gerontology: Medical Sciences, 58,* M115–M121.

Wolinsky, F. D., Stump, T. E., & Johnson, R. J. (1995). Hospital utilization profiles among older adults over time: Consistency and volume among survivors and decedents.

*Journal of Gerontology: Social Sciences, 50(2)*, S88–S100.

Wolinsky, F. D., & Tierney, W. M. (1998). Self-rated health and adverse health outcomes: An exploration and refinement of the trajectory hypothesis. *Journal of Gerontology: Social Sciences, 53B*, S336–S340.

# Fifteen

# Technological Change and Aging

## Stephen J. Cutler

The twentieth century was an era of unparalleled technological change. Revolutionary developments occurred in manufacturing, transportation, communications, information processing, and health care, among other areas. Consider the following as an illustration of the scope and rapidity of these changes. The year 2006 is the 60th anniversary of the first electronic computer, ENIAC—the University of Pennsylvania's Electronic Numerical Integrator and Computer. The computing power of this machine, which took up a large room, weighed more than 30 tons, and contained more than 17,000 vacuum tubes, is now far surpassed by inexpensive, hand-held calculators and even by the microprocessors in musical greeting cards (Birnbaum & Williams, 2000; Wulf, 2003). Miniaturization and decreasing costs have put desktop and laptop computers well within the purchasing power of large segments of the buying public (Adler, 2002).

Most observers agree that technology generally tends to be developed by young persons and aimed at a young market (Pew & Van Hemel, 2004). There are, however, signs of growing interest in the development and application of technologies specifically for the older population. Some of this interest doubtless stems from a recognition of commercial and market implications of social and demographic trends (Brink, 1997; Maney, 2004). Projections of a doubling of the size of the older (65+) population between 2000 and 2030 and of an even greater rate of increase in the numbers of the oldest-old (85+) (U.S. Census Bureau, 2003) have not escaped the attention of the business community. The purchasing power of the older population makes it a growing and attractive market. Recent trends in the direction of a "graying" of the labor force (Czaja & Moen, 2004) have been an incentive for industry to ask how technology might be better suited to the needs of older workers (Mosner, Spiezle, & Emerman, 2003). The Microsoft Corporation (2004), for example, devotes a section of its web site to the implications of how "accessible technology can help aging workers retain high productivity" (p. 1). That the prevalence of functional limitations and related health problems increases with age points to continued growth in the market for assistive and

*Handbook of Aging and the Social Sciences, Sixth Edition*

other enabling technologies. Thus, the Intel Corporation (2004) has established the Proactive Health Research Program, an initiative focussing on how technology can support aging in place among those experiencing physical and cognitive declines, meet the needs of persons with chronic health conditions, and promote wellness through primary prevention of illness.

Technological developments have fundamentally altered the fabric of social and economic life, but how have they affected older persons? Has the older population participated in and benefited from these changes? What factors are associated with technology adoption and use by older persons? The remainder of this chapter examines various facets of this nexus between aging and technology. Section I begins with a brief consideration of the state of theoretical perspectives on technological change and aging. Section II follows with an overview of ways that technology is being and can be used by older persons. Section III discusses factors associated with variation in the use of technology and considers the efficacy of interventions designed to promote technology use. The chapter concludes with a discussion of gaps that need to be addressed in future work on aging and technology.

## I. Theoretical Perspectives

Despite a longstanding substantive interest in applied dimensions of technology, theory development in social gerontology has for the most part neglected technological change. Two notable exceptions are modernization theory and environmental press theory. Although modernization theory initially emphasized the consequences of economic development for the status of older adults (Cowgill, 1972), subsequent refinements gave a prominent role to factors such as health technology, modern economic technol-

ogy, and technical training as antecedent conditions affecting the status of older persons (Cowgill, 1974). To illustrate, Cowgill suggested that improvements in health technology led to gains in longevity and to population aging. Intergenerational competition for jobs, resulting from population aging, was among the factors fostering the development and institutionalization of retirement, which in turn contributed to the declining status of older persons.

The role of technology is also implicit, if not explicit, in various versions of environmental press and person-environment fit theories (e.g., Lawton & Nahemow, 1973). From this perspective, adaptive technologies are among the types of environmental modifications that may be used in response to declining physical or cognitive abilities. Difficulty in climbing stairs, for example, can be compensated for by a mechanical stair lift.

These examples notwithstanding, the role of technology has been at best on the periphery of social gerontological theory. As Mollenkopf (2004) notes, "... a comprehensive theoretical approach for understanding the dynamic relationship between secular changes in society and technology, on the one hand, and human aging, on the other, is still to be developed" (p. 62). It is beyond the scope of this chapter to propose an inclusive theoretical perspective on technology, either as a causal factor (i.e., its impact on older persons and on the aging process) or as an outcome variable (i.e., variation in the adoption and use of technology). One starting point, however, draws on what might be referred to as "lag" theories. The concept of "structural lag" (Riley, Kahn, & Foner, 1994), for instance, speaks to a mismatch between the changing capabilities of older persons and societal opportunity structures. A case in point is suburbanization, a process predicated on the use of the automobile as a means of personal transportation. With the aging of suburbs and the aging in place of its residents, dependence on mobility via personal transportation is becoming increasingly problematic for the older population. Yet, changes in the transportation infrastructure in suburban areas have lagged far behind changes in the mobility needs of older suburban residents (Burkhardt, 2000).

A variation of structural lag is what Lawton (1998) refers to as "individual lag." Whereas structural lag suggests that social structures and social institutions fail to keep pace with changes in individuals' abilities, individual lag occurs when social structures and environments change more rapidly than peoples' abilities. Lawton cites as examples the challenges of programming a VCR or of high speed, congested highways that may tax an older person's reduced reaction time.

Lag is of value in understanding other facets of the relationship between aging and technological change. Ogburn (1964), in his theory of "cultural lag," points to a potential discrepancy in the rates of change of material and nonmaterial aspects of culture. Material aspects of culture are technological solutions to problems of human existence, and nonmaterial aspects (e.g., values, norms, and sanctions) are the "social" solutions. If one function of nonmaterial aspects of culture is to provide a set of cultural prescriptions to guide the development and deployment of technology, problems arise when technological change outpaces change in relevant nonmaterial dimensions. An imbalance in rates of change results in a kind of "anomie," a period of normative indeterminacy in the appropriateness of using available technologies. Thus, our ability to sustain life through the availability of advanced medical technology continues to be accompanied by a lack of resolution about when it is proper to use such technology, as in the case of tube feeding for persons in the final stages of Alzheimer's disease (Post, 2001; see

also Chapter 24). Because advanced medical technology is in short supply and expensive, vigorous debates have emerged about justice and the fairness of employing various criteria, including age, as bases for allocating scarce health care resources (Binstock & Post, 1991; see also Chapter 25). As a final example, recent developments in genetic testing have raised anew questions about how to balance obligations to protect the confidentiality of patient information with obligations entailed by a duty to warn of inherited health risk (Offit, Groeger, Turner, Wadsworth, & Weiser, 2004).

The notion of lags directs attention to other aspects of the development and adoption of technology. Rogers' (2003) theory of the diffusion of technology addresses variation in rates of adoption. What is popularly referred to as the "digital divide" is an outcome of forces leading to variation, or lags, in rates of becoming "wired," with age and cohort effects being among these forces. And the notion of lags will be of heuristic value in yet another context later in the chapter in considering how responsive gerontology as a field of study has been to technological change.

## II. Overview of Applications

Space constraints preclude a comprehensive cataloguing of technological devices and products, both those currently available and those in the design and development phases. Rather, the focus here is on generic uses that older adults can and do make of various technologies, with illustrative applications rather than a definitive listing.

### A. Social Interaction, Social Integration, and Social Support

Just as the telegraph and telephone did historically, recent developments in communications technology are having profound effects on social interaction. As Adams noted (1998), the advent of the Internet has contributed to the demise of territorially delimited interaction. "Communities" of interest, friendship, and support can be developed and sustained, unfettered by geographical constraints. Email, instant messaging, Internet telephony, two-way video communications, news groups, and chat rooms enable persons to reestablish, initiate, maintain, or extend social relationships (Blit-Cohen & Litwin, 2004). Although some findings suggest that Internet use at home detracts from time spent with friends and family (Nie, Hillygus, & Erbring, 2002), other studies conclude that "... the Internet provides a sphere for social interaction, for people to meet others with similar interests, and for the creation of social cohesion" (Quan-Haase, Wellman, Witte, & Hamptom, 2002, p. 318). The bulk of the evidence suggests that Internet usage is associated with heightened interaction and increased community and political involvement (Howard, Rainie, & Jones, 2002; Katz & Rice, 2002).

The Internet is of particular relevance to older adults who wish to be in contact with family and friends living at great distances or for those who are isolated because of mobility limitations (Czaja & Lee, 2003). Research consistently shows that the primary way online older adults use the Internet is for email, including intergenerational communication with children and grandchildren (Landsdale, 2002). Although only 22% of older Americans had access to the Internet between 2003 and 2004, 94% of these wired seniors used the Internet for email (Fox, 2004).

Internet-based communication also has special relevance to caregivers and others seeking social support (see, e.g., Roberts [2004] on how the Internet is being used for bereavement support). Caregiving demands may preclude attending support groups. Online groups give caregivers the flexibility to overcome constraints imposed by time and by distance, and the asynchronous character of the communication does not require that other members of the network be immediately available. Numerous online support groups exist, and approximately 13% of caregivers in a 2004 survey reported using the Internet to look for support or advice from other caregivers (National Alliance for Caregiving & AARP, 2004).

Research on the effects of participating in online support groups is scant (Morgan, 2004), but the limited evidence suggests that such access is beneficial. Bass, McClendon, Brennan, and McCarthy (1998) report that a computer support network for family caregivers of persons with Alzheimer's disease was associated with a reduction in caregiver strain, especially for caregivers with more informal support and for spousal caregivers. Evaluation of a computer-telephone integrated system for family caregivers has shown that participants value communication with other caregivers and find the online discussion groups to be beneficial (Czaja & Rubert, 2002). When this system was combined with family therapy, significant reductions in depressive symptoms were observed (Eisdorfer et al., 2003). Mahoney, Tarlow, and Jones (2003) noted that a computer-mediated automated interactive voice response intervention was associated with reductions in bothersome aspects of caregiving, anxiety, and depression, particularly among low mastery caregivers. Although these findings are suggestive, more research is needed, especially studies comparing outcomes of online support with more traditional forms of social support.

## B. Self-Enhancement and Information Gathering

New technologies are particularly well suited to accessing sources of information. This is again true of the Internet, a process facilitated by the availability of powerful search engines. The value of this aspect of technology to older adults is demonstrated by findings showing that information gathering is another of the major uses of the Internet. For example, surveys (Fox, 2004) indicate that 82% of older, online persons have used a search engine to find information.

Prominent among the types of information sought is information about health (Morrell, 2002), with 66% of wired older persons having sought health or medical information (Fox, 2004). That older adults make heavy use of the Internet to gather health-related information is understandable given the relationship between age and prevalence of health problems, but we know little about the specific purposes of information seeking. Is it used for self-diagnosis, as a supplement to information supplied by a health care provider, as a self-care substitute in place of consultation with a health care provider, or for some combination of these (and other) reasons?

By virtue of their flexibility, new technologies also have the potential to contribute to the intellectual enrichment of older persons (Adler, 2002). Distance learning courses offered via two-way interactive television and online courses open up educational opportunities for older adults who may be unable to enroll in traditional courses (Schneider, Glass, Henke, & Overton, 1997). At present, however, older adults are only half as likely as the general population (22% vs. 46%) to be enrolled in any form of adult education and lifelong learning courses (Kim, Hagedorn, & Williamson, 2004). Furthermore, data from a 1999 national survey showed that less than 1% of persons 65 and older had enrolled in any type of distance learning course during the prior year (National Center for Education Statistics, 2000).

Several concerns have been expressed about older persons using the Internet for information gathering. One issue is the accuracy and reliability of available information. This applies not only to health-related information (Silberg, Lundberg, & Musacchio, 1997) but, as Schulz and Borowski note (see Chapter 20), information pertaining to investment strategies and financial planning is often inaccurate. Second, navigating web sites to access desired information poses challenges for older users because web sites are rarely designed to take into account typical cognitive, sensory, and physical changes that accompany aging (Mead, Lamson, & Rogers, 2002). And, third, the sheer amount of material available may quickly create a situation of information overload (Czaja & Lee, 2001).

## C. Monitoring and Surveillance

Newly emerging technologies have the capacity not only to facilitate information gathering by older adults, but also to transmit information about their status and conditions (Nebeker, Hurdle, & Bair, 2003; Tamura, Togawa, Ogawa, & Yamakoshi, 1998). Such applications are particularly relevant because efforts to slow the rate of growth of health care costs have resulted in a shift in the locus of care from the hospital to the home and other community-based settings (Kaye & Davitt, 1999). With "telehealth" and "telemedicine" applications (Whitten, 2001, 2004), technology can provide the means to monitor a person's condition and provide data against which departures from baseline conditions can be identified and appropriate responses initiated. Information about parameters of health status can be collected in the home and transmitted both to health care providers and to family or other informal caregivers, including those who reside at some distance from the older person (Dishman, Mathews, & Dunbar-Jacob, 2004).

Elements of monitoring and surveillance are a central part of efforts underway in the development of "smart" houses. Projects at the Georgia Institute of Technology (2004) and the University of Florida (2003), among others (Rogers, Mayhorn, & Fisk, 2004), are attempting to harness the power of technology to monitor conditions in the home environment, movement through the house, health status, and needs for self-care (Mann, 2003). Other technology can detect wandering from the home. Sensors can indicate when doors have been opened when they should not have been, and Global Positioning System technology has the potential to track and locate cognitively impaired persons who have wandered and become lost.

Concerns about the intrusiveness of such devices have been raised, as have issues about privacy and confidentiality (Cantor, 2004; Lefton, 1997). The limited evidence available suggests that older persons are willing to permit information to be provided to others if it enhances their sense of safety and security. In a study of smart home technology, Melenhorst, Fisk, Mynatt, and Rogers (2004) report that " ... older adults felt intrusion as a potential threat and a drawback associated with Aware Home technology prototypes, but deemed it negotiable if counterbalanced by the fulfillment of needs they perceived and recognized" (p. 270).

## D. Assistive and Enabling Technologies

Various assistive devices have long been available to enable persons to cope with the effects of disabling conditions. Assistive technology can range from low technology devices, such as canes and walkers, to high technology applications such as the stair climbing wheel chair, recently approved by the U.S. Food and Drug Administration (2003), " ... that relies on a computerized system of sensors, gyroscopes and electric motors to allow indoor and outdoor use on stairs,

as well as on level and uneven surfaces" (paragraph 1). Sources of variation in the use of assistive devices are examined in Section III, but three points can be noted here.

First, because activities of daily living (ADL) and instrumental ADL impairments associated with chronic conditions become more prevalent with increasing age (see Chapter 3), we would expect use of assistive devices to be widespread among the older population. Data from the 1994 National Health Interview Survey on Disability (NHIS-D), the most recent, detailed NHIS inquiry into assistive devices, show that 2% of the noninstitutional population 65+ were using anatomical devices, 15% mobility devices, 10% hearing devices, and 1% vision devices (not including eyeglasses and contact lenses) (Russell, Hendershot, LeClere, Howie, & Adler, 1997). Use is likely to be understated by such point prevalence data, however, because they fail to provide information about transitions into and out of the use of assistive devices. Then, too, nursing home residents who have higher rates of disability are excluded from the NHIS surveys. Among older adults with one or more ADL limitations, it is estimated that close to two-thirds use some form of assistive device (Agree & Freedman, 2000).

Second, the use of assistive devices may be among the factors contributing to declining rates of chronic disability among the older population. Several investigators note that the use of assistive devices has increased at the same time that the prevalence of chronic disability has declined (Manton, Corder, & Stallard, 1993a, 1993b; Russell et al., 1997). Verbrugge and Sevak (2002) reported that equipment use can reduce disability, although Spillman (2004) cautioned that the use of devices may contribute to positive changes in *self-perceptions* of disability independent of actual changes in health.

Third, there is evidence that the use of assistive devices is cost effective and may reduce demands on caregivers. Agree and Freedman (2000, 2003), for example, noted that users of assistive technology are less likely to report a need for personal assistance and that simple devices can serve as a substitute for informal caregivers. Similarly, Allen, Foster, and Berg (2001) found that the use of simple devices such as canes and walkers may serve as a substitute by reducing reliance on both informal and formal care.

Future developments in assistive and enabling technology may come in the form of robotics (Kaye & Davitt, 1999). The Nursebot project, a collaborative undertaking between Carnegie Melon University and the Universities of Pittsburgh and Michigan, has as its objective the development of ". . . mobile, personal service robots that assist elderly people suffering from chronic disorders in their everyday life" (Carnegie Mellon University, n.d.). "Honda, Mitsubishi and scientists at the Korean Institute of Science and Technology are designing machines to help old or disabled people move from room to room, fetch snacks or drinks, operate the television, and even call the doctor when needed" (The gentle rise of the machines, 2004). Aibo, a robot developed by Sony, is being used in Japan as part of therapy sessions with dementia patients (Kageyama, 2004). Efforts to design and develop robots to serve as personal care assistants and do routine physical tasks in home and institutional settings are in their infancy, but may come to play a more prominent role.

## E. E-commerce

Forms of online commerce range from the direct electronic deposit of checks, to ordering goods and services over the Internet, to paying bills and conducting other financial transactions electronically. Direct deposit services benefit eld-

ers who are concerned about the security of mailed checks, about their personal safety when going to a bank to deposit checks, or those for whom getting to a bank is difficult because of mobility limitations. As of January 1999, 75% of Social Security and SSI recipients had these funds electronically deposited (U.S. Social Security Administration, n.d.).

Being able to shop for and purchase goods and services online has several advantages. It provides access to goods and services for those with impaired mobility; shoppers are not limited by time of day or day of the week as e-commerce sites are available continuously; and there are no geographical constraints on businesses that can be accessed. Because older people take longer to process information (Brown & Park, 2003), online purchases may also present less time pressure than would the same transaction done in person or over the phone.

As convenient as online commerce may be, only a small percentage of all older persons use e-commerce for shopping and buying, although such usage is increasing. Recent surveys of older Internet users (Fox, 2001, 2004) showed that 47% had bought a product online in 2003–2004 compared with 36% in 2000, and 41% had made a travel reservation compared with 25% in 2000. There was little change in the percentage buying or selling stocks (13% vs. 12%) or participating in online auctions (9% vs. 8%), but banking online had increased over this period from 8% to 20%.

## F. Technology in the Workplace

The implications of technological change for older workers are considerable. The nature of the workplace itself is changing (Czaja & Moen, 2004) as an increasing share of jobs require some knowledge of computers. As of 2001, 57% of employed adults used a computer at work (U.S. Department of Commerce, 2002). In addition, sectors of the labor force that are projected to show high rates of growth (e.g., management, business, and financial occupations; professional and related occupations) tend to be those with high rates of computer use (Hecker, 2004; Mosner et al., 2003). Then, too, the long-term historical trend toward earlier retirement seems to have been reversed since 1990, and there are indications that workers plan to stay in the labor force longer than previously. Between 1990 and 2003, the labor force participation rates of males 60 to 64 years old increased from 55% to 57%, from 26% to 33% among those 65 to 69 years old, and from 15% to 19% among males 70 to 74 years old (Bureau of Labor Statistics, 2004; see also Chapter 12). Reported intentions appear to be consistent with these changing labor force participation rates. Thus, a 2003 AARP survey of Baby Boomers found that 79% planned to participate in the labor force in some manner during retirement (AARP, 2004)

Older workers are often thought to be at a disadvantage because they lack experience with newer forms of technology. They are assumed to have greater difficulty learning tasks associated with new technology or to be unable to learn them at all. Retraining programs are considered to be less effective and more expensive than for younger people. Yet, numerous studies have demonstrated that older workers are both willing to learn how to use new technology and are capable of acquiring the needed skills (Czaja, 2001). The learning curve may be slower, and training programs should be designed to take account of cognitive, sensory, and physical changes accompanying aging. When such steps are instituted, research shows that older workers are able to function effectively in workplaces with changing technological environments (Czaja & Moen, 2004). Moreover, retaining older workers despite retraining costs is ultimately cost effective because of

their lower rates of absenteeism and turnover (Czaja, 2001).

## G. Transportation and Mobility

As of 2002, 90% of nondisabled older persons drove, as did 60% of older persons with one or more disabilities (Sweeney, 2004). Being able to drive is both a symbol of independence and a key determinant of a person's capacity to access goods and services and engage in various forms of social interaction and participation (Eisenhandler, 1990; Marottoli, Mendes de Leon, Glass, Williams, Cooney, & Berkman, 2000). The cessation of driving, with negative effects on the well-being of some elders (Marottoli et al., 1997), is often due to physical, cognitive, and sensory changes (Ball & Owsley, 2000; Satariano, MacLeod, Cohn, & Ragland, 2004). An analysis of "driving life expectancy" showed that 70- to 74-year-old male drivers would need alternative sources of transportation for seven years and 70- to 74-year-old female drivers for ten years (Foley, Heimovitz, Guralnik, & Brock, 2002). Furthermore, older persons living in suburban and rural areas are less likely to have alternative means of transportation when an automobile is unavailable (U.S. Department of Transportation, 2003).

Technology has the potential not only to reduce barriers to continued driving, but also to enhance the safety of older (and other) drivers. Examples of intelligent transportation systems include in-vehicle routing and navigation systems, in-vehicle safety advisory and warning systems, and collision warning systems (Hanowski & Dingus, 2000). Vehicle design can address common changes that occur with aging. Wide-angle, rear-view systems can compensate for difficulties older drivers have in looking behind them. Better headlight design can make night driving easier, and auditory warning systems can take into account hearing changes that typically accompany aging.

Drivers of all ages would benefit from changes in highway and roadway design, changes informed by knowledge of the characteristics of older drivers. Larger and more visible signage, better illumination at intersections, earlier warnings about traffic lights and stop signs, and longer entrance and exit ramps on highways would contribute to the ease and safety of driving for all drivers (Meyer, 2004; U.S. Department of Transportation, 2003).

## III. Factors in the Use of Technology by Older Persons

The previous section described various uses of technology by older persons and, data permitting, the extent to which they do so. This section examines sources of variation in technology use, with special focus on age differences and how to account for them. The section concludes with a consideration of the efficacy of interventions to promote the use of technology.

### A. Age Differences in Patterns of Usage

There are two principal patterns of age differences in technology use. The first reflects increasing use of technology with age, a pattern typically resulting from health conditions that become more prevalent with advancing age. In the second pattern, age is negatively associated with technology use, with older persons tending to be late adopters of new technology (Rogers, 2003).

A number of studies have examined age patterns in the use of assistive devices. A consistent finding is that use—especially of mobility, hearing, and vision devices—increases with age. Rates at which mobility devices are used by persons 65 years and older are 4.4 times higher than among persons 45 to 64, hearing device use is 5.2 times higher, and vision device use is 3.2 times higher

(Russell et al., 1997). Data from the 2002 NHIS showed that 20% of older adults (65+) used special equipment or assistive devices to aid them in their usual activities compared with 6% of persons 45 to 64 years old (National Center for Health Statistics, 2003). This pattern of increasing use with age persists *within* the older population, even after a variety of relevant demographic, socioeconomic, and health variables are controlled (Agree, Freedman, & Sengupta, 2004; de Klerk, Huijsman, & McDonnell, 1997; Hartke, Prohaska, & Furner, 1998).

In contrast, other technology modalities show declining prevalence of use with age. Despite trends over time toward increasing computer and Internet use by older persons (U.S. Department of Commerce, 2002), numerous studies point to the persistence of age differences. Based on the most recent Current Population Survey (CPS) of computer availability and Internet use, the data in Table 15.1 show that older adults are less likely to live in households that have a computer, are less likely to have used the

#### Table 15.1
Computer Access and Computer and Internet Use, by Age: 2003

| Age | Computer in household (% yes) | Used computer at home (% yes) | Used Internet anywhere (% yes) |
|---|---|---|---|
| 20–29 | 68 | 90 | 70 |
| 30–39 | 75 | 88 | 71 |
| 40–49 | 77 | 83 | 69 |
| 50–59 | 72 | 81 | 64 |
| 60–69 | 58 | 74 | 44 |
| 70–79 | 40 | 65 | 25 |
| 80+[a] | 25 | 45 | 11 |

**Source:** *Current Population Survey Supplements: 2003 Internet and computer use data* [Data file]. Bureau of Labor Statistics, & U.S. Bureau of the Census, 2004. Retrieved November 27, 2004, from http://www.bls.census.gov/cps/computer/2001/sdata.htm
[a]The 2003 Current Population Survey data are top coded for age at 80 and older.

computer if there is one, and are far less likely to have made use of the Internet at any location (Bureau of Labor Statistics & U.S. Census Bureau, 2004). Similar age differences were found in surveys of 15 European nations (Norris, 2001). Attempts to determine whether these differences can be accounted for by compositional factors associated with age (e.g., socioeconomic, demographic, and health variables) show that the differences persist, albeit reduced in magnitude, after relevant variables are controlled (Cutler, Hendricks, & Guyer, 2003).

Although computer and Internet use are prime examples of the negative relationship between age and technology use, similar results are seen for other modalities. Rates of both ATM and cell phone use are lower among older persons than among their younger counterparts (Horrigan, 2003; Rogers, Cabrera, Walker, Gilbert, & Fisk, 1996). For example, a 2003 AARP survey showed that only 27% of persons 65 and older had cell phone service, compared with 50% of persons 50 to 64 and 55% of persons 18 to 49 (Baker & Kim-Sung, 2003). Whether such age differences are due to age effects, cohort effects, or some combination is an important question, but one best considered after examining other sources of variation among older persons.

## B. Psychological and Human Factors Determinants

The greatest attention to the impact of technology on the lives of older adults has come from behavioral scientists in general and from those working in the human factors, ergonomics, and gerotechnology traditions in particular. Human factors research is broadly concerned with identifying impediments to technological use and designing technological interfaces that take these factors into account to make technology accessible to all users. In addition to examining problems with product design and instructions, human factors research has focused on three general classes of obstacles associated with age changes and age differences: (1) cognitive functioning, (2) sensory functioning, and (3) motor functioning. It is impossible to provide a detailed review of this literature here (see, e.g., Burdick & Kwon, 2004; Charness & Schaie, 2003; Pew & Van Hemel, 2004; Rogers & Fisk, 2001), but a few examples will suffice.

Although there is considerable variability, older persons typically perform less well than younger persons on tasks involving short-term and working memory, and they tend to be slower in completing other cognitive tasks (Brown & Park, 2003; Hedden & Park, 2001). Consider the implications of these differences for ease of using automated telephone voice menu systems. The longer the message and, in particular, the greater the number of options to be retained in one's memory, the more difficult are such systems for older users (Sharit, Czaja, Nair, & Lee, 2003). Auditory changes with aging, as in the frequency with which sounds can be discriminated, and changes in vision, such as decreasing transparency of the lens of the eye, have clear design implications (Schieber, 2003). Charness (1998), for example, showed that high-frequency auditory signals from a computer are responded to less quickly by older persons and that changes in the level of luminance have a greater impact on the task performance of older than of younger workers. Motor functioning in older adults may be slower because of differences in fine motor coordination or to conditions such as arthritis that impair motion. As a consequence, the use of a computer mouse or a trackball has been shown to be more difficult for older adults, especially with smaller on-screen targets (Czaja & Lee, 2002; Stronge, Walker, & Rogers, 2001).

## C. Social-Psychological Factors

The role of social-psychological factors has been far less systematically studied and is less well understood, although scattered evidence indicates that such variables are a source of differences in technology adoption and use. In examining attitudes about computer use, Czaja and Sharit (1998) found that age was associated with less comfort, control, and efficacy. Similarly, Ellis and Allaire (1999) found a negative relationship between age and computer interest. An examination of ATM use noted that perceived control and perceived user comfort were associated with greater use (Darch & Caltabiano, 2004). For assistive devices, Roelands, Van Oost, Depoorter, and Buysse (2002) found support for a model hypothesizing that assistive device use is a function of intentions to use these devices, which in turn are associated with general attitudes about device use, self-efficacy, and subjective norms about how others perceive the use of assistive devices. Gitlin, Schemm, Landsberg, and Burgh (1996) also found positive attitudes toward assistive device use to be a significant predictor, and that perceived need was a stronger predictor than objective need.

In addition to one's own attitudes, expectations of others may contribute to age differences. In a vignette study comparing perceptions of how likely a 25-year-old would be to enroll in a computer course and complete it successfully versus a 70-year-old, Ryan, Szechtman, and Bodkin (1992) found expectations to be lower for the older adults. They conclude that "to the extent that behaviors of young and old are influenced by this societal expectation, the opportunities and inclination of older adults to access computer technology would seem to be limited" (p. 99). A related finding comes from the work of Gitlin, Luborsky, and Schemm (1998) who, in qualitative analy-

ses, found that the potential use of assistive devices evoked concerns about social identity, stigma, and biographical management.

## D. Socioeconomic and Demographic Factors

The effects of socioeconomic and demographic factors depend on the particular type of technology being considered. In the realm of information technology, socioeconomic and demographic variables play a key and consistent role in explaining variation in access to and use of computers and the Internet. Among older persons, data from the 2003 CPS survey show that availability and use tends to be lower among women and persons who are widowed, among persons with lower incomes and education levels, and among those who have one or more disabilities; however, many of these characteristics are correlated with each other. Results from logistic regression analyses show that gender differences in the availability of a computer at home, in using that home computer, and in having used the Internet anywhere become nonsignificant when other variables are controlled. The effects of the remaining predictors continue to be significant for the three measures of computer availability and use.

The other form of technology about which we have the most extensive data concerns assistive devices. Here findings show that need variables (i.e., number and severity of limitations) are consistently the best predictors of assistive technology use (see, e.g., Agree et al., 2004; Mathieson, Kronenfeld, & Keith, 2002; Verbrugge & Sevak, 2002). As noted previously, increasing age is also generally associated with assistive technology use. Beyond these two characteristics, predictors vary from study to study and as a function of the way in which assistive technology use is measured. For instance,

Hartke et al. (1998) found that education, marital status, and income are unrelated to assistive device use after controlling for health status, but that males are significantly more likely than females to be users of devices, whereas females are more likely to be users of multiple devices. Mathieson et al. (2002), on the other hand, found after controlling for health that being female or having income plus Social Security increased the odds of using mobility equipment regardless of the number of types used, but that higher levels of education decreased the odds of using a single device (although education was unrelated to using multiple devices).

E. Age versus Cohort Effects

To what extent are age differences in technology use a product of age effects or cohort effects? Put another way, might processes of cohort succession and cohort change diminish if not eradicate age differences in the future, or will processes accompanying intra-cohort aging lead to the persistence of age differences?

On the one hand, it is reasonable to conclude that some portion of observed age differences in technology use is due to the operation of cohort effects. One of the most important factors in how attitudes shape technology use is experience (e.g., Charness, Kelley, Bosman, & Mottram, 2001). In school and workplace settings, as well as at home, both the young and middle-age persons have had much greater exposure to information technology than current cohorts of older persons. The proliferation of cell phones and familiarity with automated systems such as ATMs among young and middle-age persons likely means that these and related skills will be brought with them to their later years. Furthermore, adopting and using new technology is related to socioeconomic factors, especially education and income. That future cohorts of

older persons will certainly have higher levels of educational attainment and perhaps greater levels of economic security also suggests that age differences may diminish in coming years.

On the other hand, certain forms of technology use are associated with chronic health conditions, and it seems unlikely that age differences in chronic illnesses that call for the use of assistive devices will disappear. The use of medical technology in home care and in nursing home settings will likely continue to be related to age. Then, too, if the types of cognitive, sensory, and motor changes that human factors researchers have been interested in persist, these may lead to the continuation of age gradients. Additional features that are typically part of revised or new versions of technology can often add to their complexity. Until the objectives embodied in transgenerational and universal design (Pirkl, 1995) are realized, changes that accompany normal aging may work against adoption and use of tomorrow's new or enhanced, but more complicated, technologies just as these changes have worked against use of today's technologies by older persons.

F. Can Interventions Help?

Because it seems to be more difficult for older persons to learn how to use new technologies and their learning curve is slower, with more mistakes, many investigators have examined whether interventions might reduce age differences in the acquisition of technological skills. These studies have reached two general and important conclusions. First, with appropriate instruction and training, older persons can indeed learn the skills needed to master new technologies (Jamieson & Rogers, 2000; Kramer, Bherer, Colcombe, Dong, & Greenough 2004). Despite ageist stereotypes (Ryan et al., 1992), the evidence consistently demonstrates that older adults are capable of learning new technologies. Second, these studies also demonstrate that attitudes toward technology are malleable and modifiable. With supportive environments and with training configured in a manner consistent with what is known about optimum learning conditions for older persons, experience and success in using technology are associated with a shift toward more favorable attitudes. Direct experience with and knowledge of computers, for example, has consistently been shown to reduce anxiety and to promote computer comfort, control, efficacy, and interest (Czaja & Sharit, 1998; Ellis & Allaire, 1999; Jay & Willis, 1992). How best to configure the learning environment so as to minimize age differences in the time it takes to acquire skills and reduce the number of errors is beyond the scope of this chapter (see, e.g., Willis, 2004). The essential point is that age differences that are rooted in psychological and social psychological determinants of technology use are modifiable, even if socioeconomic determinants may be less so.

## IV. Conclusions

As this chapter makes clear, technological developments have the potential to greatly enhance the well-being of older persons, compensate for health and mobility impairments, and promote social interaction and social support. Yet, it is also evident that much remains to be accomplished in understanding the role and challenges of technology in the lives of older adults. As indicated earlier, technology has been largely neglected by gerontological theory. One approach to theory development was proposed drawing on the concept of "lags," but far more theoretical attention to technology as both a causal and an outcome variable is clearly needed.

Areas where further research is needed have been noted throughout the chapter.

Let me suggest three additional lacunae here. First, and on a fundamental level, I would argue that social gerontological research has not kept pace with technological change, that gerontological research on technology has itself been beset by lags. Take as an example the longstanding interest in patterns of intergenerational interaction. A major thrust of this research has been to document that geographic mobility and other aspects of family dynamics do not lead to pronounced declines in intergenerational contact. Rather, the pattern is more accurately described as "intimacy at a distance" (Rosenmayr & Kockeis, 1963). Thus, the Second Longitudinal Study on Aging, conducted as part of the NHIS as recently as 2000, includes items on the frequency of seeing children and other relatives, friends, and neighbors, as well as the frequency of talking with them on the phone (National Center for Health Statistics, 2000). Although email has been available for several years and despite the fact that we know email is the feature of computer technology most widely used by older persons, this form of connectivity has yet to be included among items asked in the NHIS data. As Adams and Stevenson (2004) recently observed, "Surveying the literature on technology as a relationship mediator serves to demonstrate how slowly researchers have changed their perspectives to adapt to recent changes...." (p. 369).

Second, the review of studies of factors leading to variation in technology use among the older population shows that this research has generally been domain specific. We have studies of computer use, Internet use, ATM use, assistive device use, driving, and so on. A focus on a particular domain is understandable given the complexities within any particular technology domain, but this approach makes it difficult to systematically compare variation and predictors across domains. Especially valuable in furthering our understanding of the role of technology in the lives of older adults would be a comprehensive "technology audit," one that also includes an extensive battery of relevant socioeconomic, demographic, health, psychological, and social psychological variables. Only in this manner will we be able to achieve the comparability necessary to examine intra- and inter-domain variation in technology use and in the effects of predictors across domains.

Finally, fascination with the potential of technological wizardry must be tempered by an appraisal of how accessible these developments will be to sizeable segments of the older population. Technology can be expensive and beyond the financial reach of many older persons. The potential benefits of "smart" houses are impressive, but more fundamental for many older individuals are basic housing issues of availability, affordability, and adequacy (Cutler & Hendricks, 2001). Navigational systems, already available in high-end automobiles, may make it easier to reach destinations safely. These systems may benefit some segments of the older population, but for many others the availability, accessibility, and cost of *any* form of transportation is a more immediate issue. Thus, for persons living on limited, fixed incomes, the fruits of technological change may prove to be inaccessible, thereby creating and/or perpetuating a "technological divide" as a further form of social inequality within and between age groups.

## References

AARP. (2004). *Baby boomers envision retirement II: Survey of baby boomers' expectations for retirement*. Retrieved October 18, 2004, from http://research.aarp.org/econ/boomers_envision_1.pdf

Adams, R. (1998). The demise of territorial determinism: Online friendships. In R. Adams & G. Allan (Eds.), *Placing friendship in context* (pp.153–182). Cambridge: Cambridge University Press.

Adams, R., & Stevenson, M. (2004). A lifetime of relationships mediated by technology. In F. Lang & K. Fingerman (Eds.), *Growing together: Personal relationships across the life span* (pp. 369–393). Cambridge: Cambridge University Press.

Adler, R. (2002). *The age wave meets the technology wave: Broadband and older Americans*. Retrieved October 15, 2004, from SeniorNet web site: http://www.seniornet.org/downloads/broadband.pdf

Agree, E., & Freedman, V. (2000). Incorporating assistive devices into community-based long-term care: An analysis of the potential for substitution and supplementation. *Journal of Aging and Health, 12*, 426–450.

Agree, E., & Freedman, V. (2003). A comparison of assistive technology and personal care in alleviating disability and unmet need. *The Gerontologist, 43*, 335–344.

Agree, E., Freedman, V., & Sengupta, M. (2004). Factors influencing the use of mobility technology in community-based long-term care. *Journal of Aging and Health, 16*, 267–307.

Allen, S., Foster, A., & Berg, K. (2001). Receiving help at home: The interplay of human and technological assistance. *Journal of Gerontology: Social Sciences, 56*, S374–S382.

Baker, C., & Kim-Sung, K. (2003). Consumer concerns about the quality of wireless telephone service. *AARP Public Policy Institute, In Brief Number 73*. Retrieved October 18, 2004, from http://research.aarp.org/consume/dd89_wireless.html

Ball, K., & Owsley, C. (2000). Increasing mobility and reducing accidents of older drivers. In K. Schaie & M. Pietrucha (Eds.), *Mobility and transportation in the elderly* (pp. 213–250). New York: Springer.

Bass, D., McClendon, M., Brennan, P., & McCarthy, C. (1998). The buffering effect of a computer support network on caregiver strain. *Journal of Aging and Health, 10*, 20–43.

Binstock, R., & Post, S. (Eds.). (1991). *Too old for health care? Controversies in medicine, law, economics, and ethics*. Baltimore: Johns Hopkins Press.

Birnbaum, J., & Williams, R. (2000). Physics and the information revolution. *Physics Today, 54*, 38–42.

Blit-Cohen, E., & Litwin, D. (2004). Elder participation in cyberspace: A qualitative analysis of Israeli retirees. *Journal of Aging Studies, 18*, 385–398.

Brink, S. (1997). The twin challenges of information technology and population aging. *Generations, 21*(3), 7–10.

Brown, S., & Park, D. (2003). Theoretical models of cognitive aging and implications for translational research in medicine. *The Gerontologist, 43* (Special Issue I), 57–67.

Burdick, D., & Kwon, S. (Eds.). (2004). *Gerotechnology: Research and practice in technology and aging*. New York: Springer.

Bureau of Labor Statistics. (2004). *Labor force statistics from the Current Population Survey: Customized tables*. Retrieved November 27, 2004, from http:// www.bls.gov/cps/

Bureau of Labor Statistics & U.S. Census Bureau. (2004). *Current Population Survey Supplements: 2001 Internet and computer use data* [Data file]. Retrieved November 27, 2004, from http://www.bls.census.gov/cps/computer/2003/sdata.htm

Burkhardt, J. (2000). Limitations of mass transportation and individual vehicle systems for older persons. In K. Schaie & M. Pietrucha (Eds.), *Mobility and transportation in the elderly* (pp. 279–298). New York: Springer.

Cantor, M. (2004). Privacy, ethics, and caregiving technology for older adults. *Public Policy and Aging Report, 14*(1), 6–9.

Carnegie Mellon University (n.d.). *Nursebot project: Robotic assistance for the elderly*. Retrieved October 21, 2004, from http://www-2.cs.cmu.edu/~nursebot/web/scope.html

Charness, N. (1998). Ergonomics and ageing: The role of interactions. In J. Graafmans, V. Taipale, & N. Charness (Eds.), *Gerontechnology: A sustainable investment in the future* (pp. 62–73). Amsterdam: IOS Press.

Charness, N., Kelley, C., Bosman, E., & Mottram, M. (2001). Word-processing training and retraining: Effects of adult age, experience, and interface. *Psychology and Aging, 16*, 110–127.

Charness, N., & Schaie, K. (Eds.). (2003). *Impact of technology on successful aging*. New York: Springer.

Cowgill, D. (1972). A theory of aging in cross-cultural perspective. In D. Cowgill & L. Holmes (Eds.), *Aging and modernization* (pp. 1–13). New York: Appleton-Century-Crofts.

Cowgill, D. (1974). Aging and modernization: A revision of the theory. In J. Gubrium (Ed.), *Late life: Communities and environmental policy* (pp.123–146). Springfield, IL: Charles C. Thomas Publisher.

Cutler, S., & Hendricks, J. (2001). Emerging social trends. In R. Binstock & L. George (Eds.), *Handbook of aging and the social sciences* (5th ed., pp. 462–480). San Diego: Academic Press.

Cutler, S., Hendricks, J., & Guyer, A. (2003). Age differences in home computer availability and use. *Journal of Gerontology: Social Sciences, 58*, S271–S280.

Czaja, S. (2001). Technological change and the older worker. In J. Birren (Ed.), *Handbook of the psychology of aging* (5th ed., pp. 547–555). San Diego: Academic Press.

Czaja, S., & Lee, C. (2001). The Internet and older adults: Design challenges and opportunities. In N. Charness, D. Parks, & B. Sabel (Eds.), *Communication, technology, and aging: Opportunities and challenges for the future* (pp. 60–78). New York: Springer.

Czaja, S., & Lee, C. (2002). Designing computer systems for older adults. In J. Jacko & A. Sears (Eds.), *Handbook of human-computer interaction* (pp. 413–427). Mahwah, NJ: Lawrence Erlbaum.

Czaja, S., & Lee, C. (2003). The impact of the Internet on older adults. In N. Charness & K. Schaie (Eds.), *Impact of technology on successful aging* (pp. 113–133). New York: Springer.

Czaja, S., & Moen, P. (2004). Technology and employment. In R. Pew & S. Van Hemel (Eds.), *Technology for adaptive aging* (pp. 150–178). Washington, DC: National Academies Press.

Czaja, S., & Rubert, M. (2002). Telecommunications technology as an aid to family caregivers of persons with dementia. *Psychosomatic Medicine, 64*, 469–476.

Czaja, S., & Sharit, J. (1998). Age differences in attitudes toward computers. *Journal of*

*Gerontology: Psychological Sciences, 53,* P329–P340.

Darch, U., & Caltabiano, N. (2004). Investigation of automatic teller machine banking in a sample of older adults. *Australasian Journal on Ageing, 23,* 100–103.

de Klerk, M., Huijsman, R., & McDonnell, J. (1997). The use of technical aids by elderly persons in the Netherlands: An application of the Andersen and Newman Model. *The Gerontologist, 37,* 365–373.

Dishman, E., Mathews, J., & Dunbar-Jacob, J. (2004). Everyday health: Technology for adaptive aging. In R. Pew & S. Van Hemel (Eds.), *Technology for adaptive aging* (pp. 150–178). Washington, DC: National Academies Press.

Eisdorfer, C., Czaja, S., Loewenstein, D., Rubert, M., Argüelles, S., Mitrani, V., & Szapocznik, J. (2003). The effect of a family therapy and technology-based intervention on caregiver depression. *The Gerontologist, 43,* 521–531.

Eisenhandler, S. (1990). The asphalt identikit: Old age and the driver's license. *International Journal of Aging and Human Development, 30,* 1–14.

Ellis, R., & Allaire, J. (1999). Modeling computer interest in older adults: The role of age, education, computer knowledge, and computer anxiety. *Human Factors, 41,* 345–355.

Foley, D., Heimovitz, H., Guralnik, J., & Brock, D. (2002). Driving life expectancy of persons aged 70 years and older in the United States. *American Journal of Public Health, 92,* 1284–1289.

Fox, S. (2001). *Wired seniors: A fervent few, inspired by family ties.* Retrieved October 15, 2004, from Pew Internet & American Life web site: http://www.pewinternet. org/pdfs/ PIP_Wired_Seniors_Report.pdf

Fox, S. (2004). *Older Americans and the Internet.* Retrieved October 15, 2004, from Pew Internet & American Life web site: http://www.pewinternet.org/pdfs/PIP_Seniors_Online_2004.pdf

Georgia Institute of Technology. (2004). *The aware home.* Retrieved October 21, 2004, from http://www.cc.gatech.edu/fce/ahri/

Gitlin, L., Luborsky, M., & Schemm, R. (1998). Emerging concerns of older stroke patients about assistive device use. *The Gerontologist, 38,* 169–180.

Gitlin, L., Schemm, R., Landsberg, L., & Burgh, D. (1996). Factors predicting assistive device use in the home by older people following rehabilitation. *Journal of Aging and Health, 8,* 554–575.

Hanowski, R., & Dingus, T. (2000). Will intelligent transportation systems improve older driver mobility? In K. Schaie & M. Pietrucha (Eds.), *Mobility and transportation in the elderly* (pp. 279–298). New York: Springer.

Hartke, R., Prohaska, T., & Furner, S. (1998). Older adults and assistive devices: Use, multiple-device use, and need. *Journal of Aging and Health, 10,* 99–116.

Hecker, D. (2004). Occupational employment projections to 2012. *Monthly Labor Review, 127,* 80–105.

Hedden, T., & Park, D. (2001). Culture, aging, and cognitive aspects of communication. In N. Charness, D. Parks, & B. Sabel (Eds.), *Communication, technology, and aging: Opportunities and challenges for the future* (pp. 81–107). New York: Springer.

Horrigan, J. (2003). *Consumption of information goods and services in the United States.* Retrieved October 15, 2004, from Pew Internet & American Life web site: http://www.pewinternet.org/pdfs/PIP_Info_ Consumption.pdf

Howard, P., Rainie, L., & Jones, S. (2002). Days and nights on the Internet. In B. Wellman & C. Haythornthwaite (Eds.), *The Internet in everyday life* (pp. 45–73). Malden, MA: Blackwell.

Intel Corporation. (2004). *Exploratory research anticipation: Proactive health.* Retrieved October 20, 2004, from http://www.intel.com/research/prohealth/

Jamieson, B., & Rogers, W. (2000). Age-related effects of blocked and random practice schedules on learning a new technology. *Journal of Gerontology: Psychological Sciences, 55,* P343–P353.

Jay, G., & Willis, S. (1992). Influence of direct computer experience on older adults' attitudes toward computers. *Journal of Gerontology: Psychological Sciences, 47,* P250–P257.

Kageyama, Y. (2004, April 11). In gadget-loving Japan, robots give hugs, therapy. *USA*

*Today*. Retrieved October 18, 2004, from http://www.usatoday.com/tech/news/ tech innovations/2004-04-11-robot-helpers_x.htm

Katz, J., & Rice, R. (2002). Syntopia: Access, civic involvement, and social interaction on the net. In B. Wellman & C. Haythornthwaite (Eds.), *The Internet in everyday life* (pp. 114–138). Malden, MA: Blackwell.

Kaye, L., & Davitt, J. (1999). *Current practices in high-tech home care.* New York: Springer.

Kim, K., Hagedorn, M., & Williamson, J. (2004). *Participation in adult education and lifelong learning: 2000–01 (NCES 2004–050).* U.S. Department of Education, National Center for Education Statistics. Washington, DC: U.S. Government Printing Office.

Kramer, A., Bherer, L., Colcombe, S., Dong, W., & Greenough, W. (2004). Environmental influences on cognitive and brain plasticity during aging. *Journal of Gerontology: Medical Sciences, 59*, M940–M957.

Lansdale, D. (2002). Touching lives: Opening doors for elders in retirement communities through e-mail and the Internet. In R. Morrell (Ed.), *Older adults, health information, and the World Wide Web* (pp. 133–151). Mahwah, NJ: Lawrence Erlbaum.

Lawton, M. (1998). Future society and technology. In J. Graafmans, V. Taipale, & N. Charness (Eds.), *Gerontechnology, A sustainable investment in the future* (pp. 12–22). Amsterdam: IOS Press.

Lawton, M., & Nahemow, L. (1973). Ecology and the aging process. In C. Eisdorfer & M. Lawton (Eds.), *Psychology of adult development and aging* (pp. 464–488). Washington, DC: American Psychological Association.

Lefton, A. (1997). Confidentiality and security in information technology. *Generations, 21*(3), 50–52.

Mahoney, D., Tarlow, B., & Jones, R. (2003). Effects of an automated telephone support system on caregiver burden and anxiety: Findings from the REACH for TLC intervention study. *The Gerontologist, 43*, 556–567.

Maney, K. (2004, February 10). Tech firms want to help elderly—and cash in. *USA Today*, p. 3B.

Mann, W. (2003). Assistive technology. In N. Charness & K. Schaie (Eds.), *Impact of tech-nology on successful aging* (pp. 177–187). New York: Springer.

Manton, K., Corder, L., & Stallard, E. (1993a). Changes in the use of personal assistance and special equipment from 1982 to 1989: Results from the 1982 and 1989 NLTCS. *The Gerontologist, 33*, 168–176.

Manton, K., Corder, L., & Stallard, E. (1993b). Estimates of change in chronic disability and institutional incidence and prevalence rates in the U.S. elderly population from the 1982, 1984, and 1989 National Long Term Care Survey. *Journal of Gerontology: Social Sciences, 48*, S153–S156.

Marottoli, R., Mendes de Leon, C., Glass, T., Williams, C., Cooney, L., & Berkman, L. (2000). Consequences of driving cessation: Decreased out-of-home activity levels. *Journal of Gerontology: Social Sciences, 55*, S334–S340.

Marottoli, R., Mendes de Leon, C., Glass, T., Williams, C., Conney, L., Berkman, L., & Tinetti, M. (1997). Driving cessation and increased depressive symptoms: Prospective evidence from the New Haven EPESE. *Journal of the American Geriatrics Society, 45*, 202–206.

Mathieson, K., Kronenfield, J., & Keith, V. (2002). Maintaining functional independence in elderly adults: The roles of health status and financial resources in predicting home modifications and use of mobility equipment. *The Gerontologist, 42*, 24–31.

Mead, S., Lamson, N., & Rogers, W. (2002). Human factors guidelines for web site usability: Health-oriented web sites for older adults. In R. Morrell (Ed.), *Older adults, health information, and the World Wide Web* (pp. 89–107). Mahwah, NJ: Lawrence Erlbaum.

Melenhorst, A., Fisk, A., Mynatt, E., & Rogers, W. (2004). Potential intrusiveness of aware home technology: Perceptions of older adults. *Proceedings of the Human Factors and Ergonomics Society, 48*, 266–270.

Meyer, J. (2004). Personal vehicle transportation. In R. Pew & S. Van Hemel (Eds.), *Technology for adaptive aging* (pp. 253–281). Washington, DC: National Academies Press.

Microsoft Corporation (2004). *Aging and accessible technology*. Retrieved October 20, 2004, from http://www.microsoft.com/enable/aging/default.aspx

Mollenkopf, H. (2004). Aging and technology—Social science approaches. In D. Burdick & S. Kwon (Eds.), *Gerotechnology: Research and practice in technology and aging* (pp. 54–67). New York: Springer.

Morgan, R. (2004). Computer-based technology and caregiving for older adults: Exploring the range of possibilities and beyond. *Public Policy and Aging Report, 14*(1), 1–5.

Morrell, R. (Ed.). (2002). *Older adults, health information, and the World Wide Web*. Mahwah, NJ: Lawrence Erlbaum.

Mosner, E., Spiezle, C., & Emerman, J. (2003). *The convergence of the aging workforce and accessible technology*. Retrieved October 18, 2004, from Microsoft Corporation web site: http://www.microsoft.com/enable/aging/convergence.aspx

National Alliance for Caregiving & AARP. (2004). *Caregiving in the U.S.* Retrieved October 18, 2004, from http://www.caregiving.org/04finalreport.pdf

National Center for Education Statistics. (2000). *National Household Education Survey of 1999: Adult Education Interview* [Data file]. Available from http://nces.ed.gov/nhes/dataproducts.asp#1999dp

National Center for Health Statistics. (2000). *Questionnaires, datasets, and related documentation*. Available from the National Health Interview Survey web site: http://www.cdc.gov/nchs/about/major/nhis/quest_data_related_doc.htm

National Center for Health Statistics. (2003). *2002 National Health Interview Survey: Sample adult person section* [Data file]. Available from http://www.cdc.gov/nchs/about/major/nhis/quest_data_related_doc.htm

Nebeker, J., Hurdle, J., & Bair, B. (2003). Future history: Medical informatics in geriatrics. *Journal of Gerontology: Medical Sciences, 58*, M820–M825.

Nie, N., Hillygus, D., & Erbring, L. (2002). Internet use, interpersonal relations, and sociability. In B. Wellman & C. Haythornthwaite (Eds.), *The Internet in everyday life* (pp. 215–243). Malden, MA: Blackwell.

Norris, P. (2001). *Digital divide: Civic engagement, information poverty, and the Internet worldwide*. Cambridge: Cambridge University Press.

Offit, K., Groeger, E., Turner, S., Wadsworth, E., & Weiser, M. (2004). The 'duty to warn' a patient's family members about hereditary disease risks. *Journal of the American Medical Association, 292*, 1469–1473.

Ogburn, W. F. (1964). *On culture and social change*. Chicago: University of Chicago Press.

Pew, R., & Van Hemel, S. (Eds.). (2004). *Technology for adaptive aging*. Washington, DC: National Academies Press.

Pirkl, J. (1995). Transgenerational design: Prolonging the American dream. *Generations, 19*(1), 32–36.

Post, S. (2001). Tube feeding and advanced progressive dementia. *The Hastings Center Report, 31*(1), 36–42.

Quan-Haase, A., Wellman, B., Witte, J., & Hampton, K. (2002). Capitalizing on the net: Social contact, civic engagement, and sense of community. In B. Wellman & C. Haythornthwaite (Eds.), *The Internet in everyday life* (pp. 291–324). Malden, MA: Blackwell.

Riley, M., Kahn, R., & Foner, A. (Eds.). (1994). *Age and structural lag: Society's failure to provide meaningful opportunities in work, family, and leisure*. New York: Wiley-Interscience.

Roberts, P. (2004). Here today and cyberspace tomorrow: Memorials and bereavement support on the web. *Generations, 28*(2), 41–46.

Roelands, M., Van Oost, P., Depoorter, A., & Buysse, A. (2002). A social-cognitive model to predict the use of assistive devices for mobility and self-care in elderly people. *The Gerontologist, 42*, 39–50.

Rogers, E. (2003). *Diffusion of innovations* (5th ed.). New York: Free Press.

Rogers, W, Cabrera, E., Walker, N., Gilbert, D., & Fisk, A. (1996). A survey of automatic teller machine usage across the adult life span. *Human Factors, 38*, 156–166.

Rogers, W., & Fisk, A. (Eds.). (2001). *Human factors interventions for the health care of older adults*. Mahwah, NJ: Lawrence Erlbaum.

Rogers, W., Mayhorn, C., & Fisk, A. (2004). Technology in everyday life for older adults. In D. Burdick & S. Kwon (Eds.), *Gerotechnology: Research and practice in technology and aging* (pp. 3–17). New York: Springer.

Rosenmayr, L., & Kockeis, E. (1963). Propositions for a sociological theory of ageing and the family. *International Social Science Journal, 15*(3), 410–426.

Russell, J., Hendershot, G., LeClere, F., Howie, L., & Adler, M. (1997, November 13). *Trends and differential use of assistive technology devices: United States, 1994* (Advance Data from Vital and Health Statistics No. 292). Retrieved October 15, 2004, from: http://www.cdc.gov/nchs/data/ad/ad292.pdf

Ryan, E., Szechtman, B., & Bodkin, J. (1992). Attitudes toward younger and older adults learning to use computers. *Journal of Gerontology: Psychological Sciences, 47,* P96–P101.

Satariano, W., MacLeod, K., Cohn, T., & Ragland, D. (2004). Problems with vision associated with limitations or avoidance of driving in older population. *Journal of Gerontology: Social Sciences, 59,* S281–S286.

Schieber, F. (2003). Human factors and aging: Identifying and compensating for age-related deficits in sensory and cognitive function. In N. Charness & K. Schaie (Eds.), *Impact of technology on successful aging* (pp. 42–84). New York: Springer.

Schneider, E., Glass, S., Henke, M., & Overton, J. (1997). Distance learning in gerontology: The future is here. *Generations, 21*(3), 46–49.

Sharit, J., Czaja, S., Nair, S., & Lee, C. (2003). Effects of age, speech rate, and environmental support in using telephone voice menu systems. *Human Factors, 45,* 234–251.

Silberg, W., Lundberg, G., & Musacchio, R. (1997). Assessing, controlling, and assuring the quality of medical information on the Internet: Caveant lector et viewor—let the reader and viewer beware. *Generations, 21*(3), 53–55.

Spillman, B. (2004). Changes in elderly disability rates and the implications for health care utilization and cost. *The Milbank Quarterly, 82,* 157–194.

Stronge, A., Walker, N., & Rogers, W. (2001). Searching the World Wide Web: Can older adults get what they need? In W. Rogers & A. Fisk (Eds.), *Human factors interventions for the health care of older adults* (pp. 255–269). Mahwah, NJ: Lawrence Erlbaum.

Sweeney, M. (2004). *Travel patterns of older Americans with disabilities* (Working Paper 2004-001-OAS). Retrieved November 1, 2004, from Bureau of Transportation Statistics web site: http://www.bts.gov/programs/bts_working_papers/2004/paper_01/pdf/entire.pdf

Tamura, T., Togawa, T., Ogawa, M., & Yamakoshi, K. (1998). Fully automated health monitoring at home. In J. Graafmans, V. Taipale, & N. Charness (Eds.), *Gerontechnology: A sustainable investment in the future* (pp. 280–284). Amsterdam: IOS Press.

The gentle rise of the machines. (2004, March 11). *The Economist.* Retrieved October 18, 2004, from http://www.economist.com/scence/tq/displaystory.cfm?story_id=2476972

University of Florida. (2003, November 19). *UF 'smart home' demonstrates the concept of automated elderly help and care.* Retrieved October 21, 2004, from http://www.napa.ufl.edu/2003news/smarthouse.htm

U.S. Census Bureau. (2003). *Statistical abstract of the United States, 2003* (123rd ed.). Washington, DC: U.S. Government Printing Office

U.S. Department of Commerce. (2002, February). *A nation online: How Americans are expanding their use of the Internet.* Retrieved October 15, 2004, from: http://www.ntia.doc.gov/ntiahome/dn/anationonline2.pdf

U.S. Department of Transportation. (2003, November). *Safe mobility for a maturing society: Challenges and opportunities.* Retrieved October 18, 2004, from: http://www.fta.dot.gov/CCAM/SafeMobility.pdf

U.S. Food and Drug Administration. (2003, August 13). *FDA approves stair-climbing wheelchair.* Retrieved October 21, 2004, from http://www.fda.gov/bbs/topics/NEWS/2003/NEW00933.html

U.S. Social Security Administration. (n.d.). *Social Security online: Direct deposit.* Retrieved October 21, 2004, from http://www.ssa.gov/deposit/DDFAQ898.htm

Verbrugge, L., & Sevak, P. (2002). Use, type, and efficacy of assistance for disability. *Journal of Gerontology: Social Sciences, 57,* S366–S379.

Whitten, P. (2001). The state of telecommunication technologies to enhance older adults' access to health services. In W. Rogers & A. Fisk (Eds.), *Human factors interventions for the health care of older adults* (pp. 121–146). Mahwah, NJ: Lawrence Erlbaum.

Whitten, P. (2004). Evidence regarding patient and provider perceptions and health indicators for telehome health. *Public Policy and Aging Report, 14*(1), 19–21.

Willis, S. (2004). Technology and learning in current and future older cohorts. In R. Pew & S. Van Hemel (Eds.), *Technology for adaptive aging* (pp. 209–229). Washington, DC: National Academies Press.

Wulf, W. (2003). Higher education alert: The information railroad is coming. *Educause Review, 38*(1), 12–21.

# Sixteen

# Religion and Aging

Ellen Idler

## I. Background

Religion was one, if not *the most*, prominent area of inquiry for the classical theorists in the social sciences. Emile Durkheim's *Suicide* and *Elementary Forms of the Religious Life* (1965/1915), Max Weber's *Protestant Ethic and Spirit of Capitalism* (1958/1904) and *The Sociology of Religion* (1964/1922), and William James' *The Varieties of Religious Experience* (1978/1901) are testimony to the centrality of religion as an institution and as an influence on thinking in turn-of-the-century Europe and the United States. In many ways the social force of religion was at the core of their reasoning about the influence of the social world on individual consciousness and behavior. On the other hand, consideration of the social force of individual and societal aging came later, commonly dated to Karl Mannheim's introduction of the concept of age-based social groups in his essay "The Problem of Generations" (1952/1927). Other seminal theoretical works on aging relevant to religion include Erik Erikson's eight stages of psychosocial develop-

ment in the book *Childhood and Society* (1950) and Matilda White Riley's theory of age stratification outlined in *Age and Society* (Riley & Foner, 1968–1972).

The purpose of this chapter is to describe social scientific thinking and research on religion and aging with both an individual- and a societal-level approach. The individual or micro-level focuses on the aging individual's experience of religion in small social groups, through the life course, and especially during late life; we examine patterns of religious involvement and their impact on health and quality of life. An adequate account of religion and aging must also consider the societal or macro-level; the changing age structure of populations affects all social institutions, including religious ones. Thus we also consider cohort differences and the impact of rapidly aging populations on religious institutions. As this is the first time a full chapter on religion and aging has appeared in the *Handbook*, it seems appropriate to map the terrain of the intersection of the sociologies of religion and aging, in themselves two vast areas of

*Handbook of Aging and the Social Sciences, Sixth Edition*

scholarship, by returning to the classics of social scientific thinking. The more usual approach for chapters in the *Handbook* is to review the (mostly contemporary) research literature as it exists; for topics that have had the benefit of chapters in an earlier *Handbook*, this will appropriately focus on a summary of recent research developments. For a chapter without such precedent, however, there is the opportunity, even the obligation, to plot out a research map in which the terrain is well explored in some areas, but still a wilderness in others.

## A. Early Sociologies of Religion

In Durkheim's work on religion, there are at least two ideas relevant to aging. The first is that the integration (social support) and regulation (social control) functions provided by religious groups appear to protect individuals' physical health and mental well-being, as the "sufficiently intense collective life" of Catholicism protected turn-of-the-century European Catholics from committing suicide (1951, p. 170). Second, Durkheim draws attention to the importance of ritual practices that promote the continuity and collective consciousness of social and religious groups over time (1965), suggesting an accumulation of experience of regularly repeated religious rituals over the life course of the individual, and also the relevance of religious ritual to life course transitions. From Weber we take the idea that specific religious beliefs have psychological consequences for human motivation (1958), suggesting that the differing beliefs of the world's religions, particularly concerning aging and the aged, may have specific consequences for those older persons whose late lives are lived out in those communities. Weber also makes a fascinating distinction between "religious virtuosi" and the religion of ordinary people (1964); many of the contemporary religious virtuosi we would

think of—Pope John Paul, Mother Theresa, the Dalai Lama, Maggie Kuhn— are older persons whose spirituality is heightened by their long years of selfless service to others. James' ideas provide us with some understanding of the beneficial effects of religion on psychological well-being; he argued that all religious feelings begin with a sense of wrongness that is righted by connection with higher powers. Individuals sense that the better part of themselves is connected with *more* of the same spiritual, transcendent quality, and that this material world we live in is only a small part of a larger spiritual universe to which it is connected. Consciousness of this connection yields the psychological consequences of a new "zest for life" that "overcomes temperamental melancholy and imparts endurance to the Subject" (1978, p. 486). For James, of course, this is a transient solution he ironically calls "healthy-mindedness"—"Old age has the last word" he writes; it reveals "the worm at the core" (1978, p. 150).

Thus the early social science perspective on religion offers us aging-related ideas about the importance of the specific content of particular religious beliefs, the significance of temporally cyclical rituals, the essential setting of the religious collectivity as the site for the performance of ritual practices, the idea of spiritual and religious development over long lifetimes, and the potential resources for psychological well-being provided by internal spiritual states, particularly in times of loss and sadness.

## B. Early Sociologies of Aging

There are also important, if indirect, suggestions for the study of religion in the work of early scholars of aging. Mannheim's essay on generations originated the concept of the age-based social group, and the importance of common historical experience (including, potentially, common experience of religious events and changes) in imparting a generational consciousness to such age-based groups, a process that is heightened during periods of rapid social change (1952). Erikson's well-known stages of adult development make little direct reference to religion, but the themes of identity, generativity, and integrity provide many suggestions for social scientific thinking about religiousness through the life course (1950). Finally, Riley and Foner's age stratification perspective offers a systematic way of understanding the dynamic processes of individual aging and cohort succession, an important engine for social change and mechanism for understanding change and adaptation in religious institutions (1968).

Thus the early theorists of age and aging also provide concepts and insights for the study of religion. The importance of cohort differences in religious belief and involvement, the role of religion in fostering individual psychosocial development through the life course, the impact of processes of secularization and religious revival in societies with different age structures, and the effect of changes in population age structure on religious institutions are all suggested by adapting their work to focus on religion.

## C. Reviews of Religion and Aging

Although there has been no prior chapter on religion in the *Handbook of Aging and the Social Sciences*, there are a number of important early reviews of research literature on religion and aging. In 1960, Paul Maves, also the author of an article on religious concerns of older adults for the first (1961) White House Conference on Aging, wrote a lengthy chapter for the *Handbook of Social Gerontology* entitled "Aging, Religion, and the Church" (1960); it appeared as the concluding chapter of the book. Maves had pioneered work on services for the aging for the National

Council of Churches, hence the chapter has a strong theme of practical theology, and is limited to U.S. institutional religion. It reviews mid-century research on the religious participation of older people, including that of David Moberg, who wrote a dissertation on religion and personal adjustment in old age in 1951, and was one of the first sociologists to focus directly on religion and aging (Moberg, 1953). Maves concluded that there will be a considerable impact of an aging population on religious bodies, and that these institutions will in turn play a major role in "the resolution of problems raised by aging" (Maves, 1960, p. 745). A second early review of literature on aging and religious roles (Vol. 1, 1968) accompanied Riley and Foner's development of age stratification theory (Vol. 3, 1972). They found a "substantial" amount of research (approximately 40 studies meeting their criteria for empirical research of adequate quality) on religious identification, attendance, religious associations, personal observances, beliefs, the importance of religion, its impact on life satisfaction, and societal implications, but they observed that most of the evidence is quite limited because it comes from cross-sectional studies with nonrepresentative samples. The research is " . . . generally inadequate to support any full analysis of the complex factors apparently confounding the relationship between aging and religion" (1968, p. 483). Four years later, a review of empirical articles in the sociology of religion and the aged found 55 articles in all volumes of 140 social science journals (Heenan, 1972); research topics clustered into church participation, religion and the personal adjustment of the aged, the meaning of religion to older persons, and religion and death. The author concluded, controversially, that there may have been little cross-fertilization between gerontologists and sociologists of religion, as both are "low status subdisciplines" and "the aged are not the most attractive subjects to study" (1972, p. 174).

In 1982, an annotated bibliography by Fecher (1982) appeared, containing approximately 500 articles and books, of which 114 articles reported empirical research on religious observance and internal religious beliefs. The others are descriptive or practice-oriented articles on organized religion in the service of older adults, spiritual ministration to older individuals, and miscellaneous topics. Fifteen years later, to update Fecher's bibliography, Levin (1997) reviewed research on religion and aging in 16 gerontology, sociology, and religion journals, identifying 73 additional empirical studies. By 1997, Levin was able to conclude that, "If religion was once a marginal topic in aging research, it is no longer," and he approvingly noted that "religious research" in gerontology has frequently emphasized multiethnic or racial minority samples, has included multiple measures of the complex construct of religion, has focused on the effects of religious involvement on a wide variety of health and well-being outcomes, and is increasingly using longitudinal research designs (1997, pp. 31–32).

More recently, the subject of religion and aging appears to have captured the interest of authors from a broad array of disciplinary backgrounds, works that usually include some social science perspective. In the last 10 years, books with titles such as *Aging and God* (Koenig, 1994), *Aging, Spirituality, and Religion: A Handbook* (Kimble, McFadden, Ellor, & Seeber, 1995) and a second volume of the same title appearing in 2003 (Kimble & McFadden, 2003), *Spirituality and Aging* (Jewell, 1999), *Religion, Belief, and Spirituality in Late Life* (Thomas & Eisenhandler, 1999), *Perspectives on Spiritual Well-Being and Aging* (Thorson, 2000), and *Keeping the Faith in Late Life* (Eisenhandler, 2003) are being produced for diverse audiences of academics,

clergy, parish workers, caregivers, families, and older persons themselves. Moreover, our search of social science databases using the terms *aging* with *religion, religiosity, or spirituality* for this chapter yielded 43 additional empirical studies appearing since 1997 in peer-reviewed journals, updating the 1997 Levin article.

These literature reviews and broad works on the subject form the basis for this review; it is a steady, if modest, stream of social science research on religion and aging that has been growing for more than half a century. Like much of the research on aging and social institutions reviewed by Riley and Foner (1968), the early research was not strong methodologically. And like most social science research, it has improved dramatically, with the public availability of large, longitudinal data archives including measures of religious attitudes and behavior and with increasing methodological training and sophistication on the part of researchers.

## D. Plan for the Chapter

In the following sections we review research literature in eight areas relevant to religion and the aging of individuals and societies. We begin with a short review of aging-relevant beliefs in the world's religions, including important teachings regarding aging, and any special roles for the aged in religious rituals. Then we examine the literature on religious involvement and aging across the life course, with particular attention to the importance of religion during life course transitions commonly occurring in old age. Next, we focus on cohorts, Baby Boomers among them, and their differences in religious involvement. Then, we turn to the process of societal aging and its impact on religious institutions in countries around the world with the largest older populations. We then examine the large body of literature on the impact of religious involvement in late life on physical and emotional well-being. Next, we look at studies of congregation and clergy care for older adults, at religious sponsorship of institutions for the care of the old. Finally, we close with a look at what we might learn from some ethnographies of older people in religious communities. The existing research on religion and aging is unevenly distributed among these eight areas; generally speaking, there is far more at the micro-level of individual experience and far less at the macro-level of aging societies. But interesting questions are raised everywhere.

## II. Views of Aging in the World Religions

Any review of religion and aging should begin by underscoring that religion is not one thing but many—that complex and *distinct* belief systems make religions what they are. Religious faiths and practices are about making behaviors conform to beliefs; as the beliefs are different from one religion to another, so are the resulting behaviors. As these beliefs by definition concern ultimate things, they inform believers' views about birth and death, and the living and aging that implicitly take place in between. There are numerous statements of beliefs about aging in many of the world's faith traditions from theological or historical perspectives (see Jewell, 1999; Kimble et al., 1995; Kimble & McFadden, 2003; Thomas & Eisenhandler, 1999), suggesting that much could be learned about the accompanying behaviors, with systematic study. Hindus, for example, have an explicit set of beliefs regarding the four stages of life (*ashramas*) experienced by those in the Brahman, warrior, or merchant castes. The first is the student stage, beginning in early puberty, during which one's primary duty is to study and

learn. The second stage begins with marriage and is the stage of the householder, fully engaged in the pleasures, duties, and success of raising a family, working at a vocation, and serving the surrounding community. The third stage is that of retirement, which begins at the appearance of the first grandchild, and when the earthly pleasures of the householder begin to wane; social obligations are reduced and spiritual pursuits become more important. Finally there is the stage of renunciation, or *sannyasa*, "one who neither hates nor loves anything" (Smith, 1991, p. 53). These stages of life are lived out in the repetitive cycle of birth and death and rebirth. The emphasis on withdrawal from activities and pleasures in old age allows the older person to concentrate on the spiritual life and to approach death without anxiety, as it is merely a passage into the next life (Firth, 1999; Kemp & Bhungalia, 2002).

A second Eastern wisdom tradition with elaborated beliefs about the role of older persons is Confucianism, with its teachings about the Five Constant Relationships (Smith, 1991; Thang, 2000). These five include relationships between parent and child, husband and wife, elder sibling and younger sibling, older friend and younger friend, and ruler and subject. It is significant that three of the five relationships basic to society fall within the family, and also that age differences are specified in three. A further principle of Confucian thought is Respect for Age. The young should serve and honor the old, not only because the young will themselves be old some day and need to be taken care of, but also because age brings with it wisdom, experience, and an increasingly spiritual nature.

By contrast with these two Eastern traditions, the Western, monotheistic religions of Judaism, Christianity, and Islam have placed much less emphasis on the veneration of old age as a time for the contemplative, spiritual life, and much more value on youth, activity, change, and control over the environment. At least 30 individuals are recorded in the Old Testament as having lived for more than 100 years, but only three are described as having a "good old age," and these were not especially long-lived: Abraham (Genesis 25:8), Gideon (Judges 8:32), and David (I Chronicles 29:28). One passage in Ecclesiastes states: "Remember your Creator in the days of your youth, before the bad times come and the years draw near when you will say, 'I have no pleasure in them,' before the sun and the light of day give place to darkness, before the moon and the stars grow dim, and the clouds return with the rain" (12:1-2). At the same time, the Biblical commandment to honor one's parents underlies all attitudes toward older adults, including both family obligations and the Jewish community's provision of social services for its older citizens (Olitzky & Borowitz, 1995; see also Address, 2003; Isenberg, 2000).

Similarly, there is no unambiguous Christian theology of aging, although there is no shortage of commentaries on the subject (Christiansen, 1995; Hauerwas, Stoneking, Meador, & Cloutier, 2003; Kimble, 2000). The individualism of the Protestant ethic, with its value on work as the highest form of praise for God, was a strong influence on colonial American culture and institutions, and eventually bore the fruit of the decline of respect for older adults, as argued by a number of historians (Cole, 1986; Haber & Gratton, 1994). At the same time, Christians believe that human life is created in the image of God, and that through the example of the life, suffering, and death of Jesus Christ, individuals can find meaning in many of the painful and tragic circumstances that befall human beings, particularly in old age.

Like Judaism and Christianity, Islam, the third of the Abrahamic faiths, places comparatively little emphasis on teachings regarding the old; the narratives in the Qu'ran of the old age of Abraham, Moses, Jacob, and Zachariah contrast the infirmity of old age with the constant glory and power of Allah. The Qu'ran teaches that old age will "overtake and destroy a person in the same way that even a flourishing and well-watered orchard will be burned up by a scorching whirlwind" (Thursby, 2000, p. 159). The aged Muslim is expected to contribute to society as long as physically possible; there is no expectation of or allowance for withdrawal and contemplation. Elders, especially parents, are commanded to be treated with respect, particularly at the very end of life, again placing respect for age within the context of family relationships.

Even the most cursory survey of rituals or rites of passage for the major world religions shows that many are in fact age-specific, having as their primary purpose the signification of the passage of individuals from one phase of the life course into the next (Breuilly, O'Brien, & Palmer, 1997). These transitions, however, almost exclusively occur early in the life course; baptisms, circumcisions, confirmations, coming-of-age rituals, and marriages have all occurred by young adulthood. Very few mark transitions to old age, or even to middle age, or give special place to older members of the family or religious group. Hinduism is an exception, where there is a ceremony marking the entrance to the last stage (*sannyasa*) that strips the believer of his worldly goods and familial or social identity, to permit complete dedication to spiritual enlightenment (Thursby, 2000). Another exception is the Jewish *Seder*, the ritual meal commemorating the *Pesach* and exodus of the Hebrew people from bondage in Egypt, during which the eldest male member of the family has the seat of honor, along with the duty of asking the youngest member of the family a set of ritual questions (Achenbaum, 1995). Certainly there are rites for the dying in all of the worlds' religions, but these would be performed regardless of the age of the dying person, as would bereavement and mourning rituals.

The teachings and rituals regarding old age in the world's religions thus suggest there would be differences, and yet there are few comparative empirical works addressing beliefs regarding aging in the world religions. Some rare exceptions are studies by Mehta (1997), comparing the impact of religious beliefs on the aging experiences of a group of older Hindus, Sikhs, Christians, and Muslims in Singapore; Imamoglu (1999), comparing the beliefs of older Turks and Swedes; and Mantzaris (1988) who examined the role of religion in determining attitudes toward older persons among 700 Muslims, Christians, and Hindus in Durban, South Africa. Doctrinal beliefs may have surprising or even counterintuitive manifestations in the "lived religion" of actual believers and communities even in such seemingly non-negotiable (and age-relevant) matters as the belief in life after death (Greeley & Hout, 1999). Without social scientific research from a comparative perspective, it must remain an unsubstantiated assertion that the experience and perception of aging is affected by the religious beliefs of the community in which it takes place, as well as an open area for research.

## III. Religious Involvement and Aging Across the Life Course

### A. Age-Related Patterns of Participation

By contrast with research on the world religions' beliefs about aging, research on religious involvement and individual aging is plentiful, at least in the United States, and it could easily have been the subject of this entire chapter. The theoretical perspectives guiding this research have tended more toward the life span developmental perspective deriving from

Erikson (McFadden, 1999), in particular Fowler's stages of faith development which to some degree correspond with life stages (Fowler, 1981) or the activity versus disengagement theories originating with the Duke Longitudinal Study and the Kansas City Study of Adult Life (Palmore, 1970; Cumming and Henry, 1961), and much less toward the life course perspective that derived from the earliest U.S. longitudinal studies: the Oakland Growth Study, the Berkeley Guidance Study, and the Terman Study (Elder, 1998). One reason for this may be the tendency of the life course perspective to focus on life transitions and entry into and exit from roles (George, 1993). A one-sentence summary of the research in this section would be that religious involvement remains stable or increasing until late life; therefore, a role that is most often entered in early childhood and exited at death could be overlooked by an analytical framework that focuses on timing, sequencing, and duration of roles or periods of the life course. Life course research has been much more about process and change than it has been about steady states.

Religious involvement is a complex construct. Participation in organized worship activities is by far the most frequently studied of its dimensions and has been tracked by national and international polls for decades (Princeton Religion Research Center, 2003), but various forms of private observances such as prayer and electronic media (Hays, Landerman, Blazer, Koenig, Carroll, & Musick, 1998; Levin & Taylor, 1997) and more subjective dimensions of spirituality and religious beliefs are also important (Atchley, 2000; Freund & Smith, 1999; Thorsen, 2000). In cross-sectional, nationally representative U.S. data, persons 65 years and over attend religious services significantly more frequently than younger adults; engage in private religious activities such as prayer, reading sacred texts, and meditating significantly more often; and report significantly higher levels of subjective religious experience, such as having had life-changing religious experiences, having daily spiritual experiences, using religion to cope with life crises, and thinking of themselves as religious or spiritual persons (Idler et al., 2003).

But cross-sectional studies do not provide evidence of changes with age, even when age differences are apparent. Some fascinating retrospective studies have found increasing, decreasing, and/or stable accounts of religiousness over the life course (Hays, Meador, Branch, & George, 2001; Ingersoll-Dayton, Krause, & Morgan, 2002; Wuthnow, 1999), but recall of early life events may be influenced by selection effects and later life conditions, and such studies are therefore somewhat limited. Bahr (1970) described four possible models of the longitudinal relationship between aging and religious attendance: (1) a traditional model, with a decline in attendance from 18 to 30, and then a sharp and continuing increase after that; (2) a stability model, in which childhood levels of attendance are maintained throughout the life course at whatever level was established early on; (3) a family-cycle model, with an increase in attendance coinciding with family formation and childrearing, and a decline beginning in middle age; and (4) a disengagement model, in which attendance declines after age 50, no matter what pattern had been established before that.

Stronger data to test these models come from survey data showing trends by cohort over relatively long periods. Age-period-cohort analysis of U.S. data from 1939 to 1969 shows a strong period effect of a rise in church attendance for the 1950s and early 1960s for all age cohorts, but no consistent age effect (Wingrove & Alston, 1974); for U.S. data from 1972 to 1986, the results show steadily increasing attendance with aging (Chaves, 1989);

from 1972 to 1991 the data show increasing attendance with age until age 70, and then a small decline (Ploch & Hastings, 1994); and most recently, from 1980 to 1992, a period effect from 1988 to 1992, and a significant and nonlinear increase of attendance with age, with the biggest increase coming between ages 18 and 30 (Argue, Johnson, & White, 1999). Thus, with this moving window of survey data, a succession of researchers most often find increases in U.S. attendance rates with age; however these trend analyses do not follow single individuals over time, and as samples of the adult population, they contain relatively small numbers of older adults, especially very old persons.

In studies that focus specifically on older populations and use longitudinal or repeated measures designs, a decline in attendance at service in very late life is frequently detected (Ainlay, Singleton, & Swigert, 1992; Blazer & Palmore, 1976). This decline is associated with declining health and functional ability (Benjamins, Musick, Gold, & George, 2003; Hays et al., 1998). Over time data are less available for dimensions of religiousness other than attendance; the few studies available have also tended to focus on older populations. The Duke Longitudinal Study of Normal Aging found declines with age in attendance at religious services, but simultaneous stability or even slight increases in religious beliefs over a 20-year follow-up (Blazer & Palmore, 1976). Data from the Duke site of the Established Populations for the Epidemiologic Study of the Elderly (EPESE) found no increase in religious media use to coincide with health-related declines in service attendance (Hays et al., 1998). Idler and Kasl (1997b), with New Haven EPESE data, found correlations in the range of .61 to .63 between an index of subjective religiousness at baseline and the same measure 3, 6, and 12 years later; a subset of this same sample interviewed during their last 12 months of life found a decline in attendance at services from the respondent's level of attendance 3 years previously, but small increases in already high levels of subjective religiousness (Idler, Kasl, & Hays, 2001).

Studies of adult and older adult samples also found important differences by race and gender. Women consistently show higher levels than men for both organizational and nonorganizational religiousness, in early and middle adulthood, and old age as well, and in U.S. and international samples (Cornwall, 1989; de Vaus & McAllister, 1987; Miller & Stark, 2002). Within U.S. samples, Black Americans and Mexican Americans repeatedly demonstrate higher levels of formal participation and private activities and beliefs (Markides, 1983; Taylor, Chatters, & Levin, 2004), suggesting that religion provides an especially prevalent source of support for aged women, Hispanics, and African Americans. Analysis of the National Survey of Black Americans shows that African-American women and older African Americans are the most likely to feel that the church has helped the condition of African Americans and, presumably, people like them (Taylor, Thornton, & Chatters, 1987).

Religious participation, then, appears strongly related to age, in a way that does not exactly fit any of the models proposed by Bahr decades ago. The relationship might best be described as a nonlinear increase in religiousness over the life course, with the steepest increase in early adulthood, and only a brief period of health-related decline in the immediate period before death for public participation in worship services, but no decline in subjective religiousness. This research, however, comes almost entirely from U.S. studies, with its particular mix of faith traditions and overall high levels of religious participation. Comparative international survey data sources such as the World Values Survey show (only incidentally if one looks for it in the tables) that older age is a strong cross-sectional predictor of higher attendance at services and religious beliefs (Campbell & Curtis, 1994), but we found no comparative international articles that addressed the issue directly. The study of the relationship of religiousness to universal human processes of aging, then, remains a wide-open and promising area for comparative research.

## B. Religious Involvement During Life Event Transitions

Transitions in the life course from one role or status to another are frequently marked by religious rituals. Normal, on-time transitions such as births or marriages are usually celebratory occasions marked by family gatherings, feasts, and often religious services in which the individuals making the transition are the focus of attention. Other important role transitions may be due to losses—of health or loved ones—and these are precisely the role transitions that mount in old age. Religious coping with these events often involves ritual practices to provide comfort, understanding, and meaning, and to relieve the stress of the transition (Pargament, 1997), especially in situations where changes are irrevocable (Mattlin, Wethington, & Kessler, 1990). Rituals use words and actions to legitimize and formalize the individual's passage from one status to another (Fried & Fried, 1980; van Gennep, 1960). Rituals in the world's religions, especially those for the most tragic and significant events of bereavement and death, have a bewildering diversity and specificity (Breuilly et al., 1997; Parkes, Launguani, & Young, 1997). Religious rituals recall the traditional meanings embedded in the faith and the social institution that embodies it; they link the immediate sensory experiences of the individual undergoing the ritual to the generations preceding him or her in this passage through a particular sacred time and space (Berger, 1967; Durkheim, 1965). The repetition of experience of these rituals, through one's own life course and through sharing in the life course transitions of others, in the religious community provides a continuing sense of the meaningfulness of life at its major turning-points. And because these rituals are shared, that is, experienced repeatedly in the context of an ongoing social group, they permit anticipation of one's own future significant life events and socialize individuals into culturally appropriate emotional expressions and behaviors. They also provide a strong statement of the abiding permanence and solidarity of the religious group, even when an individual member is lost.

In conclusion, late twentieth-century research, primarily conducted in the United States, appears to show that both attendance at religious worship services and the more subjective and private dimensions of religiousness increase with age and are maintained at high levels until near the end of life. At the same time, an increasing number of losses for which religious rituals are relevant occur in late life: of health and functioning, of work and community roles, and, of importance, the deaths of spouses, close friends, and siblings. Any potential causal connection between these two patterns would be restricted to industrialized societies with long life expectancies, that is, where most deaths occur in old age and are not spread randomly throughout the life course. Data on patterns of religiousness in old age in other countries where the achievement of old age is less universal are needed.

## IV. Cohort Differences in Religious Involvement

The description of aging effects in religiousness is relatively clear-cut by comparison with the much more debated research findings regarding cohort effects. Although age, cohort, and period effects are conceptually distinct, they are analytically inseparable (because any two determine the third) and, more important, they often appear in reality in complex interactions. Thus there is a lively debate in the U.S. social science literature over whether trends in religious attendance in late twentieth-century America represent period effects of secularization or religious revival, or cohort effects that play into those trends (Chaves, 1989; Firebaugh & Harley, 1991; Hout & Greeley, 1987).

Cohort effects are theoretically derived from Mannheim's early twentieth-century essay on generations, in which he argues that events have an impact on the later lives of those who live through them, particularly those who are young at the time and who form a sense of generational consciousness by experiencing important historical events in early adulthood (Mannheim, 1952). In the late twentieth century, the generation of note is the large post-World War II cohort whose size was fueled by high fertility, rising population health levels, and a rapidly growing economy, and whose young adulthood coincided with the Vietnam War period of rapid social change, social movements, and political upheaval. Earlier analyses of data collected in the 1960s to 1980s may not have detected cohort differences because the postwar Baby Boom cohort was still in adolescence or early adulthood. More recent analyses have questioned why church attendance rates are not increasing, when Baby Boom cohort members should by middle age be experiencing the aging effects of increase in religiousness. Miller and Nakamura (1996) argued that aging effects are being offset by cohort differences, with Baby Boomers showing substantially lower attendance patterns than pre-World War II cohorts. Thus the apparent period effect of secularization may be driven by the successive replacement of high-attendance pre-World War II cohorts with low-attendance post-World War II Baby Boomers.

Of course attendance at services is only one dimension of religiousness, but the thread of cohort differences runs through other indicators as well. Younger U.S. cohorts are less likely than older ones to express confidence in religious institutions (Hoffman, 1998). Jewish Baby Boomers are more likely than pre-World War II cohorts to say that Judaism is not very important to them (Waxman, 2001). On the other hand, there are suggestions that something other than simple secularization is at work: Baby Boomers are less likely than pre-World War II cohorts to say they are "religious and spiritual" or "religious only," but they are *more* likely to say they are "spiritual only" and still equally likely to say they are neither religious nor spiritual (Marler & Hadaway, 2002). An American Association for Retired Persons (AARP) survey found that fewer than half, 47%, of Baby Boomers were satisfied with their religion/spiritual life, and that this was an area in which they hoped to make positive changes in the next five years (Keegan, Gross, Fisher, & Remez, 2002). Wade Clark Roof has been a longtime student of the religious and spiritual life of Baby Boomers (Roof, 1993). From a series of large surveys and in-depth interviews he concluded that broad changes in American religious culture are being driven by the large Baby Boom generation, whom he calls a generation of seekers, who are looking for religious and spiritual goods in the spiritual marketplace that is our diverse, pluralistic, multicultural society (Roof, 1999).

Mannheim's insights should also lead us to expect religious differences by cohort in many parts of the world where there is or has been rapid social change. The fall of the Soviet Union, the rapid evolution of the economy in China, the expansion of the European Union, rapid industrialization in the developing world, not to mention religious strife in the Middle East and South Asia, all set potential social conditions for cohort differences in religiousness in those countries that may eventually be the cause of further social change. International cross-sectional differences by age in religious attendance and beliefs reported by Campbell and Curtis (1994) represent an aggregate pattern that is no doubt hiding cohort differences in some countries where the young are more observant than the old, and others where the reverse is true. Another suggestive report of data from the World Values Survey (Inglehart & Baker, 2000) shows change over the time period 1981 to 1998 in 38 societies that were assessed on the dimension of "traditional" (a dimension largely determined by religious content) versus secular/rational. Countries such as China, Brazil, Estonia, Russia, Turkey, and Argentina became notably more traditional during that period, whereas Poland, Japan, East Germany, Switzerland, Canada, and others became considerably more secular. Still other countries changed very little on that dimension. As in other sections of this review, there is a need for much more international, comparative research with existing survey data sources.

## V. Societal Aging and Its Impact on Religious Institutions

This section draws on the age stratification perspective (Riley & Foner, 1968) to consider religion from the perspective of the aging of entire societies and the institutions within them. Demographically, societies with low birth rates and low mortality rates also have long and increasing life expectancy. These are aging societies, whether we identify them by changes in median age, mean age, percent of population over 65, number of centenarians, age dependency ratio, or other population statistics. Religion has rarely been considered from the societal aging standpoint. In this section we raise topics for research on the demographic characteristics of the world's most and least religious countries, the religiousness of the world's oldest societies, and the aging of religious institutions in the United States and around the world.

As noted previously, data sources exist for research on world religion from a demographic perspective but they have not been used in this way. The International Social Survey Program (ISSP), a German-led, cross-national collaboration for survey research in 31 countries primarily in North America and Europe, has run surveys focusing specifically on religion in 1991 and 1998 (http://webapp. icpsr.umich.edu/cocoon/ICPSR-STUDY/06234.xml). The U.S.-based World Values Survey (WVS) (http://wvs. isr.umich.edu), first fielded in 1981, has four waves of data from representative national surveys of the basic values and beliefs from more than 80 countries. In one suggestive analysis of WVS data, countries were classified as traditional versus secular-rational (on a scale in which "Religion is very important in R's life" and "R believes in Heaven" are the two highest-loading items) (Inglehart & Baker, 2000). Among the 65 societies so classified, Puerto Rico, Venezuela, Ghana, Nigeria, and Colombia (in that order) are most traditional (religious), and Germany, Japan, Sweden, Norway, and Denmark are the most secular. Life expectancy in these two groups is also quite different, as is the percentage of the population over age 60; Japan has the world's highest life expectancy (81.9 years at birth), and only Italy has (slightly) more people over age 60 (24.5%) than Japan (24.4%) and Germany (24.0%) (World Health Organization, 2002). Nigeria and Ghana both have extremely low life expectancies of less than 60 years, and

none of the most traditional countries have more than 8% of their population over age 60. These country-level statistics on religiousness and age are paradoxical, given the consistent findings regarding aging and religiousness in the United States (which ranks near the middle but in the more "traditional" half of the WVS distribution). Although religiousness increases with age in the United States (as we saw earlier) and is associated positively with age cross sectionally at the individual level in pooled WVS data (Campbell & Curtis, 1994), at the country level, the opposite relationship holds. The world's oldest countries are, quite consistently, the least religious. The secularism of the world's oldest societies has been noted in the press in articles about the contrast between the age distributions of Europe's fervent young Muslim immigrants and its graying, white, and only nominally Christian native populations (Ferguson, 2004; Smith, 2004).

The age stratification perspective encourages us to also consider the aging of religious institutions in societies and institutions. The passage of time is marked not by the aging of individuals, but by the succession of cohorts, or individuals of the same age moving through the age strata of the institution. The process of cohort succession depends on the constant infusion of new cohorts entering an institution. When those cohorts become small or stop entering altogether, institutions are radically changed and can cease to exist. Perhaps the most extreme example of this process is the Shaker religion, which began in England in the late eighteenth century. Believers migrated to the United States and successfully established communities throughout New England and the Midwest during the nineteenth century. Because it was a celibate community, it relied for growth and existence on conversions of adults; and, in fact, the Shakers prospered for almost a hundred years, until the mid-nineteenth century (Bainbridge, 1982).

When conversions ceased, the population of Shakers declined, communities merged and were abandoned (Stein, 1992). Today only a small number of very old Shaker women and men reside in the last community in Maine (Skees, 1998).

From this institutional perspective, at the global level, there are no data sources for estimating and comparing the age of adherents of the world's major religions, as they cross national and continental boundaries. At the country level, it would be possible where government record-keeping includes religion in census data or international surveys to identify respondents by their specific religion. Again, there is little published research, and we have only a small number of examples of the comparative and changing age composition of religions, even within nation states. In the United States, the mainline Protestant denominations have had a higher proportion of older members since mid-century (Riley & Foner, 1968), a difference that has increased as existing members aged and new members joined in smaller numbers (Feder, 1993). Israel overall has a relatively young age composition as a result primarily of high fertility rates and high immigration rates; however, birth rates are higher in the Muslim population and more uneven among Israeli Jews, who also have lower mortality rates (Rebhun & Waxman, 2004). Age compositions of religious groups are an important and underutilized lens through which to view religious change and conflict in societies around the world; they should be considered more often.

Still at the level of the religious institution, but moving to the smaller unit of the local congregation, there has been little systematic research that considers the aging of membership. Ammerman (1997), reporting on a survey of 23 U.S. Protestant congregations, reports that about 15% describe their membership as "primarily elderly," with few young adults or chil-

dren, membership of less than 150, and a shrinking size. Cnaan's study of 297 religious congregations in the United States and Canada showed that the greater the proportion of members in the congregation over age 65, the lower membership growth was likely to be and the lower the fiscal value of the services provided to the community (Cnaan, 2002). But aging in religious institutions is often not considered at all; a major sociological interpretation of the rise and fall of American religious groups failed to mention age (Finke & Stark, 1992).

The aging membership of one particular religious institution in the U.S. has been noted repeatedly: the aging of Roman Catholic religious orders (Cave, 2004; Ebaugh, 1993). The Fecher (1982) bibliography lists more than 20 articles from social science and religion periodicals on the aging of nuns and priests, signaling that this was a concern decades ago. Finke and Stark (1992) mentioned the declining numbers of Catholic brothers and sisters but overlook the aging of this population. A recent look inside an aging U.S. religious order is provided by the Nun Study, a well-known epidemiological study of Alzheimer's disease among the School Sisters of Notre Dame (Snowdon, 2001). The pictures of the sisters in their wheelchairs, aging in place in a beautiful convent that has been their home since late adolescence, speak louder than words could about the fragility of this social institution.

## VI. Impact of Religious Involvement on Health in Late Life

On this topic there has been an immense amount of research, much of it quite recent. Religion is generally found, in well-designed longitudinal population-based and clinical studies, to be related to better physical and mental health, but there are many complexities in the association. Fortunately there are a number of reviews of the literature (Koenig, 1998; Koenig, McCullough, & Larson, 2000; Schaie, Krause, & Booth, 2004 and others cited later), because it is not possible to adequately summarize such a large number of studies in the short space allotted here. For a descriptive review, we refer the reader to these and other comprehensive and systematic literature reviews and instead approach the literature on the impact of religion on health in late life through a set of broad themes.

## A. Health Research Considering Religion Is Derived Directly from Classical Sociological Traditions

The study of health and religion is not a new research question, although the recent deluge of research might make it seem entirely contemporary. Durkheim's *Suicide* (1951) was a forerunner of modern social epidemiology, in which the distribution of health and disease in a population is studied according to the population members' social characteristics and resources. Two early reviews of research in the 1960s to 1980s found many studies comparing cross-sectional disease or mortality rates in specific religious groups such as the Mormons or Seventh-day Adventists (Jarvis & Northcott, 1987; Levin & Vanderpool, 1987) with other populations, as Durkheim did. More recent research is longitudinal and based on the individual as the unit of analysis, but here again Durkheimian theory provides theoretical frameworks for much of the thinking about potential causal mechanisms (Idler, 2001).

## B. Religion Is Many Things, but Is Often Treated as One Thing

Early research treated religion as many separate faiths and compared disease and death rates at the group level. Later work,

beginning with the Alameda County Study (reviewed in House, Landis, & Umberson, 1988), used survey data at the individual level, measured self-reported religious participation, and usually had only a single indicator of attendance as the measurement of religiousness. In these studies "religiousness" is treated as a continuum scale characteristic of individuals, and whether they are Protestant, Hindu, or Muslim is of no consequence. Thus, much of what we know about religion and health from the studies of the past two decades is limited to this one particular dimension, and yet many other dimensions are potentially relevant, including private behaviors such as prayer, subjective feelings of religious identity, religious history, conversion experiences, forgiveness, congregational support, daily spiritual experiences, beliefs, commitment, religious struggle, consolation, and certainly religious affiliation (Hill & Pargament, 2003; Idler et al., 2003).

## C. Health Is as Complex a Concept as Religion, and Different Dimensions of Religion May Be Relevant at Different Points as Physical and Mental Health and Illness Are Experienced Across the Life Course

All-cause mortality has been the most highly studied physical health outcome. A meta-analytical review concluded that "religion has a nontrivial, favorable association with all-cause mortality" (McCullough, Hoyt, Larson, Koenig, & Thoresen, 2000, p. 220). Another careful review of the associations between multiple dimensions of religiousness and multiple dimensions of health found that the "evidence is strongest and most consistent for a protective effect in healthy people . . . church/service attendance protects against death" (Powell, Shahabi, & Thoresen, 2003, p. 48). The authors found less compelling evidence that religion in any dimension helps people recover from illness more quickly. Another review, however, found that religion has a moderating effect on the mental health consequences of stressful life events. In other words, among those suffering serious adverse events such as illness or trauma, religiously involved respondents had lower levels of depression than those without such resources (Smith, McCullough, & Poll, 2003). Moreover, an early review finds that the relationship between religion and subjective well-being in adulthood is stronger for older than for younger adults (Witter, Stock, Okun, & Haring, 1985). Yet another review of studies of patients at the end of life found that religious persons exhibit higher levels of well-being and show lower rates of depression and suicide compared with nonreligious persons (Van Ness & Larson, 2002). What we know about rates of attendance at religious services is that they decline in late old age, but measures of subjective religiousness remain steady. The simultaneous increasing prevalence of chronic disease and disability suggests that the conclusions of these last three reviews are especially relevant to understanding the impact of religion on health in old age.

## D. There Are Many Potential Causal Pathways for an Association Between Religion and Health

Discussions of the pathways by which religion might affect health minimally list four: through physiology, health behaviors, social support, and coping or the provision of meaning. Direct biological pathways from religious states, particularly those induced by meditation, to health by way of cardiovascular, neuroendocrine, and immune function, are supported by epidemiological and experimental studies (Seeman, Dubin, & Seeman, 2003). A second important pathway is through the social control effect

religion has on behaviors such as smoking, exercise, alcohol use, sexual activity, or drug use. In each case religion has the effect of reducing or eliminating behaviors that increase risk for some of the major causes of mortality in the United States (e.g., Idler & Kasl, 1997a). A third pathway operates through the greater amount of social support potentially and actually received by persons who have social networks that are larger because they include religious congregations (e.g., Ellison & George, 1994). A fourth pathway has been derived from the function of religion to provide consolation, understanding, meaning, and routes to forgiveness during times of suffering or conflict. This is the stress-buffering mechanism, where religion, often in the form of rituals, is called on in times of need or crisis (e.g., Bosworth, Park, McQuoid, Hays, & Steffens, 2003; Ferraro & Kelley-Moore, 2000). It is significant that there are so many potential mechanisms through which religion might affect health. Mediational analyses typically sharply reduce, but do not entirely eliminate, the main effect (Powell, Shahabi, & Thoresen, 2003).

## E. Social Control Is at Least as Important as Social Support

The "friendly" Durkheimian social support functions of integration, inclusion, helping, confiding, emotional closeness, reducing loneliness, assistance with tasks, and caregiving have been featured in the research on religion and health (e.g., Krause, Ellison, Shaw, Marcum, & Boardman, 2001). The strict, socially controlling, rule-enforcing, behavior-regulating, boundary-setting, even punishing, stigmatizing, and sanctioning Durkheimian functions of religion, however, may be just as important in affecting health in a positive way, albeit not as warm and friendly. These functions are more likely to come to light in studies of specific religious groups with strong control over health-relevant behaviors, such as the Mormons and Seventh-day Adventists, but may play a more subtle role in religious groups across the spectrum.

## F. Can Religion Do Harm as Well as Good?

Much less has been written about negative dimensions of religiousness such as doubt (Krause, Ingersoll-Dayton, Ellison, & Wulff, 1999) or religious struggle (Pargament, Koenig, Tarakeshwar, & Hahn, 2001), or negative effects of religion on health (Contrada, Goyal, Cather, Rafalson, Idler, & Krause, 2004). More research is needed in this area, but from the first, Durkheim foresaw the possibility that, in unusual circumstances, there could be an excess of social integration or social regulation. In *Suicide* (1951), Durkheim raised the possibility that society can exert too much force on individuals, causing suicide rates to increase, just as they increase when there is too little social influence, as is the case in most modern societies. Thus there is a theoretical framework for understanding such effects and some supporting literature, but these findings have remained exceptions to the predominant pattern of positive effects of religion on health.

## G. Religion Likely Has a Cumulative Effect on Health Across the Life Course, Which Makes It Harder to Study

Studies of mortality rates among Seventh-day Adventists show that the earlier the age at entry into the religion, the lower the mortality from cardiovascular disease (Fønnebø, 1992). Prevention of smoking, learning good dietary habits, getting regular exercise, and many other important health habits associated with religiousness may be established in adolescence (Wallace & Forman, 1998) and may

reduce risk for associated diseases for the entire life course. Thus cumulative effects of good health practices and social support facilitated by lifelong religious practice should result in increasing differentiation of religion-related health by the time individuals reach old age. The selection effects of higher levels of mortality among those with lower levels of religiousness, however, will act in a countervailing way to reduce differentiation in old age, because less religious individuals will have already died. Studies of religion and health in older populations should more explicitly recognize this.

## H. Research Has Led to Controversy about Clinical Implications

This area of research and subsequent advocacy on religion and health has unquestionably generated a great deal of controversy. In a series of articles, critics have raised questions about the methods and findings of the major studies and have also criticized the recommendations that have been made by some to incorporate spiritual counseling by physicians into the usual practice of medical care (Sloan, Bagiella, & Powell, 1999; Sloan & Bagiella 2002). Rebuttals have been offered (Koenig et al., 1999; Miller & Thoresen 2003) and it seems likely that the debate will go on even as the research accumulates. Whether and in what context physicians should introduce questions of religion or spirituality into patient care will remain a complicated issue in our increasingly religiously diverse society.

## I. What Are the New Research Questions?

Religion is a feature of both individuals and communities, although they have not been studied jointly. There is a tremendous potential for future research to merge the two approaches of studying the effects of religiousness at the group level and the individual level, by using hierarchical linear models that can adjust simultaneously for individual-level characteristics, and the characteristics of aggregates. In addition, there should be further research on the influence of religiousness on specific causes of death (e.g., Hummer, Rogers, Nam, & Ellison, 1999), particularly those causes for which the risk factors are well understood and potential causal pathways can be tested.

## VII. Congregation and Clergy Care for Older Adults

As noted previously, some congregations have aging memberships; however, virtually all congregations have some old members. Indeed, the religious congregation is one of the very few social institutions in any society that is completely age-integrated; the family is the only other widespread example. Religious congregations are places where people of all ages, from newborns to the frailest older individuals, come or are brought regularly, for the same purpose; there is no other comparable public institution. These regular meetings produce long-standing relationships, shared beliefs and values, social networks of strong and weak links, conduits of information about the community, and opportunities for caregiving and care receiving. For the young, they provide adult and aged role models. For older adults they provide otherwise scarce nonfamily intergenerational ties with energetic babies and small children, rapidly developing teenagers, and young parents.

Many congregations and their clergy reach out to their aging members through providing transportation to worship services and social occasions, making large-print publications and hearing assist devices available, visiting and taking communion to shut-ins and the hospital-

ized, and praying with and for them (Cnaan, 2002). Some congregations have parish nurses, sometimes paid, sometimes volunteering, to provide health services and health education to their members, a movement that was started in Illinois in the early 1980s by Dr. Granger Westberg (Smith, 2003; Westberg, 1990). Another congregation-based movement to provide services for the aging is the Shepherd's Centers, begun by Dr. Elbert Cole in 1972. These are interfaith associations of older people, meeting in a church, synagogue, or mosque, who provide educational and in-home services to other older persons in their communities (Seeber, 1995). Through their formal and informal services to the aging, both inside congregations and in the larger community, religious groups perform the functions of *mediating structures*, a term coined by Peter Berger and Richard Neuhaus (1977). Mediating structures are small-scale social institutions that provide one face to the private life of individuals and one face to the larger society. They are independent of the state and yet provide many social services and benefits to their own communities that are attuned to the cultures and needs of particular constituencies. Among disadvantaged racial and ethnic minority communities in the United States, the church, synagogue, or mosque may be the most stable and important institution in the community. In the case of older persons, whose primary and long-term needs may be for assistance in daily tasks, a friendly visit, or spiritual support, congregation-based services may be more accessible, acceptable, and readily asked-for than services from any other source. Although there are fine systematic studies of congregation-provided services by Ammerman (1997) and Cnaan (2002), none have focused on services for older adults and the paradoxical problem of increased need and diminished resources in aging congregations.

Other important services for older persons with strong religious purpose include hospital-based chaplaincy services, hospice care, and the many nursing, old age, and continuing care retirement communities that have been founded by religious organizations. Religious bodies have had a history of founding and supporting sometimes quite innovative institutions for the care of older adults, but this is a history that has not been written (see Haber & Gratton, 1994, pp. 222–223, note 51; Maves, 1960). As has been true throughout this chapter, there is a considerable need for further research in this area that could have substantial policy implications.

## VIII. Communities of Memory: Ethnographies of Old Age in Religious Communities

Elderly people help us to see human affairs with greater wisdom, because life's vicissitudes have brought them knowledge and maturity. They are the guardians of our collective memory, and thus privileged interpreters of that body of ideals and common values which support and guide life in society.

Pope John Paul II
"Letter to the Elderly" 1999

Religious congregations are communities of memory, reliving and recreating their collective religious experiences as they worship and perform ritual observances together on a daily, weekly, or annual basis. Older members of congregations have memories that stretch back through time, through times of war and times of hardship, through peace and plenty, and through crises and uncertainty. Those memories of historical events are overlaid with the events of private life: the joy of grandparenthood, the rewards and frustration of work, the pride and struggles of parenthood, the intimacy and partnership of marriage, and even further back to adolescence and childhood. For older persons with lifelong religious observances, a

thread sews through all these seasons, providing accumulating continuity and deepening memories.

For those who have lived long lives in a single community, these observances may even take place in a single setting and therefore be even more intensely continuous. The religious and spiritual lives of older persons in such long-lived communities of memory are worth knowing about; they may achieve the status of Weber's religious virtuosi, simply by virtue of practice. Our best views of these lives come, not from the quantitative survey research on which we have mostly relied for evidence in this review, but from the close-up, qualitative, ethnographic, and interview approaches. There is a genre of books about the experience of religion in long-lived communities, and they make instructive reading. We have already mentioned a recent account of the Shakers (Skees, 1998) told through the eyes of a young visitor to the community. The small remaining number of this celibate sect live and work in the last remaining Shaker community, in austerely elegant buildings whose halls are lined with the portraits of those who have gone before. We have also mentioned the 678 members of the School Sisters of Notre Dame who have participated in the Nun Study, a groundbreaking epidemiological study of Alzheimer's disease, the disease of memory in a community of memory (Snowdon, 2001). Another study of two communities of older Lutheran women, one in the Blue Ridge Mountains of Virginia and one in northern Germany, showed, in the women's own words, their living memories of family and friendships, the inseparability of individual lives from the community, and their resilient spirituality (Ramsey & Bleiszner, 1999). One final example is the classic 1979 work by Myerhoff, an anthropologist who immersed herself in a community of older immigrant Jews in southern California. Her account of the practice of religion, particularly when practiced in the language of childhoods that were lived in a faraway land and a faraway time, has the effect of showing just how far the thread can reach. She also shows the effectiveness of religion in constituting new communities in old age, in this case a Jewish community center formed to serve a group of otherwise socially isolated and impoverished immigrants. As a group, such close-up portraits help us see lived religion in the context of daily lives that have gone on for 80, 90, or even 100 years. It is difficult to name any other aspect of those lives that would have changed so little.

## IX. Conclusion

This has been at best a cursory summary of the intersection of two vast fields of scholarship, religion and aging. We have examined aging-related beliefs in the world's faith traditions, and change and stability in religiousness as individuals grow older; the idea that cohorts may differ in their patterns of religiousness over time; the impact of societal aging on religious groups; the impact of religious involvement on the health and well-being of older persons; congregational and clergy care for older persons in their own and other communities; and some in-depth studies of special religious communities of the extremely aged. As our society and others around the world continue to age, the potential for such groups to exist increases because more and more of us will live into our eighties and nineties. Of this we can be sure: all of the future research in this field will take place against a backdrop of rapidly aging populations in the United States and abroad. Whether future generations will age with the same experiences of religiousness and support from religious communities is much less certain and deserves careful study.

## References

Achenbaum, W. A. (1995). Age-based Jewish and Christian rituals. In M. A. Kimble, S. H. McFadden, J. W. Ellor, & J. J. Seeber. (Eds.), *Aging, spirituality, and religion: A handbook* (pp. 201–217). Minneapolis: Fortress Press.

Address, R. (2003). Making decisions at the end of life: An approach from sacred Jewish texts. In M. A. Kimble & S. H. McFadden, (Eds.), *Aging, spirituality, and religion: A handbook.* (Vol. 2, pp. 345–354). Minneapolis: Fortress Press.

Ainlay, S. C., Singleton, R., & Swigert, V. L. (1992). Aging and religious participation: Reconsidering the effects of health. *Journal for the Scientific Study of Religion, 31,* 175–188.

Ammerman, N. T. (1997). *Congregation and community.* New Brunswick: Rutgers University Press.

Argue, A., Johnson, D. R., & White, L. K. (1999). Age and religiosity: Evidence from the three-wave panel analysis. *Journal for the Scientific Study of Religion, 38,* 423–435.

Atchley, R. C. (2000). Spirituality. In T. Cole, R. Kastenbaum, & R. E. Ray (Eds.), *Handbook of the humanities and aging* (2nd ed.) (pp. 324–341). New York: Springer.

Bahr, H. M. (1970). Aging and religious disaffiliation. *Social Forces, 49,* 59–71.

Bainbridge, W. S. (1982). Shaker demographics 1840–1900: An example of the use of U.S. Census enumeration schedules. *Journal for the Scientific Study of Religion, 21,* 352–365.

Benjamins, M. R., Musick, M. A., Gold, D. T., & George, L. K. (2003). Age-related declines in activity level: The relationship between chronic illness and religious activities. *Journal of Gerontology: Social Sciences, 58B,* S377–S385.

Berger, P. L. (1967). *The sacred canopy: Elements of a sociological theory of religion.* New York: Doubleday.

Berger, P. L., & Neuhaus, R. J. (1977). *To empower people: The role of mediating structures in public policy.* Washington D.C.: American Enterprise Institute for Public Policy Research.

Blazer, D., & Palmore, E. B. (1976). Religion and aging in a longitudinal panel. *The Gerontologist, 16,* 82–85.

Bosworth, H. B., Park, K. S., McQuoid, D. R., Hays, J. C., & Steffens, D. C. (2003). The impact of religious practice and religious coping on geriatric depression. *International Journal of Geriatric Psychiatry, 18,* 905–914.

Breuilly, E., O'Brien, J., & Palmer, M. (1997). *Religions of the world.* New York: Transedition Limited.

Campbell, R. A., & Curtis, J. E. (1994). Religious involvement across societies: Analyses for alternative measures in national surveys. *Journal for the Scientific Study of Religion, 33,* 215–229.

Cave, D. (2004). Coming to America, and to nuns' rescue. *New York Times,* Sept. 3, B1,5.

Chaves, M. (1989). Secularization and religious revival: Evidence from U.S. church attendance rates. *Journal for the Scientific Study of Religion, 28,* 464–477.

Christiansen, D. (1995). A Catholic perspective. In M. A. Kimble, S. H. McFadden, J. W. Ellor, & J. J. Seeber. (Eds.), *Aging, spirituality, and religion: A handbook* (pp. 403–416). Minneapolis: Fortress Press.

Cnaan, R. A. (2002). *The invisible caring hand.* New York: New York University Press.

Cole, T. R. (1986). "Putting off the old": Middle-class morality, antebellum Protestantism, and the origins of ageism. In D. D. Van Tassel and P. N. Stearns (Eds.), *Old age in a bureaucratic society* (pp.49–65). Westport, CT: Greenwood.

Contrada, R. J., Goyal, T. M., Cather, C., Rafalson, L., Idler, E. L., & Krause, T. J. (2004). Psychosocial factors in outcomes of health surgery: The impact of religious involvement and depressive symptoms. *Health Psychology 23,* 227–228.

Cornwall, M. (1989). Faith development of men and women over the life span. In S. J. Bahr & E. T. Peterson (Eds.), *Aging and the family* (pp. 115–139). Lexington, MA: Lexington Books.

Cumming, E., & Henry, W. (1961). *Growing old.* New York: Basic Books.

De Vaus, D., & McAllister, I. (1987). Gender differences in religion: A test of the structural location theory. *American Sociological Review, 52,* 472–481.

Durkheim, E. (1951/1898). *Suicide.* New York: Free Press.

Durkheim, E. (1965/1915). *The elementary forms of the religious life.* New York: Free Press.

Ebaugh, H. R. (1993). *Women in the vanishing cloister: Organizational decline in Catholic religious orders in the United States.* New Brunswick, NJ: Rutgers University Press.

Eisenhandler, S. A. (2003). *Keeping the faith in late life.* New York: Springer.

Elder, G. H. (1998). The life course as developmental theory. *Child Development, 69,* 1–12.

Ellison, C. G., & George, L. K. (1994). Religious involvement, social ties, and social support in a southeastern community. *Journal for the Scientific Study of Religion, 33,* 46–61.

Erikson, E. H. (1950). *Childhood and society.* New York: Norton.

Fecher, V. J. (1982). *Religion and aging: An annotated bibliography.* San Antonio, TX: Trinity University Press.

Feder, D. (1993). The decline of mainline Protestant churches. *Human Events, 53,* 17.

Ferguson, N. (2004). Eurabia? *The New York Times Magazine,* April 4, 13–14.

Ferraro, K. F., & Kelley-Moore, (2000). Religious consolation among men and women: Do health problems spur seeking? *Journal for the Scientific Study of Religion, 39,* 220–234.

Finke, R., & Stark, R. (1992). *The churching of America, 1776–1990: Winners and losers in our religious economy.* New Brunswick, NJ: Rutgers University Press.

Firebaugh, G., & Harley, B. (1991). Trends in U.S. church attendance: Secularization and revival, or merely lifecycle effects? *Journal for the Scientific Study of Religion 30,* 487–500.

Firth, S. (1999). Spirituality and ageing in British Hindus, Sikhs and Muslims. In A. Jewell (Ed.), *Spirituality and ageing* (pp. 158–174). London: Jessica Kingsley Publishers.

Fønnebø, V. (1992). Mortality in Norwegian Seventh-day Adventists 1962–1986. *Journal of Clinical Epidemiology, 45,* 157–167.

Fowler, J. W. (1981). *Stages of faith: The psychology of human development and the quest for meaning.* San Francisco: Harper.

Freund, A. M., & Smith, J. (1999). Content and function of the self-definition in old and very old age. *Journal of Gerontology: Psychological Sciences, 54B*, P55–P67.

Fried, M. N., & Fried, M. H. (1980). *Transitions: Four rituals in eight cultures.* New York: Penguin.

George, L. K. (1993). Sociological perspectives on life transitions. *Annual Review of Sociology, 19*, 353–373.

Greeley, A. M., & Hout, M. (1999). Americans' increasing belief in life after death: Religious competition and acculturation. *American Sociological Review, 64*, 813–835.

Haber, C., & Gratton, B. (1994). *Old age and the search for security: An American social history.* Bloomington: Indiana University Press.

Hauerwas, S., Stoneking, C. B., Meador, K. G., & Cloutier, D. (Eds.). (2003). *Growing old in Christ.* Grand Rapids, MI: William Eerdmans.

Hays, J. C., Landerman, L. R., Blazer, D. G., Koenig, H. G., Carroll, J. W., & Musick, M. A. (1998). Aging, health, and the 'Electronic Church.' *Journal of Aging and Health, 10*, 458–482.

Hays, J. C., Meador, K. G., Branch, P. S., & George, L. K. (2001). The Spiritual History Scale in four dimensions (SHS-4): Validity and reliability. *The Gerontologist, 41*, 239–249.

Heenan, E. F. (1972). Sociology of religion and the aged: The empirical lacunae. *Journal for the Scientific Study of Religion, 12*, 171–176.

Hill, P. C., & Pargament, K. I. (2003). Advances in the conceptualization and measurement of religion and spirituality. *American Psychologist, 58*, 64–74.

Hoffman, J. P. (1998). Confidence in religious institutions and secularization: Trends and implications. *Review of Religious Research, 39*, 321–343.

House, J. S., Landis, K., & Umberson, D. (1988). Social relationships and health. *Science, 4965*, 540–545.

Hout, M., & Greeley, A. M. (1987). The center doesn't hold: Church attendance in the United States, 1940–1984. *American Sociological Review, 52*, 325–345.

Hummer, R. A., Rogers, R. G., Nam, C. B., & Ellison, C. G. (1999). Religious involvement and U.S. adult mortality. *Demography, 36*, 273–285.

Idler, E. L. (2001). Religion and health. In N. J. Smelser & P. B. Baltes, (Eds.), *International encyclopedia of the social and behavioral sciences* (pp. 13037–13040). Amsterdam: Elsevier.

Idler, E. L., & Kasl, S. V. (1997a). Religion among disabled and nondisabled persons I: Cross-sectional patterns in health practices, social activities, and well-being. *Journal of Gerontology: Social Sciences, 52B*, S294–S305.

Idler, E. L., & Kasl, S. V. (1997b). Religion among disabled and nondisabled persons II: Attendance at religious services as a predictor of the course of disability. *Journal of Gerontology: Social Sciences, 52B*, S306–S316.

Idler, E. L., Kasl, S. V., & Hays, J. C. (2001). Patterns of religious practice and belief in the last year of life. *Journal of Gerontology: Social Sciences, 56B*, S326–S334.

Idler, E. L., Musick, M. A., Ellison C. G., George, L. K., Krause, N., Ory, M. G., Pargament, K. I., Powell, L. H., Underwood, L. G., & Williams, D. R. (2003). Measuring multiple dimensions of religion and spirituality for health research. *Research on Aging, 25*, 327–365.

Imamoglu, E. O. (1999). Some correlates of religiosity among Turkish adults and elderly within a cross-cultural perspective. In Thomas, L. E. & Eisenhandler, S. A. (Eds.), *Religion, belief, and spirituality in late life.* (pp. 93–110). New York: Springer.

Ingersoll-Dayton, B., Krause, N., & Morgan, D. (2002). Religious trajectories and transitions over the life course. *International Journal of Aging and Human Development, 55*, 51–70.

Inglehart, R., & Baker, W. E. (2000). Modernization, cultural change, and the persistence of traditional values. *American Sociological Review, 65*, 19–51.

Isenberg, S. (2000). Aging in Judaism: 'Crown of Glory' and 'Days of Sorrow.' In T. Cole, R. Kastenbaum, & R. E. Ray (Eds.), *Handbook of the humanities and aging* (2nd ed.) (pp.114–141). New York: Springer.

James, W. (1978/1901). *The varieties of religious experience.* Garden City, NY: Doubleday.

Jarvis, G. K., & Northcott, H. C. (1987). Religion and differences in morbidity and mortality. *Social Science and Medicine, 25*, 813–824.

Jewell, A. (Ed.). (1999). *Spirituality and ageing*. London: Jessica Kingsley Publishers.

Keegan, C., Gross, S., Fisher, L., & Remez, S. (2002). *Boomers at midlife: The AARP Life Stage Study*. Washington, DC: AARP.

Kemp, C., & Bhungalia, S. (2002). Culture and the end of life: A review of major world religions. *Journal of Hospice and Palliative Nursing, 4*, 235–242.

Kimble, M. A. (2000). Aging in the Christian tradition. In T. Cole, R. Kastenbaum, & R. E. Ray (Eds.), *Handbook of the humanities and aging* (2nd ed.) (pp. 142–154). New York: Springer.

Kimble, M. A., & McFadden, S. H. (2003). *Aging, spirituality, and religion: A handbook* (Vol. 2.). Minneapolis: Fortress Press.

Kimble, M. A., McFadden, S. H., Ellor, J. W., & Seeber, J. J. (1995). *Aging, spirituality, and religion: A handbook*. Minneapolis: Fortress Press.

Koenig, H. G. (1994). *Aging and God*. New York: Haworth.

Koenig, H. G. (Ed.). (1998). *Handbook of religion and mental health*. San Diego, CA: Academic Press.

Koenig, H. G., Idler, E. L., Kasl, S. V., Hays, J., George, L. K., Musick, M., Larson, D. B., Collins, T., & Benson, H. (1999). Religion, spirituality, and medicine: A rebuttal to skeptics. *International Journal of Psychiatry in Medicine, 29*, 123–131.

Koenig, H. G., McCullough, M. E., & Larson, D. B. (2001). *Handbook of religion and health*. Oxford: Oxford University Press.

Koenig, H. G., Smiley, M., & Gonzales, J. (1988). *Religion, health, and aging*. New York: Greenwood.

Krause, N., Ellison, C. G., Shaw, B. A., Marcum, J. P., & Boardman, J. D. (2001). Church-based social support and religious coping. *Journal for the Scientific Study of Religion, 40*, 637–656.

Krause, N., Ingersoll-Dayton, B., Ellison, C. G., & Wulff, K. M. (1999). Aging, religious doubt, and psychological well-being. *The Gerontologist, 39*, 525–533.

Levin, J. S. (1997). Religious research in gerontology, 1980–1994: A systematic review. *Journal of Religious Gerontology, 10*, 3–31.

Levin, J. S., & Taylor, R. J. (1997). Age differences in patterns and correlates of the frequency of prayer. *The Gerontologist, 37*, 75–88.

Levin, J. S., & Vanderpool, H. Y. (1987). Is frequent religious attendance really conducive to better health?: Toward an epidemiology of religion. *Social Science and Medicine, 24*, 589–600.

Mannheim, K. (1952/1927). *Essays on the sociology of knowledge*. New York: Oxford Univ. Press.

Mantzaris, E. A. (1988). Religion as a factor affecting the attitudes of South African Indians towards family solidarity and older persons. *The South African Journal of Sociology, 19*, 111–116.

Markides, K. S. (1983). Aging, religiosity and adjustment: A longitudinal analysis. *Journal of Gerontology, 38*, 621–625.

Marler, P. L., & Hadaway, C. K. (2002). 'Being religious' or 'being spiritual' in America: A zero-sum proposition? *Journal for the Scientific Study of Religion, 41*, 289–300.

Mattlin, J. A., Wethington, E., & Kessler, R. C. (1990). Situational determinants of coping and coping effectiveness. *Journal of Health and Social Behavior, 31*, 103–1122.

Maves, P. B. (1960). Aging, religion, and the church. In C. Tibbitts (Ed.), *Handbook of social gerontology: Societal aspects of aging* (pp. 698–749). Chicago: University of Chicago.

McCullough, M. E., Hoyt, W. T., Larson, D. B., Koenig, H. G., & Thoresen, C. (2000). Religious involvement and mortality: A meta-analytic review. *Health Psychology, 19*, 211–222.

McFadden, S. H. (1999). Religion, personality, and aging: A life span perspective. *Journal of Personality, 67*, 1081–1104.

Mehta, K. K. (1997). The impact of religious beliefs and practices on aging: A cross-cultural comparison. *Journal of Aging Studies, 11*, 101–115.

Miller, A. S., & Nakamura, T. (1996). On the stability of church attendance patterns during a time of demographic change: 1965–1988. *Journal for the Scientific Study of Religion, 35*, 275–284.

Miller, A. S., & Stark, R. (2002). Gender and religiousness: Can socialization explanations be saved? *American Journal of Sociology, 107*, 1399–1423.

Miller, W. R., & Thoresen, C. (2003). Spirituality, religion, and health. *American Psychologist, 58*, 24–35.

Moberg, D. O. (1953). Church membership and personal adjustment in old age. *Journal of Gerontology, 8*, 207–211.

Myerhoff, B. (1979). *Number our days.* New York: Dutton.

Olitzky, K. M., & Borowitz, E. B. (1995). A Jewish perspective. In M. A. Kimble, S. H. McFadden, J. W. Ellor, & J. J. Seeber. (Eds.), *Aging, spirituality, and religion: A handbook* (pp. 389–402). Minneapolis: Fortress Press.

Palmore, E. (Ed.). (1970). *Normal aging: Reports from the Duke Longitudinal Study.* Durham, NC: Duke University Press.

Pargament, K. I. (1997). *The psychology of religion and coping: Theory, research, practice.* New York: Guilford.

Pargament, K. I., Koenig, H. G., Tarakeshwar, N., & Hahn, J. (2001). Religious struggle as a predictor of mortality among medically ill elderly patients. *Archives of Internal Medicine, 161,* 1881–1885.

Parkes, C. M., Laungani, P., & Young, B. (Eds.). (1997). *Death and bereavement across cultures.* London: Routledge.

Ploch D. R., & Hastings, D. W. (1994). Graphic presentations of church attendance using General Social Survey data. *Journal for the Scientific Study of Religion, 33,* 16–33.

Pope John Paul II. (1999). Letter to the elderly. http://www.vatican.va/holy_father/john_paul_ii/letters/documents/hf_jp-ii_let_01101999_elderly_en.html

Powell, L. H., Shahabi, L., & Thoresen, C. E. (2003). Religion and spirituality: Linkages to physical health. *American Psychologist, 58,* 36–52.

Princeton Religion Research Center. (2003). *Emerging trends.* Princeton, NJ: Author.

Ramsey, J. L., & Blieszner, R. (1999). *Spiritual resiliency in older women.* Thousand Oaks, CA: Sage.

Rebhun, U., & Waxman, C. I., (Eds.). (2004). *Jews in Israel.* Waltham, MA: Brandeis University Press.

Riley, M. W., & Foner, A. (1968–1972). *Aging and society* (Vols. 1–3). New York: Russell Sage.

Roof, W. C. (1993). *A generation of seekers: The spiritual journeys of the Baby Boom generation.* San Francisco: Harper.

Roof, W. C. (1999). *Spiritual marketplace: Baby Boomers and the remaking of American religion.* Princeton, NJ: Princeton University Press.

Schaie, K. W., Krause, N., & Booth, A. (Eds.). (2004). *Religious influences on health and well-being in the elderly.* New York: Springer.

Seeber, J. J. (1995). Congregational models. In M. A. Kimble, S. H. McFadden, J. W. Ellor, & J. J. Seeber. (Eds.), *Aging, spirituality, and religion: A handbook* (pp. 253–269). Minneapolis: Fortress Press.

Seeman, T. E., Dubin, L. F., & Seeman, M. (2003). Religiosity/spirituality and health: A critical review of the evidence for biological pathways. *American Psychologist, 58,* 53–63.

Skees, S. (1998). *God among the Shakers: A search for stillness and faith at Sabbathday Lake.* New York: Hyperion.

Sloan, R., & Bagiella, E. (2002). Claims about religious involvement and health outcomes. *Annals of Behavioral Medicine, 24,* 14–21.

Sloan, R., Bagiella, E., & Powell, T. (1999). Religion, spirituality, and medicine. *Lancet, 353,* 664–667.

Smith, C. S. (2004). Racial tensions puncture Corsica's picturesque setting. *The New York Times,* August 26, A3.

Smith, H. (1991). *The world's religions: Our great wisdom traditions.* San Francisco: Harper.

Smith, S. D. (2003). *Parish nursing: A handbook for the new millennium.* New York: Haworth.

Smith, T. B., McCullough, M. E., & Poll, J. (2003). Religiousness and depression: Evidence for a main effect and the moderating influence of stressful life events. *Psychological Bulletin, 129,* 614–636.

Snowdon, D. (2001). *Aging with grace: What the Nun Study teaches us about leading longer, healthier, and more meaningful lives.* New York: Bantam Books.

Stein, S. J. (1992). *The Shaker experience in America: History of the United Society of Believers.* New Haven: Yale University Press.

Taylor, R. J., Chatters, L. M., & Levin, J. (2004). *Religion in the lives of African Americans.* Thousand Oaks, CA: Sage.

Taylor, R. J., Thornton, M. C., & Chatters, L. M. (1987). Black Americans' perceptions of the socio-historical role of the church. *Journal of Black Studies, 18,* 123–138.

Thang, L. L. (2000). Aging in the East: Comparative and historical reflections. In T.

Cole, R. Kastenbaum, & R. E. Ray (Eds.), *Handbook of the humanities and aging* (2nd ed.) (pp. 183–213). New York: Springer.

Thomas, L. E., & Eisenhandler, S. A. (Eds.). (1999). *Religion, belief, and spirituality in late life.* New York: Springer.

Thorson, J. A. (Ed.). (2000). *Perspectives on spiritual well-being and aging.* Springfield, IL: Charles C. Thomas.

Thursby, G. R. (2000). Aging in Eastern religious traditions. In T. Cole, R. Kastenbaum, & R. E. Ray (Eds.), *Handbook of the humanities and aging* (2nd ed.) (pp. 155–180). New York: Springer.

van Gennep, A. (1960). *The rites of passage.* Chicago: University of Chicago Press.

Van Ness, P. H., & Larson, D. B. (2002). Religion, senescence, and mental health: The end of life is not the end of hope. *American Journal of Geriatric Psychiatry, 10,* 386–397.

Wallace, J. M., & Forman T. (1998). Religion's role in promoting health and reducing risk among American youth. *Health Education and Behavior, 25,* 721–741.

Waxman, C. I. (2001). *Jewish baby boomers.* Albany: State University of New York Press.

Weber, M. (1958/1904). *The Protestant ethic and the spirit of capitalism.* New York: Scribner.

Weber, M. (1964/1922). *The sociology of religion.* Boston: Beacon.

Westberg, G. (1990). *The parish nurse.* Minneapolis: Augsburg.

Wingrove, C. R., & Alston, J. P. (1974). Cohort analysis of church attendance, 1939–69. *Social Forces, 53,* 324–331.

Witter, R. A., Stock, W. A., Okun, M. A., & Haring, M. J. (1985). Religion and subjective well-being in adulthood: A quantitative synthesis. *Review of Religious Research, 26,* 332–342.

World Health Organization. (2002). *Core health indicators.* http://www3.who.int/whosis/core/

Wuthnow, R. (1999). *Growing up religious: Christians and Jews and their journeys of faith.* Boston: Beacon.

# Seventeen

# Lifestyle and Aging

Jon Hendricks and Laurie Russell Hatch

Lifestyle is a defining attribute of social life and a key concept in social gerontology. Viewed as both cause and consequence, lifestyle is used as a construct to explicate preferences, modes of living, and as an indicator of social standing. Despite its pervasive usage, lifestyle remains a vexing concept, influential yet imprecise, difficult to define yet running throughout the gerontological literature.

It has long been recognized that access and opportunity, stress, and undesirable outcomes do not occur randomly. Since the pioneering research of Faris and Dunham (1939/1960), social scientists have examined the social epidemiology of all manner of positive and negative outcomes thought to reflect causation processes rooted in ongoing conditions of social life. These conditions include context and experience, socioeconomic status (SES), and social inequalities (Jasso, 2001; Turner, Wheaton, & Lloyd, 1995). Differential social circumstances are thought to yield differential lifestyles—as they provide the institutionalized linkages between micro-level and macro-level factors. Notwithstanding a national illusion that inequalities do not matter or

that class differences are shrinking, the literature is consistent: advantage generates advantage and disadvantage yields disadvantage over the life course (Dannefer, 2003). How people live determines how they age: simply put, lifestyles foreshadow old age

Underlying mechanisms implicit to lifestyles are often unarticulated and elusive. A major review of social science literature by Glyptis (1989) revealed scant empirical research centered on lifestyles per se. In the interval since, there have been few additions (Stebbins, 1997). Still, the concept is widely used even if it refers to little more than durable modes of living (Sobel, 1981). In their seminal *Habits of the Heart*, Bellah, Madsen, Sullivan, Swidler, and Tipton (1985) spoke of "lifestyle enclaves" in which members share and express common identities through consumption of lifestyle services or products, leisure patterns, modes of living such as retirement arrangements, and in other ways that distinguish them from nonmembers. Through lifestyles social differentiation is made apparent, group recognition made possible, and differential outcomes fashioned.

Not surprisingly, lifestyles are assumed to result from personal characteristics: individual attributes, aptitudes, capacities, the set of skills and competencies labeled human capital thought to channel individual choices. At the same time, membership in identifiable categories, including age, gender, ethnicity, social status groupings, and a host of shared circumstances that convey position, channel relationships, and circumscribe options or preferences contribute what may be termed social capital. The compilation of roles and relationships comprise a resource actors use to make their way and that shape the aging experience. Though lacking an economic metric, social capital is nonetheless palpable. In combination, social and economic capital stand as assets mobilized to fashion lifestyles instrumental in garnering opportunity or privation, affecting even mortality patterns. Among the social causes of disease identified by epidemiologists are ability to control mundane circumstances of daily life, stress, interpersonal ties, health-risk behaviors, the nature of work and so on—the same factors comprising lifestyles (Hankin, 2000; Hayward, Crimmins, Miles, & Yang, 2000; Link & Phelan, 1995; Marmot, 2004).

A goal of this chapter is to review the literature on lifestyle and aging. Our aim is to focus on work that may fuel further research and insight, not to catalog every instance where variations are attributed *en passim* to lifestyle. By identifying the strands of research addressing lifestyles, we hope to provide synergy for more productive applications. One central theme focuses on person-specific factors and behaviors stemming from human capital variables and from personal choices constitutive of lifestyles. Within this framework, psychological profiles, cognition, expressed attitudes, preferences, or behaviors are used to explain variable outcomes. There is no doubt that personality

factors and individual agency are crucial, but a unilateral focus on individuals as authors of their every action does not convey insight into group identity or collective consequences that stem from societal influences. In keeping with a more sociological perspective, a second theme highlights these broader relational resources constitutive of lifestyles. In particular, SES, and social class more broadly, are considered crucial to understanding how lifestyles are circumscribed by institutionalized conditions beyond the control of individuals. Ethnicity, gender, sexuality, and interconnections among these and other bases of group membership and identity influence individual lives.

Rather than arguing the primacy of agency or structure in explicating lifestyle and aging, a more effective approach is to consider individual behaviors and decisions, as well as social circumstances. A further goal of the chapter is to identify theoretical issues relevant to a research agenda on lifestyle and aging that simultaneously considers structure and agency, as well as their interaction. To help suggest a framework, we draw from a variety of theoretical perspectives, including phenomenology and feminist theory, and provide a model delineating how personal resources function as composite factors in creating lifestyles.

The personal resource model proffered here provides one means of bridging individualistic and societal factors generating lifestyles. In this framework, lifestyle is conceived of as contingent on the recursive, dynamic sweep of human and social capital coalescing as personal resources. Concomitants of participation in any socially defined category include access to opportunity, institutionalized experiences, values and preferences and knowledge communities that delineate ways of comprehending and behaviors constitutive of lifestyles. These ambient contextual factors provide parameters for incumbents that underpin person-environment transactions. Actors are not merely reactive; they are proactive, bringing with them an intentional agenda, as well as personal competencies and characteristics that shape lifestyles. Moen and Chermack (2005) speak of "control cycles" and the forms of capital alluded to here as perquisites in the allocation of health and well-being. As will be seen, lifestyles may be construed as resulting from a melding of what may be thought of as physiological-psychological, social-familial, and fiduciary resources.

Venturing an explication of how these resources work together to shape lifestyles will generate modifications, and that is our intent. So many facets of old age are laid at the doorstep of lifestyle differentiation that the underlying construct deserves greater attention. If lifestyles are predicates for what follows throughout life, they are deserving of explication.

## I. Defining Lifestyle

We draw from Stebbins' (1997) review of lifestyle theory and research and refer to lifestyles as distinctive attributes or recognizable patterns of behaviors reflecting shared interests and life situations incorporating related values, attitudes, and orientations that create characteristic social identities. That is, lifestyles are not merely behavioral repertoires but include corresponding attitudinal dimensions (Cockerham, Abel, & Lueschen, 1993; Stebbins, 1997). In a later section of the chapter, we suggest how this working definition of lifestyle may be modified to reflect more fully both objective (distinctive attributes or recognizable patterns of behavior) and subjective (values, attitudes, orientations, identities) dimensions.

Psychological perspectives cast lifestyles as composed of a range of psychological attributes, sensory processes, cognition, or predispositions. In general,

this literature conceives of lifestyle as contingent on personal, volitional choices. In other treatments, lifestyle stands as a proxy for access to resources, opportunity structures, and aspects of social capital such as social status and relative position that result in identifiable sets of activities or practices. There is an alternative focus in which lifestyle and successful aging, variously defined, are equated. Still another perspective uses lifestyle to refer to autonomy, control and consumption. However nuanced, lifestyle portends a structuring and pacing of the life course, signifying a variety of coherent consequences (Stebbins, 1997). For our purposes, lifestyles are both shared and relational and affect how aging unfurls. Although all facets of lifestyle are manifested through individual behavior, that is not the same as saying they originate from individual-level factors. Whether the central issue is the creation of social identity, life course trajectories, status rankings, or contingencies along the way, lifestyles are implicated. Giddens (1991) spoke to the same point in his characterization of personal regimes as institutionalized modes of behavior, reflecting individual choices as embodiments of social or cultural memberships. Within gerontology, Gordon and Longino (2000) alluded to daily practices, cum regimes, as "institutions writ small." The same characterization applies to lifestyles as representative patterns of living that frame how life is given shape.

### A. Psychological Definitions

Psychological conceptualizations of lifestyle focus on an array of individual-level attributes, activities, or behaviors underpinning patterns of experience (Stebbins, 1997). Within the purview of psychology, lifestyles are considered in light of what are labeled the three "Cs:" cognitions, conditions, and change (Walters, 1998). Cognition is commonly conceived of as mental schema or thinking patterns used to make, justify, or rationalize choices. Conditions coloring lifestyles are defined in two ways: intra- and inter-individual. The first is conceived in terms of internal states, including heredity, intelligence, or personality factors influencing how individuals engage the ebb and flow of events. Included among internal factors shaping lifestyles are sensory acuities and physical capabilities suitable for meeting challenges emerging over the life course. There is another motivational aspect: some psychologists assert individuals are driven to seek advantage and adaptation in their interaction with their milieu as part of an instinct for self-preservation or optimization. These same intrinsic factors are thought to be essential for maintaining control, autonomy, or optimism that one can respond to contingencies. These intra-individual traits, capacities, performance, temperaments, and achievements are said to result in differential outcomes, including life events, health incidents, feelings of mastery, efficacy, and the perceived gravity of consequences (Bandura, 1997).

The second facet of conditions refers to external circumstances, be they physical or interpersonal, including family, interaction partners, or social relations that undergird an individual's propensity to engage in one or another patterned form of behavior. Lewin (1939) believed that surroundings and context color all aspects of personality and adult development. Allport (1955/1968) went further, asserting that an adequate conceptualization of lifestyles grounded in environmental circumstances would obviate the need for psychological examinations of "bits and pieces of experience" (p. 32). Allport characterized lifestyle as "a mode of being in the world," while recognizing that such modes are inexorably grounded in social and physical environments. Lawton (1985) and colleagues have been particularly attentive to physical aspects of those environments and spoke of environmental press as a factor shaping lifestyles. Neugarten (1977) and others attend more closely to broadly defined sociocultural circumstances thought to shape personality and thereby characteristic modes of behavior.

The third dimension of lifestyles is concerned with change, and it, too, derives from a combination of internal psychological characteristics and in situ factors that may destabilize an individual's actual or perceived competence (Lawton, 1985). Walters (1998) asserted that these external conditions do not necessarily determine behavior but do establish parameters from which behavioral repertoires or choices are drawn and from which actors select and create lifestyles, whether construed as rational or nonreflective. Whether motivated by an existential search for control and self-efficacy, or by other aspects of personality, Walters and others conceived of lifestyles as consequences of these sorts of psychological or personality processes.

In searching for the causes of change in lifestyles, psychologists look to personalities—those patterns of thoughts and behaviors, traits, dispositional signatures, personal action constructs, or adaptive responses reflecting goals, tasks, temperament, emotionality, motivations, and so on (Hooker & McAdams, 2003; Pulkkinen & Caspi, 2002). Some see personalities as stabilizing at a fairly early age (e.g., 30 years) and remaining relatively constant thereafter (Costa & McCrae, 1994). Others see far less constancy (Small, Hertzog, Hultsch, & Dixon, 2003). In a meta-analysis of more than 150 longitudinal investigations, Roberts and DelVecchio (2000) concluded that though personality shows considerable stability over time, change is evident into the middle and later years. To the extent that personality attributes change over the life course, lifestyle will be affected.

The quest for mastery and control are important aspects of well-being and is implicated in the creation of lifestyles. The ability to exercise control over one's environment is an important element that buffers adversity. Although the specific contributions of personal control, self-actualization, self-efficacy, and adaptive capacity are debatable, scholars contend that people age with differing degrees of control, which leads to differential outcomes in such areas as sense of well-being, adaptability to environmental changes, life course trajectories, health, and ultimately life expectancy. It is said that disparities in these indicators of autonomy affect how old age is experienced and life unfolds (Andrews, Clark, & Luszcz, 2002; Bandura, 1997; Moen & Chermack, forthcoming; Pearlin & Pioli, 2003; Pulkkinen & Caspi, 2002). As Rowe and Kahn (1998), Krause (2003) and others asserted (see Zarit, Pearlin, & Schaie, 2003), the linkage between personal control and what is regarded as successful aging is widely heralded. Recognition of these linkages helps illuminate the evolution of lifestyles. Such recognition begs the question: what accounts for the development of personal control (Abeles, 2003; George, 2003)? A variety of responses are possible, but the answer lies in a combination of intrinsic factors and proximate social circumstances (Zarit & Leitsch, 2003).

Changes in lifestyle may also be volitional, linked to choices individuals make in light of motivations or in terms of perceived risk, fear, or vulnerability. Some say that aging and any corresponding losses or declining sensory capacities or physical functioning may portend lifestyle shifts. For example, Hennen and Knudten (2001), among others, concluded that escalating concerns about risk, fear, or vulnerability, whether resulting from shifting capacities or external conditions pressing in on an individual, bring lifestyle changes. As these authors asserted, decrements in either realm increase fear of victimization and presage accommodations amounting to lifestyle changes.

## B. Behavioral Factors and Lifestyles

Discussions of lifestyle as behavioral patterns generally focus on individual choices thought to affect longevity and vitality or embodying risky actions leading to detrimental consequences. Mechanic (1978) asserted that lifestyle practices include such factors as risk-taking, health behaviors, health attitudes and beliefs, and housing. Matarazzo (1983) coined the concept of behavioral pathogens to encapsulate the notion of risky lifestyles. Research, including the longitudinal UNC Alumni Heart Survey, has documented significant correlations between personality characteristics, risky behaviors, or lifestyles that stand as predicates of negative health outcomes (Siegler, Kaplan, Von Dras, & Mark, 1999). In examining the sorts of factors associated with a compression of morbidity, Hubert, Block, Oehlert, and Fries (2002) identified a gradient based on number of unhealthy lifestyle practices and a correlated slope of decline leading to death. Laditka and Laditka (2001) summarized the relationship thus: " ... when an individual makes lifestyle choices that improve health, she or he is likely to enjoy both increased longevity and better health through a larger percentage of that increased life span" (p. 52).

A recent Surgeon General's Report (cited in Pullen, Walker, & Fiandt, 2001) attributed half of all deaths each year to unhealthy lifestyles. The report asserts that eliminating lifestyle discrepancies among disparate segments of the population would have dramatic effects on differential morbidity and life expectancy. In Chapter 14, Ferraro adds a proviso that risky or health-destructive behaviors, including smoking, sedentary lifestyles, obesity, and alcohol and drug abuse, are associated with poverty or low SES. Yet, there is evidence that all such lifestyle behaviors are modifiable and that considerable variation exists.

## C. Lifestyle and Social Structure: A Relational Approach

Rather than ceding lifestyle either to proximate psychological characteristics or to behavioral choices putatively within the purview of individuals, a relational approach views individual-level factors as embedded in social contexts, relationships, and environmental circumstances, those aspects of social life generally conceived to be situational or structural in nature (Zarit & Leitsch, 2003; also see Chapter 8). For purposes of this discussion, social structure may be construed to mean institutional arrangements and organizations that stand apart from individuals, yet exercise sufficient sway over their lives to an extent that routines are more or less predictable. Those who hew strictly to a structural perspective would contend that lives are lived and experience shaped within the penumbra of structural conditions and institutionalized arrangements; there can be no other options.

A number of investigators (Avison & Cairney, 2003; Marmot, 2004; Pearlin, 1989; Turner & Roszell, 1994) have asserted that SES, social roles, and the means to mediate stressful outcomes are integral to how adversity is experienced and individuals' lives shaped. To some, SES is among the most palpable socially defining facets of lifestyles. In fact, there is resounding consensus that SES portends many aspects of a person's life, pulled together under the rubric of lifestyle. There is ample research to support the assertion that social causes associated with socioeconomic differences, which in turn are grounded in lifestyle conditions, affect virtually every aspect

of life, including morbidity and mortality (Preston & Taubman, 1994). To illustrate, in an examination of racial differences in health outcomes using two waves of the Health and Retirement Survey (HRS), Hayward et al. (2000) found substantial support for a social causation hypothesis. As Hayward and colleagues aver, ability to control everyday life circumstances, stress, social ties, diet, health-risk behaviors, the nature of work, work environments, and availability of health care revolve around cumulative and fundamental social factors rooted in socioeconomic stratification. Their study affirmed that SES, not health risk behaviors per se, explain differential mortality, differential disability, and chronic health conditions. In fact, Hayward and colleagues generalize across a number of health domains in later life, suggesting there is an inverse relationship between the accouterments of SES and poor health. They found that various factors accompanying SES explain a greater proportion of the variance in health outcomes than race or other variables. Other researchers concur that that a significant portion of the variance in exposure to stress emanates from associated social conditions and accumulated traumatic life experiences (Marmot, 2004; Turner et al., 1995). In Chapter 14, Ferraro provides insight into cascading risks and health disparities associated with cumulative disadvantage and life course inequalities associated with health-destructive behaviors.

A 1995 editorial in the *American Journal of Public Health* asserted, "There is a striking consistency in the distribution of mortality and morbidity between social groups. The more advantaged groups, whether expressed in terms of income, education, social class or ethnicity, tend to have better health than the other members of their societies. The distribution is not bipolar but graded, so that each change in the level of advantage or disadvantage is in general associated with a change in health" (Blane, 1995, p. 903). In a recent supplement to the *Journals of Gerontology: Social Science* (Zarit & Pearlin, 2005), contributors are unequivocal in maintaining that health disparities and other health-related outcomes rest firmly on SES. The relationship is complex, but access to and control over resources is thought to be one mechanism explaining differentials in the experience of stress; those same resources are constitutive elements defining lifestyles over the life course (Krause, 2003). Turner, Lloyd, and Roszell (1999) maintained there is an ineludible connection between protective psychosocial resources and relative position in the social structure. They emphasized that patterns of experience and ability to respond to whatever pressures arise are tied to personal resources actors bring to bear on their lives and what comes their way.

In observing that old age results from paths taken to get there, O'Rand and Henretta (1999) did not mean merely paths created by individual choices, but also those imposed by social and structural parameters that put boundaries around and provide scripts for individual circumstances. There is a substantial body of research that underscores the linkage between social status, health, and aging. "Where you stand in the social hierarchy—on the social ladder—is intimately related to your chances of getting ill and your length of life" (Marmot, 2004, p.1). Marmot (2004) asserted that autonomy, social connectedness, and ability to avoid stress are associated with relative positions in status hierarchies. As he noted, health and life are not separate spheres and control and autonomy, as well as ability to muster personal resources to address contingencies, are relevant to the experience of adversity, and inversely associated with relative status. Two interrelated facets of SES, income and education, have been found to have consistent positive correlations with feelings of well-being, mastery, and control across the life course and both are related to lifestyles (House, Kessler, Herzog, Mero, Kinney, & Breslow, 1992).

Although SES often stands as a proxy for social class, many sociological treatments conceptualize the latter as more inclusive than SES; both are recognized as intimately linked with lifestyles. Broadly speaking, members of a social class are thought to share similar occupations, incomes, levels of education, *and* lifestyles (Marger, 2005). Sociological discussions of lifestyle are informed by Weber's (1966) contention that social class groupings create lifestyles through the supply of products, the nature of living conditions, personal life experiences, and access to opportunities. In short, membership in social classes results in recognizable styles of living and status trappings. In terms germane to social gerontology, such a claim has led to reasonable consensus that life course trajectories, biographical pacing, and the experience of aging are shaped to a large extent by the reach of social circumstances.

Although some researchers assume that comparable processes operate to shape lifestyle precursors and outcomes for members of different social and socioeconomic groups, others have focused on sources of differentiation. Ross and Bird (1994) identified differences in personal control, access to resources, and health behaviors in women's and men's lifestyles that preceded disparate health outcomes. These gender differences reflect discrepancies in personal resources and attitudes that lead to differential stress, depression, health incidents, disabilities, and accumulated insults sufficient to impair ability to maintain functionality (Ross & Mirowsky, 2002; Steverink, Westerhof, Bode, & Dittmann-Kohli, 2001).

## II. "Successful Aging" as Code for Lifestyle

In the last decade or so, the notion of lifestyles has also been coupled with the concept of "successful aging." Successful aging is customarily defined as adaptive and agentic, wherein individuals are able to "call the shots" in order to attain optimal outcomes (Pulkkinen & Caspi, 2002). The most widely referenced examination linking lifestyles and successful aging is the 10-year MacArthur study (Rowe & Kahn, 1998). The research was predicated on assumptions that aging is neither predetermined nor inflexible, and that individuals are capable of exercising personal preference and have the wherewithal to modify either environments or lifestyles. Rowe and Kahn (1998) offered prescriptions concerning senescence and effective functioning in later life and asserted that their research identifies "lifestyle and personality factors that boost the chance of aging successfully" (p. 18). They cast successful aging as a consequence of lifestyle choices of individuals qua individuals that avoid risk factors and lead to advantageous outcomes. Maladaptive lifestyles were associated with disease and disability in later life and given greater weight in shaping the experience of old age than heredity, genetic background, even certain diseases, though they recognized that lifestyle and disease are closely coupled.

Rowe and Kahn (1998) reduced successful aging to two factors: how people live and what they eat. After delineating risky behaviors associated with harmful lifestyles and urging their diminution, these writers alluded to the implications of diet and exercise, dynamic interpersonal interaction, mental stimulation, sense of efficacy, and constructive mental outlooks. On this last point, additional psychological research suggests that maintaining emotional optimism may add up to 10 years to life (Danner, Snowdon, & Friesen, 2001; Fredrickson, 2003). Rowe and Kahn also counseled people to remain actively engaged with life and connected to others, and then extended their recommendations beyond individuals per se to encompass proposals for altering societal arrangements to promote healthy lifestyles and more successful aging.

Rowe and Kahn's (1998) emphasis on personal agency lead them to assert "successful aging is dependent upon individual choices and behaviors . . . attained through individual choice and effort" (p. 37). The successful lifestyle behaviors and practices they identified have also been examined in other countries. For example, in Australia comparable behaviors were found to lead to similar effects insofar as promoting physical and cognitive functioning, performance, and coping abilities are concerned (Andrews et al., 2002).

Attempting to illuminate what is implicit in these discussions, Holstein and Minkler (2003) contend that successful aging is predicated on assumptions that everyone has autonomy and options. Their view is that social circumstances, including social status and access to resources, can facilitate or hobble adaptive responses, even perceptions that there are alternatives. They point out that options are steeped in socially prescribed parameters, such that personal choices may or may not be obvious or feasible depending on where individuals are situated. That is to say, lifestyle choices may not be within the purview of individual action; they do not play out in a vacuum, but stand as outcomes of what Sobel (1981) characterized as "the set of ordered sequences of social experiences to which the individual is subjected" (p. 50).

## III. An Agenda to (Re)Unite Structure and Agency as Constitutive of Lifestyle

The paradox of structure and agency is an enduring question in social science (Wight, 1999). The issues are central to lifestyle research, with evidence documenting the importance of *both* structured circumstances and opportunities for lifestyle outcomes, including individual choice and decision making. This puzzle of the self-structure dialectic is indeed a conundrum if lifestyle is to be given its due. A nuanced understanding of lifestyle across the life course requires more than measures of individuals' predispositions, attitudes, or competencies along with indicators of SES; it calls for an integrated perspective. As Musolf (2003) noted, "structure and agency are now becoming recognized as specious, or spurious polarities; instead, they are inextricably intertwined in a non-quantifiable dialectic constituting constraint and emergence as two salient features of everyday life. To say that humans are both shaped and shapers means structure and agency construct each other" (p. 1).

Hagestad and Dannefer (2001) avow that gerontologists seldom include explicit attention to agency and that the concept is "often equated with choice and self-expression and sometimes with efficacy" (p. 14). This point also is apropos of discussions of lifestyle or structure, including those found in social gerontology. Structure often is equated with objective features of the social world beyond the control, and often outside the ken of individuals, but these implications are seldom spelled out in ways that foster further investigation.

This tacit assumption conflates structure and agency with objectivity and subjectivity and confounds structure and agency with micro- and macro-level phenomena. Whereas structure often is associated with macro-level social institutions and their effects on individuals and groups, agency typically is associated with individuals; however, social collectivities beyond the individual also "act" (Ritzer, 1996). Burns (1986), among others, asserted that organized groups, organizations, and even nations act as human agents. On the other hand, although discussions of agency typically focus on individuals as actors, perceptions, and even language usage, are "structured," and thereby contour thoughts and actions. Sobel (1981) spoke of structural arrangements as "reference generators" for those generalizations individuals make as they construct meanings or justify actions. In turn, actors' transactions and interactions create and re-create structural arrangements. Giddens (1984) believes "structural properties . . . exist only insofar as forms of social conduct are reproduced chronically across time and space" (p. xxi). The relationship is reciprocal; actors are swayed by structural considerations and the collective action of successive cohorts provides the impetus for structural transformation.

A fruitful research agenda on lifestyle and aging requires integration of macro- and micro-level factors and sources of agency creating lifestyles, and recognition of dialectical processes that inform how structure and agency play out for individuals and groups. Lifestyles represent an area wherein macro-level considerations and personal action combine to contour experience.

### A. Aspects of a Research Agenda on Aging and Lifestyle

#### 1. Recognize the Multifaceted Influence of Social Class

Numerous studies have emphasized the interrelationship of SES, social class, multiple indicators of lifestyle, and outcomes across the life course. At the same time, scholarly accounts of lifestyle and aging have been shaped by normative assumptions about lifestyle choices, as well as what constitutes successful or productive aging. Drawing from Bourdieu (1986), such understandings, and social practices generally, reflect class biases, whether or not individuals or groups are aware of them, and even when such practices do not yield proceeds in the form of material returns (Turner, 2003). As conceived by Bourdieu, capital encompasses more than money, material goods, or returns; it includes a complex intermingling of social, cultural, and symbolic capital that fashions how life unfolds. Besides capital as a pecuniary resource, additional forms of capital are pertinent to experience. In highlighting other forms of capital, Holstein and Minkler (2003) noted, "the power of unexamined cultural images subtly invades consciousness even when prejudicial to the person internalizing them . . . older people try to become what culture signals as desirable without always recognizing where the pressures originate and even if those efforts are ultimately self-defeating" (p. 788).

Using Bourdieu's lens, symbolic meanings attached to "aging well," "successful aging," and other laudable patterns linked with "lifestyles" (i.e., assumptions about appropriate lifestyle choices that are thought to facilitate successful aging) are part of a broader ideology that legitimates established class perspectives. Much of the literature on successful aging and lifestyle may be biased in favor of individuals and groups with a wider array of options from which to "choose" lifestyles. Particular patterns of "individual choices" are represented as more appropriate and healthy, but that disproportionately characterize those in advantaged social positions. Beaglehole (1990) reported that individuals of higher SES are more knowledgeable about health-related behaviors, including smoking,

diet, and exercise, and that they are better able to identify adaptive responses and behaviors. Injunctions to effect "better lifestyle choices" have less resonance for poor older people in unsafe neighborhoods who have functionality problems or conditions that limit choices (Grzywacz & Marks, 2001).

Critical theorists ask, "who benefits and who is harmed by prevailing culturally normative standards?" (Holstein & Minkler, 2003, p. 789). One answer is that growing commercial endeavors targeting older consumers benefit from commodified lifestyles (Katz & Marshall, 2003). One consequence is that such efforts influence normative standards of aging well, or, at a minimum, how to remain socially acceptable in the face of numerous presumed indignities imposed by aging. Lifestyle industries, as some have termed that aspect of consumerism catering to the creation of idealized images of aging, have stressed the relative advantage of activity and consumerism as a way to ward off less appealing aspects of aging. Paradoxically, lifestyle interventions echo some of the conclusions of those examining risky lifestyles but tend to equate aging well with spending well to stave off decline (Katz & Marshall, 2003). These marketing efforts do, however, provide scripts actors use to assess their own aging.

Even though a market-driven perspective reinforces or creates "problems" associated with aging that require commodified interventions, the outcomes are not entirely exploitative. Herskovits and Mitteness (1994) observed that advertising and marketing for adult diapers, promoting a theme of "get back into life," encourage enhanced social participation and integration for those experiencing incontinence. Similar observations can be made for male potency drugs or other products that may ameliorate stigmatizing conditions. Despite the fact that marketing accentuates plights suitable for solution through purchases, it has the potential to yield tangible benefits, normalizing otherwise discrediting or isolating conditions.

More generally, marketing aimed at mining "the gold in gray" is an outgrowth of lifestyle industries plumbing new consumer niches. In the mid-1970s, Myers and Gutman (1974) imported the concept of lifestyles to the world of marketing by alluding to ways the notion of lifestyles might inform advertising strategies. Subsequently, lifestyle industries have thrived as the promotion of consumer products as accouterments of lifestyle has become big business, generating a seemingly insatiable market for the young, old, and everyone in between (Katz & Marshall, 2003).

### 2. Attend to Interconnections among Social Class, Age, Ethnicity, Gender, Sexuality

Integrating structure and agency to illuminate lifestyle must attend not only to interconnections with social class, but also age, ethnicity, gender, sexuality, and other socially defined bases of group identification and differentiation. Bourdieu's critical perspective facilitates exploration of social class and attends to the influence of class biases, but tends to downplay other important forms of capital or sources of inequality. Bourdieu focused on social classes as "social facts," with structures that are external yet integral to individual cognition and action (Turner, 2003). Certainly external constraints and opportunities matter and can be observed among all groups that are ranked hierarchically and have differential access to economic, social, cultural, and/or symbolic capital (Musolf, 2003). Such attributes become classificatory, helping to shape individual perceptions and interactions, and exerting an abiding influence over both life course and age relations.

Preconceptions underpinning prevailing conceptualizations of "positive," "productive," or "successful" lifestyle practices need to move beyond social class to include ethnicity, gender, and sexuality (e.g., Holstein & Minkler, 2003). Wray (2003) contends that common conceptions of successful aging are "based on dominant assumptions about what constitutes contentment in later life," and that the approach "denies or marginalizes the diverse ethnic and cultural experiences of older people, and correspondingly, the constellation of factors that contribute toward happiness as they grow older" (p. 514). With reference to successful aging, Holstein and Minkler (2003) commented that emphasizing personal volition and, not coincidently, blame for less-than-successful aging marginalizes many older persons, especially women. "Such a perspective may trivialize the role of gender, race, socioeconomic status, and genetics in influencing both health and broader life chances both throughout life and in old age" (Holstein & Minkler, 2003, p. 794).

### 3. Avoid Reifying Social Class and Other Bases of Group Membership

In recognizing the relevance of social class, ethnicity, gender, and sexuality in shaping opportunities and constraints throughout life, researchers must avoid reifying social class and other bases of identity or inequality. Bourdieu cautioned against conflating models of actors with real individuals interacting and making choices in a variety of contexts while facing fluid constraints and opportunities. A phenomenological perspective is helpful for illuminating how individuals perceive and act on subjective and objective components or a melding of the two (Berger & Luckmann, 1967). For Giddens (1991), personal resources are inextricably fused with how experience unfolds, and he termed the confluence of actors and social circumstances structuration—the spawning of generative and emergent outcomes tacitly shaped by conventions of interaction. No matter how elusive the linkage, it is crucial to obtain a clearer understanding of how social bonds shape perceptions and lived experiences (Dannefer, 2003).

Phenomenologists urge researchers to "bracket" their own taken-for-granted assumptions and to learn from the individuals they study (Berger & Luckmann, 1967). For our purposes here, they should actively avoid a middle-class anchoring of such constructs as lifestyle. Feminist theorists incorporate a further dimension of social relativity by adopting the perspective of disenfranchised groups. With respect to aging and lifestyle, how do individuals in disenfranchised groups perceive their own aging experiences? What constitutes "aging well" or "successful aging" for members of these groups? As Dorothy Smith (1990) asked, do these individuals experience a bifurcation of consciousness between culturally accepted representations of "healthy" or "successful" lifestyles associated with opportunities and interests of dominant groups, and their own lived experiences (Holstein & Minkler, 2003)?

Wray's (2003) study of older women illustrates how marginalized groups construct personal definitions of "quality of life" and "successful aging" distinct from those implied by prevailing models. Despite economic disadvantage and racism, Wray found that many of the women "through practices of resistance and negotiation, maintain a quality of life that is not simply dependent on access to material resources" (p. 517). They developed strategies to remain involved in personally meaningful activities despite health limitations or disabilities. Wray's research revealed strong themes of freedom, self-control, and personal agency expressed by women who would otherwise be assessed as having a poor quality of life and less-than-successful aging, by virtue of commonly accepted conceptual-

izations. Ball and Whittington (1995) proffered similar insights in an analysis of older African Americans: despite what might be considered dire circumstances, a kind of successful aging was being lived out. In highlighting such conclusions, we do not wish to minimize or negate genuine hardship faced by disadvantaged groups. On the contrary, it is crucial to consider strategies used and meanings ascribed to experience by actors themselves.

## B. Conceptualizing Lifestyle: A Personal Resource Model

The challenge is to extend explanatory frameworks that do not disconnect context, experience, and meaning-construction from distinctions associated with status groupings and other social circumstances, dynamic environmental conditions, or available resources. As actors age, experience and opportunities to adapt are contingent on resources. Consistent with Lawton's notion of environmental press and Bronfenbrenner's (1979) "ecology of human development," we maintain the resources accessible by individuals, which are part and parcel of their lifestyles, are selected and provide the wherewithal to manage environments or buffer ill effects.

Figure 17.1 represents an initial conceptualization of lifestyle in terms of a "personal resource model." The nonrecursive model proposed encompasses constitutive elements of lifestyles and helps illuminate how key aspects of lifestyle are used as individuals find themselves in one or another situation. The model also stresses the intertwining of diverse resource dimensions to highlight connections between lifestyle and individual outcomes, thereby reuniting agency and milieu, contingencies central to lifestyles. Both structural conditions and personal agency are implicit in the model.

The following discussion addresses features of the model within the framework

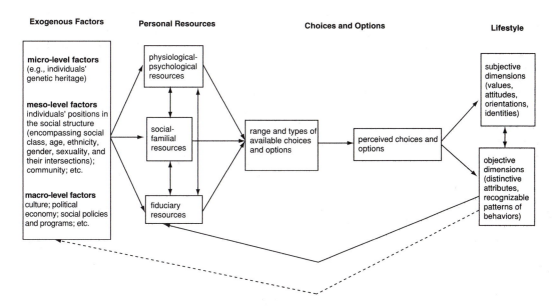

**Figure 17.1** Conceptualizing Lifestyle: A Personal Resource Model

of factors shown in Figure 17.1: exogenous factors, personal resources, choices and options, and lifestyle. We begin at the far right side of the model in order to initiate discussion with a central question raised in this chapter: What is lifestyle?

*1. Lifestyle*

Our working definition of lifestyle begins with Stebbins' (1997) conceptualization, noted earlier. Stebbins defined lifestyles as distinctive attributes or recognizable patterns of behaviors reflecting shared interests and life situations incorporating related values, attitudes, and orientations that create characteristic social identities. It may be helpful both to disaggregate and broaden this definition. Rather than encapsulating lifestyle solely as (presumably) observable "distinctive attributes or recognizable patterns of behavior," individuals' *subjective perceptions* of their behaviors or situations, and

their own identities, also are important components of lifestyle—which interleave with observable attributes and patterns of behaviors. Drawing from Stebbins, "values, attitudes and orientations" do *shape* lifestyle, but we contend that these subjective dimensions, including individuals' perceptions and identities, also can be seen as *components* of lifestyle. We refer to these as subjective dimensions of lifestyle. "Objective" dimensions of lifestyle make up the distinctive attributes or recognizable patterns of behaviors suggested by Stebbins.

Whether defined in terms of actors' perceptions, identities, and the like, or in terms of actors' recognizable attributes or patterned behaviors, operationalizations of lifestyle depend on particular manifestations of the lifestyle concept that are of interest. For example, the concept of "healthy lifestyle" may be operationalized subjectively in terms of whether individuals perceive that their lifestyle is healthy (Jolanki, 2004), or objectively in terms of specific parameters designated by the researcher (such as specified physical activity levels) (Ross & Bird, 1994); or the concept may be operationalized using both subjective *and* objective measures.

In making a distinction between subjective and objective dimensions of lifestyle, we recognize that features of the social world presumed to be objective must be perceived and labeled as such. Berger and Luckmann (1967) referred to this as "the moment of objectivation" in the social construction of reality. The dialectical relationship between subjective and objective dimensions of lifestyle is reflected in the double-headed arrow shown in the model.

### 2. Choices and Options

The range and types of choices and options available to actors help shape their lifestyles, both in terms of subjective (values, attitudes, and self-identities) and objective (recognized attributes or patterns of behavior) lifestyle dimensions. Based on the preceding discussion, actors must *perceive* that various choices and options are accessible, that they are objectively "real" in this sense, in order to act on them. Hence, effects of the "range and types of available choices" on lifestyle outcomes are filtered through individuals' "perceived choices and options," as shown in Figure 17.1.

### 3. Personal Resources

Access to key resources influences the range and types of choices that are available to individuals. Although the three dimensions of personal resources reviewed here are intertwined, they will be disaggregated for purposes of discussion.

Physiological-psychological resources, termed psychophysical capital by O'Rand (2001), refer to functional conditions, capabilities, and competencies essential for individuals to engage the ongoing flow of events. Physical health, ability to perform activities of daily living, sensory acuities appropriate for registering environmental input, and cognitive competencies essential for acquiring, processing, synthesizing, or managing environmental cues are part of the stock of physiological-psychological resources on which individuals depend. So are hearing, vision, information processing, motor performance, kinesthetic sense, sensory thresholds, and so forth that, in combination with physical health and vigor, affect an actor's autonomy. Serious erosion in any subset will impose functional limitations, compromising autonomy and ability to maintain any mode of being in the world. Control is curtailed when decrements result in cues not being perceived or responses not being possible. Functionality is integral to lifestyles and managing or taking advantage of opportunities. Physical and psychological functionality are immediate mediators of experience and therefore of lifestyles.

Social-familial resources represent those social relationships and interpersonal networks vital to experience and to coping. The linkages constitute social capital, implying actors' access to interpersonal support and exchange helpful in buffering ill effects and adaptation. Individuals may be conceived of as the intersection of a chain of relational networks, and it is from these chains that individuals perceive direction, attachment, and anchorage. Social bonds afford affirmational promise, instrumental and emotional assistance, and have pervasive effects that define experience. Although social resources are keys to physical and psychological outcomes, as well as opportunities, not all relationships are assets. Indeed, relationships that offer supportive benefits may also be sources of stress (Ingersoll-Dayton, Morgan, & Antonucci, 1997). What is crucial is how individuals perceive, integrate, and act in light of these social bonds and linkages.

Finally, the medium of exchange, whether that be money or any other barterable items, also affects how experience unfolds, as it is implicated in ability to negotiate in a desirable coin of the realm. Some fiduciary resources equate to money but other created or token currencies also serve as negotiable instruments traded to gain advantage or exercise control. Beyond their transactional value, pecuniary resources also serve as social markers, assessments of worth, and delineate circles of confidence radiating around particular actors or contexts.

In sum, these three interconnected dimensions of personal resources are constitutive of lifestyles. In this sense, personal resources are considered *both* as causal factors in the development of lifestyles or in enabling lifestyles *and* as dynamic outcomes shaped by the perceptions and behaviors that reflect lifestyle. One's "health lifestyle," for example, can influence types and levels of physiological-psychological resources available to individuals (shown in Figure 17.1 by the reverse arrow from lifestyle outcomes back to personal resource factors), which shape individuals' choices and options, which in turn are expressed in lifestyle outcomes.

Meeting one's needs or making one's way in any particular life space is contingent on an individual's inventory of each type of resource, perceptions of their adequacy, and ability to mobilize resources as need arises. Personal resources are complex, multidimensional, and interconnected, vital elements predictive of how an individual fares in life. Without an abil-

ity to engage ongoing events, without interpersonal resources on which to rely, and without sufficient fiduciary resources, life is more challenging. None of these resources are sufficient in and of themselves to ensure lifestyles or even to determine the prospects of aging, but they do interact to shape the nature of experience.

### 4. Exogenous Factors

Exogenous factors are included in Figure 17.1 to emphasize that features of the personal resource model that have been discussed thus far are not self-contained. The resources available to individuals derive from a variety of sources, traceable to phenomena at the micro-level or individual level (e.g., individuals' genetic heritage), the meso-level (individuals' social locations, including social class, age, ethnicity, gender, social class, sexuality, the intersections between these, community-level factors, etc.), and the macro-level (including cultural systems, the political-economic structure of society, extant social policies and programs, etc.). As exogenous factors, these phenomena are not explained by the variables included in the personal resource model. The reverse arrow from lifestyle outcomes to "exogenous factors" is marked with a dashed line, however, to highlight that some degree of mobility may be possible with regard to certain dimensions of individuals' social locations (e.g., social class), and that through "joint action" (Blumer, 1967), actors may influence communities and even larger social structures.

The model proffered here does not encompass all of the dimensions that shape or reflect lifestyle outcomes. In particular, the model does not incorporate an explicit temporal dimension. We recognize that personal resources, as well as individuals' lifestyle outcomes, typically are cumulative in nature, and that they are contingent on specific points in the individual and family life course, environmental conditions, and broader cultural, political-economic, social-historical contexts.

## IV. Conclusion

The path by which individuals arrive at old age is not predetermined; it is a reflection of lifestyle practices along the way. These practices derive from individual choices and behaviors, as well as from social circumstances. From these foundations both human and social capital are derived and both are integral to the aging experience. Aging is a consequence of lifestyles that are both antecedents to and concomitants of the process. Without putting too fine a point on it, the constitutive elements of lifestyle are the basis of heterogeneity found among old people. Although personal agency is important in behavior and action, the parameters of choice are set by social circumstances. Musolf (2003) asserted that social circumstances, including arrangements, relations, and practices, precede individual choice, exert enormous power and constraint over life, and are contained in the conventions of lifestyles. If we are to avoid a bifurcation of objective and subjective aspects of experience, personal choice and structural constraints must be recognized as formative of lifestyles. In turn, understanding the role of lifestyles is essential to gaining insight on how the self-structure dialectic shapes the way in which lives unfold, reflecting opportunity structures and personal action, relative position and consumption patterns.

This review highlights the need for empirical and conceptual development in the study of lifestyle and aging. An abiding question concerns the lifestyle construct: how to index it and how to assess it. Some might say that lifestyles per se are too ephemeral. Should lifestyle be conceptualized in ways that promote quantifiable, rigorous, and reliable standardized measurement? Or should it be understood phenomenologically, from the perspectives of individuals themselves? There is no doubt that sustained research efforts are needed for a more satisfactory understanding, and that even greater efforts are needed to understand linkages between lifestyle and aging. Certainly one approach need not and should not take precedence over others. With the caveat that researchers of all stripes should strive to consider the complex relationships inherent to the study of lifestyle and aging, the use of diverse conceptualizations and methodologies will fuel this agenda. There is room to spare in this multistoried undertaking.

## References

Abeles, R. (2003). Some thoughts on aging, social structures, and sense of control. In S. Zarit, L. Pearlin, & K. Schaie (Eds.), *Personal control in social and life course contexts* (pp. 23–32). New York: Springer.

Allport, G. (1968). Is the concept of the self necessary? In C. Gordon & K. Gergen (Eds.), *The self in social interaction* (pp. 25–32). New York: Wiley (original work published 1955).

Andrews, G., Clark, M., & Luszcz, M. (2002). Successful aging in the Australian longitudinal study of aging: Applying the MacArthur model cross-nationally. *Journal of Social Issues, 58,* 749–765.

Avison, W. R., & Cairney, J. (2003). Personal control and the stress process in midlife. In S. Zarit, L. Pearlin, & K. Schaie (Eds.), *Personal control in social and life course contexts* (pp. 127–164). New York: Springer.

Ball, M., & Whittington, F. (1995). *Surviving dependence: Voices of African American elders.* Amityville, NY: Baywood.

Bandura, A. (1997). *Self-efficacy: The exercise of control.* New York: Freeman.

Beaglehole, R. (1990). International trends in coronary heart disease mortality, morbidity, and risk factors. *Epidemiologic Reviews, 12,* 1–16.

Bellah, R. N., Madsen, R., Sullivan, W. A., Swidler, A., & Tipton, S. M. (1985). *Habits* of the heart: Individualism and commitment in American life. Berkeley: California Press.

Berger, P. L., & Luckmann, T. (1967). The social construction of reality. Garden City, NY: Doubleday & Co.

Blane, D. (1995). Editorial: Social determinants of health—Socioeconomic status, social class, and ethnicity. American Journal of Public Health, 85, 903–904.

Blumer, H. (1967). Symbolic interactionism: Perspective and method. Englewood Cliffs, NJ: Prentice-Hall, Inc.

Bourdieu, P. (1986). The forms of capital. In J. Richardson (Ed.), Handbook of theory and research for the sociology of education (pp. 241–258). Westwood, CT: Greenwood.

Bronfenbrenner, U. (1979). The ecology of human development. Cambridge: Harvard University Press.

Burns, T. R. (1986). Actors, transactions, and social structure. In U. Himmelstrand (Ed.), Sociology: From crisis to science? Vol. 2, The social reproduction of organization and culture (pp. 8–37). London: Sage.

Cockerham, W. C., Abel, T., & Lueschen, G. (1993). Max Weber, formal rationality, and health lifestyles. Sociological Quarterly, 3, 413–425.

Costa, P., & McCrae, R. (1994). Set like plaster? Evidence for stability of adult personality. In T. Heatherton & S. Weinberger (Eds.), Can personality change? (pp. 21–40). Washington, DC: American Psychological Association.

Dannefer, D. (2003). Cumulative advantage/disadvantage and the life course: Cross-fertilizating age and social science theory. Journal of Gerontology: Social Sciences, 58B, S327–S337.

Danner, D., Snowdon, D., & Friesen, W. (2001). Positive emotions in early life and longevity: Findings from the Nun Study. Journal of Personality and Social Psychology, 80, 804–813.

Faris, R. E. L., & Dunham. H. W. (1960). Mental disorders in urban areas. New York: Hafner. (Original work published in 1939.)

Fredrickson, B. L. (2003). The value of positive emotions. American Scientist, 91, 330–335.

George, L. (2003). Embedding control beliefs in social and cultural context. In S. Zarit,

L. Pearlin, & K. Schaie (Eds.), Personal control in social and life course contexts (pp. 33–43). New York: Springer.

Giddens, A. (1984). The constitution of society: Outline of a theory of structuration. Berkeley, CA: University of California Press.

Giddens, A. (1991). Modernity and self-identity: Self and society in the late modern age. Cambridge: Polity Press.

Glyptis, S. (1989). Lifestyles and leisure patterns—methodological approaches. In B. Filipovva, S. Glyptis, & W. Tokarski (Eds.), Lifestyles: Theories, concepts, methods and results of lifestyle research in international perspective (pp. 37–67). Prague: Academy of Sciences.

Gordon, C. C., & Longino C. F. (2000). Age structure and social structure. Contemporary Sociology, 29, 699–703.

Grzywacz, J. G., & Marks, N. F. (2001). Social inequalities and exercise during adulthood: Toward an ecological perspective. Journal of Health and Social Behavior, 42, 202–220.

Hagestad, G., & Dannefer, D. (2001). Concepts and theories of aging: Beyond microfication in social science approaches. In R. Binstock & L. George (Eds.), Handbook of aging and the social sciences (5th ed., pp. 3–21). San Diego: Academic Press.

Hankin, J. (2000). Lifestyles and health. In E. Borgatta & R. Montgomery (Eds.), Encyclopedia of sociology (pp. 1639–1643). New York: Macmillan.

Hayward, M. D., Crimmins, E. M., Miles, T. P., & Yang, Y. (2000). The significance of socioeconomic status in explaining the racial gap in chronic health conditions. American Sociological Review, 65, 910–930.

Hennen, J. R., & Knudten, R. D. (2001). A lifestyle analysis of the elderly: Perceptions of risk, fear, and vulnerability. Illness, Crisis and Loss, 9, 190–208.

Herskovits, E. J., & Mitteness, L. S. (1994). Transgressions and sickness in old age. Journal of Aging Studies, 8, 327–340.

Holstein, M. B., & Minkler, M. (2003). Self, society and the "new gerontology." The Gerontologist, 43, 787–796.

Hooker, K., & McAdams, D. P. (2003). Personality and adult development: Looking beyond the OCEAN. *Journal of Gerontology: Psychological Sciences, 58B*, P296–P304.

House, J., Kessler, R., Herzog, A., Mero, R., Kinney, A., & Breslow, M. (1992). Social stratification, age, and health. In K. Schaie, D. Blazer, & J. House (Eds.), *Aging, health behaviors, and health outcomes* (pp. 1–32). Hillsdale, NJ: Lawrence Erlbaum Associates.

Hubert, H. B., Block, D. A., Oehlert, J. W., & Fries, J. F. (2002). Lifestyle habits and compression of morbidity. *Journal of Gerontology: Medical Sciences, 57A*, M347–M351.

Ingersoll-Dayton, B., Morgan, D., & Antonucci, T. (1997). The effects of positive and negative social exchanges on aging adults. *Journals of Gerontology: Psychological Sciences and Social Sciences, 52B*, S190–S199.

Jasso, G. (2001). Studying status: An integrated framework. *American Sociological Review, 66*, 96–124.

Jolanki, O. (2004). Negotiating "healthy behavior" and its relation to old age in group discussions. Presented at the annual meeting of the Gerontological Society of America, November 19–23, Washington, DC.

Katz, S., & Marshall, B. (2003). New sex for old: Lifestyle, consumerism, and the ethics of aging well. *Journal of Aging Studies, 17*, 3–16.

Krause, N. (2003). The social foundations of personal control in later life. In S. Zarit, L. Pearlin, & K. Schaie (Eds.), *Personal control in social and life course contexts* (pp. 45–70). New York: Springer.

Laditka, S. B., & Laditka, J. N. (2001). Effects of improved morbidity rate on active life expectancy and eligibility for long-term care services. *Journal of Applied Gerontology 20*, 39–56.

Lawton, M. P. (1985). The elderly in context: Perspectives from environmental psychology and gerontology. *Environment and Behavior, 17*, 501–519.

Lewin, K. (1939). Field theory and experiment in social psychology: Concepts and methods. *American Journal of Sociology, 44*, 868–897.

Link, B., & Phelan, J. (1995). Social conditions as fundamental causes of disease. *Journal of Health and Social Behavior, 38* (supplement), 80–94.

Marger, M. N. (2005). *Social inequality: Patterns and processes* (3rd ed.). New York: McGraw Hill.

Marmot, M. (2004). *Status syndrome: How your social standing directly affects your health and life expectancy*. London: Bloomsbury.

Matarazzo, J. (1983). Behavioral health: A 1990 challenge for the health sciences professions. In J. Matarazzo, N. Miller, S. Weiss, J. Herd, & S. Weiss (Eds.), *Behavioral health: A handbook of health enhancement and disease prevention* (pp. 3–40). New York: Wiley.

Mechanic, D. (1978). *Medical sociology*. New York: Free Press.

Moen, P., & Chermack, H. (forthcoming). Gender disparities in health: Strategic selection, careers, and cycles of control. *Journals of Gerontology: Social Sciences, 60B (Special Issue II)*, 99–108.

Musolf, G. R. (2003). Social structure, human agency, and social policy. *International Journal of Sociology and Social Policy, 23*, 1–12.

Myers, J. H., & Gutman, J. (1974). Lifestyle: The essence of social class. In W. Wells (Ed.), *Lifestyle and psychographics* (pp. 235–256). Chicago: American Marketing Association.

Neugarten, B. (1977). Personality and aging. In J. Birren & K. Schaie (Eds.), *Handbook of the psychology of aging* (pp. 626–649). New York: Van Nostrand-Reinhold.

O'Rand, A. (2001). Stratification and the life course: The forms of life-course capital and their interrelationships. In R. Binstock & L. George (Eds.), *Handbook of aging and the social sciences* (5th ed., pp. 197–213). San Diego: Academic Press

O'Rand, A., & Henretta, J. (1999). *Age and inequality: Diverse pathways through later life*. Boulder, CO: Westview Press.

Pearlin, L. (1989) The sociological study of stress. *Journal of Health and Social Behavior, 30*, 241–256.

Pearlin, L., & Pioli. M. (2003). Personal control: Some conceptual turf and future directions. In S. Zarit, L. Pearlin, &

K. Schaie. (Eds.), *Personal control in social and life course contexts* (pp. 1–21). New York: Springer.

Preston, S., & Taubman, P. (1994). Socio-economic differences in adult mortality and health status. In L. Martin & S. Preston (Eds.), *Demography of aging* (pp. 279–318). Washington, DC: National Academy Press.

Pulkkinen, L., & Caspi, A. (Eds.). (2002). *Paths to successful development: Personality in the life course.* Cambridge: Cambridge University Press.

Pullen, C., Walker, S. N., & Fiandt, K. (2001). Determinants of health-promoting lifestyle behaviors in rural older women. *Family and Community Health, 24,* 49–72.

Ritzer, George. (1996.) *Modern sociological theory* (4th ed). New York: McGraw-Hill.

Roberts, B. W., & DelVecchio, W. F. (2000). The rank-order consistency of personality from childhood to old age: A quantitative review of longitudinal studies. *Psychological Bulletin, 126,* 3–25.

Ross, C. E., & Bird, C. E. (1994). Sex stratification and health lifestyle. *Journal of Health and Social Behavior, 35,* 161–178.

Ross, C. E., & Mirowsky, J. (2002). Family relationships, social support and subjective life expectancy. *Journal of Health and Social Behavior, 43,* 469–489.

Rowe, J., & Kahn, R. (1998). *Successful aging.* New York: Random House.

Siegler, I., Kaplan, B., Von Dras, D., & Mark, D. (1999). Cardiovascular health: A challenge for midlife. In S. Willis & J. Reid (Eds.), *Life in the middle: Psychological and social development in middle age* (pp. 147–157). San Diego: Academic Press.

Small, B., Hertzog, C., Hultsch, D, & Dixon, R. (2003). Stability and change in adult personality over 6 years: Findings from the Victoria longitudinal study. *Journal of Gerontology: Psychological Sciences, 55B,* P166–P176.

Smith, D. E. (1990). *The conceptual practices of power: A feminist sociology of knowledge.* Boston: Northeastern University Press.

Sobel, M. E. (1981). *Lifestyle and social structure: Concepts, definitions, analyses.* New York: Academic Press.

Stebbins, R. A. (1997). Lifestyle as a generic concept in ethnographic research. *Quality and Quantity, 31,* 347–360.

Steverink, N., Westerhof, G. J., Bode, C., & Dittmann-Kohli, F. (2001). The personal experience of aging, individual resources, and subjective well-being. *Journal of Gerontology: Psychological Sciences, 56B,* P364–P373.

Turner, J. H. (2003). *The structure of sociological theory* (7th ed.). Belmont, CA: Wadsworth.

Turner, R. J., Lloyd, D., & Roszell, P. (1999). Personal resources and the social distribution of depression. *American Journal of Community Psychology, 27,* 643–672.

Turner, R. J., & Roszell, P. (1994). Psychosocial resources and the stress process. In W. Avison & I. Gotlib (Eds.), *Stress and mental health: Contemporary issues and prospects for the future* (pp. 179–210). New York: Plenum.

Turner, R. J., Wheaton, B., & Lloyd, D. A. (1995). The epidemiology of social stress. *American Sociological Review, 60,* 104–125.

Walters, G. D. (1998). Three existential contributions to a theory of lifestyles. *Journal of Humanistic Psychology, 38,* 25–40.

Weber, M. (1966). Class, status and party. In R. Bendix & S. Lipset (Eds.), *Class, status, and power* (pp. 21–28). New York: Free Press.

Wight, C. (1999). They shoot dead horses don't they? Locating agency in the agent-structure problematique. *European Journal of International Relations, 5,* 109–142.

Wray, S. (2003). Women growing older: Agency, ethnicity and culture. *Sociology, 37,* 511–527.

Zarit, S., & Leitsch, S. (2003). Applications of personal control. In S. Zarit, L. Pearlin, & K. Schaie (Eds.), *Personal control in social and life course contexts* (pp. 281–300). New York: Springer.

Zarit, S., & Pearlin, L. (Eds.) (2005). Health inequalities across the life course. *Journal of Gerontology: Social Science, 60B (Special Issue II).*

Zarit, S., Pearlin, L., & Schaie, K. W. (Eds.). (2003). *Personal control in social and life course contexts.* New York: Springer.

# Eighteen

# Perceived Quality of Life

Linda K. George

The history of gerontology is, in many ways, the chronicle of scientific efforts to understand well-being in later life. As historians of gerontology note (e.g., Achenbaum, 1995), concern about the well-being of older adults was the driving force of early gerontological research. Indeed, the purpose of the first major, multidisciplinary studies of aging, the Kansas City Studies (Cumming & Henry, 1961; Neugarten, 1968) and the Duke Longitudinal Studies of Normal Aging (Palmore, 1970), was to identify both the nature of life quality in old age and the conditions that underpin well-being.

Although quality of life no longer dominates gerontological research, well-being remains a vital part of aging research in the social and behavioral sciences. In part this results from the desire to monitor the effects of social change, cohort characteristics and composition, and public policies on the well-being of the older population. As the measurement and our understanding of well-being have matured, however, quality of life has become part of research traditions that are beyond gerontology, but relevant to it. Two examples illustrate this point.

The U.S. Food and Drug Administration (FDA) is grappling with quality of life issues now that were below its radar screen a short decade ago. Pharmaceutical companies are now encouraged to include quality of life as an outcome in clinical trials. At the same time, however, the FDA has been unable to develop uniform criteria for interpreting quality of life claims (Lewis, 2001). Another example is provided by health economists, some of whom advocate allocating health resources in part on the trade-offs in longevity that health care consumers are willing to make to sustain life quality (e.g., Torrance, 1986). And when it comes to decisions about quantity versus quality of life, most of the relevant consumers are old.

This chapter reviews the broad landscape of research on quality of life among older adults; it is organized in five sections. The first examines the complex conceptual and definitional issues underlying research on subjective well-being, quality of life, and related constructs. Please note that after the first section, the terms *quality of life* and *subjective well-being* are used interchangeably. The

*Handbook of Aging and the Social Sciences, Sixth Edition*

second section reviews evidence that social factors are robust predictors of subjective well-being in late life. The third focuses on the psychosocial mechanisms that partially explain the links between social factors and perceptions of well-being. The fourth section takes a broader view, examining comparative studies of quality of life and the putative factors that account for cross-cultural differences. The chapter ends with suggestions for future research on subjective well-being in late life.

## I. Conceptualizing and Defining Quality of Life

Although defining and measuring quality of life (QoL) and related constructs often appear straightforward, the underlying conceptual issues are quite complex. After several decades of research, conceptual and operational consensus remains an elusive goal. There are, however, major "schools of thought" about how to conceptualize and measure QoL, each with its advocates and some degree of empirical support.

## II. Is Quality of Life an Objective or Subjective Phenomenon?

The largest bifurcation in QoL research is whether it should be conceptualized as a purely subjective assessment of personal well-being or whether more objective indicators of life conditions (e.g., health, financial status) should also be included. As Diener and Suh (1997) noted, these conceptualizations of life quality rest on distinct philosophies. Researchers who define QoL as a combination of objective characteristics and subjective perceptions take a normative stance. That is, there are implicit assumptions that scientists are competent to develop valid standards of life quality and that those standards are

universally applicable. Scholars who posit that QoL means different things to different people and rests on self-evaluation take a non-normative, experiential stance. Both strategies are strongly represented in the research literature.

Scholars who conceptualize QoL as a mixture of subjective perceptions and objective characteristics typically use multidimensional scales that yield both global QoL scores and dimension-specific scores. The SF-36 is probably the most widely-used multidimensional QoL scale (e.g., Ware & Sherbourne, 1992). The 36 items in the scale tap eight dimensions of well-being: physical activity limitations, health-related limitations in social activities, health-related limitations in normal role activities (e.g., paid labor, housekeeping), bodily pain, psychological distress and well-being, limitations in role activities resulting from emotional problems, vitality (energy and fatigue), and general health perceptions. Another multidimensional measure is the World Health Organization's WHOQOL-BREF (The WHOQOL Group, 1998), which assesses four dimensions of quality of life: physical health, psychological functioning, social relationships, and the environment. The primary advantage of this approach is the broad range of information on which summary QoL scores are based.

The competing conceptual framework posits that QoL is a purely subjective assessment of one's well-being. A corollary assumption is that, although objective life conditions may be strongly related to QoL, they are not synonymous with it. Subjective reports of QoL are ascertained using a variety of measures ranging from single-item reports of satisfaction with life to multi-item scales tapping life satisfaction or morale. One of the confusing facets of this conceptualization of QoL is that terms including *life satisfaction*, *subjective well-being* (SWB), and *morale* tend to be used interchangeably. Empirical evidence suggests, however, that measures of these concepts are highly correlated with each other and with relevant personal and social characteristics.

## III. Is "Successful Aging" the Same as Quality of Life?

During the past few decades, the term *successful aging* has appeared in the gerontological literature with increasing frequency. Are successful aging and quality of life synonymous? As used in most research, successful aging aligns more closely with the multidimensional approach than the subjective one. Indeed, it is not clear that perceptions of well-being play any part in definitions of successful aging.

Consider the definition posited by Rowe and Kahn (1998), who contend that three criteria define successful aging: low levels of disease and disability, high physical and cognitive functioning, and active engagement with life. At first glance, these characteristics seem to be uncontroversial indicators of aging well. I find this definition problematic, however, in at least two ways. First, any notion that subjective perceptions of well-being are a part of successful aging is conspicuously absent. Is an older adult successfully aging if he is disability-free, physically and cognitive intact, and generally active, but rates the quality of his life as poor? Second, this definition suggests that older adults with disability, or who experience declines in physical and cognitive function, or who cannot or do not remain active are aging unsuccessfully. This conclusion is clearly at odds with the large numbers of older adults who report high levels of well-being *despite* physical, cognitive, and/or social deficits. As Minkler and Fadem (2002) point out, taking Rowe and Kahn's definition of successful aging seriously stigmatizes and marginalizes a significant proportion of the older population.

The underlying issue here is essentially the one that underpins debates about multidimensional versus purely subjective conceptualizations of QoL: the size of the relationships between objective life conditions and perceptions of well-being. If the relationships between individuals' SWB and their objective conditions are large and consistent, joining them conceptually and operationally is justified. Rowe and Kahn would take this a step further and eliminate subjective perceptions entirely. Empirical research, however, demonstrates large mismatches between objective conditions and SWB. Among American adults of all ages, objective life conditions explain only about half of the variance in SWB (e.g., Diener, 1984). Among older adults, large proportions of disabled older adults report high levels of QoL (e.g., Pennex, Guralnik, Simonsick, Kasper, Ferrucci, & Fried, 1998) and sizeable proportions of disability-free adults report low levels of QoL (Covinksy et al., 1999). Thus, the problems with multidimensional measures are that they confound QoL with its objective antecedents and ignore the mismatches that demonstrate the need to understand the full range of factors that underlie perceptions of life quality. Definitions of successful aging such as that proposed by Rowe and Kahn are even more problematic because subjective perceptions are totally ignored.

## IV. Is Quality of Life Responsive to Changing Internal and External Circumstances?

The extent to which personal characteristics are changeable is an important and often overlooked issue in social science research. A highly stable characteristic, for example, is a poor choice as an outcome in studies that examine the effects of aging, personal experience, or social dynamics. A rapidly changing characteristic is problematic as well if it is inherently unstable or transitory. Evidence about the changeability of SWB is mixed. Longitudinal studies of SWB suggest that it is quite stable over time (Costa, Zonderman, McCrae, & Cornoni-Huntley, 1987; Fujita & Diener, 2005; Pavot & Diener, 1993; Suh, Diener, & Fujita, 1996—length of observation in these studies ranged from 2 to 17 years). Other evidence indicates that SWB changes in response to major changes in life conditions (e.g., McCrae & Costa, 1993; Mroczek & Spiro, 2005).

A related issue is whether SWB is useful for public policy. Accumulated evidence suggests that it is. Indeed, social indicators research rests on the assumption that monitoring SWB and other population parameters across societies and over time within societies is a useful strategy for determining the extent to which societies meet the needs of their members and identifying subgroups whose needs are not being met, informa-tion especially relevant to welfare policies in the broadest sense. Proponents of SWB view it as analogous to gross domestic product (GDP) and believe that policy makers should act to maximize both (e.g., Veenhoven, 1996).

## V. Determinants of Subjective Well-Being

The vast majority of research on SWB to date focuses on the relationships between objective life conditions and perceived life quality. Despite hundreds of previous studies, a consensual conceptual model of the determinants of SWB remains out of reach. Figure 18.1 is my attempt to place the identified predictors of SWB in an overall conceptual model. Although most research to date is based on cross-sectional data, the proposed model is designed to provide both a temporal and conceptual template for understanding the determinants of SWB. In addition, the model suggests that some of the determinants of SWB will be partially or totally

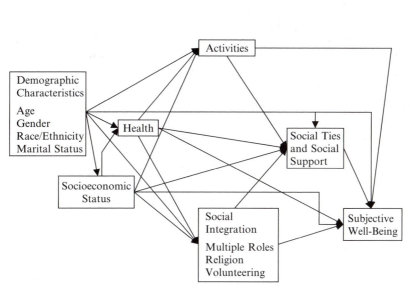

**Figure 18.1** Conceptual model of the determinants of subjective well-being.

mediated by predictors that appear in later stages of the model. Even if all of the effects of some predictors are indirect, they are meaningful determinants of SWB. Although this model has not been put to empirical test, previous research that supports it is reviewed in this section.

A cautionary note is appropriate at this point. All of the studies cited in this section are multivariate; that is, the effects of specific predictors are examined with other known or hypothesized determinants of SWB statistically controlled. But no study cited examined all the predictors included in this review.

# VI. Demographic Characteristics

## A. Age

Campbell, Converse, and Rodgers (1976) were among the first to demonstrate that older adults are more satisfied with their lives, on average, than middle-age and younger adults, a pattern that remains true (e.g., George, Okun, & Landerman, 1985). Even in samples restricted to middle-age and older persons, levels of SWB increase with age (Steverink, Westerhof, Bode, & Dittmann-Kohli, 2001; Tran, Wright, & Chatters, 1991). Mroczek & Spiro (2005), who examined 22 years of data in the all-male Normative Aging Study, reported that SWB peaked at age 65 and declined slightly thereafter. The contradiction between the cross-sectional and longitudinal studies is probably more apparent than real; even with gradual decreases in SWB during late life, levels of life satisfaction remain high.

## B. Gender

Older women report significantly lower levels of SWB than older men, as demonstrated in a meta-analysis of 300 studies (Pinquart & Soerensen, 2001). It also appears that gender interacts with age. In a study that included 146,000 adults from 65 nations, Inglehart (2002) found that women below the age of 45 reported higher levels of SWB than their male counterparts, but lower levels of SWB at age 45 and older. Pinquart and Soerensen (2001) also reported that the gender gap in SWB widens with age.

## C. Race/Ethnicity

Most investigators find that race/ethnicity is not significantly related to SWB (e.g., Campbell et al., 1976). Even when significant bivariate racial/ ethnic differences are observed, they usually disappear when socioeconomic status (SES) is taken into account (e.g., Brown, 1988; Krause, 1993).

## D. Marital Status and Marital Transitions

Married adults of all ages report higher levels of SWB than the unmarried (see Pinquart & Soerensen, 2001, for a meta-analysis based on 300 studies and Diener, Gohm, Suh, & Oishi, 2000, for an analysis based on more than 59,000 respondents in 45 countries). Nonetheless, limited evidence suggests that there is more to be learned about this relationship. George and colleagues (1985) observed an age by marital status interaction such that marital status was a less powerful predictor of SWB among persons age 65 and older than among those between 40 and 64 years old. In a study of older Swedes, Jakobsson, Hallberg, and Westergren (2004) reported that the relationship between marital status and SWB was explained by living arrangements. Specifically, living alone, rather than marital status, predicted lower SWB.

Widowhood is common in later life, especially among older women. Researchers consistently report that widowhood triggers significant declines in SWB, but that levels of life satisfaction typically rebound to pre-widowhood levels within

1 to 2 years (e.g., Lucas, Clark, Georgellis, & Diener, 2003; Mastekaasa, 1994). Similarly, after examining 22 years of data in the Normative Aging Study, Mroczek and Spiro (2005) reported that, along with changes in health, changes in marital status were the strongest predictors of changes in SWB. Based on their meta-analysis of 300 studies, Pinquart and Soerensen (2001) reported that increased rates of widowhood explain part of the gender gap in SWB during late life.

## VII. Socioeconomic Status

Among middle-age and younger adults, income is the strongest single predictor of SWB (e.g., Campbell et al., 1976); among older adults income usually ranks second in its power to explain differences in SWB. In another meta-analysis (of 286 studies), Pinquart and Soerensen (2000) reported that education and income are both strong predictors of SWB during late life, with income the stronger of the two. There are occasional exceptions to this pattern, however. For example, Bowling and colleagues (Bowling, Banister, Sutton, Evans, & Windsor, 2002), reported that SES was not a significant predictor of SWB in their sample of British older adults. Recognizing that this is an unusual finding, the authors suggested that it reflects the greater financial and health care benefits offered by the British welfare state relative to other countries, especially the United States. Satisfaction with financial resources also is a significant predictor of SWB, even with education and income statistically controlled (Jakobsson et al., 2004; Morris, 1997).

SES is a more "proximal" predictor of SWB than are demographic characteristics and plays an intervening role between some demographic characteristics and SWB. For example, some of the gender gap in SWB in late life is explained by women's lower average levels of financial resources (Pinquart & Soerensen, 2001). Similarly, bivariate differences in SWB that are occasionally observed between older African Americans and Caucasians typically disappear when SES is taken into account (e.g., Brown, 1988; Krause, 1993).

## VIII. Health

The vast majority of studies of SWB in late life find that health is the strongest single predictor (Bowling et al., 2002, in a British sample; George et al., 1985; Kirby, Coleman, & Daley, 2004; Morris, 1997; Pinquart & Soerensen, 2000, in a meta-analysis; Steverink et al., 2001, in a German sample; Tran et al., 1991, in an African-American sample; Windle & Woods, 2004). Self-rated health is the measure of health used in most studies, but some studies use functional and cognitive impairment instead.

In their 22-year study of aging men, Mroczek and Spiro (2005) found that time-varying patterns of health and marital status were the strongest predictors of changes in SWB.

Health is a much weaker predictor of SWB among young and middle-age adults than among older adults (e.g., Campbell et al., 1976; George et al., 1985). This is probably not because health is unimportant to quality of life before old age, but rather that most people take good health for granted before the increased rates of chronic illness experienced by self or peers in later life.

In line with the conceptual model in Figure 18.1, there is limited evidence that health mediates some of the effects of demographic characteristics and SES on SWB in late life (e.g., George et al., 1985; Windle & Woods, 2004).

## IX. Activities

Activities are conceptualized and measured in multiple ways, ranging from those that involve social interaction to purely physical forms of activity to detailed categories based on time-budget data (e.g., for a typical day). In general, all types of activities—social, physical, and solitary—predict higher levels of SWB in late life. This pattern is observed in both cross-sectional (e.g., Warr, Butcher, & Robertson, 2004) and longitudinal studies (e.g., Menec, 2003). Levels of activity also appear to mediate some of the relationships between basic demographic characteristics and perceived life quality. Koltyn (2001), for example, reported that differences in levels of life satisfaction observed between independent and assisted-living residents are almost totally explained by differences in levels of physical activity between the two groups.

## X. Social Integration

Social integration is usually defined as nonfamily attachments to social structure and is measured as the presence or absence of community and civic roles (e.g., Moen, Dempster-McClain, & Williams, 1989). Three types of social integration have been examined as predictors of SWB in late life: number of roles per se, religious participation, and volunteering.

### A. Multiple Roles

Research on age-heterogeneous samples consistently finds that number of roles is positively related to SWB (e.g., Barnett & Baruch, 1985; Moen et al., 1989). Although the research base is more limited, it appears that multiple roles also enhance life quality during old age (Adelmann, 1994). Similarly, loss of community roles during late life has been demonstrated to reduce SWB (Steverink et al., 2001).

Although the general pattern is clearly one in which multiple roles benefit SWB, other research demonstrates the need to examine the effects of specific roles,

rather than relying solely on role counts. There is strong evidence, for example, that acquiring the role of caregiver for an impaired older adult often results in decrements in SWB (e.g., as shown by Pinquart & Soerensen, 2003, in a meta-analysis of 84 articles). Moreover, perceived QoL appears to increase when the caregiving role ends (e.g., Bond, Clark, & Davies, 2003).

### B. Religious Participation

A sizeable body of research documents that religious participation, specifically attending religious services, is a strong, positive predictor of SWB for older adults (e.g., Ellison, Boardman, Williams, & Jackson, 2001; Morris, 1997; Warr et al., 2004). Evidence about the effects of nonorganizational forms of religious involvement is mixed. Ellison and colleagues (2001), for example, found that belief in eternal life was positively related to SWB, but that amount of time spent in private prayer was negatively related to SWB. Krause (2003) reported that finding meaning through religion benefits SWB.

In addition to having a main effect on SWB, religious involvement may enhance life quality by buffering the effects of stress. Evidence in support of the stress-buffering effects of religious beliefs was reported by Ellison and colleagues (2001) and by Kirby and colleagues (2004). The importance of religion as a source of comfort and strength during stressful times is also observed in ethnographic studies of older adults (e.g., Black, 1999).

### C. Volunteering

Although the research base is small, evidence that volunteering fosters SWB is reported in three longitudinal studies of individuals traversing late life (Morrow-Howell, Hinterling, Rozario, & Tang, 2003; Rozario, Morrow-Howell, & Hinterling, 2004; Van Willigen, 2000). In addition, Van Willigen reported that volunteering yields greater benefits for older than for middle-age adults.

## XI. Social Ties and Social Support

Overall, social relationships and social support provided by family and friends are strong predictors of SWB in late life. Several dimensions of social relationships have been studied, including number of significant others, perceived quality of social relationships, received social support, and perceived availability of social support.

In a meta-analysis of 286 studies, Pinquart and Soerensen (2000) found that both number of significant others and the perceived quality of relationships with significant others were robust predictors of SWB, with the latter being the stronger predictor. They also found that relationships with friends and with children had positive, independent effects on life satisfaction. Similarly, Adams and Jackson (2000), using data from the National Survey of Black Americans, found that contacts with friends and with family had strong, independent effects on SWB. They also observed that the effects of these factors were stronger for older than for young and middle-age participants.

Perceptions of social support are consistently strong predictors of perceived life quality during old age, and their effects are stronger than those for received social support (e.g., Bowling et al., 2002; Chappell & Reid, 2002; George et al., 1985), a pattern also observed in age-heterogeneous samples (e.g., Wethington & Kessler, 1986). In a fine-grained study of social support exchanges between German older adults and their adult children, Lang and Schutze (2002) found that receipt of emotional support and expressions of affection from their adult children were associated with higher levels of SWB, but receipt of informational support (e.g., provision of information about

health care and housing options) was associated with lower levels of SWB.

One reason that receipt of social support has weaker, or even negative, effects on SWB is that it may trigger erosion of reciprocity in relationships between older adults and their significant others. Preferences for reciprocity and decreases in SWB when reciprocity is damaged have been reported in Asian samples (Kim & Kim, 2003; Nemoto, 1998), as well as in U.S. and French samples (e.g., Antonucci, Fuhrer, & Jackson, 1990) of older adults.

As hypothesized in Figure 18.1, although evidence is scarce, it appears that social relationships, especially perceptions of high-quality social support, may partially mediate the effects of SES and health on perceived QoL (Landau & Litwin, 2001; Taylor, Chatters, Hardison, & Riley, 2001). That is, older adults who enjoy higher levels of socioeconomic resources and better health sustain higher quality social relationships, which, in turn, foster high levels of SWB.

## XII. Psychosocial Mediators of the Determinants of SWB

In addition to the template of hypothesized distal and proximal determinants presented in Figure 18.1, a largely separate body of research examines the effects of psychosocial characteristics on SWB. In this context, "psychosocial characteristics" refer to the ways that individuals cognitively appraise and process their experiences. Psychosocial characteristics are hypothesized to have both direct effects on SWB and to partially mediate the effects of objective life conditions on SWB.

## XIII. Sense of Control and Related Constructs

Sense of control refers to the extent to which individuals believe that they can control their lives. Although there are subtle differences among them, a number of other concepts, especially mastery and self-efficacy, also refer to individuals' beliefs that they are in command of their lives. There is reasonably strong evidence that sense of control is a significant mediator of the effects of objective life conditions on SWB for older adults. Bisconti and Bergeman (1999), for example, report that sense of control mediates the effects of social support on life satisfaction. Similarly, Windle and Woods (2004) found that sense of mastery largely mediated the effects of functional status and social support on SWB.

Some researchers use composite measures based on multiple psychosocial characteristics. Sharpley and Yardley (1999), for example, reported that "cognitive hardiness" mediates the effects of functional status on SWB. Cognitive hardiness was a composite measure of sense of control, self-efficacy, and sense of meaning.

## XIV. Sense of Meaning

Sense of meaning has emerged as an important psychosocial attribute in recent research. The belief that life is meaningful, despite its uncertainties and challenges, is expected to foster perceived life quality and to mediate the effects of objective life conditions on SWB. There is increasing evidence that sense of meaning is a robust predictor of SWB. With regard to its mediating effects, meaning has been found to largely mediate the effects of religious participation on SWB (Ardelt, 2003) and to partially mediate the effects of education on life satisfaction in late life (Consedine, Magai, & King, 2004).

Sense of coherence, initially conceptualized by Antonovsky (1987), is a composite measure of the extent to which individuals perceive life to be meaningful, predictable, and manageable. Nesbitt and Heidrich (2000) reported that sense of coherence mediates the relationship between functional status and SWB in a sample of older adults.

## XV. Social Comparisons

The importance of social comparisons rests on the fact that we rely on other people to serve as the "yardsticks" against which we compare ourselves. This is especially true for characteristics for which there is no alternate, objective basis of comparison. Thus, our personal assessments of the extent to which we are likeable, polite, humorous, and so forth are usually based on our evaluations of our characteristics relative to other people. A natural corollary of this process is that the people to whom we choose to compare ourselves play a pivotal role in the degree to which our assessments are ultimately positive or negative. The hypothesized link between social comparisons and SWB is straightforward: if we choose to compare our lives with those of people who are less advantaged than we are, we will have "evidence" that the quality of our lives is quite high, a process termed *downward* social comparisons. If, in contrast, we compare ourselves with those who are more advantaged than we are—that is, we use *upward* social comparisons—we are likely to view our lives negatively.

A sizeable body of research indicates that older adults are more likely to use downward social comparisons than are young and middle-age adults. In a recent study of SWB among British older adults, for example, downward social comparisons were shown to largely explain the positive relationship between age and perceived life quality (Gana, Alaphilippe, & Bailey, 2004). In another British study, based on a sample of older adults, downward social comparisons were shown to mediate the effects of multiple objective life conditions of perceived QoL (Beaumont & Kenealy, 2004).

# XVI. Discrepancy Theories

Aspiration theory has long been used to understand the conditions under which individuals view their lives in positive or negative terms. According to this theory, SWB is highest when there is little discrepancy between aspirations and achievements. Conversely, large discrepancies between one's aspirations and achievements lower SWB. Recently, this phenomenon has received increased attention by social scientists, albeit under the label of goal-discrepancy theory. Regardless of label, the central characteristic of discrepancy theory is the comparison of what one has compared to what one wants.

A sizeable body of research demonstrates that aspiration-achievement discrepancies are substantially smaller, on average, among older adults than among young and middle-age adults (e.g., Campbell et al., 1976; Ryff, 1991). Indeed, the close fit of achievements to aspirations largely explains age differences in SWB. More recently, Cheng (2004) compared goal discrepancies in three life domains—material resources, social relationships, and health—across age groups. Relative to their younger peers, older adults reported small discrepancies in material resources and social relationships but larger discrepancies in health. Despite their disadvantage in health, older adults' higher levels of life satisfaction were largely explained by their relative advantages in material resources and social relationships.

# XVII. Strategic Investments of Time and Resources

Some investigators have attempted to elucidate the strategic processes that older adults use to sustain a sense of well-being despite the losses and declines that often occur during late life, especially at advanced ages. Processes examined to date are cognitive reappraisals of one's social and personal investments, decisions about limiting investments of time and resources, and implementing those decisions. Because of the highly cognitive and intrapsychic character of these processes, they can be usefully viewed as psychosocial mediators of the relationships between objective life conditions and SWB.

Based on extensive longitudinal observations in the Berlin Aging Study, Paul and Margaret Baltes and associates (e.g., Baltes & Carstensen, 2003; Freund & Baltes, 1998) observed that the process of selective optimization with compensation (SOC) was used by older adults who were able to sustain high levels of SWB despite the onset of frailty, chronic disease, and social losses (e.g., widowhood). As losses were experienced, these older adults took mental inventory of their investments, prioritized them, discarded low priority investments, and chose to optimize their highest priority investments. When components of a high priority investment were no longer available, they created ways of compensating for the loss. Strong evidence suggests that this sequential strategy preserves SWB with a variety of other known predictors statistically controlled. Carstensen's socioemotional selectivity theory is similar to SOC, but focuses on social relationships. According to this theory, as resources and energy decline in late life, older adults drop or distance themselves from less intimate relationships and increase their emotional investments in relationships with significant others (e.g., Carstensen, 1992; Carstensen, Isaacowitz, & Charles, 1999). An important strength of research on both SOC and socioemotional selectivity is that the empirical results are based on longitudinal data.

# XVIII. A Cautionary Note

Psychosocial characteristics appear to be powerful mediators of the effects of objective life conditions on SWB. It should be kept in mind, however, that indirect effects are as conceptually relevant as direct effects. Thus, the appropriate interpretation of these studies is that objective life conditions are significant predictors of psychosocial characteristics, which, in turn, have strong direct effects on SWB.

## XIX. Cross-Cultural Comparisons

Over the last few decades, SWB has caught the attention of social indicators researchers. The primary goal of social indicators research is to identify and monitor social factors that are valid indicators of how well societies meet the needs of their members. Two basic types of issues are addressed by social indicators research: temporal variations in the same society over time and cross-cultural comparisons. Researchers in this tradition also attempt to explain temporal changes and cross-cultural differences on the basis of historical events and trends, major shifts in political and policy structures, and compositional changes/ differences in populations.

Considerable consensus has emerged for the premise that SWB is a meaningful aggregate indicator of the extent to which societies meet the needs of their members (e.g., Kahn & Juster, 2002). Despite conceptual agreement about the importance of monitoring population levels of SWB, empirical research remains scarce because of data limitations. It is only recently that measures of perceived life quality have been frequently included and, of importance, operationalized identically in population surveys outside the United States.

After more than half a century of national surveys (e.g., the General Social Survey [NORC, 2002]), it is clear that levels of SWB have been quite stable and positive in the U.S. population. Regardless of time of measurement, approximately 85% of Americans rate

their lives as "satisfying" or "very satisfying" (e.g., Campbell et al., 1976; Diener & Diener, 1996). The proportions of older Americans who report high levels of SWB are slightly greater than those reported by young and middle-age adults. Because of the stability of SWB over time in the United States, little has been learned about the social structures and processes that produce increases and decreases in SWB at the population level. It is worth noting that stability in population levels of SWB over time is not unique to the United States, but is widely observed in European countries as well (e.g., Fahey & Smyth, 2004).

Several studies compare levels of SWB across nations. Although these studies do not focus specifically on older adults, they illustrate the potential payoff cross-cultural comparisons have for understanding SWB. The most frequently investigated issue to date is the relationship between income and SWB. Not surprisingly, it is commonly observed that wealthier nations, in terms of average levels of income, have the highest levels of SWB. In arguably the most informative study to date, Fahey and Smyth (2004) examined the relationships between socioeconomic conditions and SWB among 33 European nations. They report that populations in "rich" European Countries (e.g., Germany, Denmark) have high levels of SWB with surprisingly little difference in the reports of the richest and poorest members of those societies. In contrast, population levels of SWB are substantially lower in "poor" European countries (e.g., Greece, Spain), and there are large differences in SWB between the economically advantaged and disadvantaged. It has long been observed that high levels of economic inequality within a society lead to public discontent (e.g., O'Connell, 2004). The Fahey and Smyth study suggests that this pattern applies only to societies in which the overall standard of living is low.

Kirkcaldy, Furnham, and Siefen (2004) compared levels of SWB across 30 nations. Unlike most studies to date, the nations sampled included developing as well as industrialized societies. Because of uncertainties about the equivalence of years of education across countries, the authors examined the relationships between population proportions of reading, mathematical, and scientific literacy with SWB. GDP, economic growth, and inflation rates also were included in the model. Only the three literacy measures were significant predictors of SWB, with reading literacy having the strongest effect.

A recent innovation in social indicators research is the concept of "happy life expectancy." Analogous to active life expectancy, happy life expectancy (HLE) is the estimated average number of years for which individuals report high quality of life. HLE is calculated in the same way that the more familiar active life expectancy is. Cross-sectional reports of SWB across ages are placed in a "life table," thus creating a synthetic life course pattern. Because of the focus on life expectancy, these studies are more directly linked to aging than those based on average levels of SWB. In a study using data from 48 nations, both developed and developing, Veenhoven (1996) reported that HLE is highest in northwest Europe and lowest in Africa. He found that several societal-level variables were significantly related to HLE: population affluence, democratic political systems, population levels of education, and tolerance. Diener and colleagues (Diener, Diener, & Diener, 1995) reported similar findings: HLE was significantly and positively correlated with population affluence, individualism, and human rights protections.

Finally, Diener and Suh (1998) examined the relationship between age and SWB across nations. They report that, across cultures that vary widely in political structures and economic resources, there is no evidence that older adults are less satisfied with their lives than their younger counterparts. Moreover, this pattern holds despite the fact that older adults are more disadvantaged in income, health, and marital status than young and middle-age adults.

## XX. Priority Issues for Future Research

Research on SWB during later life has a long and distinguished history. As a consequence, a great deal is already known about the conditions under which older adults experience high quality of life. The good news is that the vast majority of older adults, across a wide range of cultures, report high levels of SWB, often despite rather than as a result of objective life conditions. Moreover, SWB has been historically stable as well—at least for more than half a century in the United States. A broad range of determinants of SWB in late life have been identified, as have a number of psychosocial processes that mediate the links between objective life conditions and perceived quality of life.

Despite the immense volume of research, not all important questions about SWB have been addressed or adequately answered. I suggest that three areas of research are especially important areas for future inquiry: (1) estimating more complex, dynamic models of the determinants of SWB, (2) identifying the dynamics of SWB across the life course, and (3) pursuing more complex and targeted cross-cultural research in the social indicators tradition.

### A. Complex, Dynamic Models of SWB Determinants

As noted previously, the proposed conceptual model of the determinants of

SWB in late life presented in Figure 18.1 has never been tested in its entirety. All the predictors in the model have been demonstrated to be significantly related to SWB in previous research. But no study has reported the net or unique effects of the predictors on perceived well-being. The model proposed here is a path model and thus includes hypotheses about both indirect and direct effects of the predictors. Although some of the hypothesized mediating effects have been examined in previous research, many others have not.

The most important limitation of research on the determinants of SWB, however, is the relative neglect of temporal dynamics. A surprisingly small proportion of research on the determinants of SWB is based on longitudinal data. The proposed model is both temporal and conceptual. Research on the prospective effects of hypothesized predictors and changes in those predictors is badly needed. Although the causal direction between SWB and some of its determinants is clear in the absence of longitudinal data (e.g., SWB cannot cause age or gender), other relationships are more ambiguous (e.g., between SWB and health). The primary contribution of longitudinal analyses, however, will be the ability to test the effects of *changes* in the determinants of SWB. We know almost nothing about "how much" of a decline in health or loss of social integration, for example, is required to trigger corresponding declines in SWB.

### B. The Life Course Dynamics of SWB

Another critically important avenue for future research is the dynamics of SWB across the life course. An immense volume of research compares levels of perceived life quality across age groups in cross-sectional studies. Results consistently indicate that older adults, on average, experience levels of SWB that are at least as high as, and probably somewhat higher than, young and middle-age adults. And, as previously noted, the longitudinal studies available, with measurements spanning 2 to 17 years, report stability of SWB over time. Nonetheless, these studies fall far short of documenting the life course dynamics of perceived life quality.

A high priority for future research is studies that observe patterns of SWB over long segments of the life course. Both aggregate and more fine-grained patterns of change and stability should be identified. At the aggregate level, we need to know if there is an overall trajectory that suggests that the course of SWB is developmental. But there will undoubtedly be substantial heterogeneity in life course patterns as well. One study (the only one of which I am aware) illustrates the potential contribution of studying the life course dynamics of SWB. Using data from the Stanford-Terman Men covering 14 years (age 58 to 72), Crosnoe and Elder (2002) observed four long-term patterns of "adaptation in the later years": less adjusted (the least satisfied men), career-focused (moderate levels of satisfaction), family-focused (high levels of satisfaction), and well-rounded (high levels of satisfaction). They also identified the differing social resources and life course "turning points" that predicted adaptation style.

### C. Targeted Cross-Cultural Comparisons

Research to date that examines levels of SWB across nations is sufficient to demonstrate the potential payoff of such inquiries. But the volume of research is small (especially in comparison to social indicators such as economic productivity), conceptualization and measurement are often overly simplistic, and comparisons that focus on well-being in late life are virtually absent. Investigating research questions targeted at understanding SWB in late life is a high priority and "wide open" topic for future inquiry.

A cautionary note is in order. There are immense literatures that examine aging issues in comparative perspective. Scholars ranging from anthropologists to demographers to public policy analysts have produced important contributions to our understanding of the effects of social and cultural context on aging. What is missing, however, is linking social and economic structures, including public policies, to population levels of SWB among older adults. Social indicators researchers make a strong case for viewing SWB as important evidence of the extent to which societies meet the needs of their members. By the same token, targeting research at SWB among older adults can provide an important strategy for understanding the effects of macro-level structures and processes on the quality of late life. In addition to focusing on older adults, social indicators research could be considerably more sophisticated than is typical now. Cross-cultural research is an obvious candidate for multilevel analyses in which predictors of SWB at the individual level are nested in contextual variables at the national level.

In summary, the quest to understand the foundations of well-being in late life has been a central theme of aging research in the social sciences from the beginning and remains an essential part of the gerontological research enterprise. As is true of all vital fields, research questions change somewhat over time and analytical and measurement techniques evolve to ever higher levels of sophistication. And there is clearly important work yet to be done.

## References

Achenbaum, W. A. (1995). *Crossing frontiers: Gerontology emerges as a science.* New York: Cambridge University Press.

Adams, V. H., & Jackson, J. S. (2000). The contribution of hope to the quality of life among African Americans, 1980–1992. *International Journal of Aging and Human Development, 50,* 279–295.

Adelmann, P. K. (1994). Multiple roles and psychological well-being in a national sample of older adults. *Journal of Gerontology: Social Sciences, 49,* S277–S285.

Antonovsky, A. (1987). *Unraveling the mystery of health: How people manage stress and stay well.* San Francisco: Jossey-Bass.

Antonucci, T. C., Fuhrer, R., & Jackson, J. S. (1990). Social support and reciprocity: A cross-ethnic and cross-cultural perspective. *Journal of Social and Personal Relationships, 7,* 519–530.

Ardelt, M. (2003). Effects of religion and purpose in life on elders' subjective well-being and attitudes toward death. *Journal of Religious Gerontology, 14,* 55–77.

Baltes, M. M., & Carstensen, L. L. (2003). The process of successful aging: Selection, optimization, and compensation. In Staudinger, U. M., & Lindenberger, U. (Eds.), *Understanding human development: Dialogues with life-span psychology* (pp. 81–104). Dordrecht, Netherlands: Kluwer Academic Publishers.

Barnett, R. C., & Baruch, G. K. (1985). Women's involvement in multiple roles and psychological distress. *Journal of Personality and Social Psychology, 49,* 135–145.

Beaumont, J. G., & Kenealy, P. M. (2004). Quality of life perceptions and social comparisons in healthy old age. *Aging and Society, 24,* 755–769.

Bisconti, T. L., & Bergeman, C. S. (1999). Perceived social control as a mediator of the relationships among social support, psychological well-being, and perceived health. *The Gerontologist, 39,* 94–103.

Black, H. K. (1999). Life as gift: Spiritual narratives of elderly African American women living in poverty. *Journal of Aging Studies, 13,* 441–455.

Bond, M. J., Clark, M. S., & Davies, S. (2003). The quality of life of spouse dementia caregivers: Changes associated with yielding to formal care and widowhood. *Social Science and Medicine, 57,* 2385–2395.

Bowling, A., Banister, D., Sutton, S., Evans, O., & Windsor, J. (2002). A multidimensional model of quality of life in older age. *Aging and Mental Health, 6,* 355–371.

Brown, D., (1988). Socio-demographic vs. domain predictors of perceived stress: Racial differences among American women. *Social Indicators Research, 20*, 517–532.

Campbell, A., Converse, P. A., & Rodgers, W. L. (1976). *The quality of American life.* New York: Russell Sage Foundation.

Carstensen, L. L. (1992). Social and emotional patterns in adulthood: Support for socioemotional selectivity theory. *Psychology and Aging, 7*, 331–338.

Carstensen, L. L., Isaacowitz, D. M., & Charles, S. T. (1999). Taking time seriously: A theory of socioemotional selectivity. *The American Psychologist, 54*, 165–181.

Chappell, N. L., & Reid, R. C. (2002). Burden and well-being among caregivers: Examining the distinction. *The Gerontologist, 42*, 722–780.

Cheng, S. (2004). Age and subjective well-being: A discrepancy perspective. *Psychology and Aging, 19*, 409–415.

Consedine, N. S., Magai, C., & King, A. R. (2004). Deconstructing positive affect in later life: A differential functionalist analysis of joy and interest. *International Journal of Aging and Human Development, 58*, 49–68.

Costa, P. T., Zonderman, A. B., McCrae, R. R., & Cornoni-Huntley, J. (1987). Longitudinal analyses of psychological well-being in a national sample: Stability of mean levels. *Journal of Gerontology, 42*, 50–55.

Covinsky, K. E., Wu, A. W., Landefeld, C. S., Connors, A. F., Jr., Phillips, R. S., Tsevat, J., Dawson, N. V., Lynn, J., & Fortinsky, R. H. (1999). Health status versus quality of life in older patients: Does the distinction matter? *American Journal of Medicine, 106*, 435–440.

Crosnoe, R., & Elder, G. H., Jr. (2002). Successful adaptation in the later years: A life course approach to aging. *Social Psychology Quarterly, 65*, 309–328.

Cumming, E., & Henry, W. (1961). *Growing old: The process of disengagement.* New York: Basic Books.

Diener, E. (1984). Subjective well-being. *Psychological Bulletin, 95*, 542–575.

Diener, E., & Diener, C. (1996). Most people are happy. *Psychological Science, 7*, 181–183.

Diener, E., Diener, M., & Diener, C. (1995). Factors predicting the subjective well-being of nations. *Journal of Personality and Social Psychology, 69*, 851–864.

Diener, E., Gohm, C. L., Suh, E., & Oishi, S. (2000). Similarity of relations between marital status and subjective well-being across cultures. *Journal of Cross-Cultural Psychology, 3*, 419–436.

Diener, E., & Suh, E. (1997). Measuring quality of life: Economic, social, and economic indicators. *Social Indicators Research, 40*, 189–216.

Diener, E., & Suh, E. (1998). Subjective well-being and age: An international analysis. *Annual Review of Gerontology and Geriatrics, 17*, 304–324.

Ellison, C. G., Boardman, J. D., Williams, D. R., & Jackson, J. S. (2001). Religious involvement, stress, and mental health. *Social Forces, 80*, 215–249.

Fahey, T., & Smyth, E. (2004). Do subjective indicators measure welfare? Evidence from 33 European countries. *European Societies, 6*, 5–27.

Freund, A. M., & Baltes, P. B. (1998). Selection, optimization, and compensation as strategies of life management: Correlations with subjective indicators of successful aging. *Psychology and Aging, 13*, 531–543.

Fujita, F., & Diener, E. (2005). Life satisfaction set point: Stability and change. *Journal of Personality and Social Psychology, 88*, 158–164.

Gana, K., Alaphilippe, D., & Bailly, N. (2004). Positive illusions and mental and physical health in later life. *Aging and Mental Health, 8*, 58–64.

George, L. K., Okun, M. A., & Landerman, R. (1985). Age as a moderator of the determinants of life satisfaction. *Research on Aging, 7*, 209–233.

Inglehart, R. (2002). Gender, aging, and subjective well-being. *International Journal of Comparative Sociology, 43*, 391–408.

Jakobsson, U., Hallberg, J. R., & Westergren, A. (2004). Overall and health related quality of life among the oldest old in pain. *Quality of Life Research, 13*, 125–136.

Kahn, R. L., & Juster, F. T. (2002). Well-being: Concepts and measures. *Journal of Social Issues, 58*, 627–644.

Kim, I. K., & Kim, C. S. (2003). Patterns of family support and the quality of life of the elderly. *Social Indicators Research, 62*, 437–454.

Kirby, S. E., Coleman, P. G., & Daley, D. (2004). Spirituality and well-being in frail and non-frail older adults. *Journal of Gerontology: Psychological Sciences, 59,* P123–P129.

Kirkcaldy, B., Furnham, A., & Siefen, G. (2004). The relationship between health efficacy, educational attainment, and well-being among 30 nations. *European Psychologist, 9,* 107–119.

Koltyn, K. F. (2001). The association between physical activity and quality of life in older women. *Women's Health Issues, 11,* 471–480.

Krause, N. (1993). Race differences in life satisfaction among aged men and women. *Journals of Gerontology, 48,* S235–S244.

Krause, N. (2003). Religious meaning and subjective well-being in late life. *Journal of Gerontology: Social Sciences, 58B,* S160–S170.

Landau, R., & Litwin, H. (2001). Subjective well-being among the oldest old: The role of health, personality, and social support. *International Journal of Aging and Human Develpoment, 52,* 265–280.

Lang, F. R., & Schutze, Y. (2002). Adult children's supportive behaviors and older parents' subjective well-being. *Journal of Social Issues, 58,* 661–680.

Lewis, C. (2001). *Grappling with the quality of life: Patients, FDA, and drug companies struggle to link therapies with well-being.* Retrieved January 17, 2005, from U.S. Food and Drug Administration web site: http://www.fda.gov/fdac/features/2001/201_life.html

Lucas, R. E., Clark, A. E., Georgellis, Y., & Diener, E. (2003). Re-examining adaptation and the set-point model of happiness: Reactions to changes in marital status. *Journal of Personality and Social Psychology, 84,* 527–539.

Mastekaasa, A. (1994). The subjective well-being of the previously married. *Social Forces, 73,* 665–692.

McCrae, R. R., & Costa, P. T., Jr. (1993). Psychological resilience among widowed men and women: A 10-year follow-up of a national sample. In Stroebe, W. (Ed.), *Handbook of bereavement: Theory, research, and intervention* (pp. 196–207). New York: Cambridge University Press.

Menec, V. H. (2003). The relation between everyday activities and successful aging: A 6-year longitudinal study. *Journal of Gerontology: Social Sciences, 58B,* S74–S82.

Minkler, M., & Fadem, P. (2002). "Successful Aging:" A disability perspective. *Journal of Disability Policy Studies, 12,* 229–235.

Moen, P., Dempster-McClain, D., & Williams, R. (1989). Social integration and longevity: An event history analysis of women's roles and resilience. *American Sociological Review, 54,* 635–647.

Morris, D. C. (1997). Health, finances, religious involvement, and life satisfaction of older adults. *Journal of Religious Gerontology, 10,* 3–17.

Morrow-Howell, N., Hinterlong, J., Rozario, P. A., & Tang, F. (2003). Effects of volunteering on the well-being of older adults. *Journal of Gerontology: Social Sciences, 58B,* S137–S145.

Mroczek, D. K., & Spiro, A. (2005). Change in life satisfaction during adulthood: Findings from the Veterans Affairs Normative Aging Study. *Journal of Personality and Social Psychology, 88,* 189–202.

Nemoto, T. (1998). Subjective norms toward social support among Japanese American elderly in New York City: Why help does not always help. *Journal of Community Psychology, 26,* 293–316.

Nesbitt, B. J., & Heidrich, S. M. (2000). Sense of coherence and illness appraisal in older women's quality of life. *Research in Nursing and Health, 23,* 25–34.

Neugarten, B. L. (Ed.). (1968). *Middle age and aging.* Chicago: University of Chicago Press.

NORC (National Opinion Research Center). (2002). *General Social Survey: 1972–2000 cumulative codebook.* Retrieved June 14, 2005, from http://webapp.icpsr.umich.edu/GSS

O'Connell, M. (2004). Fairly satisfied: Economic equality, wealth, and satisfaction. *Journal of Economic Psychology, 25,* 297–305.

Palmore, E. B. (Ed.). (1970). *Normal aging: Reports from the Duke Longitudinal Studies, 1970–1973.* Durham, NC: Duke University Press.

Pavot, W., & Diener, E. (1993). Review of the Satisfaction with Life Scale. *Psychological Assessment, 5,* 164–172.

Pennex, B., Guralnik, J. M., Simonsick, E. M., Kasper, J. D., Ferrucci, L., & Fried, L. P. (1998). Emotional vitality among disabled older women: The Women's Health and Aging Study. *Journal of the American Geriatrics Society, 46,* 807–815.

Pinquart, M., & Soerensen, S. (2000). Influences of socioeconomic status, social network, and competence on subjective well-being in later life: A meta-analysis. *Psychology and Aging, 15,* 187–224.

Pinquart, M., & Soerensen, S. (2001). Gender differences in self-concept and psychological well-being in old age: A meta-analysis. *Journal of Gerontology: Psychological Sciences, 56B,* P195–P213.

Pinquart, M., & Soerensen, S. (2003). Differences between caregivers and non-caregivers in psychological health and physical health: A meta-analysis. *Psychology and Aging, 18,* 250–267.

Rozario, P. A., Morrow-Howell, N., & Hinterlong, J. E. (2004). Role enhancement or role strain: Assessing the impact of multiple productive roles on older caregiver well-being. *Research on Aging, 26,* 413–428.

Rowe, J. W., & Kahn, R. L. (1998). *Successful aging.* New York: Pantheon Books.

Ryff, C. D. (1991). Possible selves in adulthood and old age: A tale of shifting horizons. *Psychology and Aging, 6,* 286–295.

Sharpley, C. F., & Yardley, P. (1999). The relationship between cognitive hardiness, explanatory style, and depression-happiness in postretirement men and women. *Australian Psychologist, 34,* 198–203.

Steverink, N., Westerhof, G. J., Bode, C., & Dittmann-Kohli, F. (2001). The personal experience of aging, individual resources, and subjective well-being. *Journal of Gerontology: Psychological Sciences, 56B,* P364–P373.

Suh, E., Diener, E., & Fujita, F. (1996). Events and subjective well-being: Only recent events matter. *Journal of Personality and Social Psychology, 70,* 1091–1102.

Taylor, R. J., Chatters, L. M., Hardison, C. B., & Riley, A. (2001). Informal social support networks and subjective well-being among African Americans. *Journal of Black Psychology, 27,* 439–463.

Torrance, G. W. (1986). Measurement of health state utilities for economic appraisal: A review. *Journal of Health Economics, 5,* 1–32.

Tran, T. V., Wright, R., & Chatters, L. (1991). Health, stress, psychological resources, and subjective well-being among older Blacks. *Psychology and Aging, 6,* 100–108.

Van Willigen, M. (2000). Differential benefits of volunteering across the life course. *Journal of Gerontology: Social Sciences, 55B,* S308–S318.

Veenhoven, R. (1996). Happy life-expectancy: A comprehensive measure of quality of life in nations. *Social Indicators Research, 39,* 1–58.

Ware, J. E., Jr., & Sherbourne, C. D. (1992). The MOS 36-item short-form health survey (SF-36). I. Conceptual framework and item selection. *Medical Care, 30,* 473–483.

Warr, P., Butcher, V., & Robertson, J. (2004). Activity and psychological well-being in older people. *Aging and Mental Health, 8,* 172–183.

Wethington, E., & Kessler, R. C. (1986). Perceived support, received support, and adjustment to stressful life events. *Journal of Health and Social Behavior, 27,* 78–89.

Windle, G., & Woods, R. T. (2004). Variations in subjective well-being: The mediating role of a psychological resource. *Aging and Society, 24,* 583–602.

The WHOQOL Group. (1998). Development of the World Health Organization WHOQOL-BREF quality of life assessment. *Psychological Medicine, 28,* 551–558.

## Part Four

# Aging and Society

# Nineteen

# Aging and Politics

## An International Perspective

Alan Walker

This chapter examines the relationship between aging and politics, a relatively neglected topic in gerontology, and argues that it is in a state of flux globally. At the macro level of politics the liberal portrayal of older people as a deserving cause, on which the Western welfare state in all its varieties was founded, is being challenged. In some countries it has been replaced by neo-liberalism and its fundamentalist opposition to the state as a provider of welfare. At the meso and micro levels of politics, the last decade of the twentieth century saw the growth of citizens or grassroots activity among older people in Europe, although it may have already peaked by then in the United States (Binstock & Quadagno, 2001; McKenzie, 1993).

While this chapter focuses primarily on Western societies, mainly Western Europe and North America, the politics of aging is also a matter for less developed societies, and increasingly so as their age structures alter rapidly over the next 25 years. At the moment, however, political activity is mainly a luxury of older people in developed countries (Walker & Naegele, 1999). In less developed ones,

such activity is not only inhibited by the necessities of survival and/or the ravages of the AIDS/HIV pandemic but also by violence and the failure of governments to protect the human rights of, among others, older people.

This chapter starts with an overview of the new politics of aging with reference to developments at the macro and meso/micro levels. Then it discusses the limitations of the political influence and potential influence of older people and questions the popular notion of gray or senior power. Finally the chapter looks at the prospects for the macro and micro politics of aging and sets out a research agenda.

## I. The New Politics of Aging

Recent developments in the relationship between aging and politics have been characterized as the emergence of a new politics of old age (Walker, 1998, 1999). Politics is a multi-layered phenomenon involving conflict and power which, in the case of aging, is overwhelmingly concerned with resource distribution, public identities, and human rights. This neces-

*Handbook of Aging and the Social Sciences, Sixth Edition*

sarily puts the spotlight on public and social policy but does not diminish the importance of the personal identity work that older people undertake everywhere as they negotiate and shape their responses to aging. Indeed, there are important connections between public policy and identities in old age (Hendricks, 2004; Walker, 1999, 2005). In this chapter, however, we are concerned with the public issues rather than the personal ones, even when these are political. Such a distinction reflects Mills' (1970) classic sociological distinction between the "personal troubles of milieu" and the "public issues" of social structure. In the public arena, there are micro-level political activities undertaken by older people, individually or in groups, to promote their interests. Then there is a range of meso-level organizations and structures that represent the interests of older people either in the form of self-advocacy or representational politics (or a mixture of both). Finally, at the macro level, there are policies that mainly emanate from the state (including local government entities), as well as from corporations, the third or voluntary sector, and International Governmental Organizations (IGOs). A central premise of this chapter is that there is a maldistribution of power between the different levels. Looking top-down the state, the representatives of "grey capitalism" (Blackburn, 2002), and the IGOs constantly make policies that impact hugely on the everyday lives of older people However, from a bottom-up perspective, the scope for influence through micro- and meso-level participation fluctuates but remains very limited.

What is meant by the "new" politics of aging becomes clearer if we consider first the period that may be described now as the "old" politics of aging. Going back further still, the formative years of the modern politics of aging are rooted in the campaigns waged in the late nineteenth and early twentieth centuries by older people and organized labor to establish pension systems. These contributed to the introduction of public pensions, with the legislative stones being laid first in Bismarck's Germany (1889), followed by other Western European countries in the early part of the next century: 1901 in the Netherlands, 1908 in the United Kingdom, 1910 in France, 1913 in Sweden, and 1919 in Italy and Spain. The United States followed later in 1935. Although far beyond the scope of this chapter, many of the current features of national pension provision can be traced back to these early schemes. In contrast to the early history of protests and campaigns for public pensions, the post-World War II period was characterized in many countries by political passivity. This passivity arose mainly from a rather negative social construction of old age, even though some of the motivations behind this were clearly benevolent.

One key element of this negative social construction was the close identification between older people and the welfare state. All welfare states originated, wholly or partly, in the provision for old age and pension systems. They are now not only the largest item of national social expenditures but are the heart of the welfare regime found in each country. This means that the nature of a country's retirement pension system tends to have a major determining influence over the rest of the welfare state (Esping-Andersen, 1990; Walker, 2003). Welfare states were constructed at a time of relative optimism about tackling need and the prospects for the future funding of benefits. Given their economic situation and difficulty remaining employed, older people were regarded as a deserving cause for welfare spending. This was not entirely good news because it also entailed their social construction as dependent in economic terms and encouraged popular ageist stereotypes of old age as a period of poverty and frailty (Townsend, 1981, 1986; Walker, 1980).

As Binstock (1991, p. 11) has put it, older people were viewed as "poor, frail, socially dependent, objects of discrimination and, above all, deserving," and this reinforced the case for public welfare provision. There was certainly a case for action because poverty rates among older people remained high despite the introduction of pensions and other measures to assist them. For example, in the late 1960s in the United States, one in four persons age 65 and older had incomes below the official poverty line (Rix, 1999), and in the United Kingdom and Germany, it was one out of every three and one in five, respectively (Walker, 1993). Evidence such as this encouraged increases in social spending, and, in some countries, governments began concerted attempts to tackle poverty in old age. For example, in 1972, the U.S. Congress approved a 20% increase in Social Security benefits, an "average wage" index as part of the benefit level determination at the time of retirement, and an automatic cost-of-living benefit adjustment for benefits in payment status (Rix, 1999). Between 1960 and 1985, total public pension expenditures in all Organisation for Economic Cooperation and Development (OECD) countries rose significantly faster than economic output (and therefore contributed to a rising share of gross domestic product (GDP) being devoted to pensions. The influence of the three factors determining this growth—demography, eligibility, and benefit levels—was roughly equal, which implies that expansive policy decisions were taken concerning eligibility and levels of pensions and other benefits for older people (OECD, 1988a).

The other key element in the negative social construction of old age was the fact that older people were largely excluded from the political and policymaking systems by a process of disengagement whereby, on retirement, they no longer participated in formal economic structures and institutions. Thus retirement operated as a process of both social and political exclusion that detached senior citizens from some of the main sources of political consciousness and channels of representation. This exclusion contributed to a popular perception of older people as being politically passive. This then fed into age discriminatory stereotypes that portrayed older people as inactive, acquiescent, family oriented, and, therefore, disinterested in political participation.

The scientific community played its part by contributing social theories that purported to explain the social and political passivity of older people. For example, the functionalist sociological theory of "disengagement" was put forth in the early 1960s. This theory argued that old age consisted of an inevitable and mutual process of disengagement between the aging individual and other members of society (Cumming & Henry, 1961). In accordance with it, most older people would not be expected to be active participants in social and political life. The theory, however, neglected the structural processes, noted previously, that, in effect, were excluding older people from participation (Walker, 1980). Of course in every Western country there were living examples of active senior citizens who contradicted the stereotype, but this does not negate the general social construction.

Other factors also operated to limit the extent of political participation on the part of older people in the early post-World War II period. In a general political sense old age was less significant than it is today. There were fewer older people, they were less healthy, and retirement still acted as the key regulator of entry into old age. Also, in political terms, age was less salient because attention was directed chiefly at rebuilding the physical infrastructures of those countries devastated by the war and constructing the major institutions of the welfare state. Thus, in Europe at least, the politics of old age reflected the general politics of the time. Issues of conflict were dominated by traditional class and religious divisions, with corporatism containing policy conflicts within the political system.

During this postwar phase in the politics of old age, numerous pressure groups representing the interests of older people were created either at local or national levels, or at both. Often the national pressure groups represented specific sections of the older population, such as retired civil servants (e.g., in Germany). And they appeared on the political scene at different times in different countries.

In the United Kingdom most of these pressure groups date from the 1940s and 1950s, though some originated in the early part of the century. In the United States the National Council on the Aging was founded in 1950 and the American Association of Retired Persons (AARP) in 1958. In Germany the association of war victims, disabled people, and pensioners (VdK) was formed in 1917 and reestablished in the Federal Republic in 1950 (Alber, 1995).

Despite the large membership of some of the pressure groups and other organizations formed in the 1950s, 1960s, and 1970s, they were not primarily concerned with the political mobilization of the older population. Instead they chiefly spoke on behalf of older people in the policy arena. Thus the politics of old age in this period was characterized by consensus: pressure groups representing older people who bargained for public policy advances within a context of shared understanding. Generally, the groups agreed about the possibilities of politics, the assumption of progressive welfare development, and the deservingness of the case they espoused. It is not surprising therefore that this period has been described as the "bureaucratic lobby"

phase (Estes, Biggs, & Phillipson, 2003). Today things are quite different.

## II. The New Macro Politics of Aging

This "new" (but now deeply entrenched) politics of aging consists of two distinct but causally related macro and meso/micro aspects. At the macro level, policymakers began to reject the consensus on which the welfare state was based, that is, older people as the deserving poor. Instead, they began to question, more openly and frequently than hitherto, the cost of population aging. The first wave of this critical approach to welfare, particularly the public expenditure implications of pensions and health care, occurred in the mid-1970s after the world oil price shock and the fiscal crisis it contributed to (O'Connor, 1977). This was followed by a second wave of criticism in the 1980s when the macro-economic implications of pension system maturation and the financial costs of long-term care were the subject of sometimes heated debate in different countries.

For example, in the United Kingdom, the 1980s saw the change from wage to price indexation for the basic public social insurance pension. The State Earnings Related Pension was also cut substantially, and those still employed were offered tax incentives to take out private, prefunded pensions (Walker, 1991, 1993). In the United States there were parallel restrictions on the growth of Social Security and Medicare expenditures (Rix, 1999). What both countries saw in this period was a reversal of the previously politically sacrosanct status of deservingness on the part of older people and the construction of a discourse that, to a greater or lesser extent, emphasizes the "burden" of pensions on the working population. Binstock has described this reversal of fortunes for U.S. older citizens:

The expansive social policy context in which the [Older Americans Act] was created ... came to an end ... Since then, social policy retrenchment has been in vogue, and the general political environment—previously supportive of almost any policy proposals to benefit aging persons—has become increasingly hostile to older people. (Binstock, 1991, p. 11)

Sometimes this new discourse is expressed in terms of generational equity, with the scientifically flawed "dependency ratio" between older people and those of working age invariably quoted as evidence of impending doom. (As I have argued elsewhere, the power of these ratios is such that their use is impervious to counter scientific evidence [Walker, 1990a]).

Only in the United States was there a sustained public debate on generational equity that was spurred on by the creation in 1985 of the pressure group Americans for Generational Equality (AGE) (see Quadagno, 1989). The organization proved to be a front for an anti-welfare ideology, however, and signally failed to dent the support of the general public in the United States for programs for older people, support that has remained resilient (Marshall, Cook, & Marshall, 1993).

Similar discourses concerning the future costs of population aging emerged later in the other northern European countries, and this has led to modifications to most countries' pension systems. For the most part, these have been modest adjustments to the pension formulae or eligibility criteria so as to reduce long-term costs (Walker, 2003).

The crucial question for this chapter is why the United Kingdom and the United States were the first countries to implement policies designed to reduce or restrain public expenditure for welfare, pensions, and services to older people. The main answer is political ideology: it is no coincidence that during the 1980s, these policies were introduced by govern-ments holding very similar neo-liberal perspectives. The policies bear the names of their chief political advocates: "Thatcherism" in the United Kingdom and "Reaganomics" in the United States. (Australia and New Zealand followed a similar ideological path.)

The emergence of the neo-liberal "New Right" may be traced to the revision of conservative politics that took place in the 1970s mainly in Anglo-Saxon countries. This revision intertwined the previously separate strands of liberal belief in a free economy with the conservative belief in a small but strong state (Gamble, 1986). Monetarist economics was the practical tool used to implement neo-liberal thinking, and this was the justification (or scientific legitimation) for reducing the role of the state in welfare and the privatization of public interest (Walker, 1984, 1990b). Policies are always to some extent "path dependent" in that they reflect a particular country's historical legacy and institutional model. This explains why the Anglo-Saxon countries adopted neo-liberalism more readily than those of continental Europe where a social democratic tradition had been more prevalent.

Over the last 20 years, this neo-liberal ideology has been globalized by the IGOs, particularly the International Monetary Fund and World Bank, but more recently the World Trade Organization (WTO) and, to a lesser extent, the OECD (Estes & Phillipson, 2002; Walker, 1990a; Walker & Deacon, 2003). This global aspect of the macro-level new politics of old age is of increasing importance in determining the nature of provision in old age. Moreover, its power to undermine long-standing public pension and social protection systems is immense as national governments, for various reasons, fall in line with the neo-liberal consensus. Back in the 1980s, the first signs of the emerging consensus on policies for old age were already visible in two influential OECD

(1988a; 1988b) reports. These were followed by others derived from a broadly similar burden of aging discourse and advocating policy prescriptions that typically involve a reduction in public pay-as-you-go (PAYGO) and private defined benefit pension schemes and an increase in private, defined contribution ones (World Bank, 1994; OECD, 1998). In other words, an aging crisis has been manufactured as a pretext for welfare retrenchment that would be consistent with the ideological objectives of neo-liberals (Minkler & Robertson, 1991; Quadagno, 1989; Vincent, 1996; Walker, 1990a). The next logical step is the liberalization of the trade in services (including health and social care) under the WTO, which would challenge national government prerogatives to provide free services or to subsidize national not-for-profit providers (Estes & Phillipson, 2002; Walker & Deacon, 2003).

It must not be assumed that this new agenda is accepted without question by all policymakers; that is patently not the case. There are very wide variations (for example, among the Member States of the European Union [EU]) in the extent to which they have pursued the policy prescriptions dictated by this neo-liberal macroeconomic perspective. Again, the causes of this diversity are related mainly to ideology and the historical legacies of policies and institutions in different countries, including the role of organized labor in policymaking; however all governments and leading political actors now place aging cost issues high on their list of priorities. Moreover, this neo-liberal ideology has had a great impact on the countries of central and Eastern Europe, for the simple reason that the IGOs have been highly influential in determining policies on aging in these ex-communist bloc countries. There are numerous examples of these nations being "advised" to either privatize existing systems or to follow the private, prefunded, route in building pensions, often as the condition for the award of a loan (Ferge, 2002; Walker & Deacon, 2003).

## III. The New Meso and Micro Politics of Aging

At the meso and micro levels the new politics of old age consists of a rapid expansion in direct political involvement on the part of older people (including joining action groups and taking part in demonstrations). This is particularly the case in the EU, although this may to some extent be a function of the spotlight effect of research (Walker & Naegele, 1999). For example, in Germany the Senior Protection Association or "Grey Panthers" was first formed in 1975 only five years after the pioneering U.S. group with the same name (but different spelling). The U.S. Gray Panthers atrophied in the late 1980s and early 1990s, but the German Grey Panthers expanded and now have some 200 local groups (Alber, 1995). In the United Kingdom, the National Pensioners Convention (NPC) was created in 1979 and reconstituted in 1992 by an amalgamation of different preexisting grassroots and trade union groups. The NPC has around 1.5 million affiliated members in the local pensioner action groups that have mushroomed under its aegis (Carter & Nash, 1992). In Denmark in the early 1990s, a new grassroots movement of older people was established called the C Team. This group is independent of both established organizations representing older people and political parties; it arranges mass demonstrations and other actions aimed at preventing cuts in health and social services and improving provision for frail older people (Platz & Petersen, 1995). In 1992, the Italian pensioner party, the oldest such party in Europe, had its first representative elected to the regional government in Rome. A year later, seven pensioner representatives were elected to the Netherlands parliament.

These examples are sufficient to show that in a short space of time, there has been, at least as far as the EU is concerned, a mushrooming of pensioners' action groups at local and national levels and, with them, the emergence of what appears to be a newly radicalized politics of old age. Of course the new social movements among older people involve relatively few pensioners. Activism is pursued by a minority of persons in all birth cohorts, but many more older persons are now involved than in the previous consensus era and apparently more actively so (Carter & Nash, 1992; Walker & Naegele, 1999). Furthermore, the nature of political participation and representation is changing: there are more examples of direct action by senior citizens, and the new action groups are citizens' organizations composed of older people who want to represent themselves. It is too soon to say how permanent these new social movements will be. Indeed organizational instability is a familiar feature of citizens' organizations, and it is predictable that some will fail, as happened to the political party for older people in Belgium. The impact of these new forms of self-advocacy are discussed in the next section. First, how do we explain this transformation in the political participation and representation of older people?

To begin with, the growth in political action by older people is merely a reflection of the global upsurge in social movements spanning almost every element of political life (Jenkins & Klandermans, 1995). This may be seen as one facet of the transition from modernity to late modernity. On the one hand, this means the breakdown of the traditional economic and social certainties of modernity. On the other hand, it reflects the opening up of new concepts of citizenship and consumerism and new channels of political action (Harvey, 1989). The emergence of new social movements outside the familiar political institutions (political parties and trade unions) is not surprising given the profound realignments underway in the social and economic orders of the advanced industrial societies.

The interesting questions for comparative research to answer are why grassroots organizations of older people are established more easily in some countries than in others and why their sustainability varies from place to place. The factors to be taken into account are likely to include the relative openness of the political system, the strength of the civic culture, and the responsiveness of the central and local states. That the transition states of central and Eastern Europe did not mirror the growth of grassroots political activity in Western Europe emphasizes the key role played by civic culture as the wellspring of such political participation (Walker & Naegele, 1999).

Second, some of the sociodemographic developments have supported both a heightened political awareness of old age as a political issue and the likelihood that older people will participate actively. Quite simply there are more older people and, therefore, they are more visible than they were 15 to 20 years ago in social terms and in policy/political terms. Also, the cohort effects of a healthier and better educated older population have produced a potentially active pool of people in early old age.

Third, the negative changes in the macroeconomic policy context referred to earlier have had an impact on the radicalization of the politics of old age in some countries. The Gray Panthers in the United States campaigned on Social Security- and Medicare-related issues, as well as on more local ones. In Denmark, the C Team was set up to protest against cuts in public social services. The primary focus of the UK pensioners' campaigns has been government actions; both local and national campaigns have been concerned almost exclusively with cuts in pensions and social services provision and related issues. The precise impact of such policies on activism among older people obviously depends on a variety of factors, including the adequacy of welfare provision for this group in each country and the extent of the public expenditure reductions being proposed by particular governments. Thus the mobilization or activation effect of adverse public policy proposals or changes is uneven across the globe. There may also be a reciprocal relationship between the growth of social policy in the aging field and the participation of older people. For example, Campbell (2003) pointed out that, in the United States, the growth in Social Security coverage has been accompanied by a parallel rise in the political participation of older people from the 1950s to the 1990s. In the Campbell study, however, the measure of "participation" was rather basic: voting and making campaign contributions.

Fourth, the growth of political participation among older people has been openly encouraged in several countries by policymakers at both local and national levels.

## IV. Participation in Local Decision Making

Most of the participation of older people in daily life takes place at a local level, and this unit of administration is responsible, directly or indirectly, for many of the services that they receive. It is useful, however, to distinguish two different dimensions of participation in decision making at the local level. On the one hand there is the public policymaking process, which determines the general direction of services and the distribution of resources between groups. In contrast,

there are policy decisions taken at an interpersonal level, often by professionals employed by municipalities, which concern the delivery of specific services to older people.

As far as the local municipal policy-making process is concerned, the United States has had a large number of advisory committees since the 1970s. There has also been a great deal of effort over the last 20 years in different EU countries to try to improve the participation of older people. Local authorities in Austria, Denmark, France, Germany, Italy, the Netherlands, and Sweden have all established advisory boards of senior citizens (although in Germany these have no legal basis and their influence varies from one local authority to another).

Turning to the second dimension of participation in decision making at the local level, we are faced with a very complex interplay of personal and professional relationships. The health and social services are key agencies in the construction of dependency in old age (Townsend, 1981). Professional groups have been trained to regard themselves as autonomous experts, and this has had the common effect of excluding older people and their family caregivers from decision making about the services required to meet their care needs.

Pressures are building up for increased participation in decisions previously regarded as the sole province of professionals. These are coming, first, from the rise of consumerism (the transition from modernity to late modernity) and the reassertion of individualism. This social change is creating twin pressures for greater choice and for a participating voice. Second, there are grassroots pressures from service users and from informal carers. For example, in the Netherlands and the United Kingdom, caregiver organizations are calling for recognition of their right to be consulted on an equal basis with service users. Third, there are changes within professions in their orientation and practice that are beginning to question professional autonomy and that are opening up professional practice to user involvement. Together these processes are emphasising the importance of the participation of older service users and their carers.

Signs of this culture shift can be seen in some countries, notably the Scandinavian ones that emphasize rights to services. Thus Users Councils in Denmark are representing the interests of older users with regard to home care, institutional care, and other services. Even in the United Kingdom, which has a more paternalistic service tradition, user groups are being established by many local authorities (Cook, Maltby, & Warren, 2004).

There are still formidable barriers in the way of effective participation, however, and there is a long way to go before older people are genuinely empowered in the face of professional service allocators and providers. Clearly, the municipalities and other local providers have a crucial role to play in promoting a *culture of empowerment* at all levels and encouraging professionals and quasi-professionals to operate in more open and participative ways (Barnes & Walker, 1996). The challenge is greatest with regard to very frail older people (Hubbard, Tester, & Downs, 2003; Tester et al., 2004).

## V. Participation in National Decision Making

Several countries have set up national advisory boards consisting of the representatives of older people, although these are usually of only symbolic importance. There have been five U.S. White House conferences on aging—1961, 1971, 1981, 1995, and 2005—but no Administration had to follow any resolutions or positions that came out of them. France has a National Committee for Pensioners and Older People (CNRPA) and Spain a national council. The Senior Citizens Consulting Council was set up in Belgium more than 40 years ago.

National bodies such as these reflect a consensual model of policymaking and may be regarded by politically active seniors as part of a process of co-option. Nonetheless, they have probably assisted the development of the new politics of old age by both raising the profile of older people in the policymaking process and by helping to legitimize their political concerns. The Ombudsman role in Sweden is also a mechanism that raises the profile of older people's rights and, particularly with regard to frail older people, helps to include them in decision making. In the United States there are publicly financed ombudsmen in each state government, particularly focused on issues involving long-term care.

Thus the recent political participation of older people and the development of what appears to be a new citizens' politics of old age must be regarded as the consequence of two distinct impulses. From *below* there are undoubtedly pressures on the part of older people seeking a political voice; from *above*, some policymakers at local and national levels have consciously encouraged the involvement of older people.

## VI. Gray Power: Reality or Myth?

To what extent has all this involvement been translated into effective power? The evidence suggests that much of the increase in political participation witnessed in the past two decades has not led consistently to influence over events affecting older people. In fact, the ideological construction of gray power, often promoted by popular press headlines, has created a myth that sheer numbers and high voter turnout are all that matters in the battle for political influence (Binstock, 2005a; Peterson & Somit,

1994; Walker, 1991). That the matter is much more complex is illustrated by the reality that not even the world's largest pressure group for older people, the American Association of Retired Persons (AARP), with some 36 million members, is able to guarantee that the U.S. Congress will be responsive to its pleas. Described flatteringly as "the most fearsome force in politics" (Birnbaum, 1997, p. 122) and, less so, as an "800 pound gorilla" (Rix, 1999, p. 181), some observers suggest that either the heyday of its influence on national politics passed in the late 1980s or that it never existed (Binstock & Quadagno, 2001; McKenzie, 1993). Before 2003, AARP and the other representatives of older people in the United States had had little impact on the enactment or amendment of major policies such as Social Security or Medicare and were unable to prevent significant policy reforms affecting their constituency (Binstock, 1994, 2000; Day, 1998). Indeed, according to Binstock (2000, p. 24) "the political legitimacy of old-age interest groups has been eroding over the past 10 years" (cf. Campbell, 2003).

The jury is still out on the nature and magnitude of AARP's political power. It is attributed with a key role in endorsing the Republican Medicare Modernization Act (2003), a position that angered many of its members and also congressional Democrats who had seen the organization as their natural ally (Stolberg, 2003). But just how significant this was as an exercise of gray power in action is for U.S. gerontologists to verify. A tentative assessment has been made by one leading authority: ". . . its impact on this process may have been the most influential that any old-age interest group has had in U.S. politics" (Binstock, 2005a, p. 25). AARP's main role appears to be one of legitimization. It was swimming with the Republican tide backing the bill and serving its own interests as an insurance provider (more than a third of its income

comes from the sale of insurance and other products to its members), as well as seeking to establish the important principle of prescription drug coverage under Medicare. Moreover, the bill was backed by powerful vested interests in the health insurance and pharmaceutical fields plus major commercial employers (Binstock, 2005a).

The reasons that the apparently latent power of older people has not been mobilized consistently are discussed later. However, it is important to note here that the ideological construction of gray power sits closely alongside the neo-liberal myth of aging as a burden on society and serves a complementary purpose. Moreover, it may be that the various new meso-level structures of participation assembled, for example, in the EU over the last 20 years, are masking to some extent the absence of effective political power held by older people. Again, scientific evidence is required to test this hypothesis.

The formation and existence of local advisory bodies, however, does not mean that the voices of older people will actually be heard within the policymaking process or that the boards will be able to stand up for their interests, especially the interests of those of the most vulnerable. Moreover, as Verté, Ponjaert-Kristofferson, and Geerts' (1996) study of advisory councils in the Dutch-speaking part of Belgium shows, such bodies may reinforce the exclusion of some groups of older people. One of the few studies on this topic, it found that members of the advisory bodies were mainly drawn from organizations of retired people and were overwhelmingly men. When women did participate, they were rarely members of the council's executive boards.

On the positive side, there are examples of advisory councils successfully mobilizing older people and making an impact on policymaking. Moreover, there is some good evidence that it is possible to overcome the various barriers to organizing the local participation of older people. For example, in the United Kingdom, the Better Government for Older People initiative, which was established in 1997 to encourage the participation of older people in local government, consisted of 50 pilot projects, several of which reported a successful impact on decision making. A strong desire to actively engage in the local policymaking process and to have a voice in decisions affecting their lives has been demonstrated even among some of the most difficult groups to involve, such as older women from ethnic minority groups (Cook et al., 2004). It is clear though that we must be mindful about the limitations of local advisory councils. Also, the structures for local citizen participation are invariably the same and, therefore, fail to take on board inequalities among older people. Research demonstrates that participation takes many forms. This suggests that the structures created to facilitate participation must be flexible to be fully inclusive.

At the macro level it is possible that the power of pensioners is revealed in the proportion of national income allocated to pensions. Support for this hypothesis is given by the fact, noted earlier, that pure demography played a minor part in the growth of public pension expenditure in the years between 1960 and 1984 (OECD, 1988b).

Ultimately, however, the political consensus on the deservingness of older people (if not on the policies reflecting such a status) was overtaken by a neo-liberal economic one in many countries. The new consensus gradually spread from the United States, United Kingdom, Australia, and New Zealand in the early 1980s. At the same time, pensions spending stabilized and in some countries, actually declined. The change in spending growth also coincided with the growth of the older population in most OECD countries. This gives further weight to the

doubts expressed here concerning the reality of pensioner power. Furthermore, there appears to be no correlation between the level of pension expenditure and either the size of the groups representing older people or the degree of institutionalization of their right to representation. As Table 19.1 shows, the United States has the world's largest pressure group representing older people but, compared with other OECD countries, devotes one of the smallest proportions of its national income to pensions.

There is some evidence, however, that older U.S. citizens are highly responsive to threats to Social Security and that their actions have an impact on policymakers. This age group is the one frequently contacted by legislators at elections by *both* the Democratic and Republican parties (Campbell, 2003). Sweden has one of the world's most sophisticated systems of representation for older people and, although its pension spending is relatively high, it is not the highest. In fact, during the 1990s the proportion of GDP spent on pensions in Sweden actually declined by 12% (European Commission, 2002).

On balance, the available evidence suggests that gray power is a myth, and its popular promotion by policy elites and the media may have more to do with attempts to legitimize neo-liberal inspired policies intended to reduce

**Table 19.1**

Old-age Pension Spending, 2000 (as a percentage of GDP)

| | |
|---|---|
| Italy | 14.2 |
| Germany | 11.8 |
| Sweden | 9.2 |
| Finland | 8.1 |
| Japan | 7.9 |
| Netherlands | 5.2 |
| Canada | 5.1 |
| US | 4.4 |
| UK | 4.3 |

Source: OECD, 2001, p. 68

public spending on older people than any genuine examples of sustained influence over policy at the macro level. Also, although there are continuing examples of the operation of gray power in local politics, these tend to be part of the ebb and flow of pluralism rather than a sign of structured power to change resource distribution in favor of older people.

## VII. Barriers to Political Participation and Influence

Few would doubt the importance of the transformation that has taken place in the politics of old age, but it is important not to overstate what has happened. So far this change has involved only a minority of senior citizens. This suggests, at least, that the barriers to political participation may be more formidable than has been recognized generally and, perhaps, that there is no sound basis for general political mobilization among older people. There are five main impediments to such participation by older people in specifically age-related politics.

In the first place, contrary to popular perceptions, in Europe and the United States older people do not necessarily share a common interest by virtue of their age alone, which transcends all other interests (Binstock, 2000; Street, 1999; Walker & Naegele, 1999). Thus it is mistaken to regard senior citizens as a homogeneous group that might coalesce around or be attracted by a one-dimensional politics of aging. In other words, age is only one of several forms of sociopolitical consciousness such as socioeconomic status, race, gender, religion, and locality. This perspective marked a break with the long-standing tendency for social gerontologists to regard older people as a distinct and homogeneous social group cut off from their *own* status and class position formed at earlier stages of the lifecy-cle (Quadagno, 1982; Walker, 1981). Although no longer prevalent in social gerontology, this is still a view held by policymakers in many different countries and in IGOs (OECD, 1994; Walker, 1990a). As Estes (1982) has argued, a largely classless view of old age has been incorporated into public policy.

In fact, older people are just as deeply divided along social class and other structural lines as younger adults. This means that large organizations such as AARP are dealing with a diverse membership, which can cause difficulties if the organization takes a high profile stance on an issue (Lehrman, 1995; Rix, 1999) or that the competition between different organizations representing older people may diffuse potential mobilization (Douglas, 1995). The U.S. 51-member Leadership Council of Aging Organizations contains several subgroups representing trade associations, older women, ethnic groups, and disease-specific organizations (Binstock, 2005a). A fundamental fault line is gender, and this is not only consistently underplayed by policymakers but their policies are also crucial in maintaining it (Arber & Ginn, 1991; Calasanti & Slevin, 2001; Estes & Associates, 2001; Estes, 2004). The process of retirement, not aging, does impose reduced socioeconomic status on a majority of older people. Even so, retirement has a varying impact on older people depending on their prior socioeconomic status. For example, invariably there is unequal access to occupational pensions (Reday-Mulvey, 2005; World Bank, 1994). Women and other groups with incomplete employment and pensions contribution records are particularly disadvantaged in most countries (Ginn, 2003).

Second, the majority of older people remain relatively powerless politically. Traditionally the main source of working class political power has been the economic base provided by the workplace and trades union organization.

Retirement is often associated with social processes of exclusion that remove older people from their main source of income but also from potential collective political power and sources of sociopolitical consciousness. After retirement a larger portion of time is spent, on average, engaged in private and individualized home-based activities. Of course the "Fordist" model of work organization is increasingly inappropriate as a description of the late-modern, often individualized world of work (Harvey, 1989), but paid employment remains a collective activity for the majority of those in employment.

Thus, in contrast to the mobilization effect of public policy referred to earlier, detachment from paid employment may act as a dampener on political action, which deters some from political activities or creates barriers for others to surmount in order to be active. This is not to say that *interest* in politics and minimum levels of engagement, such as voting, are necessarily diminished. Political interest and engagement have been demonstrated consistently to be positively related to education and income levels (Verba, Schlozman, & Brady, 1995). Recently, however, Campbell (2003) has found that interest in Social Security is high in the United States across all education and income groups. Furthermore, Social Security-specific participation (including writing a letter, making a financial contribution, protesting and voting) is higher for low-income groups than for high-income groups. This latter finding is not surprising given that Social Security accounts for 82% of the income of U.S. older people in the lowest quintile and only 18% in the highest. But the "democratizing" effect of Social Security's universalism in the United States seems to mirror that of the classic Scandinavian citizenship welfare state (Korpi, 1983; Esping-Andersen, 1990; Palme, 1990).

Despite the apparent pressures toward bifurcation, European and U.S. research suggests that differences between younger and older voters in attitudes toward key policy issues are relatively small. This was the conclusion of a unique pan-European study of attitudes (Walker, 1993) and of an analysis of the 1996 presidential election in the United States (Binstock, 1997). In fact, it is not age as such that determines political attitudes and behaviour; rather it is ". . . the cleavages that cut across cohorts such as economic, educational, racial and ethnic, gender, and partisan divisions" (Binstock & Day, 1996, p. 364). Of course, it is obvious that some issues, such as pensions, have greater salience for older than younger cohorts.

The observation of a relationship between political efficacy and occupation dates back more than 40 years to the U.S. research by Almond and Verba (1963). Using a similar approach 20 years later, British survey analysis found that propensity for collective action is lowest among the retired and, in contrast to the employed and other groups in the labor market, retired people have a preference for personal over collective action (Young, 1984). The explanation for this passivity on the part of older people consisted of a sense of powerlessness or noncompetence, which, in turn, reflected a lack of real resources with which to gain political influence. There was, predictably, a close association between both socioeconomic group and education and subjectively assessed power. Campbell's (2003) analysis does not contradict these findings, as her focus is primarily on voting and political knowledge. In other words, minimum levels of participation, high levels of political interest, and low levels of collective action are not necessarily inconsistent.

Older people do demonstrate consistently higher political engagement than younger people in one important respect: voting. Globally, older people are more likely than younger ones to turn out in national (general) elections, and this is true for both men and women. Also the gender gap grows with age, which means that older women are more likely than older men to vote in general elections (among those 65 and over the difference is 3.7% in non-turnout levels: 13.1% for women and 16.8% for men) (Pintor & Gratschew, 2002). In both Western Europe and the United States, older people commonly record the highest turnout of all age groups in general elections (Turner, Shields, & Sharp, 2001). European data emphasize the higher turnout among older than younger people, even among those 70 and over, which averages 90% (International Institute for Democracy and Electoral Assistance [IDEA], 1999). The United States has seen a long-term growth in the portion of votes cast by older people in presidential elections (Binstock, 2000). Since 1972, those 65 and over have composed a larger share of voters than of those eligible to vote, and this gap has grown over time. The key factor in this rise is the changing turnout rates of different age groups: an increase of 6.5% among those 65 and over between 1972 and 1996 coupled with reductions in other age groups (e.g., 34.7% among 18- to 24-year-olds). In the 2004 U.S. presidential election, the senior turnout rate was 68%, compared with 54% for the electorate as a whole (Binstock, 2005b).

Third, pensioners often lack formal channels through which to exert political influence. Indeed, the political representation systems of some countries effectively exclude older people from key institutions. For example, few of the established political parties in Europe provided an organizational context for pensioners or made special efforts to include them in their machinery. The main exception is Germany, where political parties have taken steps to try to incorporate them, including a network of senior circles at district and regional lev-

els within the Social Democratic Party (Alber, 1995). Similarly, trade unions in Europe have been poor at involving ex-members and in providing continuing membership after labor force exit. Again, there are important exceptions and also signs that the trade union movement generally is becoming more aware of the need to involve older people. In Italy more than 20% of pensioners belong to the special retirement sections of the three main unions. This relatively high participation rate results from two impulses. On the one hand, older people want to defend the rights they have acquired, particularly pension rights. On the other hand, Italian trade unions have taken specific steps to increase the social and political involvement of older people (Florea, Costanzo, & Cuneo, 1995). Most other national unions in the EU lag behind their Italian counterparts, one exception being Germany: 13.3% of the 11.7 million union members are pensioners, with higher-than-average rates in the public sector and metalworkers unions (Alber, 1995).

Fourth, there are important physical and mental barriers to political participation in old age. Disability and socially disabling later life course events, such as widowhood, may further fragment political consciousness and discourage political activity. The experience of aging itself creates barriers to collective action and political participation for a minority of older people. For those with intellectual or learning disabilities who are now reaching old age for the first time, the aging process merely confirms their sociopolitical exclusion (Walker, Walker, & Ryan, 1996). Other social structural factors that militate against active political participation include poverty and low incomes, and age, gender, and race discrimination. For instance those suffering social exclusion as a result of poverty face substantial material and psychological barriers to active engagement and are among the least likely to be represented within the formal political system (Scharf, Phillipson, & Smith, 2004). This includes a small but significant proportion that live in institutions of various kinds, whose voices are usually the quietest. In addition a large number of older people, particularly women, are actively involved in caring for spouses and others in need and, therefore, may not have the physical energy and mental space to be active on the political scene as well. Despite these obvious barriers, there is political activity among low-income groups. Indeed, as noted previously, Campbell (2003) found a *higher* level of activity among low-income senior citizens than more affluent ones with regard to Social Security issues. This is possibly a function of the interaction between the significance of Social Security to pensioners and the political culture. It is a topic ripe for comparative research.

Finally, there is conservatism. It is not necessarily the case that people become more conservative as they grow older, despite the commonplace nature of that assumption (Hudson, 1980). In terms of public opinion, on most issues they differ very little from younger people in both the EU and the United States (Peterson & Somit, 1994; Walker, 1993). There is evidence, however, that older people are more conservative in certain respects than younger ones, but the reasons are not related primarily to age. Several key factors have been mentioned already, such as the removal of sources of potential influence and activity. In addition, there is a generational dimension. The present older generations have different reference points than younger people. Many of their formative years occurred between 1935 and 1955, a unique historical period in Europe and the wider world. Although the direction of party allegiance depends to some extent on age-cohort effects (Hudson & Strate, 1985), when it comes to the strength of such attachments the evi-

dence shows that, in both Western Europe and the United States, there is a uniform tendency for a disproportionate number of older people to hold strong party allegiances, an observation that was first made in the United States (Campbell, Converse, Miller, & Stokes, 1960; see also Binstock, 2000; MacManus, 1996). All of this suggests that older people are *not* more conservative in voting terms, but, rather, they have a tendency to vote for the party they have always voted for.

## VIII. Prospects for the Politics of Aging: A Research Agenda

Despite the development of a distinctly new politics of old age, with interrelated macro and meso/micro features, it is clear from the previous section that the social and economic foundations for political power and mobilization among older people remain relatively weak. This is not peculiar to old age but a demonstration that age is not, in itself, a sound basis for political consciousness. The relatively new direction of macroeconomic and social policies in developed countries is clear. Based on the available evidence, however, gray power is more hype than substance. Furthermore the aging power myth is being reproduced and amplified regularly in support of the macro level neo-liberal policy prescriptions. One reason for the apparent ease with which this myth gets translated into popular discourse is the virtual absence of scientific research on this topic (Walker, 1986). It is important to plug this research gap to better inform the public debate and, in particular, comparative research should be a priority. What should the research agenda consist of?

A topical starting point would be the behavior and preferences of the Baby Boomer generations, about which there has been a great deal of speculation including a strong element of cohort-centrism (Riley, 1992). Cross-national comparisons between Europe and the United States would be particularly fruitful. In the EU, age-based movement and political parties are likely to remain marginal features of political life. Such evidence as there is suggests that only small proportions of older people (less than one-quarter) would be prepared to join a political party based on old age (Walker, 1993). The parties that have been formed recently along these lines, such as the Grey Panthers in Germany and the U.K. Senior Citizens Party, attract only small memberships. Even in the Netherlands, one of Europe's most pluralistic political systems, the associations of older people are against the creation of an age-related political party (Rijsselt, 1995). Whereas the United States is a potentially favorable location for the development of age-based politics because, on the one hand, older Americans may be on the verge of exhibiting the "age consciousness" predicted in earlier decades (Neugarten, 1974; Cutler, Pierce, & Steckenrider, 1984; Torres-Gil, 1992) and, on the other, its pluralistic political system is highly amenable to interest group influence (Pampel, Williamson, & Stryker, 1990). Although there is little evidence in the United States to suggest that age is a potentially powerful predictor of political attitudes and behavior beyond voter turnout (Rix, 1999), Campbell's (2003) work seems to indicate a propensity for political engagement among older people not documented in Europe.

Second, it is important, therefore, to track, comparatively, changes in political involvement, nationally and locally, and its structural dimensions. Comparative research into the factors behind participation rates and the propensity for political action among older people should be a priority. Population aging will continue to raise policy questions concerning older

people higher up the political agenda, including in the developing world where the most rapid aging will occur over the next 50 years. Demographically, Europe and the United States are in different zones: Europe is the oldest region in the world, with an average fertility rate well below the replacement level of 2.1; the Untied States has a younger population, a fertility rate close to 2.1, and a high level of immigration. The aging of Europe will inevitably increase the potential for the political mobilization of older people themselves, especially if the new macro politics of old age continues to be dominated by neo-liberalism. Many of the newest and most radical pensioner groups have been formed to campaign against welfare state retrenchment dictated by neo-liberal oriented policies. The truism that "all politics is local" applies particularly to older people and, if the new grassroots politics of old age is to develop into effective gray power, then it is most likely to happen at the local level. Conflicts over local rationing of health and social care, transport, housing, crime, and public safety are potential flashpoints. The mass protests, in January 2005, by Russian pensioners against government cuts in benefits such as free transport show how quickly such campaigns can erupt.

Third, there is a major research program required on the macro-policy front where the future politics of aging look much clearer, especially since the reelection of George W. Bush in November 2004. The Transatlantic Consensus on economic globalization is likely to perpetuate its neo-liberal form, and this has predictable implications for the national and international politics of aging (Estes & Phillipson, 2002; Walker & Deacon, 2003). For example, the power of pension fund managers in the Anglo-Saxon stock market economies will be increased further; they already control more than half of the quoted equity in the United

Kingdom and the United States. This "gray capitalism" operates beyond the control of representative democracy and has demonstrated its disinterest in the welfare of both past and present pension fund contributors (Blackburn, 2002). It has also operated largely beyond the scope of gerontological research. Equally important, the global politics of aging will continue to be orchestrated by the IGOs, which are purveyors of a neo-liberal agenda in terms of both a definition of the problem—the "burden" of population aging—and the proposed "one size fits all" solutions—privatization and the reduction in the role of the state (Estes & Phillipson, 2002; Walker, 1990a). The impact of the IGOs will continue to be strongest in the former Soviet satellite and less developed countries, most of which have little or no choice but to follow IGO prescriptions in return for loans. The WTO is emerging as an immensely powerful global institution with the potential, on the one hand, to undermine established public systems of support for older people and, on the other, to prevent or greatly inhibit their introduction in transitional and less developed countries. Given their power and potential influences over the lives of older people, the IGOs have attracted too little interest from gerontologists. The replacement or minimization of the state in areas such as health and social care removes a potentially important focus for political engagement and influence. Just as the market for retail goods atomizes consumers, so markets in health and social care militate against collective representation by patients and service users. The impact of the Transatlantic Consensus on policies on aging in different countries should be a key research focus. The neoliberal prescriptions for pensions, health, and social care will continue to be represented by powerful coalitions of national and international interests as the only game in town. This suggests a future for

the macro-politics of aging that is dominated by privatization and the retreat of the state to minimal welfare functions. In a nutshell, the risks associated with old age will be increasingly individualized, a model with which the United Kingdom and United States are very familiar, as are the new democracies of central and eastern Europe (Ferge, 2002). But the politics of the implementation of this model have not been studied.

A further area for future research on the macro-policy front is how older people and their representatives respond to the increasing power of the IGOs, which means that not only is it difficult for older citizens to focus action at local level but also the source of the policies that have a potentially major impact on their lives is far removed from their influence. (The absence of representative politics at the supranational level is a huge democratic deficit.)

From the perspective of traditional welfare states and the intergenerational and inter-class solidarities on which they are based, this looks like a gloomy prospect. The outlook is also gloomy for the transitional and less developed countries whose populations are aging but who may not have the opportunity to build those solidarities. Prospects are also dim with regard to the politics of aging in terms of the democratic imperative to see healthy and vibrant political participation among all ages. But, and it must be a big BUT, things are not that straightforward, and this emphasizes the real need for comparative gerontological research to provide scientific certainty in an increasingly precarious and shifting policy context. Five potential sources of variation and research foci may be mentioned.

First, as noted earlier, social policies are demonstrably path dependent, and the extent to which economic globalization limits the freedom of nation-states to maintain existing institutions or to introduce countervailing progressive policies on pensions and health and social care, at the moment, is an open question. Of course the practical and ideological pressures to conform to neo-liberal economic globalization are powerful but, so far, the range of responses is wide and there are even less developed countries that have bucked the trend. What is clear, even to the World Bank, is that one size does not fit all. Second, the new global politics of aging may open up new arenas for discourse and, possibly, coalitions of interest and action (Estes & Phillipson, 2002; Estes, Biggs, & Phillipson, 2003). Third, the IGOs themselves are not immune to internal politics, and there has been a series of struggles about both their participation in policymaking and the nature of the policies themselves (Deacon, 2000). Fourth, perhaps there is some potential in the regional supranational bodies to resist the prescriptions of neo-liberal economic globalization. For example, the EU has attempted to combine a regional economic policy with a regional social policy agenda (European Commission, 2000). Fifth, the Madrid International Plan of Action on Ageing, 2002, offers a potential global focus for the politics of aging. Built on foundations such as human rights, it provides an alternative model to the prescriptions of neo-liberal globalization and puts the spotlight directly on the less developed countries, which will soon age most rapidly (Sidorenko & Walker, 2004).

The future politics of aging remain unclear. It will depend a great deal on how the politics of welfare develop in the coming decades and, in particular, the extent to which politicians attempt (perversely in aging societies) to take resources away from older people. It would be easy to enter the realm of speculation about the likely course of events, but what is needed instead is comparative research on the multi-layered politics of aging. The absence of such research is a gaping hole in gerontology.

## References

Alber, J. (1995). The social integration of older people in Germany. In A. Walker (Ed.), *Older people in Europe: Social integration* (pp. 111–162). Brussels: EC, DG5.

Almond, G. A., and Verba, S. (1963). *The civic culture*. Princeton: Princeton University Press.

Arber, S., & Ginn, J. (1991). *Gender and later life: A sociological analysis of resources and constraints*. London: Sage.

Barnes, M., & Walker, A. (1996). Consumerism versus empowerment: A principled approach to the involvement of older service users. *Policy and Politics, 24*(4), 375–393.

Binstock, R. H. (1991). From the great society to the aging society: 25 years of the older Americans Act. *Generations, 15*(3), 11–18.

Binstock, R. H. (1994). Changing criteria in old-age programs: The introduction of economic status and need for services. *The Gerontologist, 34*, 726–730.

Binstock, R. H. (1997). The 1996 election: Older voters and implications for policies on aging. *The Gerontologist, 37*, 15–19.

Binstock, R. H. (2000). Older people and voting participation: Past and future. *The Gerontologist, 40*, 18–31.

Binstock, R. H. (2005a). The contemporary politics of old-age policies. In R. B. Hudson (Ed.), *The new politics of old age policies*. Baltimore: Johns Hopkins University Press (in press).

Binstock, R. H. (2005b). Older voters and the 2004 presidential election. *The Gerontologist* (forthcoming).

Binstock, R. H., & Day, C. (1996) Aging and politics. In R. H. Binstock & L. George (Eds.), *Handbook of aging and social sciences* (4th ed., pp. 362–387). London: Academic Press.

Binstock, R. H., & Quadagno, J. (2001). Aging and politics. In R. H. Binstock & L. George (Eds.), *Handbook of aging and the social sciences* (5th ed., pp. 333–351). London: Academic Press.

Birnbaum, J. (1997). Washington's second most powerful man. *Fortune*, 12 May, 122–126.

Blackburn, R. (2002). *Banking on death*. London: Verso.

Calasanti, T., & Slevin, K. (2001). *Gender, social inequalities and aging*. Walnut Creek, CA: Alta Mira Press.

Campbell, A. L. (2003). *How policies make citizens: Senior political activism and the American welfare state*. Princeton, NJ: Princeton University Press.

Campbell, A., Converse, P., Miller, W., & Stokes, D. (1960). *The American voter*. New York: Wiley.

Carter, T., & Nash, C. (1992). *Pensioners forums: An active voice*. Guildford, UK: Pre-Retirement Association.

Cook, J., Maltby, T., & Warren, L. (2004). A participatory approach to older women's quality of life. In A. Walker & C. Hennessy (Eds.), *Growing older: Quality of life in old age* (pp. 149–166). Buckingham, UK: McGraw-Hill.

Cumming, E., & Henry, W. E. (1961). *Growing old, the process of disengagement*. New York: Basic Books.

Cutler, N., Pierce, R, & Steckenrider, J. (1984). How golden is the future? *Generations, 19*(1), 38–43.

Day, C. (1998). Old-age interest groups in the 1990s: Coalitions, competition, and strategy. In J. Steckenrider & T. Parrott (Eds.), *New perspectives on old-age policies* (pp. 131–150). Albany, NY: State University of New York Press.

Deacon, B. (2000). *Globalization and social policy*, UNRISD Occasional Paper 5. Geneva: United Nations Research Institute for Social Development.

Douglas, E. (1995). Professional organizations in aging: Too many doing too little for too few. *Generations, 19*(2), 35–36.

Esping-Andersen, G. (1990). *The three worlds of welfare capitalism*. Oxford: Polity Press.

Estes, C. L., (1982). Austerity and aging in the US. *International Journal of Health Services, 12*(4), 573–584.

Estes, C. L. (2004). Social security privatization and older women: A feminist political economy perspective. *Journal of Aging Studies, 18*, 9–26.

Estes, C. L., & Associates. (2001). *Social policy and aging*. London: Sage.

Estes, C. L., Biggs, S., & Phillipson, C. (2003). *Social theory, social policy and aging: A critical introduction*. Maidenhead, UK: Open University Press.

Estes, C. L., & Phillipson, C. (2002). The globalisation of capital, the welfare state and old age policy. *International Journal of Health Services, 32*(2), 279–297.

European Commission. (2000). *Social policy agenda 2000–2005*. Brussels: European Commission.

European Commission. (2002). *Social protection: Expenditure on pensions*. Brussels: EC.

Ferge, Z. (2002). European integration and the reform of social security in the accession countries. *European Journal of Social Quality, 3*(1/2), 9–25.

Florea, A., Costanzo, A., & Cuneo, A. (1995). The social integration of older people in Italy. In A. Walker (Ed.), *Older people in Europe: Social integration* (pp. 229–261). Brussels: European Commission DG5.

Gamble, A. (1986). *The free economy and the strong state*. Houndmills, UK: Macmillan.

Ginn, J. (2003). *Gender, pensions and the lifecourse*. Bristol, UK: Policy Press.

Harvey, D. (1989). *The condition of postmodernity*. Oxford, UK: Blackwell.

Hendricks, J. (2004). Public policies and old age identity. *Journal of Aging Studies*, 1–16.

Hubbard, G., Tester, S., & Downs, M. (2003). Meaningful social interactions between older people in institutional care settings. *Ageing and Society, 23*(1), 99–114.

Hudson, R. B. (1980). Old age politics in a period of change. In N. G. McCluskey & E. F. Borgatta (Eds.), *Aging and society* (pp. 147–189). London: Sage.

Hudson, R., & Strate, J. (1985). Aging and political systems. In R. H. Binstock & E. Shanas (Eds.), *Handbook of aging and the social sciences* (2nd ed., pp. 554–585). New York: Van Nostrand Reinhold.

International Institute for Democracy and Electoral Assistance (IDEA). (1999). *Youth voter participation*. Stockholm: International IDEA.

Jenkins, J. C., & Klandermans, B. (Eds.). (1995). *The politics of social protest*. London: UCL Press.

Korpi, W. (1983). *The democratic class struggle*. London: Routledge.

Lehrman, E. (1995). Health-care reform at the crossroads. *Modern Maturity*, January-February, 12.

Marshall, V., Cook, F., & Marshall J. (1993). Conflict over intergenerational equity: Rhetoric and reality in a comparative context. In V. Bengtson & W. A. Achenbaum (Eds.),

*The changing contract across generations* (pp. 119–140). New York: Aldine de Gruyter.

McKenzie, R. (1993). Senior status: Has the power of the elderly peaked? *American Enterprise, 4*(3), 74–80.

MacManus, S. (1996). *Young v. old: Generational combat in the 21st century.* Boulder, CO: Westview Press.

Mills, C. W. (1970). *The sociological imagination.* Harmondsworth, UK: Penguin.

Minkler, M., & Robertson, A. (1991). The ideology of age/race wars: Deconstructing a social problem. *Ageing and Society, 11,* 1–23.

Neugarten, B. (1974). Age groups in American society and the rise of the young-old. *Annals of the American Academy of Political and Social Science, 415,* 189–198.

O'Connor, J. (1977). *The fiscal crisis of the state.* London: St Martin's Press.

OECD (Organization for Economic Cooperation and Development). (1988a). *Reforming public pensions.* Paris: OECD.

OECD (Organization for Economic Cooperation and Development). (1988b). *Ageing populations—The social policy implications.* Paris: OECD.

OECD (Organization for Economic Cooperation and Development). (1994). *New orientations for social policy.* Paris: OECD.

OECD (Organization for Economic Cooperation and Development). (1998). *Maintaining prosperity in an aging society.* Paris: OECD.

OECD (Organization for Economic Cooperation and Development). (2001). *Ageing and income.* Paris: OECD.

Palme, J. (1990). *Pension rights in welfare capitalism.* Stockholm: Swedish Institute for Social Research.

Pampel, F., Williamson, J., & Stryker, R. (1990). Class context and pension response to demographic structure in advanced industrial democracies. *Social Problems, 37*(4), 535–550.

Peterson, S., & Somit, A. (1994). *Political behavior of older Americans.* New York: Garland.

Pintor, R., & Gratschew, M. (2002). *Voter turnout since 1945—a global report.* Stockholm: International Institute for Democracy and Electoral Assistance.

Platz, M., & Petersen, N. F. (1995). The social integration of older people in Denmark. In A. Walker (Ed.), *Older people in Europe: Social integration* (pp. 6–74). Brussels: European Commission DG5.

Quadagno, J. (1982). *Aging in early industrial society: Work, family and social policy in nineteenth century England.* New York: Academic Press.

Quadagno, J. (1989). Generational equity and the politics of the welfare state. *Politics and Society, 17,* 353–376.

Reday-Mulvey, G. (2005). *Working beyond 60.* Houndmills, UK: Palgrave.

Rijsselt, R. van. (1995). The social integration of older people in the Netherlands. In A. Walker (Ed.), *Older people in Europe: Social integration* (pp. 306–339). Brussels: EC, DG5.

Riley, M. (1992). Cohort perspectives. In E. Borgatta & M. Borgatta (Eds.), *The encyclopedia of social sciences* (pp. 52–65). New York: MacMillan.

Rix, S. (1999). The politics of old age in the United States. In A. Walker & G. Naegele (Eds.), *The politics of old age in Europe* (pp. 178–196). Buckingham: OU Press.

Scharf, T., Phillipson, C., & Smith, A. E. (2004). Poverty and social exclusion: Growing older in deprived urban neighbourhoods. In A. Walker & C. Hennessy (Eds.), *Growing older: Quality of life in old age.* Buckingham: McGraw-Hill (forthcoming).

Sidorenko, A., & Walker, A. (2004). The Madrid international plan of action on aging: From conception to implementation. *Ageing and Society, 24*(1), 147–165.

Stolberg, S. (2003). An 800-pound gorilla changes partners over Medicare. *New York Times,* November 23, wk5.

Street, D. (1999). Special interests or citizens' rights? "Senior power," social security, and Medicare. In M. Minkler & C. Estes (Eds.), *Critical gerontology: Perspectives from political and moral economy* (pp. 109–130). Amityville, NY: Baywood Publishing Company.

Tester, S., Hubbard, G., Downs, M., MacDonald, C., & Murphy, J. (2004). Frailty and institutional life. In A. Walker & C. Hagan Hennessy (Eds.), *Growing older: Quality of life in old age* (pp. 209–224). Maidenhead, UK: Open University Press.

Torres-Gil, F. (1992). *The new aging: Politics and change in America*. New York: Auburn House.

Townsend, P. (1981). The structured dependency of the elderly: The creation of social policy in the twentieth century. *Ageing and Society, 1*(1), 5–28.

Townsend, P. (1986). Ageism and social policy. In C. Phillipson & A. Walker (Eds.), *Ageing and social policy* (pp. 15–44). Aldershot, UK: Gower.

Turner, M., Shields, T., & Sharp, D. (2001). Changes and continuities in the determinants of older adults: voter turnout 1952–1996. *The Gerontologist, 41*, 805–818.

Verba, S., Schlozman, K., & Brady, H. (1995). *Voice and equality: Civic voluntarism in American politics*. Cambridge, MA: Harvard University Press.

Verté, D., Ponjaert-Kristofferson, I., & Geerts, C. (1996). Political participation of elderly in local policy. In A. Carrell, V. Gerling, C. Marking, G. Naegele, & A. Walker (Eds.), *Politische beteiligung älterer menschen in Europa* (pp. 122–140). Bonn: Bundesministerium für Familie, Senioren, Frauen und Jugend.

Vincent, J. (1996). Who's afraid of an aging population? Nationalism, the free market and the construction of old age as an issue. *Critical Social Policy, 16*, 3–26.

Walker, A. (1980). The social creation of poverty and dependency in old age. *Journal of Social Policy, 9*(1), 45–75.

Walker, A. (1981). Towards a political economy of old age. *Ageing and Society, 1*(1), 73–94.

Walker, A. (1984). The political economy of privatisation. In J. Le Grand & R. Robinson (Eds.), *Privatisation and the welfare state* (pp. 19–44). London: Allen & Unwin.

Walker, A. (1986). The politics of aging in Britain. In C. Phillipson, M. Bernard, & P. Strong (Eds.), *Dependency and interdependency in old age: Theoretical perspective and policy alternatives* (pp. 30–45). London: Croom Helm.

Walker, A. (1990a). The economic "burden" of aging and the prospect of intergenerational conflict. *Ageing and Society, 10*(4), 377–396.

Walker, A. (1990b). The strategy of inequality: Poverty and income distribution in Britain, 1979–89. In I. Taylor (Ed.), *The social effects of free market policies* (pp. 29–48). Hemel Hempstead, UK: Harvester Wheatsheaf.

Walker, A. (1991). Thatcherism and the new politics of old age. In J. Myles & J. Quadagno (Eds.), *States, labor markets and the future of old age policy* (pp. 19–36). Philadelphia: Temple University Press.

Walker, A. (1993). Poverty and inequality in old age. In J. Bond, P. Coleman, & S. Peace (Eds.), *Ageing in society* (2nd ed., pp. 280–303). London: Sage.

Walker, A. (1998). Speaking for themselves: The new politics of old age in Europe. *Education and Ageing, 13*(1), 5–12.

Walker, A. (1999). Public policy and theories of aging: Constructing and reconstructing old age. In V. Bengtson & K. W. Schaie (Eds.), *Handbook of theories of aging* (pp. 361–378). New York: Springer Publishing Company.

Walker, A. (2003). Securing the future of old age in Europe. *Journal of Societal and Social Policy, 2*(1), 13–32.

Walker, A. (2005). Reexamining the political economy of aging: Understanding the structure/agency tension. In J. Baars, D. Dannefer, C. Phillipson, & A. Walker (Eds.), *Aging, globalization and inequality: The new critical gerontology* (pp. 59–79). Amityville, NY: Baywood (forthcoming).

Walker, A., & Deacon, B. (2003). Economic globalization and policies on aging. *Journal of Societal and Social Policy, 2*(2), 1–18.

Walker, A., & Naegele, G. (Eds.). (1999). *The politics of old age in Europe*. Buckingham, UK: Open University Press.

Walker, A., Walker, C., & Ryan, T. (1996). Older people with learning difficulties leaving institutional care: A case of double jeopardy. *Ageing and Society, 16*(2), 1–26.

World Bank (1994). *Averting the old age crisis*. New York: Oxford University Press.

Young, K. (1984). Political attitudes. In R. Jowell & D. Airy (Eds.), *British social attitudes* (pp. 11–46). Aldershot, UK: Gower.

# Twenty

# Economic Security in Retirement: Reshaping the Public-Private Pension Mix

James H. Schulz and Allan Borowski

Economic security for individuals is achieved through *both* economic production and social protection. On the one hand, employment provides the goods and services that determine living standards. On the other hand, if employment stops, it often threatens that living standard and sometimes even the very survival of the people affected.

Over the years there has been a debate about the extent to which individuals should be responsible for their own welfare, as opposed to receiving social protection from private or government group programs. As observed by Theodore J. Lowi (1990), "the welfare state is a recent effort to solve the ancient and perennial problem of how to save people from starvation without lowering their incentive to work" (p. 25). Accordingly, major economic policy questions arise from the often conflicting goals of economic production and social protection.

Each prior edition of this *Handbook* has contained a chapter with detailed information about providing social protection in old age, including the operation of various public and private programs. This chapter approaches the same topic but with a different emphasis. As in prior editions, this chapter gives major attention to public and private pensions. Its focus, however, is on the dramatic shift in *pension types* currently occurring in the United States and elsewhere.

## I. What Pension Mix?

In many poor nations, the potential security of pensions is nonexistent for most of the labor force. In fact, the World Bank estimates that in 1999, only 15% of the world's population (of 6 billion) "have access to a formal system of retirement income support." (Holzmann, Packard, & Cuesta, 2001, p. 452).

In contrast, industrialized countries provide collective social protection through a combination of social assistance, public and private pensions, and/or government subsidized personal savings schemes. These countries all think that collective action is appropriate. Otherwise, individual myopia, market failures, cyclical market fluctuations, and/or technological change would result in many older individuals with inadequate income and high inequality among individuals.

A succinct rationale for Social Security is given by the U.S. Council of Economic Advisors: "Some individuals may not be capable of making the relevant retirement savings calculations themselves and may not be able to enlist the service of a financial professional to advise them" (CEA, 2004, p. 30). These risks, together with unpredictable life expectancy, are not easily insured against privately. In addition, Social Security "is unusual because it can redistribute income based on a lifetime average of earnings. By doing so, Social Security more accurately targets these transfers to people who most need the assistance" (CEA, 2004, p. 30). Thus, the critical question to be answered is not whether there should be collective social programs. Rather, it is what *mix* of programs is most appropriate?

This chapter focuses on one important aspect of that question. In recent years a major controversy has arisen over the relative merits of defined benefit (DB) versus defined contribution (DC) pension plans. DB plans promise a *specific benefit* based on a formula that typically includes years of service and (often) average earnings. DC plans promise, not a certain level of benefit, but rather *periodic contributions at a certain level* into an employee's pension account. In DC plans, the ultimate benefit is unknown because it is dependent on contributions, management fees, and investment returns. The current controversy centers around differences between DB and DC pension plans with regard to (1) coverage, (2) decision making, (3) benefit adequacy, (4) ease and cost of administration, and (5) who assumes the risks.

During the last decade, there has been a dramatic shift away from DB plans in favor of DC ones. This chapter briefly reviews the history of pensions in the United States, describes the shift in pension types that has taken place, the problems associated with DB and DC

plans, and the experience of a number of countries that rely heavily on DC plans. The chapter concludes with a review of future research priorities suggested by the shift to DC plans.

## II. Pensions in the Twentieth Century: Defined Benefit Plans Dominate

The early history of pensions in the United States is a history of DB plans. That is, most early plans covering workers were DB plans.

### A. Pensions and the Evolution of the Welfare State

In the Anglo-American nations, the nineteenth century was the era of the "poorhouse welfare state" (Rothman, 1971). A problem of early capitalism was inducing people to become "workers," that is, getting peasants to leave rural areas to provide factory manpower. To encourage the shift, community aid in times of need was generally made conditional on entry into a poorhouse, where living conditions were deliberately made almost intolerable.

With industrialization, the labor of the elderly was often not highly valued. In market economies, employers needed ways to deal with workers who *could not work* and also those that employers *did not want* to work. Thus, along with industrialization came innovative social welfare programs for older adults, starting with Germany's 1889 social insurance program. The early public old age benefits were designed as benefits for the poor. They were social assistance for the elderly (but by another name)—elderly who were for the most part indigent, unable to support themselves, and increasingly unable to get adequate support from their children.

After World War II, very different public pension programs developed. The "Social Security welfare state" was based on two principles of income distribution: universal coverage (less social assistance "targeting") and wage replacement to help maintain standards of living in a new period of life called "retirement." The transition from social assistance to Social Security occurred slowly and took various forms in different countries. At the same time, employers were also introducing their own pensions.

## B. Employer-Sponsored Pensions

Employers started pension plans for two main reasons. There was the altruistic desire to help "faithful workers" deal with economic survival when they could no longer work or, in some cases, could no longer meet the pace or physical demands of their jobs. But many employers also developed plans to promote their own interests. They used pensions to (1) help retain the most desirable workers, (2) seek greater efficiency in the workplace, (3) help adjust the company's workforce to shifting demand, and (4) facilitate (i.e., encourage) the retirement of "unsuitable" workers. Typically, pension benefits were offered on a "take it or lose it" basis. There were little or no rewards to workers who left firms for other jobs or to those workers who wanted to continue working beyond the employer's designated retirement age.

As unions emerged, still another employer use for pensions was found. Some employers incorporated pensions into a broader strategy designed to contain labor unrest and weaken the union movement. Most early company pension plans, for example, "included clauses prohibiting workers from striking on penalty of forfeiting all pension rights" (Quadagno, 1988, p. 83). The early history of private pensions, therefore, makes clear that *employer-sponsored plans were*

*basically tools of management*, one important way to assist employers in dealing with manpower issues. During the Great Depression, however, firms closed and pension plan reserves disappeared. Many workers found their future or current pension benefits gone.

In the 1940s and 1950s, employer-sponsored plan coverage began to grow again. Coverage rose from about 4 million employees in the late 1930s to roughly 20 million by 1960 (Schulz, 2001).

DB plans dominated the growth in pension coverage. By 1975, the number of workers in DB plans had reached about 27 million, compared to only 2 million in DC plans (U.S. Department of Labor, 2000). (Workers with DC coverage were predominately in small companies where the cost of administering DB plans was very high.)

### 1. The Passage of the Employee Retirement Income Security Act

With the growth of employer-sponsored pensions came problems. For example, many of the early pension plans had inadequate and inequitable vesting. Vesting refers to plan provisions that give a participant the right to receive a partial or full benefit at a designated age, regardless of whether the employee still works for the company at the age of eligibility. Vesting was virtually nonexistent in early plans; one received a pension only by staying with the company. Perhaps even worse, in many cases workers were fired just before their pension vested.

Pension rights were also lost as a result of (1) inadequate pension funding, (2) misuse of employer-controlled pension funds, and (3) the termination of plans because of plant closures, employer bankruptcy, or various other reasons. Still another problem was the fact that little or no survivor benefits were paid to most spouses.

The Employee Retirement Income Security Act (ERISA) was passed in 1974 to help deal with these problems:

- Minimum vesting standards were established.
- The government was designated to keep track of vested benefits for workers that changed jobs.
- Funding and fiduciary standards were significantly strengthened.
- A plan termination insurance program was established, run by the Pension Benefit Guaranty Corporation (the PBGC).
- Stronger plan disclosure regulations were legislated.
- Modest provisions were introduced to encourage protection of survivors.

### 2. ERISA Discourages Defined Benefit Plans

ERISA went a long way to achieving its primary goal—making sure employees received promised pension benefits. Unfortunately, this achievement came at a significant price.

As far as employers were concerned, ERISA took away one of the most important means of controlling their workforce. Pension benefits could still be used as a recruitment tool, but employers could no longer rig defined benefit plans to restrict actual pension receipt to those workers who stayed with the company and who fitted into their manpower needs.

Having lost a key manpower management tool, employers at the same time found that ERISA significantly drove up the costs of having a pension plan. First, more workers were now actually getting benefits because of better vesting provisions. Second, there was a substantial burden in added paperwork, with extensive reports to the Departments of Treasury and Labor and to the PBGC. Third, new (and steadily rising) insurance premiums were paid by companies to the

PBGC to provide benefits to workers whose plans unexpectedly terminated.

Prominent actuary Paul H. Jackson correctly predicted shortly after ERISA was passed that "the substantial impact of ERISA must, of course, result in a total reassessment by employers of the purpose and value of private pension plans... Fewer new plans will be undertaken on a purely voluntary basis—the commitment is simply too all-pervasive" (Jackson, 1977, pp. 23–24). ERISA was the beginning of the end for new private defined benefit plans.

### C. Social Security Financing: Crisis?

Social Security expenditures were about a half trillion dollars in 2003. Almost no one disputes the fact that Social Security is responsible for much of the improvement in older persons' income. Despite this success, however, there is considerable controversy over Social Security's future. The current debate revolves around three interrelated issues: (1) the financing of benefits, (2) whether future benefits should be lowered for some or all recipients, and (3) the extent to which pension planning and investment decisions should be in private hands.

Large surpluses that have accumulated in recent years are projected to decline rapidly by the middle of the century as the "Baby Boomers" retire. Without financing and/or benefit changes, future benefits will be greater than available funds.

Everyone agrees that the current Social Security system needs to be changed to deal with future financing issues. The disagreement is over how. Conservatives want to shift from the public plan DB approach to greater reliance on private DC plans, in effect taking the problem "off the government's books." But current proposals of many experts make clear that Social Security's long-term financing can be addressed in a variety of ways and that most of these ways do not require a radical change in the public/private pension mix (see, for example, Diamond & Orszag, 2004; Graetz & Mashaw, 1999; Kingson & Schulz, 1997).

### D. The Political Economy of Social Security Reform

The basic financing issues (maturation of a pay-as-you-go pension system and population aging) have been known and understood from the very beginning of Social Security's creation. Also, the transitional problem resulting from the "Baby Boom" has been known for many years.

Also well known are the potential solutions for the financing problems, along with the pros and cons for each. Choosing from among these options, however, has resulted in a major struggle between various political factions and ideologies. The nation finds itself engaged in what Pierson (1996) describes as "the politics of retrenchment and blame avoidance" (p. 145).

One of the most dramatic factors shaping current discussions is the transformation that has occurred with regard to society's view of "the elderly." Although many elderly still live close to or in poverty (see Chapter 13), in a few years the public image of the elderly has gone from one of "deserving poor" to "greedy geezers" (Binstock, 2005).

Coincident with the changed view of the elderly and controversy over how to finance Social Security, there has been renewed interest in conservatives' proposals to reduce the role of Social Security. The neo-liberal model of personal protection has been resurrected, with the current emphasis on collective provision of income in old age replaced by an emphasis on a privatized, market-based approach (see the literature survey in Gilbert, 2002).

The key to the market-oriented proposals is creation of DC plans, with money placed in individual retirement savings accounts administered and invested by private financial institutions. That is, there is a growing interest in requiring workers to assume much more responsibility and much more risk in financial preparation for retirement.

### E. National Pension Systems Are Changing

The United States and other countries continue to debate reform options. At the same time, reform is underway and many changes *have already been adopted*. Over the last couple of decades, almost every industrialized country has made significant changes in their national pension system in response to the aging of their populations. For example, the United States now taxes the Social Security benefits of higher income individuals and is gradually raising the normal retirement age for receipt of full Social Security old-age benefits.

Changes in the various countries have not followed one particular pattern. Differences in approaches result in part from variations among countries in demography, political systems, historical programs, interest group power distribution, and other social and political factors.

Myles and Pierson (2001), however, make an important distinction between demographically mature countries with traditional pay-as-you-go (earnings-related) programs and a small group of countries they call the "latecomers." The latecomers were either late to establish earning-related public pensions or never established them at all. Instead, these countries (Australia, Britain, Denmark, Ireland, the Netherlands, New Zealand, and Switzerland) rely more heavily on means-tested programs and universal flat-rate benefits.

Recent reforms in the latecomer countries have emphasized the creation of nationally mandated DC plans. In contrast, for the most part, countries with mature systems have not shifted from the traditional DB approach. Rather, reforms have concentrated on adjusting payroll taxes, changing retirement ages, modifying indexing, better targeting of benefits, and the "repackaging" of pension programs into hybrid pensions. Thus, one of the new international developments is the creation of hybrid pensions with "notional accounts" that take on some of the characteristics of DB and DC plans (see section V.C.).

## III. Pensions in the Twenty-First Century: The Rise of Defined Contribution Plans

This section looks more closely at some of the developments that have occurred related to the growing importance of DC plans. We begin with the historically important case of Chile.

### A. Chile: The Beginning of a New Approach to Public Pensions

When it was established, the Chilean DC plan was unique. "Chile [in 1981] fired a shot that was heard around the entire social security world when it privatized its long-established 'traditional' social insurance program" (Robert Myers, as quoted in Schulz, 1993, p. 51). A military government led by General Augusto Pinochet undertook radical pension reform; Chile's Social Security program was replaced with a mandatory savings scheme *administered by the private sector*. The law requires almost all wage and salary workers to participate; in reality only 62% of the economically active population does (Gill, Packard, & Yermo, 2005).

Employees in Chile are required to contribute 10% of their wages into a privately administered retirement account, selected by the worker from an officially approved group of financial management companies. Once the worker chooses a firm, the pension money is kept in a separately designated individual account. Workers, however, are allowed to move their retirement funds from one investment manager to another if they are dissatisfied with the current company's performance.

At retirement, workers can choose either to purchase a price-indexed annuity or to make "scheduled withdrawals." Also mandated as part of the overall scheme are worker-funded term life insurance and disability insurance.

The Chilean privatized approach is not cheap. The total contributions for retirement, survivors', disability, and health insurance are equal to 20% of wages, on wages up to the maximum annual amount of about $40,000 (Edwards & Edwards, 2002).

With private financial management firms competing for very large amounts of retirement funds, there is always the risk of money mismanagement or misleading claims about future returns. To reduce these and other risks, the Chilean government assumed from the beginning major supervisory and regulatory responsibility. The government also assumed the role of "payer of last resort." If the assets in a worker's personal account do not yield a benefit that is 85% of the minimum wage, the government makes up the difference.

Also, the government financially backs up the private firms. For example, it steps in to protect workers when an investment management firm goes bankrupt, when the investment manager makes extraordinarily poor investment decisions (producing very low benefits for its clients), or when a firm engages in illegal marketing or investment activities.

It is now more than 25 years since the introduction of the pension privatization in Chile. These have not been trouble-free years. The Chilean approach has been criticized from both ends of the political spectrum. Major problem areas have been (1) low coverage/participation problems, with large portions of the labor force remaining outside the system (Bonilla & Gillion, 1994; Gill, Packard, & Yermo, 2005); (2) the dilution of competition with many investment firms no longer participating, leaving participants far fewer choices among asset managers (Diamond & Valdés-Prieto, 1994); (3) reduced returns because firms have little incentive to take risks when managing funds (Kay, 2003); (4) concern, based on experience and projections, that the program is not likely to produce adequate benefits for many workers, particularly women (Korczyk, 2003); and (5) high administrative, management, and regulatory costs, resulting in a significant reduction in the ultimate pension amounts paid out (Kay & Kritzer, 2002).

It is important to note that most other Latin American countries that have adopted the Chilean approach have not introduced as many safeguards. In part, this is because extensive regulation drives up costs and lowers returns (Holzmann & Stiglitz, 2001). As a result, costs may be lower, but the risks borne by participants in these other privatized systems are higher.

## B. The 401(k) "Revolution" in the United States

As indicated previously, a dramatic change has occurred in the United States pension mix. In addition to the impact of ERISA on DB plans, there is the impact of 401(k) plans. Under the Revenue Act of 1978, section 401(k) (and 403(b) for most educational and nonprofit organizations) *employees* are permitted to make tax-deferred contributions to an employer-sponsored plan. This new section encourages employers to create DC plans. Many plans are profit-sharing plans or voluntary employee contribution plans with no employer contribution. The majority, however, are "thrift plans" where the company *matches* some portion of the employee's contribution.

The annual dollar contributions that can be made by employees into 401(k) plans are limited by law. The limit for individual employees is $15,000 (for 2006) and increases annually based on a price index. (Restrictive contribution limits apply to certain employees who earn more than $90,000 a year, and more liberal rules apply for those 50 years or older.)

There are also limits on the total amount that may be contributed to a 401(k) account from all sources combined: employer matching contributions, profit-sharing payments, or any employee contributions from after-tax compensation. For 2004, the maximum was the lesser of 100% of compensation or $41,000. (The $41,000 limit also increases using a price index.)

Participation in 401(k) plans has grown rapidly. More than 42 million workers were covered in 2000, up from 7 million in 1983 (EBRI, 2000). As participation in 401(k) plans is always voluntary, not all workers employed by businesses with such plans actually participate. Munnell and Sundén (2004) estimated that in 2001, 26% of eligible workers did not participate in 401(k) plans, down from 43% in 1988 and 35% in 1993.

The Employee Benefit Research Institute has estimated the average plan account balance in 2002 to be around $58,000 (Holden & Van Derhei, 2002). Not surprisingly, account balances generally increase with age. The same study found that the balances for persons 50 to 59, for example, averaged around $121,000.

There are a number of reasons for the dramatic 401(k) expansion. First, as discussed previously, employers have sought alternatives to highly regulated DB plans. Second, employers found that the general costs of the DB "pension promise" were not predictable (and hence not easy to budget). That is, with DB plans, employers are faced with the need to make complex actuarial projections and cope with big fluctuations in financial markets. Third, 401(k) plans have increased relative to DB plans because there has been a shift in employment from unionized industries where DB plans were common to non-unionized ones where they are comparatively rare (Gale & Orszag, 2003). Finally, employers say employees like DC plans. They vest immediately and are very "transparent," with each employee "owning" his or her personal account and receiving periodic account statements tracking its value.

## C. American IRA and Keogh Plans

Individual Retirement Accounts (IRAs) were enacted as part of ERISA. In addition, the 1974 pension reform legislation also liberalized contributions to retirement plans for the self-employed (called Keogh plans). Both postpone taxes on contributions and investment returns.

A worker can have a traditional IRA, whether or not he or she is covered by any other retirement plan; however, deductions for individuals with an employer-sponsored retirement plan are often limited. In 2001, 31% of all families in the United States owned an IRA or Keogh plan (Copeland, 2003). Accumulated money in these accounts is large, almost $2 trillion in 1997 (EBRI, 1999). The median value was $27,000 in 2001 (Copeland, 2003)

Research shows that the proportion of *lower paid* workers who take advantage of opportunities for tax-sheltered saving is much smaller than that of more highly paid persons. For example, ownership of IRA and Keogh plans varies significantly by income. In 2001, only 7% of families with incomes less than $10,000 owned a plan, compared to 67% of families with incomes of $100,000 or more. The fear

that such tax-exemption proposals would turn into tax loopholes for higher income people was the principal argument voiced in Congress against the legislation when it was proposed, and it remains a concern today.

## IV. Problems with Defined Contribution Plans

### A. Coverage and Eligibility

Private pension coverage in the United States is much lower than in many other industrial countries (Rein & Turner, 2001). The total number of workers covered under private pension plans has increased from around 10% of the private wage and salary labor force in the early 1940s to only 45% currently. This contrasts, for example, with the 90% to 91% coverage under Australia's and Switzerland's mandatory private pension program.

The creation and growth of IRAs, 401(k), and other DC plans has had no significant effect on the coverage problem. When created by Congress in 1974, IRAs were considered by many people to be a good way of expanding pension coverage. This has not happened. As indicated previously, about a quarter of employees eligible for participation in a 401(k) program do not participate. Employees at lower ages and with lower earnings are much less likely to participate (Hinz & Turner, 1998). "Procrastination and inertia emerge as important explanations both for lack of participation in 401(k) plans and for the fact that those who do participate rarely change their contributions" (Munnell & Sundén, 2004, p. 53).

### B. Lack of Informed Choice

The World Bank has raised a fundamental question: "If mandatory [pension] schemes are needed because of short-sighted workers, how can these same workers be counted on to make wise investment decisions?" (Gill, Packard, & Yermo, 2005, p. 3). DC plans shift much more pension fund decision-making responsibility to the individual. To make good decisions, individuals must be financially well informed. Competitive markets do not work well when consumers cannot manage their finances effectively.

Many research studies (e.g., GE Center for Financial Learning, 1999) have documented the limited financial knowledge of the typical investor. An Investor Protection Trust (1996) survey found that less than one-fifth of the investors were truly literate about financial matters and investing. The U.S. Securities and Exchange Commission reports that more than 50% of Americans do not know the difference between a bond and an equity (Orszag & Stiglitz, 2001). After Sweden introduced supplemental defined contribution plans, its National Audit Office reported that "many savers [have] had difficulty in selecting and managing their own portfolios" (U.S. Social Security Administration, 2004).

Employee (and employer) behavior regarding the investment of pension money in "company stock" also demonstrates how serious the problem is. Currently many DC plan participants fail to adequately diversify their holdings. Two-thirds of DC plan participants are allowed to invest in their company's stock, often encouraged by their employers. The result is that these *employees have invested 29% of their contributions in company stock*. And in companies with more than 5000 employees, the amount invested in company stock rises to 43% (Mitchell & Utkus, 2002). Unfortunately, the recent tremendous loss of retirement savings by Enron employees, mostly holding company stock, demonstrates what can happen (discussed further later).

The common response to this financial literacy problem is a call for better educa-

tion (for example, Valdès-Prieto, 2002). But the practical problems associated with this remedy are enormous. For example, Bodie (2003) reviewed help provided on the Internet to investors. He found that *every site reviewed* provided incorrect or logically flawed advice to investors wanting to follow a conservative, minimal risk strategy.

Thus, DC plans place major risk management burdens on financially unsophisticated individuals; yet adequate education in financial affairs is difficult, if not impossible, to find (assuming most people would be willing to take the time to learn). Buying advice is an option, but experience to date raises serious issues of cost and competence. There is interest, therefore, in developing ways to provide protective guarantees that shield investors from the worst possible outcomes. For example, the PBGC, established under ERISA in 1974, insures DB plans. And "guarantees" for DC plans have been adopted in several Latin American countries, Japan, and Germany. Unfortunately, as Lachance and Mitchell (2003) pointed out, such guarantees add significantly to the costs that must be paid to administer DC plans.

## C. The Adequacy of Benefits

It is difficult to talk about the adequacy of DC pensions, as there is such great variability in the benefits offered. In fact, economist Franco Modigliani, winner of a Nobel Prize, argues that instead of a predictable, guaranteed benefit, participants get something like a "lottery ticket" given the uncertain and potentially erratic performance of their portfolios (Modigliani & Muralidhar, 2004).

Simulation projections have been made to explore the benefit potential of DC plans (e.g., Munnell & Sundén, 2004; Samwick & Skinner, 2004). The simulations suggest that "people covered continuously by a 401(k) can accumulate significant retirement wealth, perhaps even more than they would have received from a traditional defined benefit plan" (Munnell & Sundrén, 2004, p. 31). Experience with *real* DC plans, however, indicates that the *actual* pension income employees receive is often much lower than the *hypothetical* simulation projections. There are many reasons for this, the main ones being that (1) significant numbers of employees do not participate in optional pension plans; (2) individuals who change jobs often do not "roll over" pension accumulations; (3) high management costs have a significantly negative impact on final payout; (4) employers sometimes reduce money matches, especially during recessions; (5) individuals frequently follow an investment strategy that is too conservative, ignoring the advice of most experts; (6) many individuals do not diversify their investment holdings, including individuals who invest large amounts in their own company's stock (often encouraged, or required, by employers); and (7) unlike traditional DB plans, most individuals take lump sums at retirement, instead of annuities, sometimes quickly spending the money.

## D. The High Costs of Defined Contribution Plans

One of the most complex and controversial issues related to comparing DC plans with other pension alternatives is the size and impact of costs related to administering DC plans. The research to date is inconclusive (see the discussion in Holzmann & Stiglitz, 2001); however, the preponderance of expert opinion sees these costs as a major problem (e.g., Claramunt, 2004; Kotlikoff & Burns, 2004).

A popular political argument made to promote DC plans in the United States is that rates of return will be much higher than one might receive under Social Security. What advocates fail to point out is that around the world, administrative and insurance fees are very large and reduce returns significantly. For example, "about half of the cumulative net (of insurance premium) contributions of the average worker [in Chile] who retired in 2000 after contributing to the system since its inception in the early 1980s went toward administrative and insurance fees" (Gill et al., p. 272). Costs are slowly falling in some countries but are still relatively high.

Bringing these costs down has been a priority of policymakers in countries with both voluntary and mandatory DC plans. As Fox and Palmer (2001) point out, one recent trend, driven by the desire to reduce administrative costs, is to have DC pension contributions transferred initially to the national government, rather than sending the funds directly to the financial manager. This has the advantage of making compliance monitoring easier and reducing costs through economies of scale in record-keeping. Additional cost containment measures include placing additional constraints on moving funds from one financial manager to another, and limiting worker choice in the number of investment options.

## E. Incompetent or Illegal Behavior by Administrators and Employers

In 1994, the investments of 10 million mutual fund shareholders in Russia's corrupt and scandal-ridden MMM Co. were wiped out almost overnight (Kaplan, 1994). Was this a unique occurrence in an unstable, unpredictable country? Not if you consider that over the years, *millions* of Americans have also lost huge amounts of money as a result of incompetent or illegal behavior by purveyors of retirement products. Examples include the savings and loan and junk bonds scandals during the 1980s, lost pensions as a result of the Enron bankruptcy in 2001, and the 2003 reports of market-timing abuses by mutual funds.

Enron had a 401(k) retirement plan for its employees, with Enron stock as the major asset held in these accounts; the company's bankruptcy reduced the value of these employees' retirement accounts to almost nothing. In 2003, 16 financial firms were implicated in a mutual fund trading scandal related to "late trading" and "market timing." These firms allowed special clients to trade after the markets had closed, to the financial detriment of other shareholders. This scandal resulted in dozens of mutual fund executives and brokers being fired or forced to resign.

Fraud and incompetence are common: (1) companies inadequately funding plans, manipulating financial reports to hide problems, and "dumping" their retirement plans on the PBGC; (2) salespeople promoting "get rich quick" schemes; (3) clients charged excessive fees and commissions; (4) brokers and financial planners incompetently investing money for clients; and (5) mutual funds and brokers engaging in illegal acts of investment and trading (such as "late trading," "market timing," and insider trading). In addition, investors face a variety of other risks when managing their monies: inflation, fluctuating interest rates, market shifts, defaults, etc. The result is that over the years, millions of workers have been seriously harmed as they have attempted to manage their money for retirement or allowed "experts" to manage it for them.

# V. International Experience with New Pension Mixes

Space constraints make it impossible for us to review all the major DC developments and experiences since Chile's initial effort. We limit ourselves to the United Kingdom, Australia, and coun-tries that are experimenting with a new approach called notional accounts. The United Kingdom and Australia are the two industrialized countries with the longest experience using national DC schemes. The notional account approach, a blend of DB and DC plans characteristics, is a recent pension innovation that is receiving a lot of attention.

## A. Privatization in the United Kingdom

In 1986, the Conservative government of Margaret Thatcher legislated radical changes in the British pension system. A "Personal Pension" option was added to the existing schemes: the flat-rate state pension, the earnings-related state supplemental pension, and "contracted out" schemes administered by private employers. The Personal Pension, a DC scheme, allows workers some investment control, primarily by allowing choice among various privately managed plans.

To this mix, the Labor government added in 2001 another new option called the "Stakeholder Pensions." Stakeholder Pensions are DC plans designed to provide private pensions to *lower earnings* workers who do not have other *private* pension coverage. The target group was 4 to 5 million workers whose earnings were between 50% and 100% of the national wage median.

Stakeholder Pensions were developed in part as a reaction to the very high administrative costs associated with Personal Pensions. The fees that can be charged for Stakeholder Pensions are limited to about 1% of assets.

Over the years, British financial managers have been able to charge whatever they wanted to recoup expenses and make profits, subject, it was hoped, to competitive market forces that would bring charges down. In fact, charges have remained very high. An initial transfer into a Personal Pension can result in costs as high as 25% of the transfer value, in addition to commissions of up to 2.5% of the annual premium. Even with the reforms introduced by the Labor government, Bateman (2001) has estimated that participants in Britain can expect to lose around 19% of their pension accumulations because of administrative costs.

Charges, however, vary enormously from company to company. Unfortunately, it has been virtually impossible for individuals to compare the cost of various competing plans; this is because charges have been imposed in a bewildering variety of ways, often disguised or presented in a misleading fashion.

Ineptness, fraud, and disinformation have dominated the history of British DC plans (Schulz, 2000). Perhaps the biggest shock to the nation came with the 1993 revelation that financial institutions were using unethical and illegal procedures to encourage workers to opt out of employer-administered plans into the Personal Pension option. Many salespersons performed inadequate analyses of clients' situations and provided biased information, virtually guaranteeing bad consumer decisions.

In reaction to this scandal, the British Securities and Investments Board mandated that all investment managers review their records, identify cases of mis-selling, and make restitution. The Board also promulgated additional standards for giving advice and new rules for providing pension information. Unfortunately, these actions did not stop these practices.

Another big problem in Britain is the complexity created by the large number of pensions. Complex provisions and rules accompany all five pension programs. The mis-selling scandal is just one result of this complex reality. Experience over the years has shown that many individuals are looking for quick and easy answers to the complex task of retirement planning and choosing from among pension options. But they are finding it difficult to get good advice.

In 2002, the British Labor Government appointed a commission to look into its growing pension problems. In its first report, the Commission called the British system the most complex pension system in the world, pointed to serious problems, and indicated the need for major changes (Pensions Commission, 2004).

## B. The Australian Approach

A large amount of global attention has been given to Australia's approach to providing pension income through DC plans. In contrast to the "voluntary" approach adopted by the United Kingdom, and the highly regulated, employee-contribution approach in Chile, Australia has *mandated* employer-funded retirement savings through privately administered pension plans called "occupational superannuation" plans.

Until the introduction of these plans, Australian retirees had relied primarily on the Age Pension, a means-tested, flat-rate government pension financed out of general revenues. Private pension plans have existed in Australia since the 1860s, but coverage has always been relatively low. In 1974, only 32% of all employees were covered by a private plan, rising to 45% in 1982. Moreover, the lump sum payouts from these plans were not viewed by many workers as money for retirement but instead as a "fringe benefit" or as deferred pay. Thus, when workers change jobs, it has been typical of them to cash out any private pension accumulations.

Before the 1980s, most employer-sponsored pension funds were DB plans; today DB plans are only about 10% of the total, with DB plans covering less than 4% of private sector workers (APRA, 2004). These current retirement income arrangements are largely the product of a reform process that began with the public recognition of population aging about two decades ago (Howe, 1981). Policy changes sought to reduce reliance on the publicly funded Age Pension while expanding and improving private pension coverage and the role played by these private plans in providing income in old age.

A major impetus to this shift was the return of a Labor Government to power in 1983. In the 1986 national wage case hearing before the Arbitration Commission (Australia's then central wage-fixing authority), the government supported organized labor's claim to allow pensions to be part of employer-employee negotiations in lieu of wage increases. (At the time unions were constrained in seeking wage increases.) The result was that pension coverage increased to almost 70% of all employees by the end of the 1980s (Borowski, 1991).

Then, under pressure from the Australian Council of Trade Unions (ACTU) to make pensions universal, the Labor government mandated pensions for almost all workers under the Superannuation Guarantee (SG) Act of 1992. All employers not already doing so were required to pay a minimum of 3% of employees' salary into individual superannuation accounts. The law specified that the level of mandatory employer (only) contributions should progressively increase. It reached 9% in 2002, where it remains. Close to 90% of workers, almost all full-time workers and three-quarters of part-time workers, now have some superannuation coverage (ASFA, 2004a; Stanford, 2003).

## 1. Superannuation Industry Structure

As a result of the SG, there has been a huge growth in superannuation fund assets, from $A40 billion ($US28 billion) in 1985 to $A565 billion ($US396 billion) today. There are about 2000 large superannuation funds in Australia, despite a continual process of fund rationalization and consolidation. Of these, 245 retail funds (typically managed by life insurance companies and other financial

institutions) hold 34% of the assets; 105 industry funds account for 11%; and about 1600 corporate funds hold 10%. The remaining superannuation assets are held in 281,000 small, self-managed, "do-it-yourself" funds (22%) and 65 public sector funds (20%) (APRA, 2004).

Australia's superannuation industry was substantially self-regulated before the mid-1980s. The SG expansion, however, was accompanied by major regulatory reforms. Despite new safeguards, some experts continue to voice concern about the security of superannuation savings. For example, Bateman (2003) concluded that the "ability of superannuation regulations to ensure the security and adequacy of retirement incomes is unclear" (p. 126).

## 2. Inadequate Income

Perhaps the most serious problem confronting future Australian retirees is the fear of inadequate income. It is generally agreed that a reasonable retirement income goal is retirement income that replaces 60% to 65% of gross preretirement earnings (Commonwealth of Australia 2002a). Most pension experts, however, think that lifetime SG contributions of 9% are almost certain to yield earnings replacement below this level. In 2002, an Australian Senate committee report concluded that SG, together with the age pension, would not meet the benchmark targets of adequacy for the majority of people on or below average incomes (Commonwealth of Australia, 2002a). Yet the issue does remain controversial. In the same report is a submission by the Australian Treasury that argues that benefits in the future will be adequate.

Although there is little agreement on the precise level of contributions required to fill any adequacy gap, major interest groups (such as the ACTU and the superannuation industry) have advocated raising the SG by an additional 6%. The government, however, has made it clear that it is not ready to support such an increase in mandatory contributions.

The government has taken some ad hoc measures to promote income adequacy. To encourage savings by low-income earners beyond the 9% SG, the government introduced, effective July 1, 2003, a matched savings program, somewhat similar to one proposed by Halperin and Munnell (1999). For the 2004–2005 financial year, the government contributed into workers' superannuation funds $A1.50 for each $A1 voluntarily contributed by workers earning up to $A28,000 (with a $A1,500 government payment maximum). Above $A28,000 the co-contribution is reduced by five cents for each dollar of income, phasing out completely at $A58,000. While an attractive scheme, it presupposes low earners have the financial wherewithal and inclination to make the required contributions.

### 3. The Tax Treatment of Superannuation

Although the inadequacy of retirement incomes is due mainly to low contributions, another important factor is the taxation of superannuation plans. In a series of legislative changes (1984, 1988, and 1996), the government substantially reduced the relatively liberal tax benefits related to superannuation plans. The result was a big reduction in the value of the benefits that would have otherwise accrued to retirees from their superannuation plans. The taxes were instituted to recoup some of the sizable forgone revenues associated with superannuation tax concessions—$A5.8 billion (or 3.3% of total revenues) in 2003 (ASFA, 2004b).

Governments in Australia have become increasingly loathe to forego these revenues. Even the Labor opposition in 2004 proposed a cut in the contribution tax of only 2 percentage points

(Weekes, 2004). But acknowledging the tax impact on the adequacy of pensions, the government, somewhat grudgingly, decreased the superannuation surcharge tax from its maximum of 14.5% to 12.5% (and then to 10% by mid-2005).

### 4. From Lump Sum to Income Stream

For some time there has been concern in Australia about lump-sum benefits being spent on nonretirement consumption, including the reduction of personal debt. The fear is that there will be a higher take-up rate of the means-tested Age Pension than would otherwise have been necessary, exacerbating the income inadequacy problem and also requiring higher levels of Age Pension expenditure. Therefore, various tax provisions have been changed to make lump sums less attractive relative to annuities. These efforts to encourage taking superannuation benefits as annuities have met with little success. Three-quarters of all retirees still opt for lump sum payments. As a result, the Senate Select Committee on Superannuation recommended in 2003 that the government should, at some future time, mandate the use of a proportion of superannuation savings for the purchase of either a lifetime or term-certain annuity in retirement (Commonwealth of Australia, 2003).

### 5. The Age Pension Still Dominates

Australia has never had a pay-as-you-go social insurance scheme. Legislated in 1908, the means-tested Age Pension was a social assistance program. However, over the years, the eligibility provisions were steadily liberalized. By the late 1970s, the Age Pension (together with the Service Pension for veterans) had become a de facto universal benefit covering about 90% of age-eligible Australians. But given economic fluctuations, demographics, and budgetary problems, recent governments have steadily tightened the eligibility criteria.

Most recently, population aging has become the main concern of many people; however, there is considerable disagreement and debate about the seriousness of the population aging issue. As of 2005, it was clear that the Liberal government, first elected in 1996, subscribed to the pessimistic outlook regarding the impact of aging on public expenditures. The Liberal government's view was reflected in two major reports that they issued: *The Intergenerational Report* (Commonwealth of Australia, 2002b) and *Economic Implications of an Ageing Population* (Productivity Commission, 2004).

There has been some further tightening of Age Pension eligibility in recent years (for example, raising the eligibility age for women). However, the major means for reducing Age Pension expenditure in the future is seen as a need to promote the expansion of private pension income.

Despite the expansion in superannuation coverage since the mid-1980s, the Age Pension remains the major source of retirement income for most Australians. About 80% of the elderly currently receive the Age Pension or the Service Pension (Tesfaghiorghis, 2001–2002). Of those, two-thirds receive a full pension and one-third receives a part pension.

More important, government projections estimate that the majority of future older Australians, people with a working lifetime of superannuation contributions, will continue to receive an Age Pension, although a smaller proportion (one-third) will rely on it for the bulk of their retirement income. By 2050, the proportion of elderly people receiving the Age Pension will have fallen by only 5%; however, the balance between full- and part-pension recipients will have reversed itself, with two-thirds receiving a part-pension and one-third receiving a full pension (Commonwealth of Australia, 2002a).

## 6. Lessons to Be Learned

A recent 12-nation study ranked Australia as least vulnerable to rising old-age dependency costs paid by government (Jackson & Howe, 2003). Australia's retirement income strategy of mandating superannuation and rolling back public income support is often held up as an approach that other countries should seek to emulate (e.g., Harris, 2004). The previous discussion, however, indicates that there is a need for further changes if Australia is to realize key retirement policy objectives. Many experts think these changes should include some combination of the following: (1) raising mandatory contributions to levels that will produce adequate retirement income, (2) reducing the superannuation "tax bite" that so seriously compromises the realization of the income adequacy objective, (3) better provisions for ensuring the safety of retirement savings held in superannuation funds, (4) ensuring that superannuation is actually used as a means of funding an income stream throughout the retirement years, and (5) reducing still further the number of people qualifying for the Age Pension.

## C. A Third Way: Notional Plans

Over the last decade, beginning with Sweden and Italy, a new model for national pensions has emerged, called the notional defined contribution approach (NDC). It blends the DB and DC approaches. Its major characteristics are:

- Like DC plans, NDC benefits are tied to contributions, with employee and/or employer contributions "credited" to an account set up for each participant; however, unlike DC plans, none of the contributions are actually deposited in these accounts.
- Retirement benefits are paid primarily using pay-as-you-go financing.

- An indexing procedure is used to increase the balances in the personal accounts (similar to returns that originate when private funds are invested in financial markets).
- At retirement, annuitized benefits are calculated based on the account balances (adjusting for changes in average life expectancy over time).
- Unlike most Social Security programs, NDC programs do not have an income redistribution component and are likely to result in greater retirement income inequality.

The driving force behind the introduction of NDC pensions in Italy, Sweden, Poland, Latvia, Kyrgystan, and Mongolia is an attempt to cope with rising pension costs, while making the benefit calculation process more transparent. The NDC approach "offers a way to shift from the defined benefit model to a less generous defined contribution model without the diversion of payroll tax revenues into funded individual accounts" (Williamson, 2004, p. 6). The approach provides an opportunity to stabilize contribution rates over a long period of time. As with regular DC plans, the size of a person's account determines generally what you get back.

Politically, the approach assists countries in the benefit retrenchment process—cloaking cutbacks with mechanistic program provisions related to notional credits, indexing procedures, life expectancy adjustments, and transitional costs relating to prior programs. At the same time, governments paradoxically hope that notional accounts will increase political support as a result of (1) what appears to be a more transparent benefit determination process, (2) personal accounts that foster a sense of ownership, and (3) the emphasis given to individual equity.

In the United States, notional accounts have been introduced in the private sector. Over the last decade, hundreds of companies have replaced their traditional DB plans with "cash balance" plans (Cahill & Soto, 2003). Because this switch results in most current older workers receiving lower pension benefits, a number of employers have been taken to court, with the plaintiffs arguing that cash balance plans have been introduced mainly to save money and discriminate against older workers.

As with other approaches to retirement income security, a NDC program is typically just one pillar of a multi-pillar approach, which includes other public and/or private income maintenance programs. It represents an interesting and important development as countries work their way through the policy challenges of determining the appropriate pension mix.

## VI. Which Way Reform?

The shift from DB plans to DC plans described in this chapter reflects two often observed policy processes. The first is that the adoption of a social policy to address a social problem during a particular era often results in new problems and challenges. These new developments invariably require the adoption of additional new policies in later years. The need for further action becomes increasingly apparent as the (usually) unanticipated consequences of the earlier policy manifest themselves. This can happen during initial policy implementation or at some later time as a result of social, economic, demographic, and/or political changes. Typically, in the course of pursuing a policy objective (such as the provision of an adequate retirement income), policymakers must confront the reality that it may conflict and/or compete with other valued objectives. For example, providing equitable tax incentives to encourage saving for retirement is likely to be costly and make budgetary problems worse. In such instances, the resulting conflicts demand that trade-offs be made between objectives, often resulting in provisions or arrangements that are "a marvel of complication" (Sass, 2004, p. 12). The need to make such trade-offs is the second policy process.

The contemporary architecture of America's retirement income system in general and, more specifically, the rise/demise of DC/DB plans can be viewed in light of these policy processes. For example, in the United States, DC plans arose in large measure out of the landmark 1974 ERISA legislation. One of the major objectives of ERISA was to secure the safety of workers' DB plan benefits. Several decades later, however, the majority of workers are no longer covered by DB plans (with PBGC protection) but by DC plans (without protection). In addition, the financial risks that were borne by employers under DB plans are now, under DC plans, effectively shifted to workers. These workers, however, often lack the financial education required to make sound investment decisions. The decline of DB plans with their explicit replacement rate-based formulas has further complicated financial planning for retirement by workers covered under the now pervasive DC plans. Further, whereas DB plan benefits were generally paid at retirement in the form of a lifetime annuity, DC plans are most often paid in lump sum form, cashed out on job change or retirement, and frequently used for other than long-term retirement income. And despite the attractiveness of DC plans (over DB plans) to employers, the dramatic shift to DC plans has had no significant effect on the extent of pension coverage. Low-to-middle income groups in particular remain either uncovered or under-covered.

Although the "pension picture" described in this chapter is a new one, it also reminds us of many longstanding challenges. In this regard, the experience

of other countries that have gone through the transition and rely heavily on DC plans is useful and should be studied by researchers interested in policies and mechanisms of old age income provision. Our discussion in this chapter just highlights what we think are some of the most important developments.

Over the last few decades, scholars have extensively researched the problems arising from DB plans, especially Social Security programs, and they have been discussed in prior editions of this Handbook. In fact, some of these problems are now used to promote the adoption of DC plans. But it is important to note that no comparable research effort has been extended to DC plans. Yet, as this chapter indicates, preliminary research indicates that the problems emerging with the DC approach are as serious or more serious than past or current problems facing DB plans. Thus, the problems we identified in Section IV are all candidates for further research.

In addition, policy research needs to look at the issues related to providing for the basic economic needs of retirement living: adequate income, manageable economic security, and options for meeting health care costs. Unfortunately, the new economic pension environment does not ensure adequate income and threatens to dramatically increase insecurity for people preparing for old age. Just as the Chilean government plays a huge role in guaranteeing DC pensions, other countries using the DC approach will have to explore and evaluate various guaranty mechanisms that are needed to protect workers from the risk of exposure to financial scandals, bear markets, overly narrow investment strategies, and administrative costs that render retirement income inadequate.

Moreover, countries cannot continue to rely on the goodwill of employers to provide pension benefits. The mandating of coverage, last seriously considered in the United States during the Carter Administration, needs to be researched and evaluated again.

Finally, we believe that policymakers should not expect workers of the future to be much less financially naive than workers today. They will also need expert help, that is, unbiased advice on investing their savings for retirement. To date, experience in country after country indicates that the financial advising industry is not performing well; in fact, the problems are horrendous, suggesting that the government should consider regulation of the industry and also suggesting the need for research in this area.

All the reforms discussed here would cost money, which brings us back again to one of the major issues, the high costs of administering DC plans. Much more research is needed to understand the reasons for these high costs and the impact government regulation (as in the case of DB plans) will have on cost.

The challenge of the new market-oriented approach to providing income in old age is great, and the implications are important. As Polanyi (1944) observed and Marx predicted, to allow income distribution to be shaped by markets alone would probably result in the self-annihilation of a society. Polanyi, when he wrote, was focused on the insecurity arising during the early years of the industrial revolution. But the critical and complex issues of that time have not gone away here in the twenty-first century.

## References

APRA (Australian Prudential Regulation Authority). (2004). *Insurance and superannuation bulletin.* Canberra: Australian Prudential Regulation Authority.

ASFA (Association of Superannuation Funds of Australia). (2004a). *How fair is Super?* Fact sheet No 6. Sydney: Association of Superannuation Funds of Australia.

ASFA (Association of Superannuation Funds of Australia). (2004b). *Taxes on Super.* Fact sheet No 4. Sydney: Association of Superannuation Funds of Australia.

Bateman, H. (2001). *Disclosure of superannuation fees and charges.* Report prepared for the Australian Institute of Superannuation Trustees. Sydney, Australia: reproduced.

Bateman, H. (2003). Regulation of superannuation, *The Australian Economic Review,* 36(1), 118–127.

Binstock, R. H. (2005). The contemporary politics of old-age policies. In R. B. Hudson (Ed.), *The new politics of old age policy.* Baltimore: Johns Hopkins University Press.

Bodie, Z. (2003). An analysis of investment advice to retirement plan participants. In O. Mitchell & K. Smetters, *The pension challenge* (pp. 19–32). Oxford: Oxford University Press.

Bonilla, A., & Gillion, C. (1994). *Private pension schemes in Chile.* Geneva: International Labour Office.

Borowski, A. (1991). The economics and politics of retirement incomes policy in Australia. *International Social Security Review,* 44(1–2), 27–40.

Cahill, K. E., & Soto, M. (2003). How do cash balance plans affect the pension landscape? *Issues in brief* #14. Newton, MA: Center for Retirement Research at Boston College.

CEA (Council of Economic Advisers). (2004). *Economic report of the president.* Washington, DC: Government Printing Office.

Claramunt, C. O. (2004). Assessing pension system reforms in Latin America. *International Social Security Review,* 57(2), 25–46.

Commonwealth of Australia, (2002a). *Superannuation and standards of living in retirement.* Canberra: Senate Select Committee on Superannuation.

Commonwealth of Australia. (2002b). *Intergenerational report 2002–03.* Budget paper no. 5. Canberra: Parliament of Australia.

Commonwealth of Australia. (2003). *Planning for retirement.* Canberra: Senate Select Committee on Superannuation.

Copeland, C. (2003). *Individual account retirement plans: An analysis of the 2001 survey of consumer finances.* Issue brief #259. Washington, DC: Employee Benefit Research Institute.

Diamond, P. A., & Orszag, P. R. (2004). *Saving social security: A balanced approach.* Washington, DC: Brookings Institution Press.

Diamond, P., & Valdés-Prieto, S. (1994). *Social security reform in the Chilean economy: Policy lessons and challenges.* Washington, DC: Brookings Institution.

EBRI. (1999). Protecting IRA balances and withdrawals. *EBRI notes* (May). Washington, DC: Employee Benefit Research Institute.

EBRI. (2000). *History of 401(k) plans.* Retrieved July 2, 2004 from http://www.ebri.org/facts/1200fact.htm

Edwards, S., & Edwards, A. C. (2002). *Social security privatization reform and labor markets: the case of Chile.* Working paper 8924. Cambridge, MA: National Bureau of Economic Research.

Fox, L., & Palmer, E. (2001). New approaches to multipillar pension systems: What in the world is going on? In R. Holzmann & J. E. Stiglitz (Eds.), *New ideas about old age* (pp. 90–132). Washington, DC: World Bank.

Gale, W. B., & Orszag, P. R. (2003). *Private pensions: Issues and options.* Discussion paper no 9. Washington, DC: The Urban Institute.

GE Center for Financial Learning. (1999). *Financial literacy project.* Retrieved June 28, 2004 from www.financiallearning.com/ge/researchstudies.jsp?c=getResearchHtml1

Gilbert, N. (2002). *Transformation of the welfare state* Oxford: Oxford University Press.

Gill, I. S., Packard, T., & Yermo, J. (2005). *Keeping the promise of social security in Latin America.* California: Stanford University Press.

Graetz, M. J., & Mashaw, J. L. (1999). *True security: Rethinking American social insurance.* New Haven, CT: Yale University Press.

Halperin, D. I., & Munnell, A. H. (1999). *How the pension system should be reformed.* Retrieved September 3, 2004 from http://www.ourfuture.org/docUploads/20010927082450.pdf

Harris, D. O. (2004). *Pension reforms and ageing populations: Lessons from Australia and the United Kingdom.* Testimony before the US Senate Special Committee on Aging. Retrieved September 3, 2004 from http://aging.senate.gov/_files/hr123dh.pdf

Hinz, R. P., & Turner, J. (1998). Why don't workers participate? In O. S. Mitchell & S. J. Schieber (Eds.), *Living with defined contribution plans: Remaking responsibility* (pp. 17–37). Philadelphia: University of Pennsylvania Press.

Holden, S., & Van Derhei, J. (2002). *Can 401(k) accumulations generate significant income for future retirees?* Issue brief #251. Washington, DC: Employee Benefits Research Institute.

Holzmann, R., & Stiglitz, J. E., Eds. *New ideas about old age security.* Washington, DC: World Bank.

Holzmann, R., Packard, T., & Cuesta, J. (2001). Extending coverage in multipillar pension systems. In R. Holzmann & J. E. Stiglitz (Eds.), *New ideas about old age security* (pp. 452–484). Washington, DC: World Bank.

Howe, A. (Ed.). (1981). *Towards an older Australia.* St. Lucia: University of Queensland Press.

Investor Protection Trust. (1996). *Investor knowledge survey 1996.* Retrieved June 24, 2004 from http://www.investorprotection.org

Jackson, P. H. (1977). Comment. In D. M. McGill (Ed.), *Social security and private pension plans: Competitive or complementary?* (pp. 23–24) Homewood, Il: Richard D. Irwin.

Jackson, R., & Howe, N. (2003). *The 2003 aging vulnerability index: an assessment of the capacity of twelve developed countries to meet the aging challenge.* Washington, DC: Center for Strategic and International Studies and Watson Wyatt Corporate Offices.

Kaplan, F. (1994. July 30). Bubble bursts for Russian investors. *Boston Globe*, 2.

Kay, S. (2003). *Pension reform and political risk.* Retrieved May, 2004 from http://www.frbatlanta.org/filelegacydocs/politicalriskandpensionreformkay.pdf

Kay, S., & Kritzer, B. (2002). Social security reform in Latin America: policy challenges. *Journal of Aging and Social Policy, 14*(1), 9–21.

Kingson, E. R., & Schulz, J. T. (Eds.). (1997). *Social security in the 21st century.* Oxford: Oxford University Press.

Korczyk, S. M. (2003). *Women and individual social security accounts in Chile, the*

United Kingdom, and Australia. AARP Policy Institute Paper 2003–09. Washington DC: AARP.

Kotlikoff, L., & Burns, S. (2004). *The coming generational storm.* Cambridge, MA: MIT Press.

Lachance, M., & Mitchell, O. (2003). Understanding individual account guarantees. In O. Mitchell & K. Smetters (Eds.), *The pension challenge* (pp. 159–186). Oxford: Oxford University Press.

Lowi, T. J. (1990). Risks and rights in the history of American governments. *Daedalus, 119*(4), 17–40.

Mitchell, O. S., & Utkus. S. P. (2002). The role of company stock in defined contribution plans. Working paper no. 9250. Cambridge, MA: National Bureau of Economic Research.

Modigliani, F., & Muralidhar, A. (2004). *Rethinking pension reform.* Cambridge, UK: Cambridge University Press.

Munnell, A. H., & Sundén, A. (2004). *Coming up short: The challenge of 410(k) plans.* Washington, DC: Brookings Institution Press.

Myles, J., & Pierson, P. (2001). The comparative political economy of pension reform. In P. Pierson (Ed.), *The new politics of the welfare state* (pp. 302–333). Oxford: Oxford University Press.

Orszag, P., & Stiglitz, J.E. (2001). Rethinking pension reform. In R. Holzmann & J. E. Stiglitz (Eds.), *New ideas about old age security* (pp. 3–31). Washington, DC: World Bank.

Pensions Commission. (2004). *Pensions: Challenges and choices.* Retrieved January 31, 2005 from www.pensionscommission.org.uk/publications/2004

Pierson, P. (1996). The new politics of the welfare state. *World Politics, 48*(2), 143–179.

Polanyi, K. (1944). *The great transformation.* Boston, MA: Beacon Press.

Productivity Commission. (2004). *Economic implications of an ageing Australia.* Canberra: The Commission.

Quadagno, J. (1988). *The transformation of old age security: Class and politics in the American welfare state.* Chicago: University of Chicago Press.

Rein, M., & Turner, J. (2001). Public-private interactions: Mandatory pensions in Australia, the Netherlands and Switzerland.

*Review of Population and Social Policy, 10,* 107–153.

Rothman, D. (1971). *The discovery of the asylum.* Boston, MA: Little Brown.

Samwick, A. A., & Skinner, J. (2004). How will 401(k) pension plans affect retirement income? *American Economic Review, 94*(1), 329–343.

Sass, S. A. (2004). Reforming the Australian retirement system: Mandating individual accounts. *Issues in brief* #2. Newton, MA: Center for Retirement Research at Boston College.

Schulz, J. H. (1993). Chile's approach to retirement income security attracts worldwide attention. *Aging International.* September, 51–52.

Schulz, J. H. (2000). *Older women and private pensions in the United Kingdom.* Waltham, MA: National Center on Women & Aging, Brandeis University.

Schulz, J. H. (2001). *The economics of aging* (7th ed.). Westport, CT: Auburn House Press.

Stanford, J. D. (2003). Is superannuation safe? The background and the issues. *The Australian Economic Review, 36*(1), 79–88.

Tesfaghiorghis, H. (2001–2002). Projections of the number of income support recipients: 1999–2051. *Australian Social Policy.* Canberra: Family and Community Services, pp. 43–78.

U.S. Department of Labor. (2000). *Private pension plan bulletin.* No. 8. Washington, DC: Pension and Welfare Benefits Administration, Office of Policy and Research.

U.S. Social Security Administration. (2004). *Sweden. International update: September 1.* Retrieved October 29, 2004 from http://www.ssa.gov/policy/docs/progdesc/intl_update/2004–09/2004–09.pdf

Valdés-Prieto, S. (2002). *Justifying mandated savings for old age.* Background paper for the regional study on social security reform. Washington, DC: World Bank.

Weekes, P. (2004, August 7). Dismal future awaits boomers. *The Age,* business section 5.

Williamson, J. (2004). Assessing the notional defined contribution model. *Issues in brief* #24. Newton, MA: Center for Retirement Research at Boston College.

Twenty-one

# Organization and Financing of Health Care

Marilyn Moon

Older Americans receive a substantial share of their health care coverage from government programs, setting seniors apart from the population as a whole. Enacted in 1965 as additions to the Social Security Act, Medicare and Medicaid offer important resources that individuals can rely on in old age. Without these protections, few Americans could afford to retire, given the costs of health care and the barriers in the private sector to obtaining reasonably priced individual coverage. But Medicare and Medicaid do not cover all the health care needs of the population over 65, despite high levels of federal and state expenditures. Because of these costly public expenditures and the implications of a rapidly aging society, Medicare and Medicaid will continue to come under scrutiny and perhaps face further major changes in the future. As such changes take place, these programs need to be viewed in the context of both meeting health care needs and offering financial protections to older Americans.

Medicare is a federal health insurance program that serves more than 97% of persons age 65 and older in the United States, providing basic protection for

their acute-care needs, although not a fully comprehensive set of benefits. Medicaid, which offers help for the aged and other specifically designated categories of low-income and low-wealth Americans, is also important for older persons because it fills in crucial gaps in Medicare coverage for this group. Medicaid, which is a joint federal/state program, supplements that coverage for about one in every seven seniors. Further, Medicaid is the only public program that helps cover the long-term care costs of older Americans (see Chapter 22). In addition, a complicated arrangement of private supplemental insurance has also evolved over time to fill in Medicare's gaps for many beneficiaries. Because of the complexities of the health care system for older Americans, this chapter does not attempt to take an international perspective, but rather focuses on experiences only in the United States.

Although in many ways Medicare has been one of the most successful public programs of the federal government, it has also faced criticism as a result of its rapid expansion. Medicare spending in 2004 stood at $297 billion (Congressional

Budget Office, 2004). From the late 1970s until 2003, Medicare was a frequent target in efforts to reduce federal spending. These efforts peaked in 1997 when the Balanced Budget Act set in motion a broad range of changes to slow Medicare's growth. In 2003, however, expansion occurred with the addition of a new prescription drug benefit. The Medicare Prescription Drug, Improvement, and Modernization Act (MMA) of 2003, discussed in detail later, will generate many changes that will substantially raise Medicare spending.

A major complicating factor in dealing with the costs of Medicare and Medicaid is the fact that their growth is attributable to the same factors generating rising costs in the rest of the health care system. Consequently, it is not only difficult but inappropriate to treat these programs as separable from the rest of the system. In the middle of the first decade of the twenty-first century, costs rose rapidly in all sectors of health care, particularly for hospital care and prescription drugs (Levit, Smith, Cowan, Sensenig, Catlin, & Health Accounts Team, 2004). Further, the size of these two public programs means that changes in payment levels or decisions about medical necessity will have impacts on all of health care spending.

## I. The Creation of Medicare and Medicaid

Medicare was established by legislation in 1965 as Title XVIII of the Social Security Act and first went into effect on July 1, 1966. The overriding goal was to provide mainstream acute health care—hospital, physician, and related services—for persons 65 years and over. This age group had been underserved by the health care system, largely because many older persons could not afford insurance. Insurance coverage as part of retirement benefits was relatively rare and insurance

companies had been reluctant to offer coverage to older persons even for those seniors who could afford it. Consequently, Medicare has contributed substantially to the well-being of America's oldest citizens. It is the largest payer of acute health care services in the United States, providing the major source of insurance for the elderly (and, since 1972, individuals who receive federal disability insurance benefits). Medicare today has given a whole generation of people access to care beyond what they had before. One of Medicare's important accomplishments is that the very old and the very sick have access to the same basic benefits as younger, healthier beneficiaries. Although there is certainly room for improvement, Medicare is insurance that is never rescinded because of the poor health of the individual.

When Medicare was implemented in 1966, it revolutionized health care coverage for persons 65 and older. For example, it almost immediately doubled the proportion of seniors with health insurance. Only about half of people in this age group had insurance before Medicare (Andersen, Lion, & Anderson, 1976). By 1970, 97% of older Americans were covered by the program, and that proportion has remained about the same ever since (Moon, 1996). Anyone 65 or over who is eligible for any type of Social Security benefit (e.g., as a worker or a dependent) receives Part A, Hospital Insurance [HI]). Part A covers hospital, skilled nursing, and hospice care and is funded by payroll tax contributions from workers and employers that are earmarked for an HI trust fund. Supplementary Medical Insurance (Part B) is available to persons 65 and over on a voluntary basis. It covers physician services, hospital outpatient services, and other ambulatory care and is funded by a combination of general revenues and beneficiary premiums. Home health care benefits are covered by both Parts A and B.

When Medicare began, it was dominated by inpatient hospital care, which accounted for about two-thirds of all spending. Indeed, most of the focus of debate before Medicare's passage was on Part A (HI). But as care has moved out of the inpatient setting, Part B (Supplementary Medical Insurance) has become a much larger share of the program (Figure 21.1). Care in hospital outpatient departments and in physicians' offices now replaces many surgeries and treatments formerly performed in inpatient settings. In addition, skilled nursing facility care and home health services, referred to as post-acute care, have also increased in importance over time as hospital stays have been shortened. When individuals leave a hospital after only a few days, post-acute care is often needed as a transition, either in a nursing facility or at home with visits from nurses or other skilled technicians. Further, some of these benefits, particularly home health, have been used for supportive or long-term care purposes, as well as post-acute skilled care. The financial incentives established by payment to health providers and by coverage of benefits have affected the mix of services used.

One original promise of the program was that it would not interfere with the practice of medicine. Payments were designed to be like standard insurance policies then in place; however, costs for the program rose rapidly almost from the beginning, and in the late 1970s, the government sought to slow spending growth in Medicare, and chose to do so largely through application of new payment policies. These both affected how much would be paid and moved payments away from per unit pricing.

Payments for hospital services, the biggest component of Medicare, were modified in the early 1980s to pay on the basis of the patient's diagnosis, regardless of length of stay in a hospital or the actual costs of a particular case. This new system encouraged hospitals to be more efficient, although it also resulted in some premature discharges. Over time, however, this payment system has been judged to be relatively successful (Moon, 1996). It has helped to encourage movement away from long inpatient stays and to more care being delivered outside of hospitals for patients of all ages.

Physician reform came later and established payments on the basis of a relative

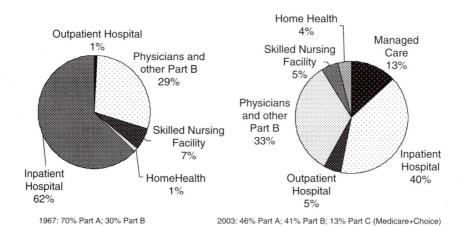

Figure 21.1   Medicare expenditures by type of service: 1967 and 2003.
**Source:** Health Care Financing Administration, 2001, and Medicare Payment Advisory Commission, 2004.

value scale, initially limiting payments to specialists and increasing them for basic primary care (Physician Payment Review Commission, 1987). Many other health care insurers now use Medicare's so-called physician relative value payment system. Both hospital and physician payments require periodic updating, and Medicare is sometimes criticized for falling behind in making adjustments in response to new medical procedures. Nevertheless, the program has been a major player affecting the delivery of care. Overall, Medicare has served as a leader, and these payment reforms have fundamentally changed the way that hospitals and doctors are paid in the United States.

The situation for Medicaid is quite different because its implementation is controlled by the states, which have wide latitude in establishing eligibility and coverage. Hence, approaches to holding the line on Medicaid spending can vary substantially across the United States. In general, however, states have relied both on keeping payments to providers very low and on requiring beneficiaries to go into managed care plans. Low payments have sometimes led to access problems when providers of services decide not to take on Medicaid patients. This effectively reduces costs both through the lower payments and through the reduced volume of services available. For example, for persons dually eligible for Medicare and Medicaid, a number of states decline to use Medicaid to pay for Medicare co-payments to physicians, thereby effectively lowering the payments doctors receive. Further, nursing home access is sometimes a problem for Medicaid patients. In terms of managed care, states cannot require the dually eligible to get services that are covered by Medicare from managed care plans, but they can restrict access to Medicaid benefits for services not covered by Medicare

if patients do not use the Medicaid managed care plans offered.

## II. The Pressures on a Public System

Although Medicare performed well relative to total health care costs in the 1980s and 1990s, the program nonetheless is often portrayed as a runaway item in the federal budget. The evidence cited for this is the higher overall growth in spending on Medicare as compared to the rest of the budget. Both Medicare and Medicaid have grown as a share of the federal budget and of the Gross Domestic Product (GDP)—the output of all goods and services produced in the United States. Medicare, however, has not grown faster than the costs of private health insurance (Boccuti & Moon, 2003; Levit et al., 2004), which does not receive the same level of skepticism as Medicare. As these programs are funded with tax dollars in an era of antitax sentiment, they get more scrutiny than health expenditures paid for by individuals or by businesses.

Further, it is largely a myth that the senior lobby has been successful in expanding Medicare (Binstock & Quadagno, 2001). Until 2003, benefits under the program had changed little. Moreover, at various points in time, regulatory and legislative changes have been used to hold down program growth.

In the early 1970s, Medicare was only 3.5% of the federal budget and by 1990 accounted for 8.6%. The percentage has grown steadily. Despite major cuts in 1997, Medicare's share totaled nearly 13% of the 2004 federal budget (Congressional Budget Office, 2004). And the new prescription drug legislation passed in 2003 has further increased the overall size of Medicare, starting with its implementation in 2006.

As a result of its growth, many policy-makers believe that Medicare may be crowding out expenditures on other domestic programs. Critics often argue that Americans will only accept a certain level of overall public spending, so if Medicare grows rapidly, it hurts other spending even if it has its own revenue source. In this argument, Medicare gets most of the attention because of the near-term increases in spending that the aging of the Baby Boom will foster. Already, the number of beneficiaries has grown faster than the population as a whole, reflecting longer life expectancies for the elderly.

Until recently, a second fiscal pressure faced by Medicare arose from the status of the Part A (HI) trust fund. Current law provides a fixed source of funding, the Federal Insurance Contributions Act pay-

roll tax, for HI. These revenues typically have not grown as fast as the level of spending, creating periodic crises when the date of trust fund exhaustion is close at hand. So far, that day of reckoning has been postponed several times by major cost-cutting efforts and an increase in the wage and salary base subject to taxation. A strong economy and the slow growth in Medicare spending in 1998 and 1999 pushed that date to 2029, based on the 2002 report of the Medicare trustees. But, as shown in Figure 21.2, the date of exhaustion of the Part A trust fund has again grown closer, as a result of higher projected spending and a less healthy economy. Yet, it remains further out than at most times in Medicare's history.

The financing issues facing Medicaid are also complicated. The concern about crowding out can be made for this

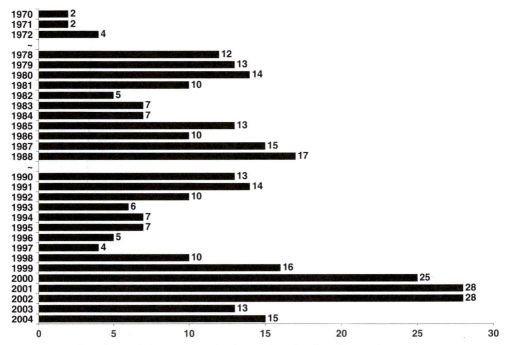

**Figure 21.2**  Number of years before HI trust fund is predicted to be exhausted.

Data not available for 1973–1977 and 1989.

**Source:** O'Sullivan, 1995, and Boards of Trustees, 2004.

program as well, especially because the constitutions of almost all states require them to balance their budgets. Moreover, states vary in the shares of their programs going to different Medicaid-eligible subgroups—and by amounts greater than would be suggested by population differences alone. Thus, they can certainly decide when to favor the old over the young, or vice versa, within the Medicaid program.

## III. How the Total System Has Evolved Over Time

Because of Medicare's limited benefits, private and public supplemental plans have developed to meet older persons' additional needs for health insurance. Four kinds of supplemental policies have evolved. As suggested previously, Medicaid, a means-tested public benefit established at the same time as Medicare, subsidizes many poor older persons through several different arrangements. Employer-based retiree insurance and individual supplemental coverage policies (termed Medigap) are provided by

private insurers. A fourth option is essentially a hybrid, in which private health plans that contract with Medicare to provide Medicare-covered services also offer at least some additional supplemental benefits. These supplemental coverages vary in quality, beneficiaries' ability to access them, and the degree to which they relieve financial burdens. A good understanding of how these supplemental plans operate and the contributions they make is essential for any analysis of the health care system facing older Americans. Figure 21.3 shows the extent and type of supplemental coverage for Medicare beneficiaries.

### A. Medicaid

Medicaid offers generous fill-in benefits for persons with low incomes and assets. Because states have latitude in establishing eligibility and coverage, however, there is considerable variation in the quality and quantity of services provided across the states. For example, Medicaid spending in 1995 on persons 65 and older ranged from $5,565 in Tennessee to $23,611 per person in the District of

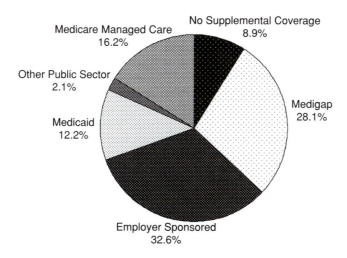

**Figure 21.3**   Sources of supplemental coverage among noninstitutionalized Medicare beneficiaries, 2001.
**Source:** Medicare Payment Advisory Commission, 2004. (Analysis of 2001 MCBS.)

Columbia. And more recently, per capita spending in 1999 for nursing facility services (used predominately by seniors) ranged from $11,095 in Arkansas to $50,963 in Alaska (Centers for Medicare and Medicaid Services, 2003). Today, two separate programs provide some benefits under the Medicaid umbrella. Basic Medicaid coverage is limited to those with the lowest incomes, generally well below the federal poverty level. For those who get these benefits, coverage is comprehensive. In addition to paying the Part B premium and relieving beneficiaries of the responsibility for co-payments and deductibles, these state-based programs all offer some type of prescription drug coverage, long-term care, and a range of other services as well.

The second set of programs under Medicaid even more directly supplement Medicare. Beginning in 1988 and varying by income, these benefits provide relief for low-income Medicare beneficiaries. The Qualified Medicare Beneficiary Program (QMB) covers Part B premiums, deductibles, and co-insurance for those whose incomes fall below 100% of the poverty level ($9,310 in 2004 for a single person). The Specified Low Income Medicare Beneficiary (SLMB) program provides Part B premium subsidies for those with incomes between 100% and 120% of the poverty level. Finally, the 1997 Balanced Budget Act created the Qualified Individuals (QI) program to cover the full premium costs for people with incomes between 120% and 135% poverty and a small portion of premium costs for those up to 175% of the poverty level (Moon, Brennan, & Segal, 1998). This last benefit has been allowed to expire.

In practice, all of these programs cover only some of the people who qualify for them. Participation rates remain low because of individuals' reluctance to seek help from a "welfare program," substantial enrollment burdens, and sometimes lack of awareness of potential eligibility.

Traditional Medicaid, for example, has never covered more than half of all elderly below the poverty line. Moreover, in 1996, only 55% of those eligible participated in QMB, and just 16% of those eligible participated in SLMB (Barents Group, 1999). Thus, Medicaid is only partially successful in ensuring comprehensive coverage to low income seniors.

In addition, the asset test for determining Medicaid eligibility, which is actually even more stringent than the income test, results in a number of individuals who would qualify on the basis of income being excluded from the program (Moon, Friedland, & Shirey, 2002). Although income limits have been increased over time, most states have asset tests that have been in place since 1987, often restricting benefits to persons with assets below $2,000 or $4,000 and couples with assets below $3,000 or $6,000. A key policy issue here is how to balance the desire to target benefits to those most in need with the goal of encouraging older Americans to save for their future needs.

## B. Employer-Sponsored Plans

Employer-based retiree health plans normally offer comprehensive supplemental insurance. Employers usually subsidize retiree premiums and establish benefits comparable to what their working population receives by filling in gaps left by Medicare. A large proportion of these plans, for example, cover prescription drugs. Thus, these plans both reduce out-of-pocket expenses and increase access to services, often without limiting provider choice. Beneficiaries in these plans have among the lowest out-of-pocket costs (Medicare Payment Advisory Commission, 2002), even though they are heavy users of care. They are thus among the best protected of all seniors.

Such plans are limited to workers and dependents whose former employer offers generous retiree benefits. Among current Medicare beneficiaries about one-third have such employer-sponsored retiree health plans (Medicare Payment Advisory Commission, 2004). And, these benefits accrue disproportionately to high income retirees. This privileged group does not need improvements in Medicare to ensure their access to care, as they are covered very well at present. In fact, this group of seniors complicates making changes in the Medicare program, as they may be opposed to anything that raises their costs. Many policymakers do not want to devote public dollars to essentially replacing benefits this group already has.

The strength of resistance to change by those with retiree insurance may decline in the future, however, because many employers are beginning to cut back benefits to control costs. They are placing more controls on the use of care, raising retiree contributions in the form of premiums or cost sharing, and even changing the benefit package. For instance, the share of those with coverage who are required to pay the full premium rose from 27% in 1997 to 40% in 1999 (Mercer, 2002).

A number of studies have tracked changes in employer behavior, each showing the same downward trend. For example, a study of large firms (with 200 or more workers who are most likely to offer such benefits) found the percentage offering retiree health benefits declined from 66% in 1988 to 36% in 2004 (Kaiser Family Foundation and Health Research and Educational Trust, 2004). Another study found similar declines from 40% to 24% for retirees over the age of 65 from 1993 to 2000 (Mercer, 2002). Although these reductions have not shown up yet in survey data on beneficiaries over the age of 65, they will likely start to have an impact on that coverage in the next several years as new retirees turn 65 without these protections. Another approach to reducing liabilities is to raise the requirements for qualifying for coverage, for example, by adding more years of employment as a condition of participation.

## C. Medigap Insurance

A traditional form of private supplemental coverage, commonly referred to as Medigap, does not lower overall out-of-pocket burdens because the premium is fully paid by the beneficiary and includes substantial administrative and marketing charges, and often, profits for the insurer (U.S. General Accounting Office, 1998). Thus, many beneficiaries have higher, not lower, financial burdens when they buy Medigap. Medigap is most useful for reducing potential catastrophic expenses for those who have high costs in a particular year. The 10 standardized plans that insurance companies are allowed to offer under federal law cover a basic package of Medicare's required cost sharing and in some cases include a limited prescription drug benefit. This form of supplemental insurance provides the least protection for beneficiaries, yet it remains popular with beneficiaries seeking to keep their out-of-pocket costs from being high in any one year.

Another issue is that Medigap premiums rose dramatically over the 1990s. Between 1992 and 1996, premium rates in Arizona, Virginia, and Ohio rose 18%, 19%, and 41%, respectively, though the majority of those rate increases took place between 1995 and 1996 (Alecxih, Lutzky, Sevak, & Claxton, 1997). National estimates for rate increases in 1999 and 2000, according to insurance experts, were 8% to 10% (Medicare Payment Advisory Commission, 2000).

Over time, Medigap plans have changed the way they price policies, also contributing to access problems. Medigap providers can sell policies that are community, issue age, or attained age rated. Companies have moved away from "community-rated" plans where the premium is the same for everyone, regardless of age. Most providers have moved to an attained age structure in which policies increase in cost rapidly as people age. This puts greater burdens on beneficiaries just as their incomes are declining. For the unwary buyer at age 65, these plans appear less costly than community-rated options (Alecxih et al., 1997). But because most beneficiaries cannot change their minds after a 6-month, open-enrollment period at age 65, they may lock themselves into a very bad deal over time. Premiums in age-rated plans can get to be so high that older persons cannot afford them. This raises issues about access to care and reduces some of the benefits from traditional Medicare, which does an excellent job of pooling risks across a large group.

## D. Private Plan Options

As noted previously, beneficiaries also can obtain additional benefits to supplement Medicare's basic package by enrolling in private health plans, termed "Medicare Advantage" in the Medicare Modernization Act of 2003. In such a case, enrollees agree to get all their coverage from the private plan, which receives a per capita payment from Medicare, rather than from a combination of traditional reimbursements for services from Medicare and private supplemental coverage. Thus far, private plans that participate in Medicare are mainly health maintenance organizations (HMOs), which restrict enrollees to a specific network of doctors and hospitals. Cost sharing is usually lower than for traditional Medicare, and some additional benefits are usually offered for less than the price of a Medigap plan. After legislative changes in 1997, however, these plans became more expensive for consumers through higher premiums and cost sharing, and many plans withdrew from Medicare altogether. The number of ben-

eficiaries enrolled in these private plans reached a peak of 16% in 1999 followed by a decline to about 12% in 2003 (Boards of Trustees, 2004). To counter this retrenchment in private plan participation, the 2003 MMA increased payments from the federal government to plans to encourage them to stay or return to offering coverage. The number of beneficiaries in Medicare Advantage is now beginning to rise.

## E. No Coverage

Finally, an increasing number of beneficiaries cannot afford any supplemental policy. As shown in Figure 21.3, about 9% of Medicare beneficiaries had no extra policy to cover what Medicare's benefit package does not. Beneficiaries who cannot afford to purchase supplemental coverage and who are not eligible for Medicaid are among the most vulnerable beneficiaries. Because they are likely to be older and with only modest financial resources, high Medicare out-of-pocket costs may prevent them from getting needed care.

Lack of supplemental coverage is associated with problems of access to care. Those who have no supplemental coverage, for example, are less likely to see a doctor in any given year, less likely to have a usual source of care, and more likely to postpone getting care in a timely fashion. For example, 21% of beneficiaries who rely on Medicare alone reported delaying care because of cost, but only 5% of beneficiaries with private coverage report delaying care (Gluck & Hanson, 2001).

## IV. Issues Surrounding Reliance on the Private Market

Claims for savings from options that shift Medicare to a system of private insurance usually rest on two basic arguments: first is the claim that the private sector is more efficient than Medicare based on the often-made claim that government is simply inefficient, and second, that competition among plans will generate more price sensitivity by beneficiaries and plans alike. Although private options are now available to beneficiaries, supporters of a private approach would go further. For example, to generate price sensitivity, privatization proposals usually call for government to limit subsidies to a share of the costs of an *average* plan, leaving beneficiaries to pay the remainder. More expensive plans would require beneficiaries to pay higher premiums.

Another particularly crucial issue in proposals to expand the role of the private sector is the treatment of the traditional Medicare program. Currently, beneficiaries are automatically enrolled in traditional Medicare unless they choose to go into a private plan. Alternatively, traditional Medicare could become just one of many plans that beneficiaries choose among, likely paying a substantially higher premium if they choose the traditional program. The MMA included a proposal to create a large demonstration of just such an approach beginning in 2011 (Boards of Trustees, 2004).

Restructuring could profoundly affect Medicare's future. In particular, the traditional Medicare program could be priced beyond the means of many beneficiaries, leaving only private plan options from which to choose. Further, if plans begin to sort into two groups of higher cost and lower cost plans, the likely result would be to segregate beneficiaries in plans on the basis of their ability to pay. This would be quite different than today where the basic program treats all beneficiaries alike. Details of a private sector approach will be important in determining the impact on both savings and beneficiaries.

## A. Inherent Advantages of Private Plans

Some supporters of a private approach assume that private plans inherently offer

advantages that traditional Medicare cannot achieve. But there is no magic bullet to holding the line on growth. Per capita spending rises because of the higher use of services, higher prices, or a combination of the two. Medicare's price clout is well known and documented, so it is difficult for private plans to do better in that area. So what about managed care's ability to control use of services? Studies of managed care have concluded that most such plans saved money by obtaining price discounts for services and not by changing the practice of health care (Strunk, Ginsburg, & Gabel. 2001). Controlling use of services represents a major challenge for both private insurance and Medicare.

A private approach has the potential to allow greater flexibility for innovation and change in coverage of benefits. This allows private insurers to respond more quickly than a large government program can to adopt new innovations and to intervene where insurers believe too much care is being delivered (Butler & Moffit, 1995). But what looks like cost-effectiveness activities from an insurer's perspective may be seen by a beneficiary as the loss of potentially essential care. Further, there are too few examples of truly innovative new techniques, organizational strategies or other contributions from private plan competition. Some managed care plans, for example, do not even have the data or administrative mechanisms to undertake care coordination (Strunk et al., 2001).

The newest type of plans suggested as an improvement for Medicare beneficiaries, preferred provider organizations (PPOs), obtain some savings through provider discounts, and also by paying very little for any patient who goes outside the network to get care. Thus, their strategy is often one of cost shifting onto beneficiaries. This may hold down PPO premiums, but from society's standpoint, would do little to help reduce overall health care costs (U.S. Government Accountability Office, 2004).

Under the traditional Medicare program, beneficiaries do not need to fear loss of coverage when they develop health problems. On the other hand, private insurers are interested in satisfying their own customers and generating profits for stockholders. When the financial incentives they face are very broad (such as receiving capitated payments), private insurers respond as good business entities should. They seek the easiest ways of holding down costs in the provision of services. Even though many private insurers are willing and able to care for Medicare patients, the easiest way to stay in business as an insurer is to seek out the healthy enrollees and avoid the sick. The incentives under the current system, with its poor adjustments for risk, push plans in that direction (Newhouse, Buntin, & Chapman, 1999). And in a market system, once that becomes the dominant approach, even insurers who would like to treat sicker patients are penalized by the market if they do so. This response helps individual insurers, but it is not good for limiting overall costs to either the federal government or to society as a whole.

Finally, private insurers will almost surely have higher administrative overhead costs than does Medicare. Private insurance, for example, tends to have administrative costs in the range of 15% (Levit et al., 2004). Insurers need to advertise and promote their plans. They face smaller risk pools than traditional Medicare, requiring them to make more conservative decisions regarding reserves and other protections against losses over time. Private plans expect to return a profit to shareholders. These factors cumulate and work against the likelihood that private companies can perform better than Medicare which has administra-

tive costs totaling about 2% of program spending (Boards of Trustees, 2004).

### B. Competition among Plans

Reform options stressing competition seek savings not only by relying on private plans but also on competition among those plans. Often this includes allowing premiums paid by beneficiaries to vary such that those choosing higher cost plans pay substantially higher premiums. The theory is that beneficiaries will become more price conscious and choose lower cost plans. This in turn will reward more efficient private insurers. But the experiences in Medicare lend considerable doubt to the notion that the theory will prove true in practice for the Medicare population (U.S. General Accounting Office, 2000). Studies on retirees show less willingness to change doctors and learn new insurance rules in order to save a few dollars each month, particularly if they have health problems.

New approaches to the delivery of health care under Medicare may generate a whole new set of problems, including problems in areas where Medicare is now working well. For example, shifting across plans is not necessarily good for patients; it is not only disruptive, it can raise costs of care. Studies have shown that having one physician over a long period of time reduces costs of care (e.g., Weiss & Blustein, 1996). And if it is only the healthier beneficiaries who choose to switch plans, the sickest and most vulnerable beneficiaries may end up being concentrated in plans that become increasingly expensive over time (Buchmueller, 2000).

Will reforms that lead to a greater reliance on the market still retain the emphasis on equal access to care and plans? For example, differential premiums could undermine some of the redistributive nature of the program that assures even low-income beneficiaries access to high quality care and responsive providers. Support for a market approach that moves away from a "one-size-fits-all" approach is a prescription for risk selection problems. If plans have flexibility in tailoring their offerings, they can, for example, raise cost sharing on benefits such as home health care which are disproportionately used by older, sicker beneficiaries. About one in every three Medicare beneficiaries has severe mental or physical health problems. In contrast, the healthy and relatively well-off (with incomes over $32,000 per year for singles and $40,000 per year for couples) make up less than 10% of the Medicare population. Consequently, anything that puts the sickest at greater risk relative to the healthy is out of sync with this basic tenet of Medicare.

If the advantages of one large risk pool (such as the traditional Medicare program) are eliminated, other means will have to be found to make sure that private insurers cannot find ways to serve only the healthy population. Although this very difficult challenge has been studied extensively, as yet no satisfactory risk adjustor has been developed (Newhouse et al., 1999). What has been developed to a finer degree, however, are marketing tools and mechanisms to select risks For example, advertising for these plans often portrays vigorous older persons, and the distribution of such materials may focus on areas where healthier beneficiaries are likely to congregate. High-quality plans that attract people with extensive health care needs are likely to be more expensive than plans that focus on serving the relatively healthy. If risk adjustors are never powerful enough to compensate plans for taking sicker patients, with health problems, who also disproportionately have lower incomes, those patients would be charged the highest premiums under many privatization reform schemes.

## V. Where Medicaid and Medicare Are Today

The MMA will create a number of crucial changes for both the Medicare and Medicaid programs. Further, the financing of the Medicare program is in considerable doubt since many of the Republicans in control of Congress and the Republican administration have both signaled a strong reluctance to providing additional resources to the program. This will likely mean that in the near future, cost containment efforts will again begin to dominate legislative activities, perhaps even threatening the viability of retaining a drug benefit under Medicare over time.

In January of 2006, a new drug program financed by a combination of beneficiary premiums (covering about 25% of costs) and general revenues (paying the other 75%) will begin. This benefit will require anyone desiring to obtain a drug benefit to enroll in a private plan. For those who remain in traditional Medicare, the plan they purchase will cover only drugs. Multiple choices may be available offering a confusing, complex set of rules including what formulary will be used (i.e., what drugs will be covered), what cost sharing will look like, what pharmacies will participate in each plan, and what premiums will be. Further, many beneficiaries are likely to end up with three sources of coverage—Medicare, private supplemental insurance, and the drug plan. On administrative grounds alone, this is likely to result in inefficiency and higher costs than necessary. Moreover, drug-only plans are risky for insurers because they are likely to selectively attract enrollees who know they will be high users of drug services. Such plans have been soundly criticized by the industry. Nearly 90% of all beneficiaries are currently in traditional Medicare, so these drug-only plans will be crucial to the success of the drug benefit.

The inadequacy of the drug benefit is also an issue. Beneficiaries are expected to spend about $1.6 trillion on drugs during the first eight years of the drug benefit. Thus, although the expected federal costs will be more than $400 billion for this period, this will still represent only a little more than one-fourth of drug spending. The difference arises because of a less than comprehensive benefit structure and the expectation that a substantial number of beneficiaries will decline to participate. For those who do participate, the federal government's share would be, on average, about 48% of drug spending. And since the beneficiary would pay one-quarter of the costs of that through a monthly premium, the effective subsidy is about 36% of costs. But in an antitax environment, it will be difficult, if not impossible, to improve the benefit.

Further, to help hold down costs to the federal government from the new drug benefit, states will be required to pay much of what they previously spent on drugs for the dually eligible (i.e., those receiving both Medicare and Medicaid). The transition of these dually eligible beneficiaries from receiving drug coverage through Medicaid to having to choose a private plan represents another major change.

Another key aspect of the 2003 legislation is the promotion of Medicare Advantage private plans in part by offering additional monies to entice new insurers to participate and new beneficiaries to enroll in them. Because evidence indicates that private plans are already overpaid on average as a result of their tendency to enroll comparatively healthy Medicare beneficiaries, private plans will be able to offer more generous benefits than before, as well as more generous benefits than traditional Medicare. If this enticement strategy works, the resulting inequities will likely hurt the very sick, who disproportionately choose to remain in the traditional options, which will not receive extra subsidies or expanded benefits.

To the extent that older persons opt to join these private plans, the equal treatment that has been an important aspect of the Medicare program is likely to erode. The rationale for moving in this direction has been based on claims that the private sector will be able to generate savings and "save" the Medicare program over time; however, the evidence does not support these claims. That is, past experience with Medicare private plans and analyses of Medicare vis-à-vis private insurance indicate that Medicare does as well as or somewhat better than the private sector at holding down costs of care (U.S. General Accounting Office, 2000; Medicare Payment Advisory Commission, 2002). Certainly, starting out by overpaying plans to get them to participate does not suggest confidence in the ability of the private sector to offer cost effective care.

## VI. Where Could We Go with the Organization and Financing of Care?

The future of Medicare has become a controversial political issue mainly because this is a large and popular public program that faces projections of rapid growth in the future. As a government program, either new revenues will have to be added to support Medicare, or its growth will have to be curtailed. Much of the problem is driven by the expected increase in the number of persons eligible for Medicare from 39 million in 2000 to 78 million in 2030 as the Baby Boom generation becomes eligible for benefits. Although the numbers covered by Medicare have already doubled since 1966, this is likely to be a more significant change because the share of the population enrolled in the program will also grow from one in every eight Americans to more than one in every five.

Making changes to Medicare that can improve its viability both in terms of its costs and in how well it serves older and disabled beneficiaries should certainly be pursued. Further, it makes little sense to look for a solution that simply turns over Medicare to the private sector. The flux and complexity of our health care system will necessitate continuing attention to this program.

What are the trade-offs from attempts to increase the role of private plans in serving Medicare beneficiaries? Any modest gains in lower costs that are likely to come from some increased competition and from the flexibility that the private sector enjoys could be more than offset by increased discrepancies in access to care between the healthy and the sick or the wealthy and the poor. The effort necessary to create in a private plan environment all the protections needed to ensure no risk selection and that all plans, including the less expensive ones, offer high quality care will be difficult to create and enforce.

## A. More Incremental Approaches

A more realistic approach would be to emphasize improvements in *both* the private plan options and the traditional Medicare program, basically retaining the current structure in which traditional Medicare is the primary option. Rather than focusing on restructuring Medicare to emphasize private insurance, the emphasis could be placed on innovations necessary for improvements in health care delivery regardless of setting. This would require, for example, that the traditional Medicare program be offered with expanded benefits to avoid the problem of generating a complex, jerry-rigged system of government and supplemental plans.

In addition, better norms and standards of care are needed if we are to provide quality of care protections to all Americans. Investment in outcomes research, disease management, and other techniques that could lead to improvements in treatment of patients will require a substantial public commitment. This cannot be done as well in a proprietary, for-profit environment where dissemination of new ways of coordinating care may not be shared.

Private plans can play a role in developing innovations on their own, but in much the same way that we view basic research on medicine as requiring a public component, innovations in health delivery also need such support. Further, innovations in treatment and coordination of care should focus on those with substantial health problems, exactly the population that many private plans avoid. Some private plans might be willing to specialize in individuals with specific needs, but this is not going to happen if the emphasis is on price competition and with barely adequate risk adjustors. Innovative plans would likely suffer in that environment; reform needs to focus on enhancing the effectiveness of private plans by rewarding such innovation. Further, the default plan—where those who do not or cannot choose or who find a hostile environment in the world of competition—must, for the time being, be traditional Medicare.

A good area to begin improvements in knowledge about the effectiveness of medical care would be with prescription drugs. Realistically, the new prescription drug benefit will require major efforts to hold down costs over time. Part of that effort needs to be based on evidence of the comparative effectiveness and safety of various drugs, for example. Establishing rules for coverage of drugs should reflect good medical evidence with higher co-pays reserved for less effective drugs, for example, or brand name drugs when equivalent generics are available. Too often, differential co-pays are established instead on the basis of the price of the drug or depending on which manufacturer offers the best discounts. Undertaking these studies and evaluations represents a public good and needs to be funded on that basis; however, no funds were made available for such an effort in the MMA and private plans, and others are reluctant to do this on their own.

Within the fee-for-service environment, it would be helpful to energize both patients and physicians in helping to coordinate care. Patients need information and support as well as incentives to become involved. Many caring physicians, who have often resented the low pay in fee-for-service and the lack of control in managed care, would likely welcome the ability to spend more time with their patients. One simple way to do this would be to give beneficiaries a certificate that spells out the care consultation benefits to which they are entitled and allow them to designate a physician who will provide those services. In that way, both the patient and the physician (who would get an additional payment for the annual services) would know what they are expected to provide. Such care would likely reduce confusion and unnecessary duplication of services that go on in a fee-for-service environment. This change should be just one of many in seeking to improve care coordination.

Additional flexibility to the Centers for Medicare and Medicaid Services (CMS) in its management and development of payment initiatives using competition also could result in long-term cost savings and serve patients well. In the areas of durable medical equipment and perhaps even some testing and laboratory services, contracting could be used to obtain better prices. This could also be done with prescription drugs if there is a repeal of the provision of the MMA that prohibits CMS from bargaining for drug prices. These are but a few of the options that ought to be considered.

## B. The Issues of Financing Medicare and Medicaid

More resources will be needed to finance Medicare over time (Gluck & Moon, 2000). This means asking beneficiaries to pay more or taxpayers to increase their contributions to Medicare or a combination of the two. It is simply not feasible to absorb a doubling of the population over the next 30 years without dealing with the financing issue. In fact, avoiding discussions of higher taxpayer revenues has already led to cost shifting onto beneficiaries, which implicitly represents a financing decision.

A wide range of mechanisms can be used to explicitly or implicitly require beneficiaries to contribute more to the costs of their care. For example, increased premiums or cost-sharing requirements can be, and have been, applied over time to shift costs onto those who use the program. The MMA included not only an increased across-the-board Part B deductible in 2005, but also provided for phasing in a higher premium for persons with annual incomes above $80,000 beginning in 2007 (Boards of Trustees 2004). As described previously, a voucher approach through private plan payments would also essentially result in cost shifting onto beneficiaries by asking them to bear a greater share of both the costs and risks of higher prices for insurance over time.

Efforts to raise the age of eligibility for the program to 67 also implicitly mean cost shifting to beneficiaries. Moreover, if individuals must then seek coverage through the private insurance market until they reach the new age of eligibility, they will quickly find that coverage is very expensive or even unavailable (Pollitz, Sorian, & Thomas, 2001). And because Medicare would be eliminating eligibility for its younger, least expensive older patients on average, the approximately 5% of people disenfranchised if eligibility age goes to 67 would save Medicare only about 2% of its costs (Waidmann, 1998).

In terms of Medicaid, it is not feasible to ask beneficiaries—who are by definition lower income—to bear a greater share of the costs of their care. Indeed, the way that Medicaid works for long-term care services is to require that individuals devote most of their incomes to the costs of institutionalization, for example, with the government then only filling in the gaps. This program will also be important to retirees who need long-term care in the future, but the crisis will come later as the costs of a Baby Boom generation in its eighties and nineties hits Medicaid. So, although less attention is currently focused on Medicaid, it too will need additional financial support over time. It is not known how well states will do in financing future needs.

What then about the costs of financing relying on greater contributions from taxpayers? This will be difficult to do in the current environment in Washington and, technically, new revenues would not have to be raised for a number of years. Doing so soon, however, would likely increase taxes most on Baby Boomers who will be drawing heavily on Medicare and Medicaid in the future. If broader revenue sources are tapped, they will affect different groups of the population depending on which sources are used. For example, payroll taxes remain relatively popular with the general public, likely because they know where the revenues raised are supposed to go; but economists criticize these taxes as raising the costs of workers to employers, discouraging employment. General revenues, the other major source of income for Medicare, are more progressive—asking higher income persons to pay more—and require that older persons, as well as the young, contribute. Medicaid relies on general revenue contributions from both the federal and state governments. Other taxes, such

as those on alcohol and tobacco, often do not bring in enough revenue to resolve the financing issues. Whatever choices are made, raising taxes is likely to be a last resort approach given the political costs often associated with such measures.

Someone will need to pay more to provide care for an aging population. Issues of fairness raise important considerations about how much beneficiaries can be asked to pay and how much should be required from others. The key issue will be how to share that burden, not whether it will increase over time, as it surely will.

## References

Alecxih, L. M. B., Lutzky, S., Sevak, P., & Claxton, G. (1997). *Key issues affecting accessibility to Medigap insurance.* New York: The Commonwealth Fund.

Andersen, R., Lion, J., & Anderson, O. W. (1976). *Two decades of health services: Social survey trends in use and expenditure.* Cambridge, MA: Ballinger Publishing Company.

Barents Group LLC. (1999). A profile of QMB-eligible and SLMB-eligible Medicare beneficiaries. Report prepared for Health Care Financing Administration, Washington DC.

Binstock, R. H., & Quadagno, J. (2001). Aging and politics. In R. H. Binstock & L. K. George (Eds.), *Handbook of aging and the social sciences* (5th ed., pp. 333–351). San Diego, CA: Academic Press.

Boards of Trustees. (2004). *2004 annual report of the Boards of Trustees of the Federal Hospital Insurance and Federal Supplementary Medical Insurance Trust Funds.* Washington, DC: U.S. Government Printing Office.

Boccuti, C., & Moon, M. (2003). Comparing Medicare and private insurance: Growth rates in spending over three decades. *Health Affairs, 22,* 230–237.

Buchmueller, T. (2000). The health plan choices of retirees under managed competition. *Health Affairs, 35,* 949–976.

Butler, S., & Moffit, R. (1995). The FEHBP as a model for a new Medicare program. *Health Affairs, 14,* 8–30.

Centers for Medicare and Medicaid Services (2003). *Health Care Financing Review: Annual Statistical Supplement, 2002.*

Congressional Budget Office. (2004). *The budget and economic outlook: An update.* Washington, DC: CBO.

Gluck, M., & Hanson, K. (2001). *Medicare chartbook.* Washington, DC: The Henry J. Kaiser Family Foundation.

Gluck, M., & Moon, M. (2000). *Financing Medicare's future: Final report of the Study Panel on Medicare's Long Term Financing.* Washington, DC: National Academy of Social Insurance.

Health Care Financing Administration. (2001). *Health Care Financing Review Medicare and Medicaid Statistical Supplement, 2001.* Baltimore, MD: U.S. Department of Health and Human Services.

Kaiser Family Foundation and Health Research and Educational Trust (2004). *Employer health benefits 2004 annual survey.* Menlo Park, CA: Kaiser Family Foundation.

Levit, K., Smith, C., Cowan, C., Sensenig, A., Catlin, A., & Health Accounts Team. (2004). Health spending rebound continues in 2002. *Health Affairs, 23*, 147–159.

Medicare Payment Advisory Commission. (2002). *Report to Congress: Assessing Medicare benefits.* Washington, DC: Medpac.

Medicare Payment Advisory Commission. (2000). *Report to Congress: Medicare payment policy.* Washington, DC: Medpac.

Medicare Payment Advisory Commission. (2004). *Report to Congress: New approaches in Medicare.* Washington, DC: Medpac

Mercer, W. (2000). *Mercer/Foster Higgins National Survey of Employer-Sponsored Health Plans, 2000.* New York: William M. Mercer, Inc.

Moon, M. (1996). *Medicare now and in the future* (2nd ed.). Washington D.C: Urban Institute Press.

Moon, M., Brennan, N., & Segal, M. (1998). Options for aiding low-income Medicare beneficiaries. *Inquiry, 35*, 346–356.

Moon, M., Friedland, R., & Shirey, L. (2002). *Medicare beneficiaries and their assets: Implications for low-income programs.* Menlo Park, CA: Henry J. Kaiser Family Foundation.

Newhouse, J., Buntin, M. B., & Chapman, J. (1999). *Risk adjustment and Medicare.* New York City: The Commonwealth Fund.

O'Sullivan, J. (1995). *Medicare: History of Part A trust fund insolvency projections.* Washington, DC: Congressional Research Service.

Physician Payment Review Commission. (1987). *Medicare physician payment: An agenda for reform.* Washington, DC: U.S. Government Printing Office.

Pollitz, K., Sorian, R., & Thomas, K. (2001). *How accessible is individual health insurance for consumers in less-than-perfect health?* Menlo Park, CA: The Henry J. Kaiser Family Foundation.

Strunk, B. C., Ginsburg, P. B., & Gabel, J. R. (2001). Tracking health care costs. *Health Affairs,* Web Exclusive, W39–W50.

U.S. Government Accountability Office (2004). *Medicare demonstration PPOs: Financial and other advantages for plans, few advantages for beneficiaries* (Rep. No. GAO-04-960). Washington, DC: U.S. General Accounting Office.

U.S. General Accounting Office. (1998). *Medigap insurance: Compliance with federal standards has increased,* GAL/HEHS-98-66, Washington, DC: U.S. General Accounting Office.

U.S. General Accounting Office. (2000). *Medicare+Choice: Payments exceed cost of fee-for-service benefits, adding billions to spending* (Rep. No. GAO/HEHS-00-161). Washington, DC: U.S. General Accounting Office.

Waidmann, T. (1998). Potential effects of raising Medicare's eligibility age. *Health Affairs, 17*, 156–164.

Weiss, L., & Blustein, J. (1996). Faithful patients: The effect of long-term physician-patient relationships on the costs and use of health care by older Americans. *American Journal of Public Health, 86*, 1742–1747.

Twenty-two

# Emerging Issues in Long-Term Care

Robyn I. Stone

Long-term care has been the subject of much analysis and debate among policymakers, providers, consumers, and researchers over the last three decades. The challenge of meeting the long-term care needs of America's chronically disabled older population will become even more salient over the next 30 to 40 years as the Baby Boom generation ages. This chapter begins with a description of long-term care—how it is defined and who needs and receives services and supports. It then reviews the "triple knot of long-term care" (Stone, 2000a)—how services are financed, where they are delivered, and by whom. The chapter concludes with a discussion of four emerging issues that the various stakeholders currently face in their efforts to be responsive to the long-term care needs and preferences of older adults and their families.

## I. Defining Long-Term Care

Long-term care is not easy to define. The boundaries between primary, acute, and long-term care have blurred (Kane, Kane, & Ladd, 1998; Stone, 2000a). Long-term care

is a variety of services and supports provided by unpaid (informal) and paid providers that concentrates on helping individuals to function as well as possible and to maintain their lifestyles in the face of disability. It frequently involves intense participation by family members, particularly wives and adult daughters, as providers and decision makers. Families are often equal beneficiaries of long-term care interventions, because care and supports provided by paid caregivers to the older person who is disabled are an important respite for the family caregiver (Stone and Kemper, 1989).

Long-term care encompasses a broad range of help with daily activities, over a long period of time, for chronically disabled people. These primarily low-tech services are designed to minimize, rehabilitate, or compensate for loss of independent physical or mental functioning. The services include assistance with basic activities of daily living (ADLs)—dressing, bathing, toileting, transferring, and eating. Services may also help with instrumental activities of daily living (IADLs), including household chores such as meal preparation and cleaning;

*Handbook of Aging and the Social Sciences, Sixth Edition*

life management such as shopping, money management, and medication management; and transportation. Services include hands-on and stand-by or supervisory human assistance, assistive devices such as canes and walkers, and technology such as computerized medication reminders and emergency alert systems that warn family members and others when an older person may be in trouble. Long-term care services also may include home modifications such as building ramps, grab bars, and easy-to-use door handles.

## A. Relationship Between Acute and Long-Term Care

The need for long-term care emerges from chronic and debilitating medical conditions that occur at birth, during various developmental stages, or from accidents. Examples are arthritis, diabetes, dementia, traumatic brain injury, and paraplegia. Often people who need long-term care also require primary and acute care when they are sick.

In 2000, the personal health care expenditures for Medicare beneficiaries with no ADL limitations (excluding nursing home residents) averaged $5,816; for beneficiaries with three or more ADL limitations, the expenditures averaged $16,425 (Centers for Medicare and Medicaid Services, 2000). Temporary, episodic services focus on curing illness or restoring an individual's health to a previous state. In contrast, the predominant strategy in long-term care is to integrate treatment and living for older adults with functional disabilities—not to undervalue health care for those getting long-term care, but to incorporate health care into the context of the functions of daily life (Kane et al., 1998).

One reason for the blurred boundaries between long-term care and various stages of medical care is the confounding of settings with services (Stone, 2000a).

More and more, acute care and high-tech rehabilitation formerly provided in hospitals are being provided in settings traditionally used for long-term care, such as skilled nursing facilities and private homes. It is difficult, therefore, to know where medically oriented care stops and long-term care begins. For example, should medication management for older adults with chronic disabilities, including the administration of injections, intravenous drug therapy, and the monitoring of adverse drug interactions, be considered long-term care or ongoing medical care?

## B. The Role of Residence in Long-Term Care

In long-term care, the place where people live, including the nature and quality of one's physical and social environment, can greatly enhance or impede a person's functional abilities, independence, and quality of life. Public policies supporting nursing home care explicitly recognize the residential needs of the long-term care population by including room and board, as well as care, in their reimbursement rates. Until recently, however, little attention was paid to the quality of the residential aspects of nursing facilities. Most were modeled after hospitals with nursing stations, long corridors, and shared rooms. Some nursing home providers, often referred to as the Pioneer Network, are engaged in "culture change" activities that are attempting to transform the physical and social environment of their facilities into a "home" environment for their residents (Weiner & Ronch, 2003).

The importance of creating a homelike atmosphere in residential care settings, including a focus on private rooms and bathrooms, was a major impetus for the expansion of adult foster homes in many states and the development of assisted living in the 1980s (Kane et al.,

1998). The quality of the physical environment also influences the extent to which disabled elders can remain in their own homes, often referred to as "aging in place." Home modifications such as grab bars in bathrooms and the installation of ramps to replace steps can make the critical difference between being able to stay at home and needing to find a more restrictive residential setting.

## C. Who Needs and Uses Long-Term Care?

The long-term care population is diverse in age and level of disability. Of the estimated 12.8 million Americans reporting long-term care needs in 1995, as measured by the need for assistance with ADLs or IADLs, 57% were over the age of 65 (National Academy on Aging, 1997). Data from 2000 highlights the fact that the need for long-term care increases substantially with age. Among those 65 to 74 years, only 1.8% needed assistance with one or two ADLs; 1.7% needed assistance with three to six ADLs. In contrast, among those 80 years or older, 8.2% needed assistance with one to two ADLs and 10.9% required help with three or more ADLs (Davis, 2004).

Data on the noninstitutionalized civilian older population in the 1998 Health and Retirement Study indicate the prevalence of moderate to severe memory impairment (a measure of cognitive ability) was 4.4% among those 65 to 69 years old, 8.3% among those 70 to 74 years old, 13.5% among those 75 to 79 years old, 20.1% among those 80 to 84 years old, and 35.8% among those 85 years or older (Federal Interagency Forum on Aging-Related Statistics, 2001). Comparing samples of older nursing home residents drawn from the 1987 National Medical Expenditures Survey and the 1996 Medical Expenditure Panel Study, Spillman, Krauss, and Altman (1997) observed an increase in the prevalence of cognitive impairment in nursing homes over the decade. Fewer nursing home residents recognized staff and a higher proportion had difficulty making decisions in 1996 compared with those in the 1987 cohort.

An estimated 1.5 million older Americans resided in nursing homes in 1997; 14% were 65 to 74 years old, 36% were 75 to 84 years old, and the remaining 50% were 85 years and older (Congressional Budget Office, 2004). Data from the National Nursing Home Survey suggest a continuing decline in the rate of use of nursing home care for the oldest old between 1985 and 1999 (Bishop, 2003). The downward trends in age-adjusted disability rates are small and cannot account for the decline in nursing home use. Rather, Bishop (2003) argued that the change is probably a function of the shifting configuration of available services, including (1) a move toward short-term post-acute care being provided in nursing homes, (2) an increase of Medicare home health and home care use, and (3) the increased use of assisted living as a substitute for nursing home placement.

Nursing home occupancy rates have been falling, and the characteristics of the residents have also been changing. The nursing home resident population was older in 1996 than in 1987; the proportion of those 85 years or older increased from 43.5% to 49.3% over the decade (Spillman et al., 1997). The later cohort also tended to be more severely disabled; one-third of the 1987 cohort had five ADL limitations compared to more than 50% in the later cohort.

Approximately 81% of older adults with ADL or IADL limitations live in the community. They tend to be much less disabled than those in nursing homes (Alexcih, 1997). Sixty percent are disabled only in IADLs. Approximately 17% are considered severely disabled, with limitations in three or more ADLs. In 1996, an estimated 1.8 million older clients received one or more home health care visits (Congressional Budget Office, 2004). Estimates for the population receiving formal, paid home care services are difficult to make because of a lack of consistent, reliable data. Data from the 1994 National Long-Term Care Survey indicate that average weekly hours of care provided to older adults living in the community rise as long-term care needs increase and that an estimated 5.3 billion hours of care are provided in a typical year (Bishop, 2003). Four-fifths of this assistance is unpaid care provided by family and friends.

The proportion of all people likely to use nursing homes at age 65 or older ranges from 39% to 49%, depending on the database. Congressional Budget Office (2004) estimates based on analyses by Spillman and Lubitz (2002) suggest that 44% of people who turned 65 in 2000 will use some nursing home care in their remaining lifetime; the estimate increases to 46% in 2020. One-third of those using such facilities will use at least three months of nursing home care and one quarter will use at least one year. In contrast, almost three out of four (72%) of people 65 or older are likely to use some type of home care service over their remaining lifetime (Alexcih, 1997). Many home care users receive care for only short periods, but a small proportion use substantial amounts of long-term care services.

## II. The Triple Knot of Long-Term Care

Policymakers and practitioners must address all three of the domains of the "triple knot" of long-term care (Stone, 2000a)—financing, delivery, and workforce—to develop and sustain a long-term care system that meets the needs of today's and tomorrow's older populations.

### A. Who Pays for Long-Term Care?

The financing of services, the first element of the triple knot of long-term care, is a patchwork of funds from the federal, state, and local levels and private dollars, primarily paid from the consumer's own pocket. In 2004, national spending on long-term care for older adults totaled about $135 billion, or roughly $15,000 per disabled older person (Congressional Budget Office, 2004). The majority of the spending is for nursing home care, although the proportion of expenditures for home and community-based alternatives has increased substantially over the past 12 years. In 1990, 21% of all long-term care dollars were spent on home and community-based services; this figure increased to 34% in 2002 (Congressional Budget Office, 2004).

For individuals with extensive long-term care needs, services can be costly. In 2002, the average annual cost of nursing home care was $52,000 for a semi-private room and $61,000 for a private room (MetLife Mature Market Institute, 2002). Care purchased outside of an institution typically is purchased in smaller increments (Friedland, 2003). Nurses hired through an agency charge between $20 and $40 per hour; the services of a personal care attendant or home care aide might cost $12 to $18 per hour through an agency or about half that amount in the "underground" market. Long-term care might be needed for three months, two years, ten years or more, with varying amounts, types, and hours of care required.

In 2004, public funds, primarily Medicaid and Medicare, accounted for approximately 60% of national long-term care spending on older adults (Congressional Budget Office, 2004). Out-of-pocket spending accounted for one-third, private long-term care insurance for 4%, and various other federal, state, and local agencies for most of the rest.

These estimates do not place a dollar value on the vast amount of unpaid care, including the value of wages forgone by informal caregivers (Stone & Short, 1990). Arno, Levine, and Memmott (1999) estimated that $196 billion a year is contributed to the U.S. health and long-term care systems by family and friends who provide care at home to people of all ages with chronic disabilities.

### 1. Medicaid

Medicaid is the nation's largest source of financing for long-term care, accounting for 35% of all long-term care spending on older adults in 2004 and 40% of spending for nursing home care (Congressional Budget Office, 2004). This jointly federal-state funded, state-administered health insurance program for the poor is required to provide coverage for nursing home care for older and disabled people who meet certain financial eligibility requirements (because they are low income and have negligible assets). In fiscal year 2003, nursing home care accounted for two-thirds of total Medicaid spending on long-term care (Burwell, Sredl, & Eiken, 2004).

Since 1970, states have been required to cover home health services for those who are eligible for Medicaid-covered nursing home care. Beginning in the mid-1970s, states have had the option to offer personal care services under their Medicaid state plans (Smith et al., 2000). In 1981, Congress authorized waivers of certain federal requirements to enable states to provide home and community services (other than room and board) to individuals who would otherwise require nursing home services reimbursable by Medicaid. Waiver services include case management, homemaker, home health aide, personal care, adult day health, habilitation, and respite care. In FY 2003, one-third of Medicaid long-term care expenditures covered home health, personal care, and home and community-based services (Burwell et al., 2004).

State spending for Medicaid long-term care per older person varies widely (Merlis, 2004). In fiscal year 2001, estimated state spending (excluding federal matching funds) ranged from $61 per older Louisianan to $1,323 per older New Yorker. Some of this variation is attributable to difference in the federal share of Medicaid spending, prevalence of disability rates among older adults, and other factors. State coverage and reimbursement policies, however, are the most important differentiating factors.

The proportion of Medicaid spending on waiver services has increased substantially from 5% in fiscal year 1991 to 22% in fiscal year 2003, but Medicaid policies (and subsequent expenditures) are still biased in favor of nursing home care despite the fact that people feel less positive about it than any other provider of health or long-term care (Friedland, 2003). In all, 45% of individuals responding to a poll on long-term care believed that people deteriorate after nursing home placement; only 12% said they would prefer a nursing home if they became unable to take care of themselves at home (The News Hour with Jim Lehrer and the Henry J. Kaiser Family Foundation/ Harvard School of Public Health, 2001). A total of 43% reported that they would find it totally unacceptable to be moved into a nursing home. In another study, one-third of people who had resided in or observed care in a nursing home for a substantial period of time reported dissatisfaction with the care that they, a family member, or a friend received in the last three years (Leatherman & McCarthy, 2002).

A number of states (Oregon, Washington, Arkansas, Maine, for example) have taken the lead in attempting to rebalance the long-term care system away from institutional care toward more home and community-based care options. It was primarily advocates from the disability movement that pushed states to take advantage of the Medicaid waiver opportunities beginning in 1981. More recently, the Supreme Court's Olmstead Decision (1999) requires that people with disabilities have the option of receiving services in the least restrictive setting. The Centers for Medicare and Medicaid Services (CMS), which administers Medicaid at the federal level, have made the waiver process very flexible and have also invested millions of dollars in Systems Change Grants to assist states in their balancing efforts. Many states also invest their own dollars in helping to strengthen the home and community-based infrastructure.

## 2. Medicare

The federal Medicare program, providing health insurance to almost all people age 65 or older and some disabled people under age 65, financed 17% of national long-term care expenditures in 2002, including 10% of nursing home care and 21% of home health care (Komisar & Thompson, 2004). Although Medicare was legislated primarily to pay for acute and primary care, the program does provide limited coverage of skilled nursing facility and home health care services to Medicare enrollees who meet certain requirements. Medicare pays for the first 20 days, and in part for an additional 80 days, of care in a skilled nursing facility after a hospital stay of at least three days. In the case of home health care, Medicare will pay for skilled nursing, therapy, and aide services for individuals who are not able to leave their homes because of their health condition and require intermittent care.

## 3. Private Insurance

For individuals, purchasing long-term care insurance is, in theory, a much more reasonable option than saving for long-term care, as one is likely to save either too much or too little, neither of which is an efficient or satisfactory strategy. As noted previously, however, private long-term care insurance financed only about 4% of the older population's long-term care in 2004. A long-term care insurance market has existed since the 1960s, but it is only since the mid-1980s that national insurance companies began developing and marketing policies nationwide. About 4.1 million persons were insured through long-term care insurance policies in 1998, compared with 1.7 million in 1992 (Scanlon, 2000, p. 10). Between 1991 and 2002, the total number of policies ever sold grew from 2.4 million to 9.2 million (Coronel, 2004). According to industry statistics, roughly 7 in 10 individual policies ever sold by the end of 2002 were still in force, and during that year insurers paid about $1.4 billion in claims. The average age of purchasers was 67 years in 2000; the average annual premium for insurance increased by 11% between 1995 and 2000, from $1,505 to $1,677 (Health Insurance Association of America, 2000).

Since 1990, the federal and state governments have instituted numerous consumer protections to guard against fraud and abuse by long-term care insurance companies. In addition, they have taken a number of actions to promote and strengthen the private long-term care insurance market. Early on, the Internal Revenue Service decided to treat the earnings on premiums collected and held by insurance companies with preferential tax treatment. The Health Insurance Portability and Accountability Act extended the tax deductibility of some premiums and tax exemptions for certain benefits to qualified insurance policies (Health Insurance Association of America, 2000). As of 1999, at least 19 states had passed tax credits or deductions for long-term care insurance policies. Some states also offered incentives to employers who contributed to the costs of a group insurance plan for their employees (Health Insurance Association of America, 2000).

In 1998, 29% of long-term care insurance policies in force were held through employer-based programs (Scanlon, 2000). Although they offer significant advantages over individual policies— lower administrative costs, less stringent underwriting, and an efficient mechanism to target to younger purchasers— relatively few employers have been willing to offer products to their employees (Friedland, 2003). In most of the plans that are offered, the policyholder pays the entire premium. It is estimated that only 6% to 9% of eligible employees take advantage of the employer-based plans (Scanlon, 2000).

As of 2000, 21 states offered private long-term care insurance to their employees (Health Insurance Association of America, 2000). In 2002, the Office of Personnel Management (OPM) began to offer access to long-term care insurance (with no employer contribution) to all federal employees, their parents, and federal retirees (Cutler, 2003). John Hancock and MetLife, the two insurers that were selected by OPM to offer insurance coverage under the Federal Long-Term Care Insurance Program, formed a joint venture called Long-Term Care Partners devoted exclusively to administering this program. It is too early to know the effects of this program, but the size of the potential pool (the large number of federal employees and retirees who could purchase) provides a unique opportunity to examine the outcomes of this initiative over time.

Why so few people have purchased long-term care insurance has been the subject of much debate (Friedland, 2003; Stone, 2000a; Murtaugh, Spillman & Warshawsky, 2001; Warshawsky, 2003). Most experts agree that, given the availability of Medicaid for the poor older population, this insurance is not appropriate or a good choice for people who do not have significant savings. Polniaszek (1997), for example, suggested that a single person ought to have at least $40,000 in liquid assets to consider purchasing insurance. The median income of long-term care insurance purchasers in 2000 was $42,400, and five out of seven buyers had liquid assets of $100,000 or more (Merlis, 2003).

People may not recognize the risk or value the coverage of that risk at the premium price, or do not see insurance as a preferred option over Medicaid (Pauly, 1990). Others may want to purchase insurance but are not able to afford it. Some studies estimate that long-term care insurance is affordable to only 10% to 20% of the older population (Scanlon, 2001). The average annual premium for a good long-term care policy ($150 daily benefit amount in any setting, 90-day elimination period, 5% compounded inflation protection, and a nonforfeiture benefit) in 2002 was $1,474 for a 50-year-old purchaser and $2,862 for a 65-year-old purchaser (America's Health Insurance Plans, 2004). Affordability is even more of an issue for married couples, where each partner must purchase individual coverage. Even with couple discounts offered by some insurers, older couples are likely to pay at least several thousand dollars annually for long-term care coverage (Scanlon, 2001).

Warshawsky (2003) identified several other barriers to the expansion of the long-term care insurance market. At current modal ages of purchase, around retirement, about a quarter of the population would be rejected by insurance companies under current underwriting criteria. These criteria exclude people with "pre-existing conditions" that have a relatively high probability of rendering individuals eligible for benefits by their becoming dependent in several ADLs or dependent on full-time supervision because of cognitive impairment. Younger purchasers could avoid exclusion through such underwriting but would pay premiums and freeze in place for a potentially lengthy period (30 to 40 years) certain modes of care that exist at the time of purchase but may not be available by the time they need to use the benefits. The typical indemnity or reimbursement-of-cost approaches are somewhat inflexible. They would also risk the dissolution of the issuing insurer at some time in the future. Furthermore, even though individual premiums are stable, state regulators can allow insurers to increase premiums for all policyholders within a class of policies issued.

## B. Where Is Long-Term Care Provided?

The second knot of long-term care policy is the delivery system. Long-term care is provided in a range of settings, depending on the recipient's needs and preferences, the availability of informal support, and the source of reimbursement. Much gerontological literature refers to a continuum of care, identifying the nursing home as the most restrictive and one's own home as the least restrictive setting in the spectrum. The literature also stresses the appropriateness of setting, assuming that a mechanism exists for judiciously matching the individual and the setting. Some researchers have challenged the "continuum" and "appropriateness" paradigms (see, for example, Kane et al., 1998; Stone, 2000a), arguing that services can be delivered appropriately in any one of these settings, depending on a constellation of individual, familial, and policy factors. However, one's own home can be as restrictive as a nursing home, if an individual is home-bound and is not getting the services that would facilitate some independence. As the Pioneer Network providers (described in more detail below) have demonstrated, a homelike environment can be created

in any setting, including a nursing home. Furthermore, appropriateness is subjective and should not be invoked to prevent individuals from making their own choices.

### 1. Nursing Home

Nursing homes—or nursing facilities, as Medicaid and Medicare refer to them—are the institutional setting for long-term care. In 2002, there were approximately 16,491 nursing homes and 1.77 million nursing beds (Cowles, 2003). Proprietary homes accounted for 65% of all facilities in 2002; 29% were nonprofit and 6% were government-sponsored. Approximately 83% of the facilities were both Medicare and Medicaid certified, and only 65,000 of all nursing home beds were uncertified.

### 2. Residential Care

"Home and community-based care" is a catch-all phrase that refers to a wide variety of noninstitutional long-term care settings, ranging from various types of congregate living arrangements to the homes of care recipients. One category of home and community-based care, residential care, includes assisted living, board and care, and adult foster homes. Residential care tends to be regarded as an option for individuals who may not need nursing home assistance but who can no longer remain in their own homes. It is often seen as a substitute for living at home and as the next step in a downward trajectory toward nursing home placement. States such as Oregon and Washington, however, have aggressively used residential care as an alternative to nursing home care and have been successful in either preventing such placement or in relocating nursing home residents to assisted living or adult foster homes (Stone and Reinhard, 2004).

The boundaries between nursing homes and residential care are far from clear. Many assisted living and board and care facilities are large buildings that strongly resemble hotels or nursing homes in physical appearance and philosophy. Other residential care options are small, homey settings that offer privacy and choice to residents. Some make services available to residents either directly or through contracts; many, however, are long on room and board and short on care (Stone, 2000a).

In contrast to nursing homes, which are licensed and regulated by the federal government because they receive significant Medicare and Medicaid reimbursement, residential care is handled by state and local jurisdictions. Consequently, there is no consensus on the definition of "residential care"; the nomenclature, as well as the nature and scope of services, varies tremendously (Mollica, 1998). Board and care homes are nonmedical community-based facilities that typically provide at least two meals a day and routine protective oversight to one or more unrelated individuals with some level of functional disability. Board and care homes are licensed and regulated under more than 25 different names; many more are unlicensed. A 10-state study of board and care homes and residents in 1993 found that 92% of licensed homes and 63% of unlicensed homes provided some level of ADL support (Hawes, Wildfire, & Lux, 1995). Most homes provided three meals a day and assistance with storage and supervision of medication.

Adult foster homes are small group residential settings housing just a few residents, typically between three and six individuals (Kane et al., 1998). This setting closely resembles a private home in the community. In the typical model, the owner of the home or someone hired by the owner lives there and provides the cooking, housekeeping, and personal care services that residents need. Most adult foster homes will be unable to care for Medicaid-eligible or other low-income

clientele with heavy levels of disability unless state regulation permits nursing functions to be done by foster care personnel without nursing licenses or unless the reimbursement is high enough to permit contracting with nurses (Kane et al., 1998, pp. 174–175). Relatively few evaluations of adult foster care have been performed, and the service modality has only recently emerged as a setting for middle-class older individuals.

Although no single definition of assisted living exists, the term tends to be used to connote a residential setting that is similar to board and care but that explicitly undertakes to provide or arrange for personal care and routine nursing services to address ADL needs (Wunderlich & Kohler, 2001). One national study of assisted living reported an estimated 11,472 facilities with approximately 650,500 beds in 1998 (Hawes, Rose, & Phillips, 1999). The researchers' definition included facilities with 11 or more beds, serving a primarily older population, providing 24-hour oversight, housekeeping, and at least two meals a day, and supplying personal assistance with at least two of the following activities: taking medications, bathing, and dressing.

When the concept was first operationalized in Oregon two decades ago, assisted living was envisioned as a setting that combined much of the high level of care provided in a nursing home with desirable features of apartment life, including private rooms and bathrooms. In practice, however, many self-described assisted living facilities have neither the service capability nor the privacy and homelike accommodations envisaged by advocates.

There are also more than 1.2 million older people, the majority of whom are now 80 years or older, living in subsidized rental housing funded through a wide variety of federal, state, and private resources. A federal commission created by the Congress to examine affordable senior housing needs and options projected that 730,000 additional subsidized rental units would be required by 2020 just to accommodate the same proportion of older residents as they do today (Commission on Affordable Housing and Facility Needs for Seniors in the 21st Century, 2002). The U.S. Department of Housing and Urban Development has taken important steps to assist states in making use of existing housing stock by providing grants to physically convert subsidized housing properties into assisted living units, as well as funding service coordinators to improve resident access to needed services. Many subsidized housing providers cobble together additional public and private resources to offer supportive and health-related services to help increasingly disabled residents remain in their apartments for as along as possible.

### 3. Adult Day Care

Another home and community-based setting is the adult day center. The number of adult day service providers has almost doubled from 2000 in 1985 to 3500 today (Wake Forest University, 2003). In all, 21% of adult day centers are based on the medical model of care, 37% are based on the social model (with no health-related services), and 42% are a combination of the two. Adult day centers provide an array of services such as therapeutic activities, health monitoring, social services, personal care services, meals, transportation, nursing services, medication management, emergency respite, and caregiver support services. Over three-quarters of the centers are not-for-profit, and 70% operate under the umbrella of a large parent organization. These programs report an average daily census of 25 at an average cost of $56 per day. The majority of these programs are open Monday through Friday for eight hours; only a fraction have evening or weekend hours.

### 4. Home Care

Most older people who need long-term care live at home, either in their own homes, with or without a spouse, or in the home of a close relative such as a daughter. In this setting, a range of home health care and home care services, paid and unpaid, may be provided. Home health care includes skilled nursing and assistance (under nurse supervision) with personal care (ADLs) and IADLs. Home care tends to be nonmedical and includes personal care and IADL assistance. The number of home health agencies rose from 8,000 in 1992 to 13,500 in 1996—a 68% increase. Nearly 62% of these agencies were proprietary and 66% of them were part of a group or a chain. More than 90% of these agencies were certified either by Medicare or Medicaid (National Center for Health Statistics, 2002).

## C. Who Provides Care?

Much long-term care, in contrast to more medically oriented services, is unpaid assistance provided by family and friends (Stone, 2000a). This has been true in the past, and despite the persistent myth of family abandonment fostered by many policymakers, it remains true today. Frontline caregivers, sometimes referred to as paraprofessional workers, dominate the much smaller group of paid providers.

### 1. Informal Care

The major long-term care provider is the family and, to a lesser extent, other unpaid "informal" caregivers. Estimates of the size of the caregiver population vary depending on the data source and the definition used. According to the 1994 National Long-Term Care Survey, a reliable data source that uses a conservative definition of hands-on or supervisory caregiving, more than 7 million Americans—mostly family members, provide 120 million hours of unpaid care to elders with functional disabilities in the community (Assistant Secretary for Planning and Evaluation & the Administration on Aging, 1998). The overwhelming majority of noninstitutionalized older adults with long-term care needs—about 95%—receive at least some assistance from relatives, friends, and neighbors. Almost 67% rely solely on unpaid help, primarily from wives and adult daughters. As disability increases, older adults receive more and more informal care. In all, 86% of older persons with three or more ADL limitations live with others and receive about 60 hours of informal care per week, supplemented by a little more than 14 hours of paid assistance.

Most older people with long-term care needs have a primary caregiver who provides the bulk of the care and obtains and coordinates help from other "secondary" caregivers, unpaid and paid. Almost 75% of the primary caregivers are women, 36% are adult children, and 40% are spouses. Given that the average age of the informal caregiver is 60 years old, the majority of primary informal caregivers do not hold paying jobs. Among the 31% who are in the labor force, two-thirds work full-time. Employed caregivers provide fewer weekly hours of assistance than nonemployed caregivers, but they still invest, on average, 18 hours per week. Two-thirds of working caregivers report conflicts between jobs and caregiving that caused them to rearrange their work schedules, work fewer paid hours, or take leaves of absence (usually unpaid) from work.

## 2. Formal Care Providers

Physicians are the primary health professionals in acute care, but nurses provide the majority of skilled services in long-term care. Physicians are directly involved in long-term care as medical directors of nursing homes or home health agencies;

they also are required to sign off on home health care plans. In 2002, approximately 1 in 10 registered nurses (RNs) were employed in long-term care (U.S. Bureau of Labor Statistics, 2004). Almost 127,000 were working in nursing homes and a little more than 111,000 were providing home health care. In contrast to RNs, one-third of all licensed practical/licensed vocational nurses (LPNs/LVNs) were employed in long-care in 2002. More than 180,000 were in nursing homes and 49,000 were providing home health care.

Long-term care nurses are typically in management/supervisory positions, as well as having responsibility for clinical care. More than 87% of RNs working full-time in nursing homes serve as director or assistant director of nursing (Institute of Medicine, 1996). Although LPNs are not allowed to assess or formally plan care, they often serve as charge nurses on the units in nursing homes. Their major responsibilities include supervising the care provided by nursing assistants, administering medications and providing therapeutic treatments to residents, and monitoring residents' conditions.

Most paid providers of long-term care are the direct care workers who are the frontline caregivers. These workers—often referred to as paraprofessional workers, certified nursing assistants, home health or home care aides, personal care workers, and attendants—deliver most of the hands-on, low-tech personal care and assistance with daily life. They are also the eyes and ears of long-term care as well as the "high touch" providers in all long-term care settings (Stone and Wiener, 2001). After unpaid caregivers, these workers are the key to helping older individuals manage long-term care needs and maintain their independence and quality of life. Nursing assistants held about 750,000 jobs in nursing homes in 1998, and home health and personal care aides held about 746,000 jobs in that same year. Like infor-

mal caregivers, the overwhelming majority of direct care workers are women.
There is great diversity among these workers. The majority (about 55%) of nursing
home and home care assistants are white;
among the remaining 45%, more than
one-third are African American and the
rest are Hispanic or Asian. Most workers
are relatively disadvantaged economically
and have low levels of educational attainment. Although these paraprofessional
workers are engaged in physically and
emotionally demanding work, they are
among the lowest paid in the service
industry, making little more than the minimum wage.

## III. Emerging Issues in Long-Term Care

A number of emerging issues in long-
term care reflect the interests of policymakers, providers, and consumers to
design a system of services that is responsive to the needs of older clients and their
families and that addresses the twin goals
of quality of care and quality of life.
These include (1) how to better integrate
acute, primary, and long-term care services for chronically disabled older people;
(2) how to develop consumer-directed
delivery systems; (3) how to develop a
committed, quality direct care workforce;
and (4) how to ensure quality in long-
term care.

### A. Integrating Acute, Primary, and Long-Term Care

People who need long-term care tend to
have multiple chronic conditions and
often require primary care and acute care
when they are sick (Feder & Lambrew,
1996; Bishop, 2003). It is important, therefore, to design care systems that recognize
and manage the multiple needs of chronically disabled older individuals. A number
of initiatives at the federal, state, and

provider levels seek to manage acute, primary, and long-term care by integrating
services in various ways. The goals for
most of these programs are to improve
continuity of care and to make more efficient use of existing resources by minimizing use of services in more expensive
settings, primarily hospitals and nursing
homes. There is no consensus on the definition of "integration," but most
observers agree that integrated services
demand the following: (1) broad and flexible benefits; (2) far-reaching delivery systems that include community-based
long-term care and care management;
(3) adoption of mechanisms that really
integrate care (e.g., care planning
protocols, interdisciplinary care teams,
integrated information systems); (4) over-
arching quality-control systems with
a single point of accountability; and
(5) flexible funding streams with incentives to integrate dollars and minimize
cost shifting (Booth, Fralich, & Saucier,
1997).

Despite the rhetoric of integration,
there has been a dearth of experimenta-
tion and successful innovation over the
last 25 years. Barriers to integration
include fragmentation of funding sources
(particularly Medicare and Medicaid),
inadequate risk adjustment methodologies to ensure that payments will cover
the costs of the most chronically disabled, and lack of knowledge, information, and training that health and
long-term care practitioners need to
offer, coordinate, and manage an array of
services (Stone, 2000a).

### 1. Federal Initiatives

Three federal demonstrations have been
conducted to test the viability and efficacy of integrated service models. The
Social Health Maintenance Organization
(SHMO), which began as a federally
funded demonstration in 1985 in four sites
(two HMOs and two community-based

organizations), provides an extra payment to a Medicare HMO acute care plan to cover long-term care services, primarily community-based care with vigorous care management, and limited short-term nursing home care. The SHMOs enroll a broad cross section of older individuals, most of whom do not need long-term care services, with the goal of redistributing service dollars to those with the greatest needs (Kane et al., 1997). The results from the evaluation were equivocal (Leutz, Greenlick, & Ritter, 1995; Newcomer, Manton, Harrington, Yordi, & Vertrees, 1995; Manton, Newcomer, Lowrimore, Vertrees, & Harrington, 1993). A second-generation SHMO program with better risk adjustment and targeted geriatric care management for all high-risk clients is currently being implemented in one health system in Nevada.

The Program for All Inclusive Care for the Elderly (PACE) began as a national demonstration funded jointly by the federal government and the Robert Wood Johnson Foundation to replicate an integrated model of care in San Francisco called OnLok. This program serves primarily low-income, chronically disabled older Medicare beneficiaries who are eligible for Medicaid and who are nursing home certifiable. Through an intensive care management approach conducted by interdisciplinary care teams, PACE programs strive to keep individuals in community care and out of nursing homes (Branch, Coulam, & Zimmerman, 1995). Providers receive a combined Medicare/Medicaid capitation payment per client and rely on the adult day care setting as the focal point for service coordination. Despite equivocal evaluation results (Branch et al., 1995; Miller, 2001), PACE organizations gained permanent Medicare provider status in 1997 with about 30 programs currently in various stages of operation.

Using Medicare and Medicaid waivers, the federal government is currently testing the EverCare model of integrated primary and long-term care in nursing homes, by enrolling nursing home residents in a risk-based HMO, with costs covered by Medicaid or private insurance. Teams of geriatric physicians and nurses provide intensive primary care services to the residents and coordinate this with the long-term care services provided by nurses and nurse assistants. Because EverCare pays for all medical services incurred by residents, there is no incentive for the nursing home provider to shift costs to Medicare by hospitalizing a resident. The federal evaluation has not yet been completed, but the program appears to save money by shortening hospital stays (Malone, Chase, & Bayard, 1993).

### 2. State Initiatives

States have also experimented with the integration of services for their chronically disabled older populations. Arizona's long-term care system is part of a mandatory Medicaid managed care program begun in the late 1980s. Medicaid acute, long-term, and behavioral health services are included in the package, but Medicare funding is not integrated. The program implicitly achieves a degree of integration at the contractor level, because Medicare services are usually delivered through the organization that provides the capitated long-term care services (Stone, 2000a).

Minnesota was the first state to receive Medicare and Medicaid waivers to integrate acute and long-term care services for older adults in seven counties. The Minnesota Senior Health Options (MSHO) program offers a package of acute and long-term care services on a voluntary basis; plans pay for community-based care, case management for high-risk patients, up to 180 days of nursing home costs, and financial incentives to minimize nursing home use and to encourage early nursing home discharges (Kane et al., 1998). Other states (Massachusetts, Maine, Florida, Texas, Wisconsin) have established integrated initiatives combining Medicaid Home and Community-Based Waiver programs with fee-for-service Medicare through various coordination mechanisms (Stone, 2000a; Miller, 2001).

### 3. Provider Initiatives

Despite the lack of financial incentives to integrate a continuum of care, some providers are attempting to create integrated service systems. In addition to the aim of providing a more seamless system for their clients, there are strong market incentives to develop such systems, including vertically integrated hospitals trying to fill beds and skilled nursing facilities looking to expand beyond traditional long-term care (Stone, 2000a).

One interesting model is the continuing care retirement community (CCRC), an organization that provides a geographically adjacent, commonly managed spectrum of care options for older adults who hope to age in place and minimize disruptive moves (Kane et al., 1998). Begun in the late 1970s as a mechanism for mostly higher income individuals and couples who preferred to invest their home equity and other resources in a campus environment to insure against the risk of needing long-term care as they aged, these entities typically include independent housing, assisted living, and skilled nursing. Today only a minority of CCRCs are true insurance products (known as Type A contracts) where the new resident or couple pays an entrance fee and a lump sum that covers all services they may require while living in the CCRC. Most CCRCs charge an admission fee and offer residential and service options on a "pay as you go" basis. All CCRC residents, however, have access to a wide array of medical, personal care, and housekeeping services, including wellness programs and other health promotion initiatives and care management efforts. Several CCRCs (for example, the Erickson Communities) have also partnered with physician groups to offer intensive primary care as an option to their residents.

### B. Developing a More Consumer-Directed System

"The 1990s may someday be referred to as the period when the health care and long-term care consumer came of age" (Stone, 2000b; p. 33). Catalyzed by younger people with disabilities who strongly oppose institutionalization and demand a range of community-based options controlled by consumers, a trend toward more consumer involvement and direction in long-term care (including nursing homes) has begun to emerge among the older adults and their families. Consumer direction begins with the ability of the individual with long-term care needs to actively choose the care and setting. This approach emphasizes privacy, autonomy, and the right to "negotiate and manage one's own risk." In addition to recognizing the preferences of many consumers, a growing number of policymakers see it as a potential way to save money through more efficient allocation of resources, fewer administrative costs, and more tailored care delivery.

### 1. Consumer Direction in Home and Community-Based Care

The major focus of consumer direction over the last decade has been in the home and community-based care arena (Stone, 2000b). Policy and program options range from consumer involvement in choosing whether they want to assume the responsibilities of consumer direction, to active participation in care planning and decision making, to the ultimate in consumer direction, providing cash benefits to beneficiaries and letting them purchase their own services and supports. Except for one program administered by the U.S. Department of Veterans Affairs, most consumer direction has occurred at the state level, through Medicaid waivers and state-funded personal assistance service programs.

Results from a 2004 online survey of state agency on aging and Medicaid directors found that 40 states reported operating a total of 62 consumer-directed home and community-based care programs that serve older persons, with the number of clients ranging from 15 to 15,000 (Infeld, 2004). The two primary funding sources are Medicaid and state general revenues and almost three-quarters of the programs require beneficiaries to meet some type of financial eligibility criteria. Programs generally reimburse providers through a fiscal intermediary or directly rather than providing vouchers or direct payments to clients.

Over the years policymakers have expressed concerns about consumer direction, particularly in terms of how appropriate the approach is for the older population and how attractive it will be to this segment of the long-term care population. These include (1) many older people are more comfortable with decisions made by professionals and prefer to have decisions made for them, (2) a large and growing proportion of older long-term care users are cognitively impaired and are not competent to make their own decisions about hiring and firing workers and purchasing services and supports, (3) older individuals and their families will not use the cash payments for care and supports but for other purposes, and (4) quality of care and safety will be jeopardized.

Researchers who have examined the impact of consumer direction, however, challenge these assumptions. One study of California's Medicaid-funded personal care program that relies primarily on independent providers (i.e., clients hire their workers privately, including paying family members) found that clients using the client-directed mode reported greater satisfaction with services, greater feelings of empowerment, and greater perceived quality of life than those who received care through an agency (Doty, Benjamin, & Mathias, 1999). No significant differences were found in client safety and unmet needs. The independent providers also reported better relationships with their clients than did the agency-based workers. A more recent randomized case/control demonstration and evaluation of consumer-direction in the Medicaid waiver program in Arkansas funded by the federal government and the Robert Wood Johnson Foundation (the Cash and Counseling Demonstration) provides further evidence that quality of life and safety are not jeopardized in the consumer-direction mode (Foster, Brown, Phillips, Schore, & Carlson, 2003). In addition, the higher than expected consumer direction take-up rates by older clients (rather than the agency-based delivery mode) counters the concern identified above that there will be no older market for this option. It is also interesting to note that in the demonstration sites where people had the option of receiving cash, many chose to use the fiscal intermediary program because they did not want to deal with the hassles of being an employer (e.g., paying for the worker's Social Security and worker compensation benefits).

## 2. Consumer Direction in Assisted Living

The trend toward consumer direction extends beyond services purchased in the home. The underlying philosophy of assisted living, for example, is to provide individuals with lifestyle and service choices that one could have in one's own home. Key characteristics that are supposed to differentiate assisted living from other types of residential care are: (1) an explicit focus on privacy, autonomy, and independence, including the ability to lock doors and use a separate bathroom; (2) an emphasis on apartment settings in which the resident may choose to share living space; and (3) the opportunity to engage in some "negotiated risk" in which the resident assumes responsibility for untoward consequences of certain individual decisions and actions (e.g., descending stairways that may lead to a fall).

As noted previously in this chapter, however, the practice does not always square with the rhetoric. Hawes and colleagues (1999) found that less than one-third of the assisted living facilities in their national sample offered high privacy. Single rooms, rather than apartments, were the most common residential unit. The researchers did note that residents of these facilities had considerably more choice than residents in most nursing homes and in the board and care homes they had investigated in a previous study. The potential for real consumer direction in assisted living may be significantly impeded by a trend toward strong state regulation and provider concerns about liability and litigation.

### 3. Culture Change in Nursing Homes

The "culture change" movement in nursing homes, spearheaded by nursing home members of the Pioneer Network, is attempting to reclaim the term *home* and to create resident-centered living spaces where older consumers' demands, preferences, and lifestyles drive the design of the physical, social, and clinical environments and decisions (Weiner & Ronch, 2003). The goal of this movement requires substantial transformation of the living and working environments within the organization (Fagan, 2003). It begins by acknowledging the centrality of the consumer (the resident) and recognition that the nursing home is "home" to that

individual. The Pioneer values and principles include the following: (1) residents receive individualized care to nurture the human spirit, (2) residents make their own decisions, (3) the facility belongs to the residents, (4) the staff follow the resident's routine, (5) the staff have personal relationships with the residents, and (6) residents and families are an integral part of the service team. This movement, exemplified by such Pioneer Network models as the Eden Alternative, Deep Culture Change, Regenerative Care, and the Greenhouse Project, has strong intuitive appeal. But the impact of these interventions on residents, staff, and costs are just beginning to be evaluated. Culture change activities will also be included in the next three-year work plan that CMS has developed for its state-level network of Quality Improvement Organizations that provide technical assistance to local providers (Nakhnikian, 2004).

### C. Developing a Committed, Sustainable Direct Care Workforce

Recruiting and, more important, retaining direct care workers has become a major issue for providers, workers, consumers, and policymakers at the state and federal levels (Stone & Wiener, 2001). Labor shortages are a chronic problem in long-term care, but since the late 1990s, concerns about high turnover and job vacancy rates in long-term care have escalated. A recent national survey of state initiatives related to the long-term care direct care workforce indicates that three-quarters of the 44 states responding see workforce as a major priority (Paraprofessional Healthcare Institute & the North Carolina Department of Health and Human Services, 2004). It is not just a question of finding "warm bodies" to fill frontline jobs in long-term care. The attitudes, values, skills, and knowledge these workers bring to their caregiving jobs; the education and training they receive; and the quality of their jobs (i.e., how they are compensated and rewarded and the way their jobs are organized and managed) significantly influence quality of long-term care—the recipients' clinical and functional outcomes and quality of life (Stone, Dawson, & Harahan, 2003).

The success of efforts to recruit, retain, and maintain a direct care workforce is dependent on a variety of interdependent factors including: (1) the value that society places on caregiving; (2) local labor market conditions, including wage levels and the degree of unemployment; (3) long-term care regulatory and reimbursement policies; (4) federal, state, and local workforce resources targeted to this sector; and (5) immigration policy (Stone & Wiener, 2001). The confluence of these factors and individual employer and employee decisions are played out in the workplace. Organizational philosophy and management style, wages and benefits, quality of the work environment, and interpersonal dynamics affect the successful development of the frontline workforce.

There is little empirical research on the effects of policy and practice interventions (Stone, 1999; Harris-Kojetin, Lipson, Fielding, Kiefer, & Stone, 2004). Most evidence has been derived from descriptive, qualitative studies conducted primarily in nursing homes. The evidence to date suggests that among the major factors influencing job satisfaction and staff retention are (1) the management style of supervisors, (2) the degree of empowerment of the frontline staff, including having proactive roles in care planning and treatment decisions, and (3) the quality of the communication between the supervisor and direct care worker and between the direct care worker and the resident/client.

At the policy level, states have experimented with a number of interventions including Medicaid "wage pass-throughs" (requiring any Medicaid reimbursement increases to go directly to the frontline workers), expanded health insurance coverage, enhanced training programs focusing on life skills and clinical knowledge, and the development of new labor pools (e.g., older workers, former welfare recipients). Providers have implemented a range of interventions including culture change activities (described previously), peer mentoring programs, career ladders for professional development and promotion opportunities, and supervisory and communication training.

The U.S. Department of Labor included the development of the direct care workforce in its recent "high economic growth" initiative, and has awarded several grants to help create and test new models of long-term care worker training, support, and professional growth. In 2003, the Robert Wood Johnson Foundation and Atlantic Philanthropies created a national program—Better Jobs Better Care (BJBC)—which awarded more than 7 million dollars to state-based coalitions in Iowa, North Carolina, Oregon, Pennsylvania, and Vermont to develop and implement practices and policies for workforce improvement; eight applied research projects were also funded. These efforts are designed to shed new light on which activities at the practice and policy levels have the most potential for improving and sustaining a quality long-term care workforce.

## D. Ensuring Quality in Long-Term Care

There is substantial evidence that long-term care quality, particularly in nursing homes, is seriously inadequate (Wunderlich & Kohler, 2001). Yet, there remains considerable disagreement about how to ensure and improve it. Stakeholder groups have tended to be polarized around rival philosophies regarding the appropriate role of government regulation, litigation, and alternative, more market-driven approaches to quality improvement (QI). At the same time, insufficient attention has been paid to the relative effectiveness of various QI strategies in achieving quality of care, quality of life, and safety, and to understanding the conditions under which they are most likely to have a positive effect on one or more of these outcomes.

The dominant model of long-term care QI is one of *command and control*, including legalistic, punitive, and sanction-oriented strategies designed primarily to deter or eliminate poor performers. Examples of such strategies are the federally required, state-operated nursing home survey and certification system, state licensing and training requirements, government actions against nursing homes and home health agencies under the False Claims Act, certificate of need programs, and private litigation. *Persuasion* or *incentive-based strategies*—less legalistic and punitive—are designed to generate both negative and positive incentives to influence providers to improve their own performance. Examples include private accreditation, public disclosure, and comparisons of quality information (e.g., state level nursing home and home care report cards, Medicaid's Nursing Home Compare), the long-term care ombudsman program, incentive payment policies, and CMS-funded technical assistance to nursing homes and home health care agencies provided by the quality improvement organization in each state. *Voluntary self-regulatory strategies* have also been initiated by providers to improve quality. Examples include "Quality First" (the grass roots, provider-based national QI activity developed by national associations representing the for-profit and not-for-profit nursing homes), continuous quality improvement strategies implemented by individual providers or groups of providers (e.g., Wellspring), periodic consumer and staff satisfaction surveys, ongoing staff education and training, adoption of best practice guide-

lines around particular clinical areas (e.g., dementia care, pain management, falls and pressure ulcer prevention), and organizational/culture change interventions.

A number of researchers and policy analysts have argued that we need to understand the relative effectiveness of the multiple strategies that are currently being used to ensure quality in long-term care (Schnelle, Ouslander, & Cruise, 1997; Kapp, 2003; Walshe, 2001). Several reviews of the impact of regulation on nursing home quality since the implementation of federal standards set forth in the Omnibus Budget Reconciliation Act of 1987 have found limited positive effects on the organizational performance of nursing homes or resident outcomes (Hawes, Mor, & Phillips, 1997; Kapp, 2003; Wiener, 2003). A review of the implementation and effectiveness of QI initiatives found that these interventions have highly variable effects depending on the circumstances under which they are used and how they are implemented (Walshe & Freeman, 2002). A meta-analysis of the long-term care QI literature found that these interventions had inconsistent effects on health outcomes of nursing home residents (Wagner, van der Wal, Groenewegen, & de Bakker, 2001).

A lot of resources have been spent at the federal, state, and provider levels with little evidence of much improvement in the quality of care, quality of life, or safety in long-term care settings. Long-term care recipients and their families will be better off, and long-term care policy will be advanced, if we can better understand what combination of interventions, introduced at what level, under what circumstances, and at what costs seem to work best to ensure quality and achieve better outcomes.

References

Alexcih, M. B. (1997). What it is, who needs it, and who provides it. In *Long-term care:*

*Knowing the risk, paying the price* (pp. 1–17), Washington, DC: Health Insurance Association of America.

America's Health Insurance Plans. (2004). *Research findings: Long-term care insurance in 2002*. Washington, DC: America's Health Insurance Plans.

Arno, P. S., Levine, C., & Memmott, M. (1999). The economic value of informal caregiving. *Health Affairs, 18*(2), 182–188.

Assistant Secretary for Planning and Evaluation and the Administration on Aging, U.S. Department of Health and Human Services. (1998). *Informal caregiving: Compassion in action*. Washington, DC: Department of Health and Human Services.

Bishop, C. (2003). Long-term care needs of elderly and persons with disability. In D. Blumenthal et al. (Eds.), *Long-term care and Medicare policy* (pp. 21–37). Washington, DC: Brookings Institution Press.

Booth, M., Fralich, J., & Saucier, P. (1997). *Integration of acute and long-term care for dually eligible beneficiaries through managed care*. Portland, ME: Muskie School of Public Service, University of Southern Maine.

Branch, L. G., Coulam, R. F., & Zimmerman, Y. A. (1995). The PACE evaluation: Initial findings. *The Gerontologist, 35*(3), 349–359.

Burwell, B., Sredl, K., & Eiken, S. (2004). Medicaid long-term care expenditures in FY 2003. Memo prepared for the U.S. Department of Health and Human Services, Centers for Medicare and Medicaid Services. Cambridge, MA: Medstat.

Centers for Medicare and Medicaid Services. (2000). Health and health care of the Medicare population, 2000. Table 4.B. Retrieved October 18, 2004, from http://www.cms.gov/mcbs/pubHHCOO.asp.

Commission on Affordable Housing and Facility Needs for Seniors in the 21st Century. (2002). A quiet crisis in America. Report to Congress submitted to the Committee on Financial Services, Committee on Appropriations, U.S. House of Representatives & the Committee on Banking, Housing and Urban Affairs, Committee on Appropriations, U.S. Senate, June 30.

Congressional Budget Office. (2004). *Financing long-term care for the elderly*. Washington, DC: Congressional Budget Office.

Coronel, S. (2004). *Long-term care insurance in 2002*. Washington, DC: America's Health Insurance Plans.

Cowles, M. K. (2003). *Nursing home statistical yearbook, 2002*. Gaithersburg, MD: Cowles Research Group.

Cutler, J. (2003). Private long-term care solutions: The government as employer. In D. Blumenthal et al. (Eds.), *Long-term care and Medicare policy* (pp. 183–190). Washington, DC: Brookings Institution Press.

Davis, K. (2004). Long-term care policy: Time for attention. Keynote address delivered at the Long-Term Care Colloquium, Annual meeting of AcademyHealth, San Diego, California, June 5.

Doty, P., Benjamin, H. E., & Mathias, R. (1999). *In-home supportive services for the elderly and disabled: A comparison of client-directed and professional management models of service delivery*. Report prepared for the Assistant Secretary for Planning and Evaluation. Washington, DC: Department of Health and Human Services.

Fagan, R. M., (2003). Pioneer network: Changing the culture of aging in America. In Weiner, A. S., & Ronch, J. L. (Eds.), *Culture change in long-term care*, (pp. 125–140). Binghamton, NY: Haworth Press.

Feder, J., & Lambrew, J. (1996). Why Medicare matters to people who need long-term care. *Health Care Financing Review, 18*(2), 99–112.

Federal Interagency Forum on Aging-Related Statistics. (2001). *Older Americans 2000: Key indicators of well being*. Hyattsville, MD.

Foster, L., Brown, R., Phillips, B., Schore, J., & Carlson, B.L. (2003). Improving the quality of Medicaid personal assistance through consumer direction. Health Affairs, March 26. Retrieved October 18, 2003 from http://content.healthaffairs.org/webexclusives/index.dtl?year=2003.

Friedland, R. B. (2003). Planning for and financing long-term care. In D. Blumenthal et al. (Eds.), *Long-term care and Medicare policy* (pp. 48–67). Washington, DC: Brookings Institution Press.

Harris-Kojetin, L., Lipson, D., Fielding, J., Kiefer, K., & Stone, R. I. (2004). *Recent findings on frontline long-term care workers:*

*A research synthesis 1999–2003*. Monograph prepared under contract #10001–0035, U.S. Department of Health and Human Services, Office of the Assistant Secretary for Planning and Evaluation. Washington, DC: American Association of Homes and Services for the Aging.

Hawes, C., Mor, V., & Phillips, C. D. (1997), The OBRA 87 nursing home regulations and implementation of the resident assessment instrument: Effects on process quality. *Journal of the American Geriatrics Society, 45,* 977–985.

Hawes, C., Rose, M., & Phillips, C. D (1999). *A national study of assisted living for the frail elderly.* Beachwood, OH: Menorah Park Center for the Aging.

Hawes, C., Wildfire, J. B, & Lux, L. J. (1995). *Regulation of board and care homes.* Washington, DC: American Association of Retired Persons.

Health Insurance Association of America (HIAA). (2000). *Who buys long-term care insurance in 2000?* Washington, DC: HIAA.

Infeld, D. (2004). Information, knowledge, attitudes and practices in consumer direction for older people—2004. Draft report presented at the advisory meeting of Promoting Consumer Direction in Aging Services. Washington, DC.

Institute of Medicine (IOM). (1996). *Nursing staff in hospitals and nursing homes: Is it inadequate?* Washington, DC: National Academy Press.

Kane, R. A., Kane, R. L, & Ladd, R. C. (1998). *The heart of long-term care.* Oxford: Oxford University Press.

Kane, R. L., Kane, R. A., Finch, M. D., Harrington, C., Newcomer, R., Miller, N., & Hulbert, M. (1997). SHMOs, the second generation: Building on the experience of the first social health maintenance organization demonstrations. *Journal of the American Geriatric Society, 45*(1), 101–107.

Kapp, M. B. (2003). At least mom will be safe here: The role of resident safety in nursing home quality. *Quality and Safety in Health Care, 12,* 201–204.

Komisar, H., & Thompson, L. S. (2004). *Who pays for long-term care?* Long-Term Care Financing Project Fact Sheet. Washington, DC: Georgetown University.

Leatherman, S., & McCarthy, D. (2002). *Quality of healthcare in the United States: A chartbook.* New York: The Commonwealth Fund.

Leutz, W., Greenlick, M., & Ritter, G. (1995). Evaluation of the Social HMO: A reply to Manton et al. *Medical Care, 33*(12)M, 1228–1231.

Malone, J. K., Chase, D., & Bayard, J. L. (1993). Caring for nursing home residents. *Journal of Health Care Benefits,* January/February, 51–54.

Manton, K. G., Newcomer, R., Lowrimore, G., Vertrees, J. C., & Harrington, C. (1993). Social health maintenance organization and fee-for-service outcomes over time. *Health Care Financing Review, 15*(2), 173–202.

Merlis, M. (2004). *Medicaid and an aging population.* Long-Term Care Financing Project Fact Sheet. Washington, DC: Georgetown University.

Merlis, M. (2003). *Private long-term care insurance: Who should buy it and what should they buy?* Washington, DC: The Kaiser Family Foundation.

MetLife Mature Market Institute. (2002). *MetLife market survey on nursing home and home care costs.* Westport, CT: MetLife.

Miller, E. A. (2001). *Federal and state initiatives to integrate acute and long-term care: Issues and profiles.* Congressional Research Service Report for Congress, RL30813. Washington, DC: Congressional Research Service.

Mollica, R. L. (1998). *State assisted living policy.* Report to the Office of the Assistant Secretary for Planning and Evaluation. Washington, DC: Department of Health and Human Services.

Murtaugh, C., Spillman, B., & Warshawsky, M. (2001). In sickness and in health: An annuity approach to financing long-term care and retirement income. *Journal of Risk and Insurance, 68*(2), 225–254.

Nakhnikian, E. (2004). *Quality improvement organizations: Recognizing direct care workers' role in nursing home quality improvement.* Better Jobs Better Care Issue Brief Number 4. Washington, DC: American Association of Homes and Services for the Aging.

National Academy on Aging. (1997). Facts on long-term care. Washington, DC. Retrieved October 5, 2004 from http://geron.org.

National Center for Health Statistics (NCHS). (2002). *An overview of nursing homes and their current residents: Data from the 1997 national nursing home survey.* Advance Data from the Vital and Health Statistics. No 311. NCHS/COC. Hyattsville, MD.

Newcomer, R., Manton, K., Harrington, C., Yordi, C., & Vertrees, J. C. (1995). Case mix controlled service use and expenditures in the social health maintenance organization demonstration. *Journal of Gerontology: Medical Sciences, 50a*(1), M35–M44.

Olmstead *v.* LC, 527 U.S. 581. (1999).

Paraprofessional Healthcare Institute and North Carolina Department of Health and Human Services. (2004). Results of the 2003 national survey of state initiatives on long-term care direct care workforce. Retrieved September 9, 2004 from http://www.direct-careclearinghouse.org/download/2003.

Pauly, M. V. (1990). The rational nonpurchase of long-term care insurance. *Journal of Political Economy, 98*(1), 153–168.

Polniaszek, S. E. (1997). Consumer issues. In Boyd, B. L. (Ed.), *Long-term care: Knowing the risk, paying the price* (pp. 129–146). Washington, DC: Health Insurance Association of America.

Scanlon, W. (2001). Long-term care: Baby boom generation increases challenge of financing needed services. Testimony before the U.S. Senate Committee on Finance, Washington, DC, March 27.

Scanlon, W. J. (2000). *Long-term care insurance: Better information critical to prospective purchasers.* GAO/T-HEHS-00-196. US. Washington, DC: General Accounting Office.

Schnelle J., Ouslander, J. G., & Cruise P. (1997). Policy without technology: A barrier to improving nursing home care. *The Gerontologist, 37*(4), 527–532.

Smith, G., O'Keefe, J., Carpenter, L., Doty, P., Kennedy, G., Burwell, B., Mollica, R., & Williams, L. (2000). Understanding Medicaid home and community services: A primer. Final report prepared under contract #HHS-100-97-0015 between the U.S. Department of Health and Human Services, Office of Disability, Aging and Long-Term Care Policy and George Washington University's Center for Health Policy Research. Washington, DC.

Spillman, B., Krauss, N., & Altman, B. (1997). *A comparison of nursing home resident characteristics: 1987–1996.* Rockville, MD: Agency for Health Care Policy and Research.

Spillman, B., & Lubitz, J. (2002). New estimates for lifetime nursing home use: Have patterns of use changed? *Medical Care, 40*(10), 965–975.

Stone, R. I. (1999). Frontline workers in long-term care: Research challenges and opportunities, *Generations, 25*(1), 49–57.

Stone, R. I. (2000a). *Long-term care for the elderly with disabilities.* New York: Milbank Memorial Fund.

Stone, R. I. (2000b). Introduction: Consumer direction in long-term care. *Generations, 24*(3), 5–9.

Stone, R. I., Dawson, S. L., & Harahan, M. F. (2003). *Why workforce development should be part of the long-term care quality debate.* Washington, DC: American Association of Homes and Services for the Aging.

Stone, R. I., & Kemper, P. (1989). Spouses and children of disabled elders: How large a constituency for long-term care reform? *Milbank Quarterly, 67*(3–4), 485–506.

Stone, R. I., & Reinhard, S. (2004). Assisted living's place in long-term care and related service systems. Paper prepared for the National Assisted Living Research Conference funded by the Agency for Healthcare Research and Quality, Crystal City, VA, June 12.

Stone, R. I., & Short, P. F. (1990). The competing demands of employment and informal caregiving to disabled elders. *Medical Care, 28*(6), 513–525.

Stone, R. I., & Wiener, J. M. (2001). *Who will care for us? Addressing the long-term care workforce crisis.* Washington, DC: The Urban Institute and the American Association of Homes and Services for the Aging.

The NewsHour with Jim Lehrer & the Henry J. Kaiser Family Foundation/Harvard School of Public Health. National Survey on Nursing Homes, 2001.

U.S. Bureau of Labor Statistics. (2004). Occupation report. Retrieved October 14, 2004, from http://www.bls.gov/EMP.

Wagner, C., van der Wal, G., Groenewegen, P. P., & de Bakker, P. H. (2001). The effectiveness of quality systems in nursing homes: A review. *Quality and Safety in Health Care, 10,* 211–217.

Wake Forest University. (2003). The role of adult day services. Retrieved September 3, 2004 from http://www.rwjf.org/news.

Walshe, K. (2001). Regulating U.S. nursing homes: Are we learning from experience? *Health Affairs, 20*(6), 129–144.

Walshe, K., & Freeman, T. (2002). Effectiveness of quality improvement: Learning from evaluations. *Quality and Safety in Health Care, 11,* 85–87.

Warshawsky, M. (2003). The life care annuity: A better approach to financing long-term care and retirement income. In D. Blumenthal et al. (Eds.), *Long-term care and Medicare policy,* (pp. 191–207). Washington, DC: Brookings Institution Press.

Weiner, A. S., & Ronch, J. L. (Eds.). (2003). *Culture change in long-term care.* New York: Haworth Press, Inc.

Wiener, J. M. (2003). An assessment of strategies for improving quality of care in nursing homes. *The Gerontologist, 43*(Special Issue II), 19–27.

Wunderlich, G. S., & Kohler, P. O. (Eds.). (2001). *Improving the quality of long-term care.* Washington, DC: National Academy Press.

Twenty-three

# Aging and the Law

Marshall B. Kapp

## I. Law as a Social Tool

Law is a social process that embodies and symbolizes important public attitudes, while at the same time influencing various actions by society. In light of these fundamental social roles, law and the legal system exert an enormous impact on the everyday lives of older persons and those who care for and about them. The introduction to this chapter briefly outlines the different types of law, sources of legal authority, and functions of the law pertinent to an aging population and those individuals and agencies who interact with it personally and professionally—a sort of "gerontological jurisprudence" or "elder civics" lesson. The following sections then discuss law as a source of elder rights, legal grounds for various forms of governmental interventions, the legal status of older persons in terms of both protection against discrimination and entitlement to preferential treatment based on age, whether the law accomplishes its intended goals for older intended beneficiaries, and the development of elder law as a recognized and distinct legal specialty.

## A. Types of Law

"The law" is not one monolithic entity, but instead is composed of several distinguishable but interwoven strands. Constitutional law emanates from the written documents that serve as the basic blueprints for the national government and the various states and localities. A constitution, and judicial interpretations of its provisions, spell out the powers and limits of a government as it relates to its citizens. The federal Constitution's Bill of Rights (the first 10 amendments) and the Fourteenth Amendment, which extended most of those rights to the state level, explicitly protect individuals against unwanted official intrusions by limiting the authority of the federal and state governments in important respects. For example, the Fourteenth Amendment's guaranty of equal protection of the laws probably would prohibit a state from enforcing a law that attempted to single out only persons above a specified age for periodic driving reexaminations as a mandatory condition of licensure.

Statutory or legislative law consists of enactments by elected federal, state, and

*Handbook of Aging and the Social Sciences, Sixth Edition*

local legislatures operating under constitutional authority. Political ideology and pragmatic considerations greatly influence how elected officials use their constitutional powers to legislate social policy. Among the numerous federal statutes of direct significance to older persons are the Social Security Act provisions on retirement and disability (see Chapter 13), Medicare and Medicaid health insurance (see Chapter 21), the Older Americans Act (OAA), various Omnibus Budget Reconciliation Acts (OBRAs), the Age Discrimination in Employment Act (ADEA) (see Chapter 12), the Americans with Disabilities Act, the Age Discrimination Act, the Employee Retirement Income Security Act (ERISA), and the Patient Self-Determination Act (PSDA). Relevant state statutes would include, among many others, those concerning guardianship, advance medical directives, and special treatment of property taxes for older landowners. Older persons are also likely to be affected by local ordinances concerning fire safety in businesses and dwellings (including assisted living facilities and nursing homes) and minimum age restrictions on who may occupy units in particular types of rental communities.

Often, legislatures pass broadly written statutes (for instance, the creation of a prescription drug subsidy for older persons in the Medicare Modernization Act of 2003). The authority to fill in the crucial specific details pertaining to the implementation and enforcement of such a broad program usually is delegated to administrative (regulatory) agencies that are part of the executive branch of government, such as the federal Department of Health and Human Services (DHHS) or state health or welfare departments. Every public program benefiting older persons is governed pervasively by rules or regulations that have been promulgated as part of the formal administrative law-making process.

Finally, common law refers to principles developed by the courts, pursuant to an evolutionary process of case-by-case adjudication, to resolve disputes and guide future conduct in situations where there are no applicable constitutional, statutory, or regulatory provisions. Contemporary laws relating, for example, to medical malpractice mainly come from the common law (although both substantive and procedural principles may subsequently have been modified by, or codified in, statutes).

## B. Sources of Legal Authority

Congress' power to legislate (and, hence, federal administrative agencies' delegated authority to regulate) in areas affecting older persons emanates from two main provisions in Article I of the U.S. Constitution. One section grants Congress the power to collect revenues through taxation and to spend those revenues to promote the general welfare. The Social Security retirement and disability programs, Medicare, and Medicaid are illustrations of government's power to bestow benefits on a specific group while at the same time imposing binding legal obligations on both program beneficiaries and their service providers; the United States Supreme Court has specifically rejected legal attacks on Congress' authority to enact the Social Security Act, which is a form of tax (income withholding) program (Steward Machine Company v Davis, 1937).

Another section of Article I empowers Congress to control interstate and foreign commerce. The Americans with Disabilities Act (ADA) and ADEA, for instance, both impose legal duties on employers and service vendors who are engaged (and almost all of them today are so engaged) in some element of interstate commerce.

State legislatures and administrative agencies attain the authority to enact statutes and publish regulations affecting older persons through two inherent governmental powers: police and *parens patriae*. The police power is a state's innate authority to act to protect and promote the general health, safety, welfare, and morals of the community. Laws authorizing involuntary commitment of mentally ill individuals who pose a serious danger to others (e.g., a demented person who subjects his neighborhood to an imminent fire hazard by leaving his stove turned on constantly) are an example of the police power in action. By contrast, *parens patriae* (literally, "father of the country") is the state's innate authority to benevolently protect people who are unable, because of disability, to fend for themselves adequately; guardianship laws, for instance, are justified on this theory.

## C. Functions of the Law

The law as a social tool serves a number of important purposes. First, legal definitions that create distinct groups solely on the basis of their members' chronological age are a clear means of establishing and delineating relative social status. As noted later in this chapter, the law can affect the social status of the elderly, either positively or negatively, by requiring others to treat them either equally or preferentially.

Second, the law may seek to prevent or mitigate potentially harmful behavior, for example by requiring automobile seatbelt use or mandating periodic vision examinations for drivers. Similarly, federal regulations require local Institutional Review Boards to evaluate and approve or disapprove (or order the modification of) risk-benefit ratios created within biomedical and behavioral research protocols involving human subjects exposed to an undue possibility of harm. An example of such a subject group would be persons with Alzheimer's disease whose desperate

families may be willing to consent to almost any experimental intervention carrying even the most remote possibility of benefit.

Third, law is a tool for creating and financing social programs, many of which are either targeted intentionally toward older persons or incidentally but disproportionately affect the elderly. Medicare and the various health and social services funded under the OAA are examples of this facet of the law.

Fourth, law is an instrument for controlling the production and distributional of particular resources; licensure statutes for professionals and businesses, as well as legislation establishing and funding specific professional education programs, illustrate this role. So, too, do certificate of need laws such as the Illinois Health Facilities Planning Act, 20 ILCS 3960/5, which require a satisfactory prior demonstration of public need for a particular health facility (for instance, a nursing home) before the facility may be built or expanded.

Fifth, laws try to ensure that consumers receive services that satisfy minimum standards of quality. Quality control is one of the chief rationales for the professional liability or malpractice tort system currently in place. It is also a justification for licensure and certification laws such as the parts of OBRA 1987 setting new minimum quality standards for nursing homes (42 U.S.C. §§ 1395i-3(a)-(h) and 1396r(a)-(h)) and home health agencies (OBRA 1987 Title IV, subpart B) receiving federal dollars for their services. Political considerations frequently influence the ways in which quality assurance laws get (or fail to get) implemented and enforced in practice. This is illustrated both by the consistent cooperation between consumer advocacy organizations, federal and state enforcement agencies, and the plaintiffs' personal injury bar, on one side, and the aggressive political lobbying efforts of the health care industry,

especially the nursing home trade associations (American Health Care Association, 2004) on the other.

Finally, law is an instrument for establishing personal rights. Legal rights may
be of two general types. Liberties, or negative rights, consist of an individual's
shield against unwanted external interference. For instance, a physician is legally
prohibited from performing surgery without the informed consent of the patient
(or the patient's surrogate) because the
patient owns a liberty right or freedom
concerning the integrity of her own body.
OBRA 1987 and its implementing regulations contain entire sections devoted to
the rights of nursing home residents (e.g.,
rights to privacy, religious practice, and
communication) against unwanted intrusions by nursing facilities or their personnel. Conversely, positive rights, or
claims, entitle an individual to demand
some affirmative benefit from someone
else. Social Security, Medicare, and
Medicaid create entitlements for designated older persons. So, too, do provisions
requiring reasonable accommodations—
that is, affirmative action, not just equal
treatment—from employers or businesses
serving disabled persons under the ADA.

## II. Law as a Source of Elder Rights

### A. Decision-Making Rights

Contemporary American society places a
great deal of emphasis on the legal (as
well as the ethical) right of all adults,
with no upper age limits, to make their
own choices regarding medical (including diagnostic, therapeutic, and research
components), residential, other personal,
and financial matters. This personal decision-making prerogative is expressed in
the legal doctrine of informed consent,
which prohibits, under the threat of civil
liability and monetary damages, third
parties (such as health or social service

providers) from doing anything to an individual without that person's permission
to do so (Annas, 2004). The informed consent doctrine applies fully to medical,
research (Kapp, 2002a), residential (Kapp,
2002b), other personal, and financial
interventions proposed in both institutional and home and community-based
settings.

The main foundation for the informed
consent doctrine is the ethical principle
of autonomy or self-determination, the
right to control one's fate. An individual's
strong interest in maintaining autonomy
over personal and financial matters
does not automatically diminish as an
invariable corollary of the aging process, despite the paternalistic attitude
(Whitton, 1997) that some people still
harbor toward the elderly as a group.

To be considered legal, a person's consent to participate in some action or to
have some action done to them must contain three elements. First, the individual's
choice about whether to accept or reject
an offered intervention or activity must
be voluntary, that is, not the product of
force or coercion. Put differently, a choice
is voluntary only if the individual had the
freedom to make a different decision if
so desired. Second, the individual needs
to have access to sufficient information about the potential service or activity proposed, hence the terminology
informed consent. The potential inter-
venor must supply the decision maker
with as much accurate, material information about the diagnosed problem or need,
alternative interventions and their implications, reasonably foreseeable risks and
benefits, and such other pertinent facts as
a reasonable decision maker in similar
circumstances would want to know to
make an intelligent choice. Third, the
decision maker must be adequately able,
cognitively and emotionally, to understand the information disclosed, weigh
and manipulate it according to a rational
thought process, and appreciate the likely

personal ramifications of alternative decisions (Kapp, 2004a). Terminology varies among jurisdictions and one's particular state statutes should always be consulted. In general, though, "competence" technically refers to a formal judicial adjudication concerning an individual's legal authority to make decisions. In contrast, "capacity" strictly speaking is a working, often implicit, evaluation of the type made all the time by helping professionals about the present functional abilities of patients/clients. Even when a person is not minimally able to make and express autonomous choices at the time, informed consent still is necessary before an intervention or action may occur, but such consent must be obtained through a surrogate or proxy decision maker.

A capable patient may prospectively designate someone to act as his or her agent or decision-making proxy for health care purposes at a future time when the principal no longer is capable. This may be accomplished by executing a springing durable power of attorney instrument, which is a form of advance medical directive that becomes effective ("springs" into action) only when a designated event such as a finding of incapacity occurs. Under the federal Patient Self-Determination Act (42 U.S.C. §§ 1395cc(a)(1) and 1396a(a)), health care providers are required, at or before the time of admission, to inquire whether the patient had previously executed an advance directive; if the answer to that inquiry is in the negative but the patient currently is capable, the Act requires the provider to offer the patient an opportunity to execute an advance directive at that time.

The doctrine of informed consent applies with full force to every adult, regardless of upper age, unless the usual presumption of decisional capacity has been rebutted or overcome under the facts of a particular case. In practice, however, the tendency of professionals to question an individual's decisional capacity no doubt increases directly with the age of the potential decision maker. In other words, despite the law, aging often is used (albeit in unspoken fashion) by health, social service, and financial professionals as an indicator of, or at least a significant risk factor for, decisional incapacity, especially when an older person rejects the professional's recommendation. This may result in decisions by health care professionals that do not carry out a patient's treatment wishes including those indicated in advance directives. This frequent chasm has been thoroughly documented empirically (SUPPORT Principal Investigators, 1995).

## B. Consumer Protection

To ensure that older individuals' personal and financial choices truly are autonomous (i.e., voluntary, informed, and capable), American society has established a substantial web of laws designed to protect consumers against the potential excesses of a completely laissez-faire, caveat emptor ("buyer beware") environment. For example, the federal Food, Drug, and Cosmetic Act prohibits pharmaceutical companies from marketing or selling to consumers drugs that have not been proven to be safe and effective for their intended uses. The Federal Trade Commission and its state counterparts protect consumers from the false advertising of products and services. However, the powers of the Food and Drug Administration and the Federal Trade Commission to regulate risky and even ineffective or fraudulent antiaging products and services, especially since Congressional enactment of the Dietary Supplement Health and Education Act in 1994, are substantially constrained (Mehlman, Binstock, Juengst, Ponsaran, & Whitehouse, 2004).

Frequently, consumer protection laws specifically identify older persons as especially vulnerable and therefore needing special protection in the marketplace. For example, statutes may include enhanced criminal penalties for committing certain fraudulent conduct when the victim is more than a specified chronological age (Starnes, 1996).

## C. Privacy

Privacy is a generic area of legal rights that affects older persons in important ways. In the course of performing their responsibilities, health, social service, and financial professionals consistently and unavoidably come into contact with very personal, often intimate information about people of all ages, including older persons. This knowledge of personal information imposes certain duties of confidentiality under common law and state and federal statutes and regulations that recognize the interests individuals possess in not having personal information publicized.. In the medical privacy arena, the most significant recent development has been the federal government's promulgation of regulations implementing the Health Insurance Portability and Accountability Act (HIPAA), 45 Code of Federal Regulations Part 164, setting out detailed requirements for health care entities regarding the protection and documentation of personally identifiable health information. Enforcing compliance with this law is the responsibility of the Department of Health and Human Services (U.S. Department of Health and Human Services, 2004).

## III. Legal Grounds for Government Interventions

There are several different ways in which state executive or judicial agencies, acting under their police or *parens patriae* powers, may intervene into the life of an older person without that person's acqui-

escence. Several of these legal mechanisms are described later.

It should be borne in mind at the same time, though, that government interventions that impinge on the personal liberties of individuals are supposed to be controlled by both legal doctrine (based on the 14th Amendment's due process liberty clause) and the ethical doctrine of least restrictive or intrusive alternative (LRA). Under this latter concept, government intrusion into personal autonomy ought not be more extensive than is necessary to accomplish a legitimate public objective. Under the LRA doctrine, a number of legal and financial mechanisms have been developed to assist vulnerable persons who are currently or prospectively decisionally impaired to exercise autonomy as long as possible, rather than to lose it prematurely. These devices, intended to provide protection against exploitation without overwhelming the individual's self-determination, include (among others) durable powers of attorney, daily money management services, joint bank accounts, and living (inter vivos) trusts.

## A. Guardianship

A court (in most jurisdictions, located administratively in the probate division) may adjudicate a person as incompetent to make decisions and appoint a guardian or conservator (terminology varies among jurisdictions) to act as this ward's surrogate decision maker (Quinn, 2004; Zimny & Grossberg, 1998). Guardianship statutes typically contain a two-pronged definition of incompetence: (1) a categorical label or clinical diagnosis (in the past, "senility" appeared in most statutes) coupled with (2) proof of actual functional impairment. In the last two decades, there has been a strong trend for states to move away from global, all-or-nothing characterizations of an individual's competence, and the creation of plenary or total guardianships that they require.

Today, state statutes recognize and authorize (and in many jurisdictions affirmatively favor) the creation of limited or partial guardianships that deprive the ward of decision-making prerogatives only in those specific areas where very serious impairment presently exists (Frolik, 2002).

Similarly, temporary guardianships that must be periodically reviewed, rather than permanent proxy appointments, currently are in favor in all state statutory schema. State statutes now uniformly contain fairly tight substantive criteria, that is, narrow definitions of incompetence. State statutes also contain procedural requirements, such as the right of the proposed ward to be present at the hearing and to have legal representation, as well as a strict burden and form of proof, relating to the appointment and monitoring of a guardian. In practice, however, courts continue to defer heavily in guardianship matters to medical affidavits and the oral and written reports of other health and social service professionals.

## B. Civil Commitment

Another form of coerced government intervention that disproportionately affects older people is involuntary civil commitment. Every state has statutory authority to confine in a public or publicly licensed mental health facility, against their will, individuals who have been diagnosed as mentally ill and proven to be dangerous to themselves or others. As long as the civil commitment process involves strict due process procedural safeguards, analogous to those found in the criminal justice system, it is not inconsistent with federal constitutional requirements (Addington v Texas, 1979). Forced pharmacological treatment of involuntarily committed patients presents an additional set of legal issues (Saks, 2002).

## C. Protective Services

State elder abuse and neglect activities represent another way in which government may become involved in the personal lives of older persons (Brandl, Dyer, Heisler, Otto, Stiegel, & Thomas, 2005). Almost every state has legislation mandating physicians and certain other professionals to report observed instances or suspected patterns of abuse or neglect of an older person to the local Adult Protective Services (APS) department. (Many statutes do not state a particular age demarcation, but encompass adult abuse generally.) Depending on the state, abuse and neglect may be defined in physical, psychological, and financial terms, and may include (controversially) patterns of self-neglect.

Even in the few states still lacking a mandatory reporting law, people who report abuse and neglect and act in good faith (i.e., honestly and not motivated by malice) are immunized by state statute against any civil liability or professional disciplinary action for defamation or breach of confidentiality. Failure to make a mandated report may expose a covered professional to criminal prosecution (in some jurisdictions at the felony level), although actual enforcement of and compliance with these mandatory reporting statutes is less than perfect (Rosenblatt, Cho, & Durance, 1996).

Adult abuse and neglect legislation also authorizes APS personnel to investigate reports from any source and, at least on an emergency basis, enter into the situation with interventions ranging from bringing in meals or immediate medical attention to forcible removal of the individual from a private home and placement in a long-term care facility. Adult abuse and neglect laws mandate reports and authorize investigations and interventions whether or not the alleged victim consents; stated differently, neither the alleged victim, nor anyone else (such as a family member or caregiver) has any standing to veto or prevent these exercises of governmental beneficence and to demand hands-off of the observed or suspected situation. Many states also have enacted separate statutes making serious criminal offenses out of acts or omissions of abuse or neglect of older persons by provider staff and mandating the reporting of suspected instances of institutional abuse and neglect. Besides authorizing APS interventions, state abuse and neglect statutes also create criminal penalties for the abuser or neglector and civil remedies for the victim, including temporary restraining or protective orders and injunctions. Protective orders may direct the wrongdoer to desist from further abuse, vacate the household, and/or pay financial compensation to the victim.

Moreover, a number of civil judgments and settlements involving large amounts of punitive or exemplary damages against long-term care providers have been based on patterns of institutional abuse or neglect (Scott, 2002). The legal theories underlying these lawsuits are battery and/or negligence.

## D. Representative Payee System

Another way in which society may intervene in the lives of older individuals without their permission and restrict their decision-making authority is through the administrative appointment of a substitute payee for a person who is regularly receiving certain government benefit payments. The substitute check handler is called a fiduciary under the Department of Veterans Affairs (VA) program and a representative payee under other government programs. Participating programs include pension and disability benefits from the VA, Department of Defense, Railroad Retirement Board, and Office of Personnel Management (for federal employees' retirement benefits). The most important group of people, in terms

of numbers and amounts of money, are the older people affected by the appointment of Social Security representative payees for benefits paid out under Old Age, Survivors, and Disability Insurance (OASDI) and the Supplemental Security Income (SSI) benefit programs to the very low income old, blind, and disabled.

## IV. Legal Status of Older Persons

As noted earlier, one function of the law is to assign social status to individuals based on their membership in particular age groups. A major question confronting lawmakers, as the ones who are responsible for formulating and implementing specific public policy choices, is the extent to which laws and policies should differ for people of different ages. Should laws affecting older people reflect the philosophy that (1) the elderly are just like the rest of the population, so that they ought to be assured equal treatment and protection against discrimination or, alternatively, the view that (2) the elderly as an identifiable group are unique in some relevant manner that compels, or at least justifies, special (i.e., preferential) treatment as compared to everyone else? Both advocates for older persons and lawmakers have been inconsistent on this matter, justifying their actions on both sets of arguments, depending on the particular issue context. The first model of aging and the law embraces liberty or negative rights: the right of the older individual to be protected against unwanted outside interference or unequal treatment. The latter position results in the legislative creation or judicial recognition of entitlements (claims) for the provision of specific benefits that may be enforced by the individual, solely because of his or her membership in a specific age category, against others in the public or private spheres.

## A. Equality and Nondiscrimination

The principles of equal or nondiscriminatory treatment are contained in many laws that may affect various aspects of older persons' lives. Prominent examples include the Age Discrimination Act, ADEA, ADA, state and local ordinances forbidding housing discrimination against the aged, and the removal of age references from most state guardianship statutes pertaining to adults.

The most straightforward illustration of a law in this category is the federal Age Discrimination Act passed in 1975. This Act, codified at 42 U.S.C. § 6102, provides: "No person in the United States shall on the basis of age be excluded from participation in, be denied the benefits of, or be subjected to discrimination under, any program or activity receiving federal financial assistance."

The ADEA, 29 U.S.C. § 621, was passed by Congress and signed into law in 1967, as a sequel to the federal 1964 Civil Rights Act (which dealt with other, non-age-based forms of discrimination). Coverage of the ADEA has been expanded by amendments several times since the original enactment. Many states have enacted their own counterparts to the federal legislation; hence, those states regulate age discrimination concurrently with the federal government.

In enacting the ADEA, Congress intended to protect people against discrimination in the workplace based exclusively on their age. The ADEA, as subsequently amended, imposes on most employers, employment agencies, and unions nondiscrimination obligations concerning hiring, termination, promotion, training, and other terms and conditions of employment or retirement. With limited exceptions for high level corporate executives and public safety officers, employers no longer can mandate that employees retire at any specified age. Unequal treatment of older workers or applicants is justified to a limited extent under the ADEA only on the basis of reasonable factors other than age, such as the inability of an individual to perform the essential functions of the position satisfactorily, or where age is a Bona Fide Occupational Qualification, as in piloting an airplane or working in public safety.

Older persons who think that they have been unfairly discriminated against may attempt to have their rights enforced through complaint to the Equal Employment Opportunity Commission (EEOC), or, if this fails, ultimately through a civil lawsuit for monetary damages and equitable relief (e.g., job reinstatement) in federal district court. In Fiscal Year 2002, the EEOC received 19,921 charges of age discrimination. EEOC also resolved 18,673 age discrimination charges in that year and recovered $55.7 million in monetary benefits for charging parties and other aggrieved individuals (not including monetary benefits obtained through litigation).

In 2004, the U.S. Supreme Court ruled on a case arising out of ambiguity in the law with regard to who the ADEA is intended to protect. In the case of General Dynamics Land Systems v Cline (2004), a group of present and former employees between the ages of 40 and 49 sued the employer under the ADEA, alleging that a collective bargaining agreement between the employer and the union, by eliminating the employer's retiree benefits health insurance coverage for workers then under age 50, impermissibly discriminated against younger workers. The Supreme Court held that the employer, by eliminating health insurance benefits for workers under 50 but retaining coverage for workers over 50, did not violate the ADEA because discrimination against the relatively young is outside the ADEA's protection.

One large group in the United States, older state and local government employees, do not enjoy the nondiscrimination protections of the ADEA. In Kimel *v* Florida Board of Regents (2000), the complicated legal issue concerned Congress' power under the 14th Amendment Equal Protection clause to create an exception to the 11th Amendment's prohibition against lawsuits being brought against the states by private citizens. But at its core, the outcome of the case hinged on proof of the extent to which older persons in the United States historically had been discriminated against in the workplace by state and local governments. In finding that the historical record of age discrimination in the public sector did not justify recognizing an exception to the 11th Amendment's sovereign or governmental immunity protections, the Court held:

Age classifications, unlike governmental conduct based on race or gender, cannot be characterized as so seldom relevant to the achievement of any legitimate state interest that laws grounded in such considerations are deemed to reflect prejudice and antipathy. Older persons, again, unlike those who suffer discrimination on the basis of race or gender, have not been subjected to a history of purposeful unequal treatment. Old age does not define a discrete and insular minority because all persons, if they live out their normal life spans, will experience it. (p. 83)

The ADA (Public Law No. 101–336, codified at 42 U.S.C. §§ 12101 et seq.) was enacted in 1990. Building on § 504 of the Rehabilitation Act of 1974 (29 U.S.C. § 794), the ADA prohibits employers, plus providers of goods and services to the public, from discriminating in their relationships with potential or actual employees, students, or customers on the basis of an individual's mental or physical disability, so long as the individual is "otherwise qualified" to participate in such a relationship and enjoy its benefits. Individuals are protected against discriminatory treatment if they have diseases or defects that significantly interfere with one or more major life functions, if they have a history of such a disability, or if others (correctly or mistakenly) perceive

them as having such a disability. Financial and equitable (i.e., orders to others to do things other than pay money) remedies are available to aggrieved parties through complaints to the EEOC and private federal lawsuits (Burke, 2002).

Of importance, however, the ADA goes further than simply prohibiting discrimination against "otherwise qualified" disabled persons. It imposes on employers and the providers of goods and services the affirmative or positive duty to make "reasonable accommodations," short of "undue hardship," when those reasonable accommodations will make the difference between a disabled person's participation in or exclusion from an activity. An example would be building a wheelchair ramp to allow a wheelchair-bound person to enter a building to purchase goods or services or to work. Older persons often will benefit from such affirmative accommodations.

Even though the ADA is not on its face targeted directly to the elderly, its coverage enables many older persons to benefit from its anti-discrimination and reasonable accommodations provisions (Barnes, 2001/2002). For instance, the Supreme Court's interpretation of the ADA in the case of Olmstead *v* L.C. (1999) has given a major boost to the development of home and community-based alternatives to nursing home placement. Every state has enacted its own counterpart to the federal ADA.

Many states and localities have enacted statutes and ordinances that prohibit discrimination in the sale or rental of housing based on the potential buyer's or tenant's age. On the federal level, Congress enacted the Fair Housing Amendments Act, 42 U.S.C. 3601, in 1994. These laws are intended to protect older persons from being involuntarily segregated away from desired housing opportunities. They have had mixed success in achieving this objective (Ziaja, 2001).

At times, the legal system itself has discriminated in a negative way against individuals on the basis of age. For instance, most state guardianship statutes used to list "advanced age" as one criterion potentially subjecting a person to a declaration of incompetence and the unwanted imposition of a surrogate decision maker. State legislative reform has largely removed this institutionalized form of age discrimination, with the intention of destroying the presumption that older persons, solely because of their age, are different from the remainder of the population.

## B. Special Needs and Preferential Treatment

In contrast to the foregoing nondiscrimination laws pertaining to the elderly is a set of laws that, paradoxically, treat older persons collectively as a group that is significantly different from, and presumptively disadvantaged in comparison with, the younger portion of the population. These latter laws represent the development, through legal processes, of programs that provide special, preferential benefits to which older persons are entitled by virtue of achieving a specified chronological age, usually plus satisfying some other qualification such as having a specific work history or present financial need. The movement toward group claims or entitlements, predicated on the presumption of unique needs resulting from old age, has been quite successful (Hudson, 1997). It is exemplified by laws establishing the Social Security retirement system and other public pension programs, Medicare, Supplemental Security Income, social services (including legal services) under the OAA, government housing subsidies for the elderly, and expedited hearings for older litigants in civil lawsuits.

Title 2 of the Social Security Act (42 U.S.C. §§ 401–433), entitled Old Age, Survivors and Disability Insurance (OASDI), establishes retirement benefit payments for retirees age 62 and older (the benefit amount increasing the longer one waits to claim the benefit) who contributed to the Social Security trust fund by way of Federal Insurance Contribution Act (FICA) payroll taxes during their years of employment. This landmark exercise of Congress' taxing and spending power (Berkowitz, 1995) is discussed more fully in Chapter 13. In the same vein are legislatively established public pension programs, using advanced years as one eligibility criterion, for railroad retirees, state and local government retirees, military retirees, and veterans.

Another example of Congress' authority to collect revenues and then spend them to benefit the elderly as a group is Title 18 of the Social Security Act, created in 1965 as the Medicare program (42 U.S.C. §§ 1395 et seq.). Medicare has evolved through legislative amendment, most recently the 2003 Medicare Prescription Drug, Improvement, and Modernization Act of 2003, Public Law No. 108–173. Medicare actually is a combination of several federal entitlements (Medicare Parts A, B, C, and D) that subsidize the cost of hospital, hospice, and physician services and outpatient prescription drugs, and to a much lesser extent nursing facility and home health care, rendered to persons 65 and older who either have worked and paid FICA taxes for at least 40 calendar quarters or are spouses of persons who have paid FICA taxes for at least 40 quarters. Services may be provided by private or public health care providers. The permanently and totally disabled who qualify for the Social Security Disability Insurance program and persons with end-stage renal disease also are eligible for Medicare.

Passage of the Medicare legislation as a centerpiece of President Lyndon Johnson's Great Society initiative was predicated on a Congressional judgment (quite well founded at the time) that older persons, purely by virtue of membership in the elderly cohort, were likely to need public financial assistance to secure meaningful access to acceptable quality medical services. Put differently, advanced age was used in the Medicare legislation as a workable proxy for the inability of many older people to obtain group health insurance (and the lower rates thereby available) once they had terminated employment and were subject to be targeted for expensive individualized premiums, as well as extensive examinations for preexisting conditions. What really was created by Congress and President Johnson, as the recent politics of Medicare expansion has made undeniable, was a vast new middle class entitlement program (Rothman, 1997). This result is not inconsistent with the intent of the original architects of Medicare to use the 1965 legislation as a strategic, incremental first step toward eventual national health insurance (Berkowitz, 1995; Marmor, 1973; Oberlander, 2003), although it is at this point incomplete.

Title 16 of the Social Security Act (42 U.S.C. § 1381) established the federal SSI program in 1972, replacing a variety of "old age assistance" means-tested programs that were administered by the states under very minimal federal guidelines. Under the SSI legislation, monthly cash payments are provided to any eligible aged, blind, or disabled persons whose income and assets fall below predetermined amounts. To qualify as an aged person under SSI, an individual must be at least 65 years old.

The SSI program is an excellent illustration of the legal doctrine of federalism, or the appropriate distribution of authority between the federal (national) government and the various states. The 10th Amendment of the U.S. Constitution states: "The powers not delegated to the United States by the Constitution, nor prohibited by it to the states, are reserved to the states respectively, or to the people." Welfare traditionally was a subject reserved for state action. SSI was an exercise of Congress' taxing and spending authority (discussed earlier) to superimpose national welfare standards on the states, by essentially paying states to adopt Congressionally set standards, because preexisting state provisions and standards varied hugely among the states and were perceived by national policymakers to be deficient in many cases.

The OAA (42 U.S.C. § 3001), enacted in 1965 and subsequently amended during several reauthorization processes, provides federal funds to an extensive nationwide network of State Units on Aging (SUAs) and local Area Agencies on Aging (AAAs). In turn, these state and local entities pass these funds on to a network of thousands of providers of a variety of social services to older persons, including legal and long-term care ombudsman counseling and representation. Eligibility for most OAA-funded social services is restricted to people age 60 and older and their spouses, on the theory that membership in that age group can accurately and fairly serve as a substitute for assessing individual need. Consequently, OAA programs do not require participants to prove financial need on an individual basis. In harmony with this philosophy, federal OAA funds are distributed to SUAs largely on the basis of each state's proportion of the national population 60 years and older. Yet, numerous targeting requirements that do not directly affect an individual's eligibility for services have been included in amendments to the OAA passed since the late 1970s. For example, intrastate funding formulas developed by each state, through which SUAs distribute funds to AAAs, are required by the OAA to favor those local areas that are more heavily populated by low-income and minority elderly, as well as older persons with the greatest need for services. Similarly, providers of OAA-funded services must target low-income and minority elderly, as well as those with the greatest need for their services (Takamura, 2001; Gelfand, 1999).

Lawmakers also have assumed that at least a portion of the elderly population requires direct public financial subsidization concerning housing arrangements. Hence, Congress has legislated a variety of rent subsidy and home-owner assistance programs that use age as one criterion for eligibility (Frolik, 1996). Furthermore, many federal and state housing assistance programs that are age-neutral on their faces in effect indirectly benefit older persons disproportionately because those persons meet financial means-tested eligibility criteria.

State statutes in some jurisdictions (e.g., California) afford older persons preferred status when they appear as plaintiffs in civil litigation, by expediting their cases for trial on the court's docket. These statutes are predicated on the presumption that, absent special treatment, older persons as a group may be in danger of being disadvantaged by having their lawsuits outlive themselves. In many states, the advanced age of a crime victim is considered an aggravating factor in determining the severity of the offense and the proper punishment.

The assumption in public benefits programs that age should be treated as an automatic proxy for negative characteristics such as poverty, dependency, vulnerability, illness, and disability has been questioned, both recently (Skinner, 1997) and decades ago (Neugarten, 1982). As noted by Robert Binstock, the "compassionate ageism" that undergirded the creation of today's age-based programs actually "set the stage for tabloid thinking about older persons by obscuring the individual and subgroup differences among them" (Binstock, 1983). Richard Kalish referred to the equation of old age with failure, and hence a need for public beneficence, as "the New Ageism" (Kalish, 1979).

## V. Does the Law Accomplish Its Goals?

A large body of law, which might be termed "geriatric jurisprudence," has been created with the praiseworthy intention of benefiting the older persons toward whose lives these laws are aimed. Insufficient follow-up attention, however, has been directed to investigating whether this intention is always satisfied in actual practice, that is, whether laws that are supposed to improve the quality of older persons' lives really work to achieve that goal. Only recently have scholars begun to use the analytical lens of therapeutic jurisprudence to explore the ways in which the law in practice (as opposed to theory) can exert positive or negative effects on real older people in a variety of tangible contexts, including long-term regulation, end-of-life medical care, protection of human research subjects, guardianship and other interventions for the mentally incapacitated aged, and others (Kapp, 2003). Research to date on this question indicates that the effectiveness of the law in these areas is decidedly mixed. The research points to some successes, some failures, and many uncertainties.

To cite but one of many possible examples, most state guardianship statutes have been amended in the last two decades to ensure that proposed wards in guardianship proceedings are ensured the right of representation by legal counsel. Yet, elder law experts have noted a lack of any empirical evidence that appointment of counsel actually has increased the effectiveness of guardianship proceedings (however effectiveness may be measured) (Schmidt, 2002).

## VI. Elder Law as a Legal Specialty

Many attorneys, either by design or incidentally, deal periodically with issues and cases pertaining to older persons, whether or not the attorney has any particular educational or experiential background regarding the substance of elder law or working with older persons and their families. There was some early resistance to a field of elder law with a distinct, credentialed specialty designation. Much of this resistance came from general legal practitioners (especially those involved heavily in financial and estate planning) who have derived a significant portion of their incomes by de facto serving older clients. Currently, however, the field of elder law as a distinct, credentialed specialty designation for attorneys is burgeoning.

There are multiple explanations for the growth of this new specialty. The sheer demographics of population aging make it increasingly likely that any legal transactions or disputes will in some way involve older persons, their families, or vendors of goods or services to the elderly and their families. As noted previously, a substantial body of federal and state statutory and regulatory law has been developed to target older persons particularly, either for special protection against improper discrimination or for the receipt of cash, voucher, or in-kind public benefits. Even generic laws (e.g., the informed consent doctrine) usually take on unique twists and nuances when applied to situations involving older persons. Thus, many facets of elder law practice may be beyond the competencies of attorneys who have not undergone specific educational and experiential preparation for the unique challenges entailed in advising and/or representing the elderly and their families.

### A. The Role of Legal Advocacy

Legal advocacy may take a variety of different forms in an aging society (Kapp, 2004b). Attorneys working in private law firms may be retained, on a paid or pro bono basis, by older clients to provide advice and/or representation aimed at achieving particular desired results (e.g., successful resolution of a dispute, the securing of certain public or private benefits, or the crafting of an estate plan) for the client. By contrast, public interest attorneys primarily are concerned with advancing social change, meaning "policy change with a nationwide impact affecting large groups of people" (Rosenberg, 1991). Public interest lawyering on behalf of older persons might take the form of engaging in class action litigation on behalf of a defined group of them with a common interest in a specific outcome; alternatively, public interest legal advocacy may consist of community organizing and political mobilization focusing on achieving substantive goals or results consistent with the attorney's values about a good society (Esquivel, 1996). Additionally, attorneys may counsel and advocate for government agencies whose work affects the rights and well-being of older persons.

### B. Practice

The content of elder law is expansive. Matters falling within this ambit include (but are not limited to) advice to, and representation of, older persons, their families, and service providers regarding Social Security retirement and disability benefits; other federal and state benefits; Medicare and Medicaid (including asset sheltering and divestiture for eligibility purposes [McCauley, Day, & Hunt, 2002]); housing issues, financial management (e.g., trusts), and estate planning; medical treatment decision making and advance health care planning; judicial and nonjudicial forms of substitute decision making; elder abuse and neglect; employment discrimination; and tax counseling. Elder law practice is necessarily interdisciplinary and interprofessional in nature, entailing cooperation among the attorney, other human service providers, governmental agencies, and nonlegal advocacy and support organizations.

Elder law practice is replete with ethical challenges. For example, there is an ongoing spirited debate about the ethical propriety of attorneys assisting clients to divest themselves of financial assets to qualify for Medicaid coverage in the event that long-term care services are needed later. Critics of this practice argue that it is wrong, as a gross perversion and therefore weakening of a public program intended to benefit the most financially needy, to assist in the artificial, unnecessary impoverishment of individuals who really do not have a need for public benefits (Center for Long-Term Care Financing, 2004). By contrast, defenders of the practice of "Medicaid planning" or "asset protection" contend that elder law attorneys merely are rendering competent legal counsel in helping clients to claim benefits to which they are legally entitled, and that it would constitute professional negligence for an attorney engaged in financial and estate planning to fail to make the availability of Medicaid planning techniques known to relevant clients (Takacs, 2003). Legislative attempts, in the Health Insurance Portability and Accountability Act of 1996, to restrict the ability of attorneys to counsel clients concerning this matter have been invalidated as a violation of the First Amendment freedom of speech guaranty (New York State Bar Association v Reno, 1998).

Older individuals now are firmly entrenched as distinct legal service consumers and beneficiaries of the law. So, too, are proprietary and not-for-profit agencies that serve the aged.

## C. Education in Elder Law

For both future and present attorneys, as well as for gerontologists and others working in various capacities with older persons, educational institutions and private companies offer specialized courses and other learning opportunities in this sphere. Focused textbooks (Frolik & Barnes, 2003; Kapp, 2001) and practice handbooks (Frolik & Kaplan, 2003) have proliferated. Academic journals are published (e.g., University of Illinois College of Law's *Elder Law Journal* and Marquette University College of Law's *Elder's Advisor*). And national and state organizations (e.g., National Academy of Elder Law Attorneys, American Bar Association Commission on Law and Aging, Elder Law sections of state bars) and Internet networks such as the American Health Lawyers Association Long Term Care listserve (American Health Lawyers Association, 2004) devoted to the field have developed and grown.

## VII. Looking to the Future

A variety of challenging legal questions related to older persons and the social relevance of age and aging are likely to confront individuals, corporations, public and private agencies, and society as a whole in the coming years. Some of these questions undoubtedly will concern the impact of continued technological advances on medical decision making. Some will revolve around the continued dilemma of balancing the autonomy and safety concerns of older persons, especially as new kinds of acute and long-term care delivery settings keep developing and more people live to a point at which their own decisional capacity becomes impaired. Issues relating to the participation of older persons in the workplace and the consumer marketplace raise a panoply of possible legal concerns. Changing family roles—for example, increasing numbers of grandparents as primary caregivers for their grandchildren—will necessitate the development of innovative legal responses. Perhaps most profoundly, the growing consciousness among government, private entities, and the general public that financial and human resources to support the health care and retirement income needs of a rapidly aging population are finite, and in many senses shrinking, will challenge lawmakers and the legal system to satisfactorily balance the legitimate, but no doubt sometimes competing, interests of individual elders and other components of our society.

## References

Addington v Texas (1979). 441 U.S. 418.

American Health Care Association. (2004). Profile of the American Health Care Association. Retrieved October 8, 2004, from www.ahca.org/about/profile.

American Health Lawyers Association. (2004). Listserves. Retrieved October 8, 2004, from www.ahla.org/listserves.

Annas, G. J. (2004). The rights of patients (pp. 113–140). Carbondale, IL: Southern Illinois University Press.

Barnes, A. (2001/2002). Envisioning a future for age and disability discrimination claims. University of Michigan Journal of Law Reform, 35, 263–303.

Berkowitz, E. D. (1995). Mr. Social Security: The life of Wilbur J. Cohen. Lawrence, KS: University of Kansas Press.

Binstock, R. H. (1983). The aged as scapegoat. Gerontologist, 23, 136–143.

Brandl, B., Dyer, C. B., Heisler, C. J., Otto, J. M., Stiegel, L. A., & Thomas, R. W. (2005). Combating elder abuse. New York: Springer Publishing Company.

Burke, T. F. (2002). Lawyers, lawsuits, and legal rights (pp. 60–102). Berkeley, CA: University of California Press.

Center for Long-Term Care Financing. (2004). The realist's guide to Medicaid and long-term care. Retrieved September 24, 2004, from http://www.centerltc.org/realistsguide.pdf.

Esquivel, D. R. (1996). The identity crisis in public interest law. Duke Law Journal, 46, 327–351.

Frolik, L. A. (1996). The special housing needs of older persons. Stetson Law Review, 26, 647–66.

Frolik, L. A. (2002). Promoting judicial acceptance and use of limited guardianship. Stetson Law Review, 31, 735–755.

Frolik, L. A., & Barnes, A. P. (2003). Elderlaw: Cases and materials (3rd ed.). Charlottesville, VA: LexisNexis.

Frolik, L. A., & Kaplan, R. L. (2003). Elder law in a nutshell (3rd ed.). St. Paul, MN: West Group.

Gelfand, D. E. (1999). The aging network: Programs and services (5th ed.). New York: Springer Publishing Company.

General Dynamics Land Systems v Cline (2004). 540 U.S. 581.

Hudson, R. B. (Ed.) (1997). The future of age-based public policy. Baltimore: Johns Hopkins University Press.

Kalish, R. A. (1979). The new ageism and the failure models: A polemic. Gerontologist, 19, 398–402.

Kapp, M. B. (2001). Lessons in law and aging: A tool for educators and students. New York: Springer Publishing Company.

Kapp, M. B. (Ed.) (2002a). Issues in conducting research with and about older persons. New York: Springer Publishing Company.

Kapp, M. B. (2002b). Where will I live? How do housing choices get made for older persons? NAELA Quarterly—Journal of the American Academy of Elder Law Attorneys, 15(3), 2–5.

Kapp, M. B. (2003). The law and older persons: Is geriatric jurisprudence therapeutic? Durham, NC: Carolina Academic Press.

Kapp, M. B. (Ed.). (2004a). Decision making capacity and older persons. New York: Springer Publishing Company.

Kapp, M. B. (2004b). Advocacy in an aging society: The varied roles of attorneys. Generations, XXVIII (1), 31–35.

Kimel v Florida Board of Regents. (2000). 528 U.S. 62.

Marmor, T. R. (1973). The politics of Medicare. Chicago: Aldine Publishers.

McCauley, M., Day, P., & Hunt, L. R. (2002). Understanding elder law: Issues in estate planning, Medicaid, and long-term care benefits. Chicago: American Bar Association.

Mehlman, M. J., Binstock, R. H., Juengst, E. T., Ponsaran, R. S., & Whitehouse, P. J. (2004). Anti-aging medicine: Can consumers be better protected? Gerontologist, 44, 304–310.

Neugarten, B. L. (Ed.). (1982). Age or need? Public policies for older people. Beverly Hills, CA: Sage Publications.

New York State Bar Association v Reno (1998). 999 F.Supp. 710.

Oberlander, J. (2003). *The political life of Medicare*. Chicago: University of Chicago Press.

Olmstead v L.C. (1999). 527 U.S. 581.

Quinn, M. J. (2004). *Guardianship of adults*. New York: Springer Publishing Company.

Rosenberg, G. N. (1991). *The hollow hope: Can courts bring about social change?* Chicago: University of Chicago Press.

Rosenblatt, D. E., Cho, K. H., & Durance, P. W. (1996). Reporting mistreatment of older adults: The role of physicians. *Journal of the American Geriatrics Society, 44*, 65–70.

Rothman, D. J. (1997). *Beginnings count: The technological imperative in American health care*. (pp. 67–86). New York: Oxford University Press.

Saks, E. R. (2002). *Refusing care: Forced treatment and the rights of the mentally ill*. Chicago: University of Chicago Press.

Schmidt, W. C., Jr. (2002). The Wingspan of Wingspread: What is known and not known about the state of the guardianship and public guardianship system thirteen years after the Wingspread National Guardianship Symposium. *Stetson Law Review, 31*, 1027–1046.

Scott, E. J. (2002). Punitive damages in lawsuits against nursing homes. *Journal of Legal Medicine, 23*, 115–129.

Skinner, J. H. (1997). Should age be abandoned as a basis for program and service eligibility? Yes. In A. E. Scharlach & L. W. Kaye (Eds.), *Controversial issues in aging* (pp. 59–62). Boston: Allyn and Bacon.

Starnes, R. A. (1996). Consumer fraud and the elderly: The need for a uniform system of enforcement and increased civil and criminal penalties. *Elder Law Journal, 4*, 201–224.

Steward Machine Company v Davis (1937). 301 U.S. 548, 57 S.Ct. 883.

SUPPORT Principal Investigators. (1995). A controlled trial to improve care for seriously ill hospitalized patients: The study to understand the prognoses and preferences for outcomes and risks of treatments. *Journal of the American Medical Association, 274*, 1591–1598.

Takacs, T. (2003 Winter). The life care plan: Integrating a healthcare-focused approach to meeting the needs of your clients and families into your elder law practice. *NAELA Quarterly—Journal of the National Academy of Elder Law Attorneys, 16*, 2–8.

Takamura, J. (2001). Older Americans Act. In G. L. Maddox (Ed.), *Encyclopedia of aging* (pp. 762–765). New York: Springer Publishing Company.

U.S. Department of Health and Human Services, Office of Civil Rights. (2004). Medical Privacy. Retrieved October 8, 2004, from www.cms.hhs.gov/hipaa.

Whitton, L. S. (1997). Ageism: Paternalism and prejudice. *DePaul Law Review, 46*, 453–482.

Ziaja, E. (2001). Do independent and assisted living communities violate the Fair Housing Amendments Act and the Americans with Disabilities Act? *Elder Law Journal, 9*, 313–339.

Zimny, G. H., & Grossberg, G. T. (Eds.). (1998). *Guardianship of the elderly: Psychiatric and judicial aspects*. New York: Springer Publishing Company.

# Twenty-four

# Anti-Aging Medicine and Science
## Social Implications

Robert H. Binstock, Jennifer R. Fishman, and Thomas E. Johnson

Ambitions and attempts to control aging have been part of human culture since early civilizations (Gruman, 1966/2003). An obsession with immortality is a central theme in a Babylonian legend about the king Gilgamesh who ruled southern Mesopotamia in about 3000 BC. In the third century BC, adherents of the Taoist religion in China developed a systematic program aimed at prolonging life (Olshansky & Carnes, 2001). Through the centuries, a variety of anti-aging approaches have recurred. Among them have been alchemy, the use of precious metals (e.g., as eating utensils) that have been transmuted from baser minerals; "shunamatism" or "gerocomy" (cavorting with young girls); grafts (or injected extracts) from the testicles, ovaries, or glands of various animal species; cell injections from the tissues of newborn or fetal animals; consumption of elixirs, ointments, drugs, hormones, dietary supplements, and specific foods; cryonics; and rejuvenation from devices and exposure to various substances such as mineral and thermal springs (Gruman, 2003; Hayflick, 1994).

Anti-aging aspirations and efforts flourish today, perhaps more than ever, in the forms of (1) a commercial and clinical movement that offers anti-aging products, regimens, and treatments; and (2) research and development efforts of biogerontologists, scientists who study the biology of aging. (It should be noted, however, that most geriatricians and many biogerontologists do not perceive themselves as undertaking "anti-aging" interventions.)

The goals of the commercial and clinical anti-aging movement are essentially to extend the time its customers and patients can live without the common morbidities of aging such as wrinkling of the skin, hardening of the arteries, memory loss, muscle loss, visual impairment, and slowed gait and speech. Although biogerontologists generally share these objectives, they also have more ambitious aims. They seek to achieve what historian Gerald Gruman (2003) termed *prolongevity*, a significant extension of average human life expectancy and/or maximum life span without extending suffering and infirmity. The goals of these

*Handbook of Aging and the Social Sciences, Sixth Edition*

biogerontologists can be summarized by three paradigms.

The most conservative of these is commonly described as *compression of morbidity* (Fries, 1980). In this scenario, humans live long and vigorous lives, terminated by a sharp decline in functioning mandated by senescence, followed relatively swiftly by death. Compressed morbidity includes the possibility of increases in average life expectancy, but not in maximum life span.

A more ambitious paradigm is *decelerated aging* in which the processes of aging are slowed and average life expectancy and/or maximum life span are increased. In contrast to the compression of morbidity ideal, late-life functional disabilities are not eliminated but occur at a more advanced age than has been the case historically. It has been suggested that decelerated aging could "produce 90-year-old adults who are as healthy and active as today's 50-year-olds" (Miller, 2002, p. 155).

The most radical paradigm is *arrested aging* in which the processes of aging are reversed in adults. In contrast to slowing the rate of aging, the goal of reversing aging is to *restore* vitality and function to those who have lost them. Some scientists envision that reversal could be accomplished through strategies that remove the damage inevitably caused by basic metabolic processes and thereby attain "negligible senescence" (de Grey et al., 2002a).

The goals of the anti-aging movement and interventional biogerontologists have many social implications that will be considered in this chapter. Section I discusses the anti-aging medicine movement and its social and cultural implications. Section II examines the "boundary work" that biogerontologists have undertaken to distinguish themselves from the anti-aging medicine movement, why they seek to do so, and the responses from

the movement. Section III summarizes the areas of biogerontological research that are promising avenues for the development of effective anti-aging interventions and delineates a series of ethical and social implications of achieving prolongevity. A final section suggests future directions for research on the social implications of anti-aging medicine and science.

## I. The Contemporary Anti-Aging Movement

The use of anti-aging products in the United States, particularly dietary supplements, soared in the years after the enactment of the Dietary Supplement Health and Education Act of 1994, which relaxed regulation of such products (U.S. General Accounting office [GAO], 2001). During the same period, several dozen anti-aging books were published (e.g., Chopra, 2001). A refereed scientific publication, the *Journal of Anti-Aging Medicine*, began publishing in 1998 and several nonrefereed publications with similar sounding names also appeared (de Grey et al., 2002b). Dozens of web sites such as "Youngevity: The Anti-Aging Company" marketed products such as "The Vilcabamba Mineral Essence" to enable people to live their lives "in a state of youthfulness" (Youngevity, 2005). There are no hard statistics on the size of the overall anti-aging market in the United States, but some estimates are available. A research report prepared by a "knowledge services company," FIND/SVP (2005), estimated that the anti-aging market was about $43 billion in 2002 and could increase to $64 billion by 2007. It defines the market in terms of five categories: cosmetic treatments and surgery; exercise and therapy, food, and beverages; vitamins, minerals, and supplements; and cosmetics and cosmeceuticals. Whatever the magnitude of the market, it seems likely to grow as the Baby Boom cohort ages.

One particular element of the anti-aging movement that has directly challenged the established gerontological community is the American Academy of Anti-Aging Medicine (A4M), which proclaims that "anti-aging medicine is ushering in the Ageless Society" (A4M, 2002a). Founded in 1993 by "pioneering anti-aging physicians and practitioners" (Klatz, 1999, p. 4), A4M claims it has 11,500 members from 65 countries and receives 1.8 million hits per month on its web site (A4M, 2005). Publicly available income tax returns show that it had accumulated net assets of $3.6 million by 2003 (Guidestar, 2005).

Although A4M is not recognized by the American Medical Association or the American Board of Medical Specialties, it has established certification programs under its auspices for physicians, chiropractors, dentists, naturopaths, podiatrists, pharmacists, registered nurses, nurse practitioners, nutritionists, dietitians, sports trainers and fitness consultants, and PhDs. According to A4M, it has organized 17 international conferences on anti-aging medicine, and sponsored production of a weekly aired cable television feature called "Anti-Aging Update." A4M states that it does not sell or endorse any commercial product or promote or endorse any specific treatment, but it actively solicits and displays numerous advertisements on its web site for products and services (such as cosmetics and alternative medicines and therapies), anti-aging clinics, and anti-aging physicians and practitioners, many of them listing certification by A4M.

The president and the chairman of A4M are Chicago-based osteopaths. In the 1980s, they published books on the subject of drugs and training regimens intended to enhance performance in sports (e.g., Goldman & Klatz, 1988). Since the inception of A4M, however, they have turned to a different subject matter, publishing more than a half dozen books with such titles as *Ten Weeks to a Younger You* (Klatz, 1999), the cover of which promises "age reversing benefits of the youth hormones" such as enhancing IQ, eliminating wrinkles, increasing memory, and enhancing sexual performance.

Although what A4M terms "the traditional, antiquated gerontological establishment" (Arumainathan, 2001) may disagree with many of the organization's messages and the measures it promotes, most elements of A4M's broadly stated goals seem, on the surface, to be the same as those of many biomedical researchers and practitioners in gerontology and geriatrics. The stated mission of A4M is:

the advancement of technology to detect, prevent, and treat aging related disease and to promote research into methods to retard and optimize the human aging process.... A4M believes that the disabilities associated with normal aging are caused by physiological dysfunction which in many cases are ameliorable [sic] to medical treatment, such that the human life span can be increased, and the quality of one's life improved as one grows chronologically older. (A4M, 2005)

Most anti-aging web sites espouse similar goals.

## A. Social and Cultural Considerations

Although there has clearly been consumer interest in interventions to prevent, arrest, or reverse aging throughout human history, historian Carole Haber asks, "Why this sudden resurgence in the notion that aging is an abhorrent disease that must be eliminated?" (2001–2002, p. 13). She suggests that there may be several relatively unique social and cultural forces driving the contemporary enthusiasm for anti-aging products and services in the United States. One factor is that anti-aging interventions may have a special appeal to the large cohort of aging Baby

Boomers because they grew up in an especially youth-oriented period in mass culture. Another factor is that recent scientific discoveries seemingly have potential relevance to slowing the rate of aging in humans (see Section III). Haber attributes "the precise timing of this movement and the nature of its appeal" (2001–2002, p. 13) to a third factor, the social context of concerns about the negative economic consequences for society associated with the Baby Boom reaching old age. Cole and Thompson (2001–2002) suggest that still another factor is a consumer culture that is eager to exploit a widespread fear of decline. An additional influence, of course, is the long-term and increasing medicalization of human conditions and experiences previously considered to be nonpathological (Clarke, Shim, Mamo, Fosket, & Fishman, 2003). This phenomenon has been specifically noted in the field of gerontology as the "biomedicalization of aging" (Estes & Binney, 1989) and chronicled with respect to the sociopolitical transformation of cognitive senility into Alzheimer's disease (Fox, 1989).

The anti-aging movement, however, is hardly confined to the United States. Indeed, modern Europeans have had a strong interest in anti-aging interventions, predating the social and scientific phenomena noted by Haber. The European anti-aging movement was spearheaded in the 1960s and 1970s by a Romanian woman, Anna Aslan, who established an institute in Bucharest that offered rejuvenation therapies and an elixir called Gerovital (Robinson, 2001), which is still widely marketed. Members of the European and Asian elite, including Nikita Kruschev, visited the institute for treatments, and the Soviet Union established its own institute to study Gerovital and other chemicals. Today, according to Leslie Robert (2004), various academies and centers on anti-aging medicine can be found in France,

Germany, Belgium, and Japan, accompanied by European and Asian/Pacific organizations of this ilk. Robert suggested that one possible reason for the increasing interest in anti-aging medicine worldwide is that many health care professionals are feeling a financial pinch and are exploring alternative sources of income.

Although segments of the health care community may see anti-aging as an avenue for income, some gerontologists have expressed concern that the anti-aging movement will stigmatize and marginalize old people in general, and particularly those who "look their age" because they are not anti-aging consumers. Robert Butler, founding director of the U.S. National Institute on Aging, argued that, "Anti-aging medicine promotes and reinforces ageism because it...puts a profoundly negative connotation on the natural and inevitable occurrence of growing old, emphasizing its negative and depleting aspects" (2001–2002, p. 64). Martha Holstein (2001–2002) concurs with this view, and sees several more specific problems arising from the anti-aging movement. One problem is the emergence of sharpening class distinctions between those consumers who can afford anti-aging medicine and those who cannot. In her view, this divide will especially affect older women because they tend to be less well off economically than older men (see Chapter 13). Holstein emphasizes that older women, especially, already suffer from mean-spirited and vicious stereotypes, and that the spread of even superficial anti-aging practices, such as dying one's graying hair, marginalizes the woman who ages naturally.

## B. Protecting the Welfare of Consumers

Another area of social concerns raised by anti-aging medicine is consumer protection. Some contemporary interventions undertaken by the anti-aging movement, such as cosmetics, exercise programs, and nutritional regimens, can be beneficial, benign, and not greatly harmful in terms of economic loss to the consumer. Moreover, even if the efficacy of some interventions has not been established through conventional clinical evidence, they may have beneficial results for consumers through placebo effects.

Nonetheless, anti-aging interventions raise a number of welfare concerns for patients, practitioners, and the larger society, as set forth by Mehlman, Binstock, Juengst, Ponsaran, and Whitehouse (2004) and summarized here. Foremost is the question of safety for those older persons and aging Baby Boomers who consume them. The wares being sold and techniques being endorsed include powerful drugs that have the potential to cause serious physical and mental harm. For example, studies have indicated that some short-term anti-aging hormone treatments can have adverse effects such as diabetes and glucose intolerance (e.g., Blackman et al., 2002; Janssens & Vanderschueren, 2000), and that long-run administration of growth hormone to older persons may potentially elevate the risk of cancer (e.g., Chan et al., 1998). Similarly, hormone replacement therapy consisting of estrogen plus progestin for postmenopausal women has been shown to elevate their risks of breast cancer, coronary heart disease, stroke, and pulmonary embolism (Writing Group for the Women's Health Initiative Investigators, 2002).

In addition to issues of harm, the mere ineffectiveness of some anti-aging interventions can have deleterious consequences for the welfare of patients and consumers. Engaging in an ineffective anti-aging therapy may preclude patients from participating in other regimens that could be beneficial and waste money that could be used for helpful medical interventions. For instance, older persons may choose to undergo growth hormone treatments because they are mistakenly led to believe that this will increase their muscle strength, and thereby divert themselves from undertaking regimens such as resistance exercise training, which has been shown to increase muscle strength significantly (Blackman et al., 2002). For some treatments the sums involved can be substantial. Growth hormone treatments cost between $7,500 and $10,000 annually according to one report (Vance, 2003), and "longevity clinics" are charging as much as $2,000 per day (Pope, 2002). Granted, the majority of older people and Baby Boomers are not able to spend such sums. But even those who can buy comparatively inexpensive mineral waters and ineffective dietary supplements are caused some degree of economic harm.

To date, there are no indications that market forces are weeding out risky, ineffective, economically harmful, and fraudulent anti-aging interventions. In principle, one possible approach to achieving greater consumer protection is governmental action; however, a number of distinct barriers to effective governmental regulation of anti-aging medicine are discussed in detail by Mehlman and colleagues (2004). They argue that in view of the limited capacity of government to protect anti-aging consumers, physicians and other health care professionals, especially gerontologists and geriatricians, will need to bear a major responsibility. To this end they recommend a number of steps for self-regulation by individual physicians and by medical organizations and journals. In addition, Mehlman and colleagues (2004) pointedly challenge organized groups of gerontologists and geriatricians to undertake much more vigorous leadership than they have so far in the arena of anti-aging medicine, because professionals in these specific fields are and should be most concerned about the impact of anti-aging interventions on older adults and aging Baby Boomers. In particular, they suggest that the Gerontological Society of America and the American Geriatrics Society work separately and jointly to develop educational programs that directly embrace health care professionals who are practicing anti-aging medicine and to launch sustained campaigns of public health messages targeted to practitioners and to the general public regarding harmful, risky, and ineffective anti-aging interventions.

This strategy of disseminating public health messages has already been undertaken by several governmental entities. The U.S. Senate Special Committee on Aging (2001) has held a hearing focused on fraudulent marketing tactics for antiaging medicines. The U.S. General Accounting Office (2001) has issued a report on the physical and economic harms wrought by anti-aging products. The National Institute on Aging (NIA) has produced an "Age Page" called "Life Extension: Fact or Fiction" in which it discredits "very much exaggerated" anti-aging claims for pills containing anti-oxidants, DNA, and RNA, as well as for dehydroepiandrostene and growth hormone (NIA, 2002a). And the web site of NIA promotes a free fact sheet on "'anti-aging' miracle drugs" (NIA, 2002b) as part of "an educational effort urging consumers to use caution when it comes to 'anti-aging' hormone supplements" (NIA, 1997).

A4M has exploited these messages, particularly those issued by NIA, to actively promote itself as a challenger to the established gerontological community. In a document entitled "Intellectual Dishonesty in Geriatric Medicine—Truth versus Fallacy," it berated NIA for its public information campaign regarding anti-aging therapies, characterizing it as anti-competitive censorship and an attempt to maintain the status quo of research funding and academic interests, and to consolidate power (Arumainathan,

2001). NIA has not responded to this diatribe. Indeed, publicly, NIA has appeared to ignore A4M altogether. Although the institute lists and describes more than 250 organizations that may be helpful resources for older people, A4M is not among them (NIA, 2005). Individuals in the field of gerontology, however, have certainly responded to the marketing of anti-aging products and therapies by A4M and others.

## II. Boundary Work: Gerontologists versus Anti-Aging Medicine

In 2002, a number of gerontologists weighed in with what appeared on its face to be a public health warning about the anti-aging medicine movement. Three scientists who have undertaken research on aging for many years—Jay Olshansky, Leonard Hayflick, and Bruce Carnes (2002a)—published an article in *Scientific American* entitled "No Truth to the Fountain of Youth," in which they declared:

The hawking of anti-aging "therapies" has taken a particularly troubling turn of late. Disturbingly large numbers of entrepreneurs are luring gullible and frequently desperate customers of all ages to "longevity" clinics, claiming a scientific basis for the anti-aging products they recommend and, often, sell. At the same time, the Internet has enabled those who seek lucre from supposed anti-aging products to reach new consumers with ease. (p. 92)

They went on to assert that "no currently marketed intervention—none—has yet been proved to slow, stop, or reverse human aging, and some can be downright dangerous" (pp. 92–93). They also presented interpretations of various lines of biological research relevant to the underlying nature of aging, and their promise, or lack of promise, for slowing the progression of aging.

The *Scientific American* essay was a summary of a lengthier position statement, "The Truth about Human Aging," that had been posted a month earlier on the web site of the magazine and explicitly endorsed there by an international roster of 51 scientists and physicians. The conveners of the group then arranged for the position statement to be published in a half dozen journals throughout the world (e.g., Olshansky, Hayflick, & Carnes, 2002b). Their message also reached a very large audience when the *AARP Bulletin*, with a circulation of more than 30 million, made the *Scientific American* article the lead story in its next issue (Pope, 2002). In addition, they specifically targeted A4M by presenting it with a Silver Fleece Award for "leading the lay public and some in the medical and scientific community to the mistaken belief that technologies already exist that stop or reverse human aging" (University of Illinois at Chicago, 2002). Subsequently, the organizers of the position statement continued to criticize anti-aging products and organizations, and many others in the gerontological community have joined in to maintain an ongoing war of words on the anti-aging medicine movement, but largely in professional journals (e.g., Fisher & Morley, 2002; Perls, 2004; Wick, 2002).

Although these attacks on anti-aging medicine are presented as public health messages, they are also a manifestation of "boundary work," paralleling disputes in many other areas of science in which rhetorical demarcations are used to acquire and maintain legitimacy and power (Gieryn, 1983). Taylor (1996) observed that, "Practicing scientists, consciously or otherwise, discursively construct working definitions of science that function, for example, to exclude various non- or pseudo-sciences so as to sustain their (perhaps well-earned) position of epistemic authority and to maintain a variety of professional resources" (p. 5). Such is the case with the established community of biogerontologists and geri-

atricians, who are concerned with maintaining and enhancing their hard won, but still fragile, legitimacy as scientists. The basis of this concern is best understood in the historical context of the biogerontological enterprise.

## A. Biogerontologists' Struggle for Legitimacy

Gruman (2003) has noted that throughout most of human history efforts to achieve *prolongevity* have tended to be "relegated to a limbo reserved for impractical projects or eccentric whims not quite worthy of serious scientific or philosophic consideration" (p. 2). This observation fits rather well the perceptions of biological research on aging held by many in the scientific community until recent decades (Achenbaum, 1995). As a history of U.S. biogerontology put it in the early 1980s: "Those who would study aging in order to retard or halt the process have been considered on the fringe of biomedical research, looking for the fountain of youth...a marginal area...with so little backing from the scientific community" (Lockett, 1983, p. 5). Indeed, throughout their efforts to obtain greater funding for biogerontology and to establish a separate institute on aging at the National Institutes of Health (NIH) during the late 1960s and early 1970s, the scientific ability and legitimacy of biogerontologists were denigrated (see Binstock, 2003). The present effort of gerontologists to downplay "the fountain of youth" can be best understood in this historical context.

The creation of NIA in 1974, however, provided for worldwide biogerontology the kind of institutionalization that confers scientific stature and power (Cozzens, 1990), legitimating it both as more of a "mainstream" subject for biomedical research and as an appropriate area in which to invest sizable amounts of public funds. Since then, as will be summarized below, a number of important scientific frontiers have been opened up in biogerontology.

Nonetheless, the image of biogerontology as a legitimate and mainstream scientific pursuit is still vulnerable enough to be threatened by the anti-aging medicine movement. The position statement by the 51 scientists acknowledged, "Our concern is that when proponents of anti-aging medicine claim that the fountain of youth has already been discovered, it negatively affects the credibility of serious scientific research efforts on aging" (Olshansky et al., 2002b, p. B295). Similarly, Butler laments, "Unfortunately, anti-aging medicine is often confused with serious research. Consequently, public and private philanthropic organizations are less interested in funding serious aging research . . . ." (2001–2002, p. 64). As these comments imply, the war of words against anti-aging medicine is being waged primarily so that the image of research on aging will not become blemished once more.

## B. Ongoing Boundary Work

Not surprisingly, the various attacks on anti-aging medicine have engendered strong boundary-work ripostes from A4M. After Olshansky presented the Silver Fleece Award to the organization, A4M characterized him as "part of a 'multi-billion gerontological machine' that, without any basis in truth or fact, seeks to discredit tens of thousands of innovative, honest, world-class scientists, physicians, and health practitioners" (A4M, 2002a). In response to the position statement signed by 51 scientists, A4M set forth 10 alleged "gerontological biases" and purported to refute each of them by describing various articles and data (often in a misleading pseudoscientific fashion). In conclusion, it asserted:

Simply put, the death cult of gerontology desperately labors to sustain an arcane, outmoded stance that aging is natural and inevitable.... Ultimately,

the truth on aging intervention will prevail, but this truth will be scarred from the well-funded propaganda campaign of the power elite who depend on an uninterrupted status quo in the concept of aging in order to maintain its unilateral control over the funding of today's research in aging. (A4M, 2002b)

It is interesting to note that this attack on the gerontological establishment is directed at the very people whose research discoveries could further A4M's anti-aging mission.

The boundary work between the anti-aging medicine movement and selected members of the gerontological community continues unabated. Olshansky and his colleagues continue to present Silver Fleece Awards and critique anti-aging medicine (e.g., Olshansky, Hayflick, & Perls, 2004). A4M has attempted to curtail their activities by filing a lawsuit against them. Whether the movement or the gerontologists are gaining or losing anything through this boundary work is difficult to document empirically. Binstock (2003) suggested that the net effect of gerontologists' attacks on anti-aging medicine may be to provide the movement with far greater visibility and credibility than it might otherwise have.

## III. Anti-Aging Frontiers in Biogerontology

Even as they are attacking anti-aging medicine, many biogerontologists, encouraged by public scientific institutions such as the National Institutes of Health, are attempting to achieve anti-aging effects that parallel and exceed those espoused by the anti-aging medicine movement. In 1999, for example, two NIH institutes jointly convened a working group of more than 50 scientists to explore the possibilities for applying to humans the prolongevity effects that have been achieved in caloric restriction experiments with laboratory animals (Masoro, 2001). The group produced a substantial agenda of opportunities for research on human implications, including the goals of slowing fundamental processes of aging and extending maximum human life span. This fit right in with one of the priorities declared by NIA in its 2001–2005 official strategic plan, which is to "unlock the secrets" of aging, health, and longevity, including the identification of factors that "slow the clock" of aging (NIA, 2001). Caloric restriction is only one of many areas of biogerontological research pursuant to this facet of the strategic plan.

## A. Promising Avenues for Anti-Aging Interventions

Maximum observable life expectancy for females has risen linearly for the last 160 years; moreover, life expectancy continues to rise fastest among the oldest segment of the population, suggesting that there is little likelihood that an upper limit to life span will be reached any time soon (Oeppen & Vaupel, 2002). Biogerontological research has opened up a number of avenues that may lead to effective anti-aging interventions that accelerate these broad trends in life expectancy by specifically targeting the aging process(es).

Although there are many possible ways in which prolongevity can be achieved, such as lifestyle changes (e.g., weight loss), that improve average life expectancy, this discussion focuses on several areas of research where there is good evidence for the efficacy of more dramatic anti-aging interventions that can achieve substantial increases in average life expectancy and maximum life span. None of these interventions have been effectively applied to humans (with the possible exception of dietary restriction), but there is reason to believe that these interventions eventually may be effective for humans.

Two distinct interventions are addressed here at some length. Both have demonstrated the ability to prolong average life expectancy and maximum life span and have been widely replicated. The first of these is food restriction, which is also called dietary or calorie restriction (Masoro, 2002). The other is genetic intervention (Henderson, Rea, & Johnson, 2006; Longo & Finch, 2003; Masoro & Austad, 2006). In animal models, both of these experimental interventions have been shown to increase average life expectancy and maximum life span, and also to increase functionality in multiple physiological systems at older ages. There are also numerous interventions that offer amelioration of one, or sometimes several, causes of death and impairment in old age. Such therapeutic interventions include stem cell transplantation and peripheral gene therapy, as well as more conventional medical interventions that have been in the clinic for decades for treating heart disease, Alzheimer's disease, and cancer (Hadley, Lakatta, Morrison-Bogorad, Warner, & Hodes, 2005; Weiner & Selkoe, 2002), among others. Although these may not intervene directly into the fundamental causes of aging, some argue that an engineering approach that directly targets a range of problems can ultimately succeed in arresting aging (de Grey et al., 2002a). Note also that research on the biology of aging has anti-aging implications regardless of whether aging is interpreted as a disease or not.

### 1. Caloric Restriction

Caloric restriction (CR), also known as dietary restriction or food restriction, is a reduction in caloric intake while still maintaining sufficient intake of vitamins and other essential nutrients. Hundreds of studies have shown that a regimen of 20% to 60% reduction in calories leads to substantial increases in both average life expectancy and maximum life span in a variety of species, but especially in rodents. Most important, CR also lowers mortality rates and slows many of the physiological problems associated with aging (Mair, Goymer, Pletcher, & Partridge, 2003). Despite the almost 70 years of research into the effects of CR, the mechanisms of action are still unknown, but significant advances are being made into understanding the molecular and physiologic etiology (Rikke, Yerg, Battaglia, Nagy, Allison, & Johnson, 2004; Roth, Mattison, Ottinger, Chachich, Lane, & Ingram, 2004). There is a significant possibility that small molecules in the form of oral pharmaceuticals (CR mimetics) may be able to elicit the effects of dietary CR without the need for continual restriction of food intake (a dietary practice that seems unlikely to be appealing to many individuals in the developed world) (Ingram et al., 2004). Several companies are currently working in this area including GeroTech, LifeGen, and others (Pollack, 2003).

## 2. The Hayflick Limit and Stem Cells

Most cells in the human body have a finite proliferative potential, known as the Hayflick limit (after its discoverer). Moreover, most cells cannot be stimulated to "dedifferentiate" and to yield new cell types even in laboratory settings; however, a special type of cell, known as a stem cell, seems to have almost unlimited proliferative potentials (Atala, 2004). More important, stem cells have the ability to form many distinct cell types and even to correct organ level deficits. Even more potential is expected from embryonic stem cells. Although federal funding for research on embryonic stem cells has been restricted by the Bush administration because of its "right to life" concerns (see Hall, 2003), California, Massachusetts, and other states have undertaken initiatives to fund such research within their jurisdictions. Stem cells are being used in many areas of anti-aging research. It seems almost certain that such research will continue to proliferate and that it has a distinct possibility of having an impact in compressing morbidity.

## 3. Genetic Targets

The greatest revolution in biogerontological thinking about aging and the possibility of intervening to reverse aging has been the discovery that mutating a single gene can lead to a more than twofold extension of both average life expectancy and maximum life span in animal models. Using such approaches in several invertebrate species, but especially in the nematode Caenorhabditis elegans (C. elegans), numerous anti-aging/longevity targets have been discovered with relative ease (Henderson, Rea, & Johnson, 2006; Longo & Finch, 2003). This approach has been extended to mice where altering any one of several genes has been found to lead to life extension (Tatar, Bartke, & Antebi, 2003). These interventions lower the age-related rates of increase in mortality (Johnson, Wu, Tedesco, Dames, & Vaupel, 2001). Genetic methodology is sufficiently developed that one can identify literally hundreds of genes that lead to extended longevity in these species (Science of Aging Knowledge Environment, 2005). The identification of mammalian longevity/anti-aging genes provides obvious targets for intervention into human aging.

## 4. Pharmacological Interventions

It is commonplace in modern pharmacological research to use genetic strategies to identify protein targets for pharmacological intervention via small, stable, bioactive molecules (drugs) that can be taken orally or injected into the body. Such small-molecule drugs then can be developed to target the protein encoded by the identified mutant gene or otherwise modify the function of that protein and thus mimic the action of mutations that lead to life extension in model systems. Numerous companies such as Elixir Pharmaceuticals, founded by two eminent molecular geneticists (Lenny Guarante and Cynthia Kenyon), and GenoPlex (a presently inactive company founded by one of the authors, T.E.J.), embarked on just such enterprises. Dozens of companies are currently in this market (Pollack, 2003).

There are currently no drugs in clinical trials for human life extension; moreover, there are potential problems in getting drugs for life extension validated when the only marker of effectiveness is life extension. Nevertheless, the huge potential return on investment will continue to drive research in this area. An astounding discovery is that small molecules, such as resveratrol, which are found in red wine and medicinal herbs, can prolong life (Sinclair, 2005). These compounds have been shown to rescue neuronal dysfunction promoted by polyglutamine, a model of human Huntington's disease, in both *C. elegans* and in neuronal cells (Parker et al., 2005). Because resveratrol is already in clinical trials as an anti-cancer drug, it may well be the first drug approved that has clinically proven therapeutic value in increasing longevity and slowing at least some of the diseases of aging.

The NIA regards the area of anti-aging interventions as sufficiently promising to make an investment in monitoring such interventions in a multisite preclinical study designed to test the efficacy of interventions on life extension in the mouse (Warner, Ingram, Miller, Nadon, & Richardson, 2000). Four interventions are currently being tested under NIA funding: aspirin and an ibuprofen derivative (both anti-inflammatory agents with only limited evidence for an anti-aging effect); hydroxyl PBN, a possible antioxidant demonstrated to prolong life and func-

tionality in rodent models (Carney et al., 1991); and nordihydroguairetic acid, a resveratrol-like compound. Ten other compounds are currently being evaluated for a second wave of tests (Warner, personal communication to T.E.J., May 2, 2005). (For more detailed information regarding anti-aging science, see a companion volume in this *Handbooks of Aging* series, the *Handbook of the Biology of Aging* [Masoro & Austad, 2006], and Post and Binstock [2004]).

## B. Ethical and Social Implications

Even as some of the outcome claims of the commercial and clinical anti-aging movement seem far fetched, the pro-longevity results of effective anti-aging interventions envisioned by some biogerontologists are astounding. Richard Miller (2002, p. 164), while discussing the potentialities of CR research, suggested that it may be possible through decelerated aging to "increase the mean and maximal life span by about 40 percent, which is a mean age at death of about 112 years for Caucasian American or Japanese women, with an occasional winner topping out at about 140 years." Aubrey de Grey, a leading proponent of achieving arrested aging through strategies that remove the damage inevitably caused by basic metabolic processes, asserted that it is "inevitable, barring the end of civilization, that we will eventually achieve a 150-year mean longevity" (2002, p. 369).

Although achievement of such biogerontological visions may seem improbable, history shows how developments in biomedical science—like the cloning of mammals—can catch society unawares by accomplishing what seemed to be "The Impossible" (Bonnicksen, 2002). Consequently, a number of bioethicists, gerontologists, and a variety of social commentators are actively discussing the implications of achieving prolongevity, thereby renewing a dialogue that Gruman

(2003) has chronicled as dating back through several thousand years.

A longstanding concern about pro-longevity, of course, has been that it would come with a cost of extended morbidity and senescence as exemplified by the immortal, demented, deformed, and miserable Struldbruggs portrayed in *Gulliver's Travels* (Swift, 1726/1991). Numerous studies, however, have shown that those interventions that extend average life expectancy and maximum life span in various animal models also provide increased resistance to a variety of environmental stressors and promote increased health and functionality at advanced ages in all instances studied (Finkel & Holbrook, 2000; Johnson et al., 2002). Thus, the search for anti-aging interventions to extend average life expectancy and maximum human life span is not likely to result in prolonging senescence and morbidity, a most undesirable outcome.

Nonetheless, a major issue in the contemporary dialogue regarding pro-longevity is whether its pursuit is desirable. Some bioethicists, such as Arthur Caplan (2004) and John Harris (2000), see no coherent ethical objections to the pursuit of substantially increased life spans. Philosopher Christine Overall (2003) not only rejects various arguments against prolongevity, but also strongly endorses a social policy of promoting life extension. She embraces the prospect of many additional healthy years because they would afford opportunities to overcome the injustices of class, race, and gender biases. Similarly, biogerontologist David Gems (2003) argued that longer life will facilitate a richer and fuller life (although he worries that power could be concentrated into fewer hands because those who wield it will give way more slowly to death and disease). Bioethicist Stephen Post (2004) endorses interventions that would decelerate aging because they would lessen the years of dementia and other chronic diseases experienced in old age. Psychologist Paul Baltes (1997), while recognizing serious ethical issues, regards compression of morbidity through genetic intervention as an essential component for completing the "life span architecture" of human development, a positive balance of gains and losses in advanced old age.

In sharp contrast are the views of political theorist Francis Fukuyama (2002) and philosopher/physician Leon Kass (2003), chairman of the U.S. President's Council on Bioethics, who believe that pro-longevity is undesirable because it would be unnatural and thereby undermine valued aspects of human nature. Kass (2001) argued that even if the average life expectancy were increased by only 20 years, we would lose the benefits that finitude confers: (1) interest and engagement in life, (2) seriousness and aspiration, (3) beauty and love, and (4) virtue and moral excellence. Building on these long-held views, Kass set the agenda for the President's Council to issue a report in 2003 that expresses some dim views regarding prolongevity, including a strong critique of the potential societal implications:

If individuals did not age, if their functions did not decline and their horizons did not narrow, it might just be that societies would age far more acutely, and would experience their own sort of senescence—a hardening of the vital social pathways, a stiffening and loss of flexibility, a setting of the ways and views, a corroding of the muscles and the sinews. (Presidents's Council on Bioethics, 2003, p. 197)

Like Kass, bioethicist Daniel Callahan has long been an opponent of prolongevity. In a prominent book published in 1987, he proposed, for both economic and philosophical reasons, that life-extending health care be categorically denied to people 80 years or older because they have already lived out their natural, "biographical" life span (Callahan, 1987). The only deaths that he regards as "premature" are those that occur before age 65 (Callahan, 2000).

Biogerontologist Leonard Hayflick (1994) fears the societal implications of slowing or arresting the aging process such as worldwide overpopulation and its consequences, but many other biogerontologists who are engaged in efforts to decelerate aging or to arrest aging do not believe that such concerns warrant a halt to the quest for prolongevity (e.g., de Grey et al., 2002a; Miller, 2002). Indeed, as Stephen Hall (2003) makes clear in his book, *Merchants of Immortality: Chasing the Dream of Human Life Extension*, scientists and entrepreneurs will persist in their efforts to combat aging as well as disease, with or without government funding, and with or without the approval of bioethicists, philosophers, and other critics.

Consequently, other commentators have confronted the possibility that prolongevity will be achieved through one means or another, and have delineated a number of possible social and ethical issues that need attention. Juengst, Binstock, Mehlman, and Post (2003a) briefly summarized the major categories of issues involved, as follows:

Is aging as we have known it a human experience to be encouraged or discouraged, from the point of view of the public good? If longer healthy life is an unalloyed social benefit, how should it be distributed? Serious ethical issues would arise if antiaging interventions were not universally available, but were distributed in response to status (economic, social, or political), merit, nationality, or other criteria. If access to antiaging interventions were unlimited, radical societal changes would take place in virtually every social institution. (p. 1323)

Some of these issues, and others, have been addressed over the years. Anthropological, economic, ethical, kinship, legal, psychological, sociological, and policy implications of major increases in life expectancy and life span were explored in a compendium edited by gerontologist Mildred Seltzer (1995). Bioethicist Chris Hackler (2001–2002) has posited a doubling of the human life span and devoted a paragraph or two to considering what

things might be like in each of a number of sectors: marriage, the family, work, careers, the penal system, ecological consequences of global overpopulation, and approaches to distribution and regulation of anti-aging technologies. Ethicist Audrey Chapman (2004) has discussed possible implications of extended life span for social justice. Political scientist Binstock (2004) has considered what politics might be like in the "long-lived society" populated by the "prolonged old." Bioethicist Eric Juengst (2004) has examined issues concerning the moral commitments of the medical profession that will need to be addressed as anti-aging technologies emerge from the laboratory.

These speculative discussions of the potential social and ethical consequences of substantially increasing average life expectancy and maximum life span have only been disseminated in venues that do not reach wide audiences. Yet, success by biogerontologists in achieving their prolongevity goals will make the ramifications of most other current biomedical policy issues, such as the ethics of research on embryonic stem cells, seem relatively minor. In recognition of this, Juengst et al. (2003a) have suggested that NIH, which has been providing its cachet and public funds for anti-aging research, has the responsibility of generating a sustained and widespread public dialogue on the implications of that research. Ultimately, they argued, social questions that biogerontology is provoking involve civil values that can only be identified, weighed, and ranked through democratic deliberation.

## IV. Issues for Future Research

The issues raised by these various forays into the land of the prolonged old and the "extended old" are provocative and challenging, and they can be thoughtfully and imaginatively informed by what we know about these social and ethical arenas to date. In the nature of the case, however, they are not amenable to contemporary empirical research because the very existence of a substantial population of very old and healthy people in the future would certainly alter social ecology by changing almost every institution with which we are now familiar. The features of a long-lived society can be subjected only to imagination and debate (see Moody,2001–2002; Stock & Callahan, 2004). Yet, amenable to research and analysis are the contemporary social implications of (1) the consumption of anti-aging medicine, (2) how the anti-aging medicine movement and biogerontologists present and represent themselves, (3) the social context of anti-aging medicine and science, and (4) anti-aging medicine and biogerontology as emergent areas of specialty and discipline.

## A. Anti-Aging Consumers

One phenomenon that is virtually unstudied is the behavior and attitudes of anti-aging consumers. Empirical evidence can be collected from consumers regarding how they think about, consume, and experience contemporary anti-aging products and treatments. How do they define anti-aging therapies? Why they are interested in them (if indeed they are)? How do these interventions become incorporated into people's lives? What do they regard as "successful" outcomes from using them? Have they experienced "success"?

Another area for investigation is consumer attitudes about prolongevity. Although there may be a rhetorical divide between the anti-aging medicine movement and biogerontologists, do consumers perceive any important difference between them? If genetically based anti-aging interventions to achieve substantial prolongevity do become available, how willing would consumers be to try them?

## B. The Politics of Presentation

The ways in which the anti-aging movement and biogerontology present themselves to consumers, other clinicians, the research community, funding agencies, and the general public have interesting social implications. There are several rhetorical strategies for defining anti-aging products, therapies, and research. For example, A4M clinicians present anti-aging interventions as *medical treatments* for the maladies that are commonly associated with aging. They thereby claim for their services all the cultural moral authority and professional autonomy of medical attempts to combat disease and address conventional health care needs. Because this treatment construct requires reinterpreting the aging process as fundamentally pathological, this strategy has generated a renewed debate within gerontology, geriatrics, and the philosophy of medicine over the nosological status of senescence as humans have experienced it to date (e.g., Blumenthal, 2003). In contrast to characterizing anti-aging efforts as treatments, some elements of the anti-aging movement present their interventions as ways people can *enhance* their lives by "staying young," or restoring mental and physical capacities that decline with age. As Juengst, Binstock, Mehlman, Post, and Whitehouse (2003b) point out, because anti-aging enhancements are envisioned as attempts to improve on human form and function, they provoke criticism that they are unnatural and therefore unethical (e.g., see Kass, 2003). Politically, however, the use of enhancement rhetoric takes the enterprise out of the realm of biomedicine, thereby freeing it from control by the medical profession and governmental regulatory bodies.

A third rhetorical position is to characterize anti-aging interventions as *prevention*. Like vaccinations, the argument goes, anti-aging interventions do manipulate a perfectly normal biological process, but with the legitimate aim of forestalling the chronic health problems associated with aging for as long as possible. This presentational strategy seems to be the most widely embraced within mainstream biogerontology and by its funding institutions. Biogerontologists portray themselves as "the good guys who favor preventive medicine and medical research [and want] to prevent late-life illness" (Miller, 2002, p. 172). This presentation of the anti-aging enterprise skirts the controversies about whether aging is a disease that needs treatment and whether enhancement is unethical (Juengst & Ponsaran, 2004).

An important line of empirical research is to trace how these rhetorical strategies affect developments in the field. What are their differential impacts on policies? Empirical tracking of such developments will make it possible to address important questions. Does defining anti-aging research as a route to effective prevention of disease and disability secure greater public funding for biogerontological research? Hayflick believes that it will, as demonstrated by his repeated call for greater allocation of NIA monies to biological research by arguing that aging is the single biggest risk factor for the diseases associated with old age (e.g., Hayflick, 2004). If the anti-aging medicine movement continues to portray itself as treating aging, will organized medicine attempt to assert control over it, or will it engage in boundary work as have the biogerontologists and geriatricians? To the extent that anti-aging interventions are portrayed as enhancements, will there be a political movement to curtail them?

## C. Social Context

Scientific developments do not occur in a social vacuum separate and apart from society but rather as part of it, influenced by and influencing cultural ideas of life,

death, and the nature of the world we live in (e.g., Downey, Dumit, & Traweek, 1997). In this case, anti-aging medicine and science both reflect and help to create our popular and cultural understandings of aging, wellness, sickness, and mortality. (Of course, this is not meant to suggest that there is a single, monolithic understanding of aging that transcends culture, but rather that there are different degrees and types of articulation between scientific notions and various cultural beliefs. It is the specifics of this articulation that are worthy of further exploration.) Social and cultural factors such as the aging of the baby boomers, the continuing authority that medicoscientific knowledge carries for explaining life experiences, and the elaboration of medical interventions to treat an ever-expanding array of human conditions have shaped the anti-aging arena. Just as anti-aging medicine and science are shaped by broader forces, however, they in turn have an impact on social institutions, regulatory bodies, and the political and economic climate. There are rich avenues for empirical research on such questions as: Who is funding anti-aging research? What scientific, ethical, economic, and political differences flow from public and private sector support for this research? What do the supporters of research gain from it?

## D. Disciplinary Emergence

The development of biogerontology as a field requires ongoing study in the tradition of sociological and historical scholarship on the emergence of new disciplines in science and medicine (e.g., Achenbaum, 1995; Cozzens, 1990). As evidenced previously, the field of biogerontology is still fragile enough for its leaders to engage in boundary work to maintain and enhance its legitimacy and funding. Empirical research on the discipline's efforts to develop and thrive would add to our general understanding of science as a political and social endeavor. Tracking the development of biogerontology may also throw light on how the science and politics of the anti-aging arena shape our popular and cultural understandings of aging, wellness, sickness, and mortality. In addition, it could reveal how endeavors in anti-aging science and their applications may reshape the broader gerontological enterprise in its approaches to the study of aging.

## Acknowledgments

Support for Robert H. Binstock's preparation of this chapter was provided by the National Institute on Aging and the National Human Genome Research Institute, grant 1R01AGHG20916, Eric T. Juengst, Principal Investigator. Thomas E. Johnson's work has been supported by grants from the National Institutes of Health, and by gifts from the Ellison Medical Foundation and the Glenn Foundation for Medical Research.

## References

Achenbaum, W. A. (1995). *Crossing frontiers: Gerontology emerges as a science.* New York: Cambridge University Press.

A4M (American Academy of Anti-Aging Medicine). (2002a). *The fleecing of academic integrity by the gerontological establishment.* Retrieved June 13, 2002, from http://www.worldhealth.net/html/fleecing_of_academic_integrity.htm

A4M (American Academy of Anti-Aging Medicine). (2002b). *Official position statement on the truth about aging intervention.* Retrieved June 13, 2003, from http://www.worldhealth.net/html/truth.html

A4M (American Academy of Anti-Aging Medicine). (2005). *The American Academy of Anti-Aging Medicine.* Retrieved May 31, 2005, from *http://www.worldhealth.net/p/96.html*

Arumainathan, S. (2001). *Intellectual dishonesty in geriatric medicine—truth versus fallacy: A4M sets the record straight on a campaign of disinformation challenging the facts of the science of anti-aging medicine.* Retrieved November 3, 2003, from http://www.worldhealth.net/resources/IntellDishonesty.PDF

Atala, A. (2004). Tissue engineering and regenerative medicine: Concepts for clinical application. *Rejuvenation Research, 7*(1), 15–31.

Baltes, P. B. (1997). On the incomplete architecture of human ontogeny: Selection, optimization, and compensation as foundation of developmental theory. *American Psychologist, 55,* 366–380.

Binstock, R. H. (2003). The war on "anti-aging medicine." *Gerontologist, 43,* 4–14.

Binstock, R. H. (2004). The prolonged old, the long-lived society, and the politics of age. In S. G. Post & R. H. Binstock (Eds.), *The fountain of youth: Cultural, scientific, and ethical perspectives on a biomedical goal* (pp. 362–386). New York: Oxford University Press.

Blackman, M. R., Sorkin, J. D., Munzer, T., Bellantoni, M. F., Busby-Whitehead, J., Stevens, T. E., Jayme, J., O'Connor, K. G., Christmas, C., Tobin, J. D., Steward, K. J., Cottrell, E., St. Clair, C., Pabst, K. M., & Harman, S. M. (2002). Growth hormone and sex steroid administration in healthy aged women and men: A randomized controlled trial. *Journal of the American Medical Association, 288,* 282–292.

Blumenthal, H. T. (2003). The aging/disease dichotomy: True or false? *Journal of Gerontology: Medical Sciences, 58A,* M138–M145.

Bonnicksen, A. L. (2002). *Crafting a cloning policy: From Dolly to stem cells.* Washington, DC: Georgetown University Press.

Butler, R. N. (2001–2002). Is there an "anti-aging" medicine? *Generations, 25*(4), 63–65.

Callahan, D. (1987). *Setting limits: Medical goals in an aging society.* New York: Simon and Schuster.

Callahan, D. (2000). Death and the research imperative. *New England Journal of Medicine, 342,* 654–656.

Caplan, A. L. (2004). An unnatural process: Why it is not inherently wrong to seek a cure for aging. In S. G. Post & R. H. Binstock (Eds.), *The fountain of youth: Cultural, scientific, and ethical perspectives on a biomedical goal* (pp. 271–285). New York: Oxford University Press.

Carney, J. M., Starke-Reed, P. E., Oliver, C. N., Landum, R. W., Cheng, M. S., Wu, J. F., & Floyd, R. A. (1991). Reversal of age-related increase in brain protein oxidation, decrease in enzyme activity, and loss in temporal and spatial memory by chronic administration of the spin-trapping compound *N-tert*-butyl-α-phenylnitorne. *Proceedings of the National Academy of Sciences USA, 88,* 3633–3636.

Chan, J. M., Stampfer, M. J., Giovannucci, E., Gann, P. H., Ma, J., Wilkinson, P., Hennekens, C. H., & Pollak, M. (1998). Plasma insulin-like growth factor I and prostate cancer risk: A prospective study. *Science, 279,* 563–566.

Chapman, A. R. (2004). The social and justice implications of extending the human life span. In S. G. Post & R. H. Binstock (Eds.), *The fountain of youth: Cultural, scientific, and ethical perspectives on a biomedical goal* (pp. 340–361). New York: Oxford University Press.

Chopra, D. (2001). *Grow younger, live longer: 10 steps to reverse aging.* New York: Harmony Books.

Clarke, A. E., Shim, J. K., Mamo, L., Fosket, J. R., & Fishman, J. R. (2003). Biomedicalization: Technoscientific transformations of health, illness, and U.S. biomedicine. *American Sociological Review, 68,* 161–194.

Cole, T. R., & Thompson, B. (2001–2002). Anti-aging: Are you for it or against it? *Generations, 25*(4), 6–8.

Cozzens, S. E. (1990). Autonomy and power in science. In S. E. Cozzens & T. F. Gieryn (Eds.), *Theories of science in society* (pp. 164–184). Bloomington, IN: Indiana University Press.

de Grey, A.D.N.J. (2002). Gerontologists and the media: The dangers of over pessimism. *Biogerontology, 1,* 369.

de Grey, A.D.N.J., Ames, B. N., Andersen, J. K., Bartke, A., Campisi, J., Heward, C. B., McCarter, R.J.M., & Stock, G. (2002a). Time to talk SENS: Critiquing the immutability of human aging. *Annals of the New York Academy of Science, 959,* 452–462.

de Grey, A.D.N.J., Gavrilov, L., Olshansky, S. J., Coles, L. S., Cutler, R. G., Fossel, M., & Harman, S. M. (2002b). Antiaging technology and pseudoscience. *Science, 296,* 656.

Downey, G. L., Dumit, J., & Traweek, S. (Eds.). (1997). *Cyborgs and citadels: Anthropological interventions in emerging sciences, technologies and medicines.* Santa Fe, NM: School of American Research Press.

Estes, C. L., & Binney, E. A. (1989). The biomedicalization of aging: Dangers and dilemmas. *Gerontologist, 29,* 587–596.

FIND/SVP. (2005). *New anti-aging market creates opportunities for marketers.* Retrieved May 31, 2005 from http://www.findsvp.com/about/2003-04-08antiaging.cfm

Finkel, T., & Holbrook, N. J. (2000). Oxidants, oxidative stress and the biology of ageing. *Nature, 408,* 239–247.

Fisher, A., & Morley, J. E. (2002). Antiaging medicine: The good, the bad, and the ugly. *Journal of Gerontology: Medical Sciences, 57A,* M636–M639.

Fox, P. (1989). From senility to Alzheimer's disease: The rise of the Alzheimer's disease movement. *Milbank Quarterly, 67,* 58–102.

Fries, J. F. (1980). Aging, natural death and the compression of morbidity. *New England Journal of Medicine, 303,* 130–136.

Fukuyama, F. (2002). *Our posthuman future: Consequences of the biotechnology revolution.* New York: Farrar, Straus & Giroux.

Gems, D. (2003). Is more life always better? The new biology of aging and the meaning of life. *Hastings Center Report, 33*(4), 31–39.

Gieryn, T. F. (1983). Boundary-work and the demarcation of science from non-science: Strains and interests in professional ideologies of scientists. *American Sociological Review, 48,* 781–795.

Goldman, B., & Klatz, R. (1988). *The "E" factor: Ergogenic aids, the secrets of new-tech training and fitness for the winning edge.* Chicago: Elite Sports Medicine Publications, Inc.

Gruman, G. J. (2003). *A history of ideas about the prolongation of life.* New York: Springer Publishing Company. (Original work published in 1966.)

Guidestar. (2005). *U.S. Income tax return of the American Academy of Anti-Aging Medicine for 2003, Internal Revenue Service form 990.* Retrieved May 26, 2005, from http://www.guidestar.org/Documents/2003/364/087/2003-364087310-1.9.pdf

Haber, C. (2001–2002). Anti-aging: Why now? A historical framework for understanding the contemporary enthusiasm. *Generations*, 25(4), 9–14.

Hackler, C. (2001–2002). Troubling implications of doubling the lifespan. *Generations*, 25(4), 15–19.

Hadley, E. C., Lakatta, E. G., Morrison-Bogorad, M., Warner, H. R., & Hodes, R. J. (2005). The future of aging therapies, *Cell*, 120, 557–567.

Hall, S. S. (2003). *Merchants of immortality: Chasing the dream of human life extension.* New York: Houghton Mifflin Company.

Harris, J. (2000). Intimations of immortality. *Science*, 288, 59.

Hayflick, L. (1994). *How and why we age.* New York: Ballantine Books.

Hayflick, L. (2004). "Anti-aging" is an oxymoron. *Journal of Gerontology: Biological Sciences*, 59A, 573–578.

Henderson, S. T., Rea, S. L., & Johnson. T. E. (2006). Dissecting the processes of aging using the nematode *Caenorhabditis elegans*. In E. J. Masoro & S. N. Austad (Eds.), *Handbook of the biology of aging* (6th ed.), pp. 352–391. San Diego: Academic Press.

Holstein, M. B. (2001–2002). A feminist perspective on anti-aging medicine. *Generations*, 25(4), 38–43.

Ingram, D. K., Anson, R. M., de Cabo, R., Mamczarz, J., Zhu, M., Mattison, J., Lane, M. A., & Roth, G. S. (2004). Development of calorie restriction mimetics as a prolongevity strategy. *Annals of the New York Academy of Science*, 1019, 412–423.

Janssens, H., & Vanderschueren, D.M.O.I. (2000). Endocrinological aspects of aging in men: Is hormone replacement of benefit? *European Journal of Obstetrics and Gynecology and Reproductive Biology*, 92, 7–12.

Johnson, T. E., Wu, D., Tedesco, P., Dames, S., & Vaupel, J. W., (2001). Age-specific demographic profiles of longevity mutants in *Caenorhabditis elegans* show segmental effects. *Journals of Gerontology: Biological Sciences*, 56A, B331–B339.

Johnson, T. E., de Castro, E., de Castro, S. H., Cypser, J., Henderson, S., Murakami, S., Rikke, B., Tedesco, P., & Link, C. (2002). Longevity genes in the nematode *Caenorhabditis elegans* also mediate increased resistance to stress and prevent disease.

*Journal of Inherited Metabolic Disease*, 25, 197–206.

Juengst, E. T. (2004). Anti-aging research and the limits of medicine. In S. G. Post & R. H. Binstock (Eds.), *The fountain of youth: Cultural, scientific, and ethical perspectives on a biomedical goal* (pp. 321–339). New York: Oxford University Press.

Juengst, E. T., Binstock, R. H., Mehlman, M. J., & Post, S. G. (2003a). Antiaging research and the need for public dialogue. *Science*, 299, 1323.

Juengst, E. T., Binstock, R. H., Mehlman, M. J., Post, S. G., & Whitehouse, P. J. (2003b). "Anti-aging medicine" and the challenges of human enhancement. *Hastings Center Report*, 33(4), 21–30.

Juengst, E. T., & Ponsaran, R. S. (2004). Normal aging, disease prevention, and medical ethics. *Public Policy & Aging Report*, 14(2), 14–18.

Kass, L. R. (2001). L'chaim and its limits. Why not immortality? *First Things*, 13, 17–24.

Kass, L. R. (2003). Ageless bodies, happy souls. *The New Atlantis* (1), 9–28.

Klatz, R. (Ed.). (1999). *Ten weeks to a younger you.* Chicago: Sport Tech Labs, Inc.

Lockett, B. A. (1983). *Aging, politics, and research: Setting the federal agenda for research on aging.* New York: Springer Publishing Company.

Longo, V. D., & Finch, C. E. (2003). Evolutionary medicine: From dwarf model systems to healthy centenarians? *Science*, 299, 1342–1346.

Mair, W., Goymer, P., Pletcher, S. D., & Partridge, L. (2003). Demography of dietary restriction and death in *Drosophila*. *Science*, 301, 1731–1733.

Masoro, E. J. (Ed.). (2001). Caloric restriction's effects on aging: Opportunities for research on human implications. *Journal of Gerontology: Biological Sciences*, 56A (Special Issue 1).

Masoro E. J. (2002). *Caloric restriction: A key to understanding and modulating aging.* Amsterdam: Elsevier Science.

Masoro, E. J., & Austad, S. N. (2006). *Handbook of the biology of aging* (6th ed.). San Diego: Academic Press.

Mehlman, M. J., Binstock, R. H., Juengst, E. T., Ponsaran, R. S., & Whitehouse, P. J. (2004).

Anti-aging medicine: Can consumers be better protected? *Gerontologist, 44,* 304–310.

Miller, R. A. (2002). Extending life: Scientific prospects and political obstacles. *Milbank Quarterly, 80,* 155–174.

Moody, H. R. (2001–2002). Who's afraid of life extension? *Generations, 25*(4), 33–37.

NIA (National Institute on Aging). (1997). *Media campaign cautions consumers about "anti-aging" hormone supplements.* [NIH news release, April 1.] Retrieved July 3, 2002, from http://www.nia.nih.gov/news/pr/1997/04%2D01.htm

NIA (National Institute on Aging). (2001). *Action plan for aging research: Strategic plan for fiscal years 2001–2005.* Retrieved May 31, 2005, from http://www.nia.nih.gov/AboutNIA/StrategicPlan/ResearchGoalB/Subgoal1.htm

NIA (National Institute on Aging). (2002a). *Life-extension. Science or science fiction?* Retrieved July 8, 2002, from http://www.nia.nih.gov/health/agepages/lifeext.htm

NIA (National Institute on Aging). (2002b). *Looking for the fountain of youth?* Retrieved July 3, 2002, from http://www.nia.nih.gov/health/ads/fount1.git

NIA (National Institute on Aging). (2005). *Resource directory for older people.* Retrieved May 26, 2005 from http://www.nia.nih.gov/HealthInformation/ResourceDirectory.htm

Oeppen, J., & Vaupel, J. W. (2002). Broken limits to life expectancy. *Science, 296,* 1029–1031.

Olshansky, S. J., & Carnes, B. A. (2001). *The quest for immortality: Science at the frontiers of aging.* New York: W. W. Norton.

Olshansky, S. J., Hayflick, L., & Carnes, B. A. (2002a). No truth to the fountain of youth. *Scientific American, 286*(6), 92–95.

Olshansky, J. S., Hayflick, L., & Carnes, B. A. (2002b). Position statement on human aging. *Journal of Gerontology: Biological Sciences, 57A,* B292–B297.

Olshansky, J. S., Hayflick, L., & Perls, T. T. (Eds.). (2004). *Anti-aging medicine: The hype and the reality. Journal of Gerontology: Biological Sciences* (special publication). Washington, DC: The Gerontological Society of America.

Overall, C. (2003). *Aging, death, and human longevity: A philosophical inquiry.* Berkley, CA: University of California Press.

Parker, J. A., Arango, M., Abderrahmane, S., Lambert, E., Tourette, C., Catoire, H., & Neri, C. (2005). Resveratrol rescues mutant polyglutamine cytotoxicity in nematode and mammalian neurons. *Nature Genetics, 37,* 349–350.

Perls, T. T. (2004). Anti-aging quackery: Human growth hormone and tricks of the trade—more dangerous than ever. *Journal of Gerontology: Biological Sciences, 59A,* 682–691.

Pollack, A. (2003, September 21). Forget Botox. Anti aging pills may be next. *New York Times,* Section 3, pp. 1, 10.

Pope, E. (2002). 51 top scientists blast anti-aging idea. *AARP Bulletin, 23*(43), 3–5.

Post, S. G. (2004). Establishing an appropriate ethical framework: The moral conversation around the goal of prolongevity. *Journal of Gerontology: Biological Sciences, 59A,* B534–B539.

Post, S. G., & Binstock, R. H. (Eds.). (2004). *The fountain of youth: Cultural, scientific, and ethical perspectives on a biomedical goal.* New York: Oxford University Press.

President's Council on Bioethics. (2003). *Beyond therapy: Biotechnology and the pursuit of happiness.* New York: Harper Collins Publishers.

Rikke, B. A., Yerg, J. E., Battaglia, M. E., Nagy, T. R., Allison, D. B., & Johnson, T. E., (2004). Quantitative trait loci specifying the response of body temperature to dietary restriction. *Journal of Gerontology: Biological Sciences, 59A,* B118–B125.

Robert, L. L. (2004). The three avenues of gerontology: From basic research to clinical gerontology and anti-aging medicine. Another French paradox. *Journal of Gerontology: Biological Sciences, 59A,* 540–542.

Robinson, J. (2001). *Noble conspirator: Florence S. Mahoney and the rise of the National Institutes of Health.* Washington, DC: The Francis Press.

Roth, G. S., Mattison, J. A., Ottinger M. A., Chachich, M. E., Lane, M. A., & Ingram, D. K. (2004). Aging in rhesus monkeys: Relevance to human health interventions. *Science, 305,* 1423–1426.

Science of Aging Knowledge Environment. (2005). *Genes/interventions (database).*

Retrieved April 30, 2005 from http://sageke.sciencemag.org/cgi/genesdb

Seltzer, M. M. (Ed.). (1995). *The impact of increased life expectancy: Beyond the gray horizon.* New York: Springer Publishing Company.

Sinclair, D. (2005). Sirtuins for healthy neurons. *Nature Genetics, 37,* 339–340.

Stock, S., & Callahan, D. (2004). Point-counterpoint: Would doubling the human life span be a net positive or negative for us either as individuals or as a society? *Journal of Gerontology: Biological Sciences, 59A,* B554–B559.

Swift, J. (1991). *Gulliver's travels.* New York: Knopf Everyman's Library. (Original work published in 1726.)

Tatar, M., Bartke, A., & Antebi, A. (2003). The endocrine regulation of aging by insulin-like signals. *Science, 299,* 1346–1351.

Taylor, C. A. (1996). *Defining science: A rhetoric of demarcation.* Madison, WI: University of Wisconsin Press.

U.S. GAO (General Accounting Office). (2001). *Health products for seniors: "Anti-aging" products pose potential for physical and economic harm.* Washington, DC: U.S. Government Printing Office, GAO-01-1129.

U.S. Senate Special Committee on Aging. (2001). *Swindlers, hucksters and snake oil salesmen: The hype and hope of marketing anti-aging products to seniors.* Hearing held in Washington, DC, September 10.

University of Illinois at Chicago (2002). *Silver Fleece Awards target anti-aging hype.* [Office of Public Affairs, News Release, February 12.] Retrieved June 21, 2002, from http://tigger.uic.edu/htbin/cgiwrap/bin/newsbureau

Vance, M. L. (2003). Can growth hormone prevent aging? *New England Journal of Medicine, 348,* 779–780.

Warner, H. R., Ingram, D., Miller, R. A., Nadon, N. L., & Richardson, A. G. (2000). Program for testing biological interventions to promote healthy aging. *Mechanisms of Ageing and Development, 115,* 199–208.

Weiner, H. L., & Selkoe, D. J. (2002). Inflammation and therapeutic vaccination in CNS diseases. *Nature, 420,* 879–884.

Wick, G. (2002). Anti-aging medicine: Does it exist? A critical discussion of anti-aging health products. *Experimental Gerontology, 37,* 1137–1140.

Writing Group for the Women's Health Initiative Investigators. (2002). Risks and benefits of estrogen plus progestin in healthy postmenopausal women: Principal results from the Women's Health Initiative randomized controlled trial. *Journal of the American Medical Association, 288,* 321–333.

Youngevity. (2005). *Youngevity product highlights.* Retrieved May 29, 2005, from http://youngevity.com/brochure/brochure_p1.htm

Twenty-five

# Aging and Justice

Martin Kohli

This chapter focuses on justice between age groups and generations. A *Handbook of Aging* obviously asks for such a focus. But more generally, this dimension of justice has become one of the major issues of contemporary societies. In the history of most Western welfare states, the key "social question" to be solved was the integration of the industrial workers, in other words, the pacification of class conflict. This was achieved by giving workers some assurance of a stable life course, including retirement as a normal life phase funded to a large extent through public pay-as-you-go contribution systems or general taxes (Kohli, 1987). In the twenty-first century, class conflict seems to be defunct and its place taken over by generational conflict (Bengtson, 1993; Kaufmann, 2005). The new prominence of the latter is due both to the evolved patterns of social security, which have turned older adults into the main clients of the welfare state, and to the demographic challenge of low fertility and increasing longevity.

Such an assertion needs to be qualified in two ways. First, it should be noted that conflict or competition between young and old over scarce resources is by no means new. As is discussed later, it is a common theme in historical and anthropological accounts of premodern societies as well (see Foner, 1984; Williamson & Watts-Roy, 1999). With the evolution of the modern welfare state, however, the form and arena of this conflict have changed. Second, and more important for our present concerns, it remains essential to assess the extent of the generational cleavage per se and the extent to which it masks the continued existence of the class cleavage between wealthy and poor (or owners and workers). In other words, to what extent have the new *inter*generational conflicts really crowded out traditional *intra*generational ones? There are moreover other cleavages that are usually categorized as "new" dimensions of inequality (in distinction to the "old" ones of class), such as those of gender and ethnicity (or "race").

Parts of this chapter are an expanded and revised version of the arguments presented in Kohli (2004).

Issues of justice play a prominent role in adjudicating conflicts and legitimizing their solutions along all these cleavages. Modern democratic polities, evolving under conditions of individualized participation in public affairs, increasingly depend on broad cognitively based acceptance by their citizenry and thus rely on commonly shared (universal or local) sources of legitimacy such as those provided by justice ideas.

Justice as used here should not be equated with the world of law. I will not go into the discussions, for example, of how age boundaries are legally regulated and to what extent these regulations are constitutionally valid (see Igl, 2000, for a perspective from Germany), nor of the legal framework against discrimination on the grounds of age (see Chapter 22). These problems are related to the arguments developed here insofar as they rely on the same general set of ideas about the fair division of the life course and construction of age groups. Setting the age boundary of retirement is tantamount to deciding which ages are institutionally expected to gain their living from participation in the labor market, and which ages have access to public pensions. But it would go beyond the scope of the present chapter to cover these issues—even more so as they present major differences among national legal regimes.

The first two sections of this chapter discuss the two basic concepts: age and generation on the one hand, justice on the other. As to age and generation, I will show that most problems are situated not at the level of age groups but of generations or cohorts, and then outline my own distinctions between (various types of) societal and family generations in order to frame the issue of generational equity. As to justice, the focus is less on normative conceptions than on the perspectives of empirical justice research: as analysis of attitudes and

values, as institutional analysis, and as discourse analysis. In the third section, the discourse on and institutional anchoring of generational equity are reviewed. The fourth section presents the distributive outcomes in terms of income shares and poverty risks of different age groups, and the fifth, the patterns of public attitudes and beliefs concerning justice among generations, the role of the state and other possible providers of social security, and the acceptability of various reform proposals. A brief final section returns to the issue of intergenerational versus intragenerational conflict, and discusses the link between the public and the private generational "contract."

Wherever possible this chapter relies on comparative arguments and findings among the economically advanced nations of the OECD world. The emphasis is on European conceptualizations and sources where the comparative perspective has (by necessity) been given more prominence. The U.S. literature is not fully reviewed, but is included for comparison, both with regard to institutional specifics and empirical dimensions of resource distribution and attitudes.

## I. Age and Generation

Aging is relevant to justice concerns not so much in terms of the process of individual aging as in terms of the aggregation of individuals into age groups and generations or cohorts as socially delimited entities. And, as will be seen, age groups per se are not really problematic; it is the differentiation into generations that creates the major problems in terms of distributive justice. During the last two decades, they have usually been addressed as the problem of *generational equity*.

It needs to be emphasized that age groups are not given but socially constructed through the institutionalization of the life course. "The elderly" as a category are today directly predicated on the institutionalized age boundary of retirement. Changing this boundary would create different relative sizes of age groups, and thus change the distributional balance. Raising it has therefore become one of the main avenues in the current reform or retrenchment of pension systems. Such changes, however, are difficult to implement because these age boundaries, although socially constructed, are not freely available to political intervention; they are linked to basic structural properties of welfare states and labor markets (e.g., seniority wage systems) and stabilized through deeply entrenched biographical orientations and expectations (see Kohli, 1994).

In all modern societies, the elderly are the main recipients of public income transfer programs, while children, even when taking child allowances and the costs of schooling into account, are to a large part financed privately by their parents. Such unequal allocation of public resources among age groups may be considered "unfair" or ineffective if, for example, its outcome is that one group is consistently worse off than another. In principle, however, an unequal treatment of age groups is perfectly legitimate. The reason is that age is not a fixed characteristic (see Daniels, 1988, p. 18). Age groups are to be viewed not as entities with fixed membership but with regularly changing membership, with all individuals progressing through the life course from one to the next according to an institutionalized schedule.

With generations this is not the case. The concept of generation can be defined with regard to society or to family: two levels which are usually analyzed separately but need to be treated in a unified framework (Kohli, 1996; Kohli & Szydlik, 2000). At the level of the family, generation refers to position in the lineage. At the societal level, it refers to the aggregate of persons born in a limited period (i.e., a birth cohort according to demographic parlance) who therefore experience historical events at similar ages and move up through the life course in unison. One cannot leave a societal generation or birth cohort in this formal sense; they are fixed-membership entities. In a title such as *Justice between age groups and generations* (Laslett & Fishkin, 1992), the *and* thus stands for a major conceptual and empirical problem.

Under what conditions and to what extent this common sociohistorical location experienced by a birth cohort throughout its life leads to a shared consciousness of being a generation and to a common mobilization as a societal actor has been the subject of intense argument and research. What is clear, however, is that the concept of generation is a key to the analysis of social dynamics. In the sequence of generations, families and societies create continuity and change with regard to parents and children, economic resources, political power, and cultural hegemony. In all of these spheres, generations are a basic unit of social reproduction and social change—in other words, of stability over time as well as renewal (or sometimes revolution).

In some "simple" traditional societies without centralized political power and class-based social stratification, age and gender are the basic criteria for social organization and the distribution of rights and duties. The most obvious type are the societies, found mostly in East Africa, based on formal age classes or age-sets, as they are sometimes called (Bernardi, 1985). A subtype of particular relevance to the present chapter are those societies in which the basis is not age but generation, that is, position in the family lineage. Here, the sequence of generations in the family directly conditions the position of the individual in the economic, political, and cultural sphere (Müller, 1990). In modern societies, these features of social organization have been differentiated and are now institutionalized in separate spheres; however, they need to be linked at least conceptually, so that shifts in the relative importance of these spheres may be detected. There are indications, for instance, that in the West, the main arena of intergenerational conflict has shifted from the political and cultural to the economic sphere. The political cleavage between generations has turned into a cleavage over the distribution of public resources.

As these brief remarks show, the idea of conflict or competition between young and old is by no means new. But it may have taken on a new form of institutionalization in the modern era, with its emphasis on societal dynamics and progress through the replacement of old by new generations. In political and cultural terms, a case in point is the youth movements at the beginning of the twentieth century. They celebrated and mobilized youth as the vanguard of cultural and political change, and even as a higher form of human existence, necessarily at war against the adult world (Wohl, 1979). The contemporary history of the conflict dates from the institutionalization of age-based social security (Williamson & Watts-Roy, 1999). In the United States, it was the passage of the Social Security Act in 1935 that brought the distribution of resources between young and old—the conflict that later came to be known under the term of *generational equity*—into public focus.

## II. Justice: Empirical and Normative Perspectives

Empirical social science research on distributive justice (issues of procedural and retributive justice are not covered here) comes mostly in two variants which can usefully be differentiated along two dimensions: that of small-group contexts versus whole societies and that of attitudes versus behavior (Miller, 1992, 1999; Swift, Marshall, Burgoyne, & Routh, 1995). The first variant is that of social psychology, and more recently, of economics: experimental studies of behavior in terms of distributing rewards at the micro-level. The second variant is that of sociology and political science: survey studies of attitudes or beliefs about the fairness of the distribution of resources across whole societies. It is with this second variant that the present chapter is concerned.

Public beliefs about whether social arrangements are just play an increasing role today. Processes of societal individualization have reduced the power of traditional loyalties and at the same time raised the level of expectations toward democratic polities. In this situation the reference to and conflict over basic principles of justice becomes critical. This is especially the case now that, in all advanced societies, the institutional patterns of resource distribution are under stress, and the public agenda is dominated less by the prospect of giving new benefits to the citizenry than by the retrenchment of existing ones (Liebig, Lengfeld, & Mau, 2004).

Public issues of aging are, above all, issues of social security and the welfare state. This may be the arena where the reference to principles of justice is most marked, because it is here that the problems of the societal distribution of resources are to be resolved (Liebig et al., 2004). The welfare state directly bases its legitimacy on principles of just distribution, and therefore its legitimacy is especially dependent on whether it is perceived as fulfilling these principles.

Justice beliefs and attitudes are thus critical because, at the collective level, they condition the public acceptance of welfare state reforms (and by that, the latter's political fate). Moreover, they are critical because, at the individual level, they affect compliance with the taxes and contributions imposed by the welfare state.

It must be noted, however, that the relevance of attitudes may be questioned on two grounds. The first is the possibility that the opinions of ordinary people will be unsystematic and contradictory. The second is that it is not clear to what extent beliefs are in line with actual behavior, and that expressed beliefs may reflect social desirability (Swift et al., 1995). These are both potentially serious drawbacks to empirical justice research in the sociological style. This is especially clear in relation to the large body of scholarship in the philosophy or political theory of justice, that is, in the normative arguments on what is to be considered just on what grounds. The relation between empirical and normative work has so far been tenuous at best. Among the practitioners of the former there is at least some awareness of theories of justice, whereas among the practitioners of the latter, there is little interest in the other side. The widespread disregard and even contempt of empirical justice research by philosophers and political theorists is aptly expressed by the anonymous British referee of the *International Social Justice Project* cited by Swift et al. (1995), who considers it "a waste of time to survey the views of people who are not in a position to judge the issues" (p. 17). This disregard of course does not do justice to the role of popular beliefs as a source of political legitimacy. For some theorists it remains moreover essential to ground a theory of justice for a democratic state on some consideration of the beliefs of the people who make up the democratic constituency. As an example, Elster (1992) asserts that "theories of justice need empirical foundations" (p. 192). What exactly the latter should be and how they should inform theories of justice remains a complex issue (see Swift et al., 1995, for a lucid

overview), but any empirical foundations presuppose a good answer to the two potential drawbacks.

The first one, about the inconsistency of popular opinion, is not special to the field of justice. It is a common experience for researchers aiming to measure attitudes (or related concepts) that their respondents will agree with many different statements simultaneously, including contradictory ones (e.g., Kohli & Künemund, 2003). But this need not be the end of the story. On the one hand, attitude statements in surveys, even if worded closely to specific situations, are never fully defined; they always leave room for definition of what precisely they mean to say. It may be possible in many instances to reconstruct the meaning of seemingly contradictory items so that the contradiction vanishes. On the other hand, even if we accept that ordinary people do not spend as much energy and intelligence as political theorists would on the logical structuring of their beliefs, there is a range of psychometric procedures to get at the underlying or latent meaning of answers to a set of attitude items. According to psychometric standards the common practice by many sociologists to base their interpretations on single-item answers is problematic, even though in many instances (and in this chapter as well) it may be unavoidable because the survey in question does not include full batteries of items.

The most ambitious comparative measurement of the cognitive space of justice beliefs so far is the already mentioned *International Social Justice Project* (Kluegel, Mason, & Wegener, 1995). A careful analysis of the large number of attitude items in different formats collected here (Swift et al., 1995) shows that these beliefs are indeed reasonably well structured, both in terms of internal consistency and of external validation according to plausible sociodemographic differences such as gender, education, class, and political preference. The three main factors common (in varying degrees) to the three countries under investigation (West Germany, Britain, and the United States) are equality of outcomes, justified inequality, and need—the factors that also usually result from systematic discussions of distributive justice, or from reconstructions of the criteria embodied in welfare institutions. People consistently use these different criteria for different situations. In all three societies, people thus organize their normative judgments "around established and coherent principles of justice" (Swift et al., 1995, p. 35).

The second potential drawback may be thornier. The attitude versus behavior conflict has been the subject of a long research tradition in social psychology that, as discussed by Swift et al. (1995), has culminated in "general agreement that attitude, no matter how assessed, is only one of the factors that influence behavior" (Ajzen & Fishbein, 1980, p. 26), but not much more. Given the contextual (societal and situational) variation in which individuals act, however, it may be unreasonable to expect more. The conclusion may also be stated in more positive terms, aptly summarized by Swift et al. (1995): "attitudes do not determine behavior, but they do provide relatively enduring predispositions to action, albeit leading to different behavioral outcomes in different concrete circumstances" (p. 41). One of the methodological consequences is that when surveying attitudes, it is essential to phrase them so as to represent situated behavioral choices or dilemmas as closely as possible. Moreover, they should be complemented by direct measures of behavior, such as voting on relevant issues (e.g., Bonoli, 2004).

Miller (1999), in his far-ranging discussion of the principles of social justice in political philosophy as well as in empirical research, addresses both problems simultaneously. His aim is "to discover the underlying principles that people use when they judge some aspect of their society to be just or unjust, and then to show that these principles are coherent" (p. ix). He again asserts that popular judgments are indeed coherent but that different principles are used in different contexts. Yet the coherent expression of justice beliefs in behavior depends on what he terms the "circumstances of social justice," a state of affairs that presupposes morally bounded societies, a set of institutions with predictable distributive outcomes, and an agency capable of regulating them. It is especially the first of these presuppositions that is becoming problematic today under the double pressure of globalization and multiculturalism.

The perspective of justice research at the level of attitudes may be contrasted to the perspective of institutional analysis (Liebig et al., 2004). Justice research as institutional analysis aims to describe or to reconstruct the principles embodied in institutions such as those of the welfare state. The interest in such an analysis is threefold: first, institutions have differential chances of survival according to the plausibility of the moral principles they rely on; second, they can themselves be read as moral statements of the purposes that a state or society aims at; and third, they may in turn influence public attitudes by highlighting certain principles and discarding others (V. H. Schmidt, 1995). There is now a substantial body of comparative research on the justice ideas institutionalized in different welfare states (e.g., Rothstein, 1998), and more specifically, pension regimes (e.g., Palme, 1990). Goodin, Headey, Muffels, & Dirven (1999) go one step further by confronting institutional justice principles with empirical distributive outcomes, following a longstanding tradition of "critique of ideology" but with an emphasis on a sophisticated empirical analysis. Another way to pursue institutional analysis is to focus on how distributive judgments are made and implemented in empirical social settings (e.g., Elster, 1992; V. H. Schmidt, 2000). Studies of decision-making in situations, such as granting access to medical treatment or higher education, show that these processes are often "local," with little reference to over-arching standards of justice.

More recently, a third perspective of justice research has become prominent, that of discourse analysis (e.g., Leisering, 2004). It examines the semantics of justice as they emerge (or are shaped) in public discourse on the distribution of resources, and in turn influence the public perception of these issues. It may also examine the structure of beliefs held and communicated by specific political actors (e.g., Reeher, 1996). Discourse can be understood as "policy discourse," a form of systematic communication from above, used by governments (or other agents in charge) to argue the case of institutional change. Vivien A. Schmidt (2000) has demonstrated that such discourse has indeed been effective in facilitating popular acceptance of change, especially in the present circumstances of the politics of retrenchment where "policy initiatives that go against the narrow self-interest of electoral majorities succeed more often than one would expect" (p. 230). It is a tantalizing issue to what extent a successful policy discourse can be motivated and designed in a purely strategic way. In any case, however, just as the welfare state could not exist without the support of strong normative arguments and moral convictions, discursive attempts to gain support for retrenchment must convincingly appeal to values, including those values of solidarity on which the traditional welfare state was built. As Schmidt shows, "no major and initially unpopular welfare-state reform could succeed in the medium term if it did not also succeed in changing the underlying definition of moral appropriateness" (p. 231).

Discourse can also be understood more broadly, in the sense of "discursive politics" characterizing the democratic process as such. As Rothstein (1998) argues, democratic institutions "force participants to defend their positions publicly. Those taking part must therefore justify their actions in moral terms. . . . Democracy thus acquires a special moral logic, which differs in part from the logic of other institutions (such as the market)" (p. 117). This is most succinctly stated in the currently popular concept of "deliberative democracy."

What are the substantive results emerging from the literature on distributive justice? Given the complexity that our brief discussion has hinted at, it may come as a surprise that there seems to be convergence on some broad conclusions. There are three basic principles by which distributive outcomes are justified: need, merit or desert (usually based on work performance), and equality (usually based on citizenship status). In addition to need and merit as criteria to justify an unequal distribution, one may also invoke the incentive criterion—inequality serving to motivate people to perform better so that in a positive-sum game everyone will be better off in the end. These principles operate at the level of normative theories (e.g., Miller, 1999), at the level of popular beliefs (e.g., Forma & Kangas, 1999; Swift et al., 1995), and at the level of welfare state institutions (e.g., Leisering, 2004; Palme, 1990; Rothstein, 1998). Their salience varies between countries, between groups of persons, and between the parts of the welfare state, but together they seem to exhaust most of the conceptual and empirical space of distributive justice.

For the specific topic of justice between age groups and generations, it is first of all necessary to analytically separate these two dimensions. As Daniels (1988) has shown, inequality among age groups, based, for example, on needs perceived to be different, does not violate justice principles (as unequal treatment based on other "morally irrelevant" traits such as gender or race would). The reason is that while we (usually) do not change our gender or race, we do change our membership in age groups by the simple process of aging. Thus, the fact that we successively live through all the stages of life makes treating them differently morally acceptable. (For more precision, the argument has to take into account differential longevity structured along relevant sociodemographic group characteristics. Indeed the question of whether groups with shorter life expectancy—e.g., lower vs. higher status groups, or men vs. women—should help finance the benefits for those living longer has become a pressing issue of relating *inter*generational with *intra*generational equity.) There may be grounds for justifying a distribution according to the different needs of age groups—e.g., children vs. adults or old people. They are institutionalized in practices such as income equivalence scales, which often assume lower costs for children (but usually do not differentiate among adults of different ages). On the other hand, there may be reasonable political decisions to allocate more resources to children—more precisely, families with children—because, for example, of a perceived need to invest in a society's future (see Esping-Andersen, Gallie, Hemerijck, & Myles, 2002; Esping-Andersen & Sarasa, 2002; Preston, 1984). There is also the heavily discussed issue of singling out age groups by ascribing them different levels of "merit," such as through rationing access to some forms of medical treatment for older persons (see Callahan, 1987). Usually, however, it is most appropriate to have equality across age groups. The "prudential life span account" proposed by Daniels (1988) as a normative standard seems to ultimately favor equal outcomes. And

indeed it can be observed that special benefits for one age group (e.g., free or subsidized access to public transports or cultural events) are usually legitimized in terms of making up for the disadvantaged economic situation of this group rather than of different needs.

The domination of the equality criterion is even clearer for the distribution across generations. It may be questionable how far into the future (or into the past) the standard of equality should be extended, but there is little ground for legitimizing any other distributional standard. The intergenerational sharing of burden and rewards is just or fair to the extent that each successive generation can expect to receive the same treatment as the preceding and following ones when it moves up through the stages of life. In such a world, financing the elderly during one's earning years through a pay-as-you-go system is not problematic because one can expect to reap the same benefits in one's retirement funded by the next generation (a pattern often called *indirect* or *sequential reciprocity*). Problems arise "only" to the extent that such equality of treatment is not given, which, in the real world, is unfortunately rather the rule than the exception. Criteria of need or merit come into play with reference to *intra*generational justice, as, for example, with the idea that the pension system should conserve the level of income that the individual achieved when in the labor force (merit), or conversely, that it should ensure a basic income floor (need). The first of these ideas is central to the welfare states of the "conservative" regime type, the second to both the "social-democratic" (universalist) and "liberal" (residual) types. Most welfare states have some combination of the two, as when an income-maintaining pension system is complemented by a minimum guaranteed pension for those below a certain threshold.

## III. Generational Equity: Discourse and Institutions

During the last two decades, these issues have usually been debated under the term *generational equity* (see the detailed overview by Williamson & Watts-Roy, 1999; also Binstock & Quadagno, 2001; Cook, 2002). During the 1960s and 1970s the United States enjoyed a period of expansion of Social Security for elderly under the banner of what Binstock (1983) described as *compassionate ageism*. This idea of the elderly as discriminated against, poor, and in need of public support proved to be "an effective rhetorical device... [that] helped sell social policies that increased the share of societal resources" allocated to the elderly (Williamson & Watts-Roy, 1999, p. 10). The turn away from compassion for the old had to do with the success of these policies in changing their economic situation (see later), with changing demographics, and with the economic downturn of the early 1970s. But these changes in the "real world" needed again to be discursively focused and packaged to become politically effective. This was achieved not least by a number of conservative think tanks and foundations. The media have become the central arena for the construction of political meaning, favoring through their rhetorics not only individual actors but also "flamboyance, simplification, polarization, and the related styles that emphasize the crisis nature of social problems" (Williamson & Watts-Roy, 1999, p. 26).

Generational equity refers to "the argument that the elderly have been the recipients of an unfair distribution of public resources for income, health care, and social services" (Binstock & Quadagno, 2001, p. 343), and that this comes at the expense of the nonaged population, especially children. As Williamson and Watts-Roy (1999) show, this idea has been anything but new, but its growth into a full-blown political discourse can be dated to 1984, with, on the one hand, Preston's (1984) influential comparison of the well-being of children and the elderly, and on the other, the founding of Americans for Generational Equity (AGE).

From the United States the discourse has been imported to the United Kingdom and to the European continent (see Attias-Donfut, & Arber, 2000) where institutionalization has been slower but with more current weight, such as with the German Stiftung für die Rechte zukünftiger Generationen (Foundation for the Rights of Future Generations) founded in 1996. The different patterns of debate in Europe can be attributed to its institutions, as well as to its discursive traditions. In fact there are also major differences within Europe. As Vivien A. Schmidt notes, intergenerational justice has become a recurrent theme "only in those Continental countries with pay-as-you-go, earnings-related pensions, where the problems of funding remain significant—for example, in Germany, Austria, Italy, Belgium, and France—and not the Netherlands or Switzerland" where pensions are to a larger extent privatized (V. A. Schmidt, 2000, p. 302).

The discourse of generational equity has clearly been one of the more effective ones in shaping the public agenda of welfare retrenchment over the last two decades. Its effectiveness in changing popular attitudes and beliefs has so far been less impressive, as is shown later. The political consequences drawn by the proponents of generational equity go in the direction of reducing public spending for the elderly (e.g., by privatizing [parts of] old-age security, reducing the benefits, and increasing the retirement age). Other demands include age-based rationing for some types of medical care and age tests for a range of issues such as driving or even voting. The demands are often grouped under the term *sustainability*, which links the long-term survival of social security schemes to issues in the domain of ecology.

Although the general idea of keeping the world intact for future generations is readily accepted, the more specific demands have drawn intense criticism. Among the scientific community of gerontology and the associational community of old age concerns, the generational equity demands have become a common rallying point for repudiation and indignation, and an easy occasion for claiming the scientific and moral high ground. The proponents of generational equity have accordingly been hit by a range of counter-statements from public or scientific associations for the elderly, such as the volume from the Gerontological Society of America (Kingson, Hirshorn, & Cornman, 1986), which proposed a competing frame, that of generational interdependence, or the volume from the AARP, formerly the American Association of Retired Persons (Cohen, 1993).

These counter-statements have indeed made a strong case, pointing out that the expansion of old-age security should be seen as a success that, far from unduly privileging the elderly, has only given them their due share by finally bringing them up to par with the active population (Hudson, 1999). Moreover, improving their well-being does not necessarily come at the expense of other population groups. The argument of a zero-sum game in the distribution of resources between young and old can be criticized on three grounds: first, children and older adults depend on different institutions for their economic well-being (Easterlin, 1987; see later); second, if seen in a comparative perspective, higher public spending on children and older adults are not mutually exclusive (Pampel, 1994); and third, children and older adults are linked through intergenerational family ties so

that resources flowing to one side profit the other as well (Kingson et al., 1986; Kohli, 1999).

Finally, the institutional alternatives to public social security are less convincing than they are discursively made to look. For example, privatizing old age pensions through a fully funded system will not solve the problem of lower returns, for returns from private funds depend equally on the domestic economic product at the time they are cashed in (except if the funds are invested in more dynamic economies abroad). The costs of private funds—in other words, the profits to be made for the financial industry—are often much higher than those of public administration. Predictably, a mature privatized system such as that of Chile is now facing these problems.

In the United States, reframing the discourse of generational equity as an "entitlement crisis" has also been less than convincing (Quadagno, 1996). It suffered its first blow at the disappearance of the federal budget deficit in the late 1990s. In the meantime, the deficit has skyrocketed again under the combined pressure of the Bush administration's tax cuts and the costs of war. (For the latter there are obvious parallels to the early 1970s.) It remains to be seen whether the current administration's attempts to resurrect the entitlement crisis frame by putting the blame for the deficit on social security will succeed even in the absence of supporting numbers.

European welfare states, however, have been less fortunate. Here, the issues of generational equity have become an important part of the broader efforts toward welfare retrenchment (Esping-Andersen et al., 2002; Pierson, 2001). This is due to the tightening of public finances under the pressures of Europeanization and globalization, but also to the increasingly bleak demographic outlook. Demography is not destiny (and presenting it as such may be another form of ideology), but it does create a major challenge in terms of population aging. This challenge goes beyond the economically advanced societies of the OECD. It is, however, largest for some of the latter that have shown a persistent pattern of low fertility.

The joint impact of low fertility, increasing life expectancy, and relatively early exit from the labor force will drive up the contribution rates or drive down the income replacement level of pensions, especially (but not only) in the welfare states of Southern and Continental Europe and Scandinavia with their extensive pay-as-you-go (contribution- or tax-based) pension systems. Immigration (see United Nations Population Division, 2000), increasing female labor force participation, and an increase in the retirement age limit will all provide some financial relief, but the demographic numbers are such that the issues will remain critical. The current conflicts over pension "reform" or, more to the point, pension retrenchment, are taxing these societies' capacities for finding viable political compromises to their limits (see Myles, 2002).

Some proponents of generational equity argue that the window of opportunity for implementing these reforms is closing because the older population increasingly dominates the political arena by its sheer voting weight (see Binstock, 2000). They see a point of no return when the power of the elderly will be such that they will be able to block any attempt at reducing their benefits. In a formal analysis for Germany, Sinn, and Uebelmesser (2002) have projected the median age of voters and the "indifference age" as the age of the cohort that is affected neither positively nor negatively by a pension reform. The assumption is that reform will be feasible if, and only if, the median voter favors it (2002, p. 155). The authors concluded that until 2016, a reform can be democratically enforced because a majority of the voters will still be below the indifference age;

2016 is "Germany's last chance." After that year, it will be a gerontocracy.

Such a model is of course highly mechanical; it presupposes that voting shares fully translate into specific policies, and that people's votes are based only on their current individual position, which is manifestly not the case. Pampel (1994) has shown that from 1959 to 1986, the effects of population aging on public spending in OECD countries varied according to whether a country had class-based corporatism and strong leftist parties. Population aging has resulted in higher spending on pensions and the aged relative to spending on families and children only in countries (such as the United States) without these features. Self-interested mobilization by age is thus more likely in countries which do not have class-based institutions that emphasize *intra*generational over *inter*generational cleavages and conflicts (see Chapter 19).

If political action is not purely interest-based, this creates room for discourse based on justice ideas. According to Daniels' (1988) argument presented previously, intergenerational sharing of burden and rewards is just or fair to the extent that each successive generation can expect to receive the same treatment as the preceding and following ones when it moves up the through the stages of life. Unfortunately, the real world never quite conforms to this ideal. The most drastic departure from it may be illustrated by Thomson's (1989) account of the development of the welfare state in New Zealand. According to Thomson, it has been the result of the political activity of a specific generation which first created a youth-state with housing subsidies and benefits for young families, and then over its own life course turned it into a welfare state for the elderly. New Zealand's welfare state thus would have represented one generation's success in exploiting its preceding and succeeding ones.

Although such blatant political exploitation of the public "generational contract" seems to be the exception rather than the rule, there are other sources of discontinuity. As mentioned previously, the most obvious one today is demography. An interesting proposal for coping with the changing size of successive cohorts is the *fixed relative position* model (as set out by Myles, 2002, based on Musgrave, 1986) where "contributions and benefits are set so as to hold constant the ratio of per capita earnings of those in the working population (net of contributions) to the per capita benefits (net of taxes) of retirees" (p. 141). This allows for proportional risk sharing: "As the population ages, the tax rate rises but benefits also fall so that both parties 'lose' at the same rate" (Myles, 2002, p. 141). In other words, the distribution of resources among age groups agreed on in a society is stabilized so that it remains identical for each successive cohort, thus fulfilling the condition for Daniels' (1988) justice standard.

Problems of equity arise in the *intra*generational dimension as well. The relation of the "old" issues of inequitable distribution (or poverty, or exclusion) along class lines and of the "new" ones such as those based on generations remains problematic. The discourse on intergenerational equity may function as an ideology, that is, as a way to divert attention away from the still existing problems of poverty and exclusion *within* generations. If welfare systems are redesigned as a consequence of demographic change, these problems may be exacerbated in surprising ways. An example is the proposed rise in the age of retirement. Given that longevity is socially stratified, a rising retirement age would disadvantage the less well off because an additional year of employment represents a larger proportional loss for someone with a shorter life expectancy (Myles, 2002). This may be one reason why raising the retirement age

proves to be so broadly unpopular, as indicated next.

## IV. Generational Equity: The Empirical Record

Most of the claims of generational equity focus on the distribution of resources between the young and the old. As mentioned previously, one line of research examines the input side: welfare state spending targeted to different population groups, among them, the young and the old, and how it is brought about by welfare state institutions (e.g., Pampel, 1994). This concerns not only the large redistributive programs, such as old age income security or health insurance, but also arrangements only partially organized or subsidized by the state such as long-term care (see Anttonen, Baldock, & Sipilä, 2003). An important extension is that of generational accounting, which includes both contributions and spending, and tries to establish long-term balances for each successive cohort (e.g., Kotlikoff, 1992).

A direct comparison between spending on the elderly and on children and youth, however, would be misleading. In modern welfare states, incomes and services for older adults are to a large extent publicly financed, whereas those for the young are still mostly borne by their families. The one exception is the educational system, but even if it is included in a broader conceptualization of the welfare state the transfer shares for the young and the old are still uneven. In low-fertility countries there is now a heightened emphasis on the need for public financial aid and services for families with children, but the projected increase remains far below the large transfer programs directed at the elderly.

The more straightforward way of validating the claims of the generational equity debate is to assess the output side: the outcome of market distribution and state redistribution in terms of the economic well-being of the young and the old. That this is indeed the outcome of state activity *and* market processes poses an interesting problem of causal attribution and should caution us not to treat the well-being of children and the elderly simply as the result of a zero-sum game. What Easterlin (1987) remarked in response to Preston's (1984) argument needs to be heeded today as well: "the divergent trends in poverty rates of children and the elderly chiefly reflect two different and largely independent causes. Whereas the improved status of the elderly is largely attributable to government action…, the rise in the poverty rate of children is, to an important extent, a result of market forces" (Easterlin, 1987, p. 195). If there is a trade-off between the two, it is probably more nation-specific than universal; in other words, it is conditioned by specific institutional arrangements (Pampel, 1994). Esping-Andersen & Sarasa (2002) recently tried to refute the zero-sum view on the grounds that it is premised on an overly static analysis. They attempt to identify "a win-win policy model that simultaneously ensures child and elderly welfare" in the sense that "social investments in children now will have strong and positive secondary effects in terms of helping maintain welfare guarantees for the elderly in the future. The key lies in minimizing child poverty" (p. 5) which in most countries would be surprisingly affordable. On the other hand, there are attempts today to show that high contributions for public programs such as pensions do indeed lower the market incomes of younger cohorts, and moreover have negative consequences for economic growth, and thus for future market incomes; but this link remains tenuous as long as distributional issues are not taken into account.

With this caution about causal attribution in mind, we now turn to a descriptive account of the economic well-being of the elderly relative to other age groups. Table 25.1 shows that from the mid-1980s to the mid-1990s, children have lost ground in some countries, and that their income position is considerably below that of the active population. The income position of older adults has indeed improved in most countries but also remains below that of the active population, particularly in the United Kingdom with its "residual" welfare state. Moreover, the position of those above age 75 is clearly less favorable than that of the "young old."

Another perspective is that of poverty. As shown by Table 25.2, poverty rates among children and the elderly vary massively among nations. The "liberal" cluster of welfare states (where the share of private pensions is larger) has generally higher poverty rates among both groups of dependents, with some interesting exceptions (Canada and Switzerland). Regarding the evolution of poverty across 25 years in West Germany (Table 25.3), the elderly have improved their lot, but only to the general population level, whereas the situation of children has worsened to a level considerably less favorable than that of the general population. Similar results for the United States between 1960 and 1995 have been presented by Johnson and Smeeding (1998). It should be noted that this may reflect some structural changes, such as more single parents and fewer children to mothers with higher education. It is obvious from these results that, in terms of generational equity (as well as of pronatalist incentives), families with young children should indeed be the target of supplementary welfare efforts; but the results give no reason to strip the elderly of (part of) their current benefits.

**Table 25.1**
Relative equivalent disposable incomes, by age groups
Average income of entire population = 100

| | Children | Young | Young adults | Adults | Older adults | Younger senior citizens | Older senior citizens |
|---|---|---|---|---|---|---|---|
| | Age 0–17 | Age 18–25 | Age 26–40 | Age 41–50 | Age 51–65 | Age 65–75 | Age 75+ |
| Canada, 1985 | 88 | 102 | 103 | 116 | 110 | 91 | 84 |
| Canada, 1995 | 88 | 100 | 100 | 114 | 114 | 99 | 95 |
| France, 1984 | 95 | 102 | 106 | 112 | 103 | 86 | 82 |
| France, 1994 | 95 | 97 | 100 | 115 | 109 | 94 | 82 |
| Germany, 1984 | 93 | 98 | 102 | 113 | 109 | 85 | 81 |
| Germany, 1994 | 91 | 96 | 99 | 118 | 110 | 93 | 77 |
| Hungary, 1991 | 99 | 109 | 103 | 119 | 96 | 81 | 77 |
| Hungary, 1997 | 93 | 111 | 104 | 109 | 104 | 88 | 81 |
| Italy, 1984 | 90 | 107 | 106 | 106 | 108 | 82 | 78 |
| Italy, 1993 | 89 | 103 | 105 | 109 | 108 | 85 | 82 |
| Sweden, 1983 | 101 | 71 | 105 | 119 | 119 | 91 | 70 |
| Sweden, 1995 | 99 | 60 | 100 | 120 | 127 | 96 | 78 |
| U. K., 1985 | 90 | 114 | 105 | 124 | 105 | 74 | 72 |
| U. K., 1995 | 86 | 112 | 106 | 123 | 108 | 80 | 74 |
| United States, 1985 | 82 | 99 | 104 | 118 | 121 | 99 | 84 |
| United States, 1995 | 84 | 94 | 102 | 118 | 124 | 99 | 82 |

**Note:** For calculating relative income changes, population shares have been kept constant at the beginning of the period.
**From:** Förster & Pearson, 2002 (based on a questionnaire sent out by the OECD to national representatives).

**Table 25.2**
Poverty rates (in percent) by country for total population, children and the elderly

| Country | Total population | Children (–18) | Elderly (65+) |
|---|---|---|---|
| Australia, 1994 | 14.3 | 15.8 | 29.4 |
| Austria, 1995 | 10.6 | 15.0 | 10.3 |
| Belgium, 1997 | 8.2 | 7.6 | 12.4 |
| Canada, 1997 | 11.9 | 15.7 | 5.3 |
| Denmark, 1997 | 9.2 | 8.7 | 6.6 |
| Finland, 1995 | 5.1 | 4.2 | 5.2 |
| France, 1994 | 8.0 | 7.9 | 9.8 |
| Germany, 1994 | 7.5 | 10.6 | 7.0 |
| Italy, 1995 | 14.2 | 20.2 | 12.2 |
| Netherlands, 1994 | 8.1 | 8.1 | 6.4 |
| Spain, 1990 | 10.1 | 12.2 | 11.3 |
| Sweden, 1995 | 6.6 | 2.6 | 2.7 |
| Switzerland, 1992 | 9.3 | 10.0 | 8.4 |
| U.K., 1995 | 13.4 | 19.8 | 13.7 |
| United States, 1997 | 16.9 | 22.3 | 20.7 |

**Note:** Poverty rates refer to 50% of median equivalence income.
**From:** Jesuit & Smeeding, 2002 (based on the Luxembourg Income Study).

**Table 25.3**
Poverty rates (in percent) by age in West Germany,
1973–1998

| Age | 1973 | 1983 | 1998 |
|---|---|---|---|
| Less than 6 years | 8.0 | 11.5 | 15.9 |
| 7 to ca. 13 years | 7.6 | 9.9 | 15.3 |
| ca. 14 to ca. 17 years | 4.2 | 7.3 | 14.9 |
| ca. 18 to 24 years | 4.6 | 12.0 | 13.3 |
| 25 to 54 years | 4.0 | 5.8 | 9.6 |
| 55 to 64 years | 6.2 | 4.9 | 7.5 |
| 65+ years | 13.3 | 11.9 | 10.9 |
| All | 6.5 | 7.7 | 10.9 |

**Note:** Poverty rates refer to 50% of mean equivalence income.
**From:** Becker & Hauser, 2003 (based on the German Survey of Income and Consumption).

# V. Attitudes Toward the Public Generational Contract

What are the popular attitudes and beliefs in terms of justice between age groups and generations? In addition to a range of national studies on attitudes toward welfare reform and generational equity, there are now several cross-national surveys that lend themselves to comparative studies. The most comprehensive, in terms of the number and range of nations covered, is the *International Social Survey Program* (*ISSP*, e.g., Andreß & Heien, 2001; Blekesaune & Quadagno, 2003; Hicks, 2001; Smith, 2000; Svallfors, 2004). This is a yearly survey with additional topical modules repeated at larger intervals, which currently comprises almost 40 countries (including most Western and Central European ones, as well as Canada, Mexico, and the United States). More restricted in scope but sometimes offering more detailed measurements are the *Eurobarometer* (e.g., European Commission, 2004; Kohl, 2003a, 2003b; Walker & Maltby, 1997), a regular European Union survey covering its member and candidate states, which also has changing topical modules, and special surveys such as the *International Social Justice*

*Project* (*ISJP*), (see Kluegel et al., 1995) or the *International Survey of Economic Attitudes* (*ISEA*) (see Forma & Kangas, 1999).

Most attitude studies up to now show a level of acceptance of welfare policies that is much higher than the discourse on generational equity would lead us to think, with pensions being the most popular part the welfare state. There is some differentiation along the age dimension, but much less than one would expect from an interest-based model of political preference.

One set of questions is about which one among the different institutional systems or "pillars" of the welfare mix should provide social security. On the issue of whose responsibility it should be to provide a decent standard of living for the old (*ISSP* 1996, see Hicks, 2001), an overwhelming majority in all countries say that this should (definitely or probably) be the government's responsibility: from 84% in Japan and 86% in the United States to fully 96% in the United Kingdom and 97% in Italy. The proportion of those stating that this should definitely be so increases over the life course, but even among those under age 30, it ranges between 38% (in Canada) and 69% (in Italy), while among those over 65, the range is from 42% (in the United States) to 81% (in Sweden). As Hicks (2001) concludes, this "is not large enough to signal any intergenerational rift" (p. 8). Contrary to what the lively public discourse in the United States would suggest, the age gap is almost nonexistent in this country.

As Figure 25.1 shows, in the four countries for which consistent time series from 1985 to 2001 are available (West Germany, Italy, the United Kingdom, and the United States), support fell slightly until 1996, but again much less than the public emphasis on "reform" in the sense of retrenchment would lead us to believe. Since 1996 it has even slightly increased again in three of the four countries, especially the United States. It seems

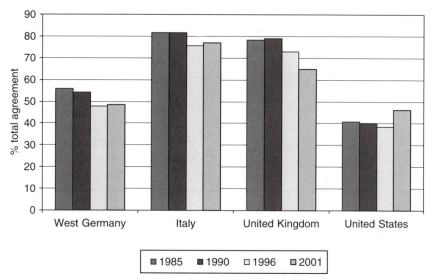

**Figure 25.1**   Views on responsibilities for a decent standard of living for the old, 1985–2001.
Percentage indicating that it should definitely be the government's responsibility to provide a decent standard of living for the old
**From:** Hicks, 2001 (based on *ISSP* 1985–96), and author's calculations (based on *ISSP* 2001).

plausible to conclude that when old-age security is perceived to be in danger, the responsibility of the state is affirmed more stringently.

A second question concerns the desired extent of public spending for old age security (see Hicks, 2001, p. 11). The question wording takes pains to avoid making the response too easy by signaling that "much more" spending might require a tax increase, but even so, between 7% (in Canada) and 27% (in the United Kingdom) say "much more," and between 21% and 51% say "more." The large majority of the rest opt for "same," between 1% and 8% for "less," and only between 0% and 2% for "much less." Clearly, there is very little support for cutting old age benefits, and considerable support for expanding it.

Table 25.4 presents the data according to age groups. The desire to expand government spending on pensions increases somewhat with age, but less than expected, with the two North American

countries even going in the opposite direction. Bivariate results such as these may obviously reflect compositional changes other than age. There is, for example, a gender gap (not shown in the table), largest in Sweden and smallest in Japan (see Hicks, 2001, p. 20), with women having a higher preference for more public spending than men, which is partly behind the higher preference in the older age groups. More multivariate analyses will be needed to separate the various effects.

There is thus little evidence for the widely presumed loss of legitimacy of public social security, and especially pension provisions. Most people "favour existing arrangements—whatever they happen to be. That is a realistic view in light of the success of those policies" (Hicks, 2001, p. 4). What needs also to be noted, however, is a widespread loss of confidence that these existing arrangements will continue. It is in this sense of empirical prediction rather than political

**Table 25.4**
Views on public retirement spending, 1996

| | Age group | | | | |
|---|---|---|---|---|---|
| | Under 30 | 30–39 | 40–49 | 50–64 | 65+ |
| Canada | 34.8 | 23.4 | 24.6 | 30.5 | 20.5 |
| Germany | 45.5 | 41.6 | 41.6 | 48.4 | 51.7 |
| Italy | 55.8 | 60.4 | 65.8 | 65.8 | 75.6 |
| Japan | 54.6 | 48.0 | 53.9 | 57.9 | 60.9 |
| Sweden | 41.7 | 51.3 | 51.9 | 59.8 | 66.8 |
| United Kingdom | 63.3 | 79.2 | 79.7 | 79.8 | 87.1 |
| United States | 55.0 | 51.0 | 45.7 | 48.9 | 45.2 |

Percentage indicating they would like to see more, or much more, government spending on retirement benefits (being asked to remember that, if you say "much more," it might require a tax increase to pay for it)
**From:** Hicks, 2001 (based on the International Social Survey Program).

preference that the public generational equity discourse has been effective.

A special *Eurobarometer* module of fall 2001 (as analyzed by Kohl, 2003a, 2003b; see European Commission, 2004) provides a more recent description of EU public opinion on these matters, with detailed indications on specific pension goals and policy options. Goals refer to the normative foundations of pension policies as seen by the citizens, in other words, to their underlying value orientations, and in particular their ideas of social justice (European Commission, 2004, p. 44). The two most popular goals are prevention of poverty (92% agree with the statement that "the primary goal of a good pension scheme should be to protect elderly people against the risk of poverty") and provision of basic social rights in the form of a guaranteed minimum pension (90%). Maintaining one's living standard (88% agreement that "a good pension system should allow everybody to maintain an adequate standard of living relative to their income before retirement"), greater equality among the elderly (84%), and the pay-as-you-go principle (81%) are also supported by more than four-fifths of the population.

Country differences in these normative preferences are not very marked. "There seems (to be) a broad consensus amongst

European citizens concerning the goals of pension policies and even about the prioritisation of certain goals" (European Commission, 2004, p. 7). This is held to be good news for the proponents of a common EU social policy, showing that "the value orientations and the social policy attitudes of citizens in the EU member countries do not fall as far apart as the institutionalised forms of social security do (especially in the field of pensions)" (p. 7). It should be noted, however, that other studies have shown a clear correspondence between welfare state regime types and attitudes such as towards redistribution (e.g., Svallfors, 1997).

As to age differences, the support for most of the statements shows an age trend in the expected direction. "The magnitude of this age effect, however, is not very significant" (Kohl, 2003a, p. 14). The strongest age difference concerns the pension entitlements of homosexual couples, and this is clearly not an age effect related to economic (self-)interest but a cohort effect related to value change.

Figure 25.2 shows support for three alternative proposals for balancing revenues and expenditures of public pension schemes. To raise awareness of the costs of each option, the trade-offs were explicitly mentioned in the alternatives posed: (1) current benefit levels should be

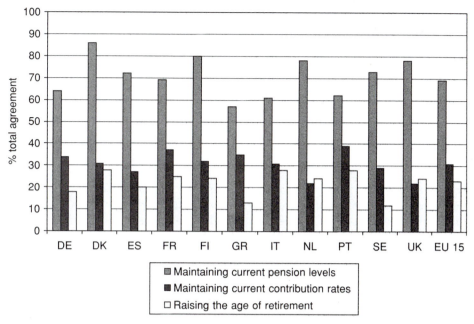

**Figure 25.2** Support for pension policy alternatives, 2001
**From:** Kohl, 2003b (based on Special Eurobarometer 161).

maintained, even if this means increasing contribution rates or taxes; (2) contributions should be maintained, even if this means lower pension benefits; and (3) the age of retirement should be raised so that people work longer and spend less time in retirement. The first option, maintaining current pension levels, gains majority support in all EU member states. In the EU as a whole, 30% strongly agree and 38% slightly agree with this statement, whereas only 5% strongly disagree and an additional 15% slightly disagree. In contrast, the second option, maintaining current contribution rates, is supported by only 31% and disapproved by a majority of EU citizens (53%).

The third alternative, raising the age of retirement, is clearly the least popular. Only 23% approve it, while there is strong disagreement by 40% and slight disagreement by an additional 29%. If working longer turns out to be inevitable, such a policy will have to overcome considerable popular resistance. It may be

true, as Hicks (2001) maintains, that there is "no opposition to working later in principle: people would like to work at older ages if the work were enjoyable" (p. 17; see Kohl, 2003b, p. 14, for a similar point). Apart from the issue of how widely available such enjoyable jobs are, however, there is also the issue of control and choice. Raising the age of retirement would mean a longer dependency on whatever the labor market offers, and fewer resources for freely choosing between work and retirement. Does this mean that ordinary people are so stubborn that they will never give up their privileges? This is clearly not so. It means that they will have to be convinced that their sacrifices are necessary, that institutional retrenchments will be implemented with circumspection, and that they will be balanced by labor market reforms in favor of older workers.

The first option (maintaining current benefit levels) places the burden mostly on the taxpayers or the active labor force, the second (maintaining current contribution rates even at the expense of lower pensions), on the pensioners. Again, however, this does not translate into massively different rates of support by age. There is some tendency for pensioners (76%) to prefer the first option more often than the "active" population (i.e., those in the labor force), but even among the latter, a strong majority (66%) support maintaining current benefit levels even at the cost of rising contributions. Raising the retirement age is rejected by 69% of the retired, as well as the nonretired part of the population.

These results demonstrate that the distributional conflict among generations is much less pronounced than is presumed (or advertised) by the proponents of generational equity. This is true even for the more recent measurements. We may be on the brink of change, but, if so, it does not yet show in the available data.

## VI. The Public and the Private Generational Contract

How is it to be explained that age (and/or cohort) effects remain so modest? The best answer seems to be through the generational interdependence frame that has been raised in opposition to that of generational equity (Williamson & Watts-Roy, 1999). It emphasizes burden-sharing and solidarity between the generations and also more tangible forms of support. On the other hand, it highlights problems of intragenerational equity as well. For the young, the institutionalization of income-maintaining retirement pensions means that they are freed from any expectation of income support toward their parents. They can moreover count on services such as grandparenting, and in many cases, they can also expect material support. The public resource flow to older adults has enabled the latter to transfer resources to their offspring in turn.

Recent research on *inter vivos* family transfers demonstrates that such transfers are considerable, that they occur mostly in the generational lineage, and that they flow mostly downwards, from the older to the younger generations (Kohli, 1999). There may be expectations of reciprocity, or other strings attached, but by and large parents are motivated by altruism or feelings of unconditional obligation, and direct their gifts to situations of need. For Germany, our survey in 1996 showed that 32% of those above age 60 made a transfer to their children or grandchildren during the 12 months before the interview, with a mean net value of about 3700 €. Thus, part of the public transfers from the active population to the elderly was handed back by the latter to their family descendants. The aggregate net *inter vivos* transfers by the the the elderly amounted to about 9% of the total yearly public pension sum. This link needs to be qualified, but the overall pattern is clear: The public generational contract is partly balanced by a private one in the opposite direction. The family transfers function to some extent as an informal insurance system for periods of special needs. Even more important in monetary terms are bequests. They are more frequent and much higher in the upper economic strata, but now also increasingly extend into the middle and lower ranks.

## VII. Conclusion

Our discussion has shown that the potential for distributional conflicts among generations certainly exists and is fueled by the current challenges of public finances and demography. The discourse of generational equity, however, overstates the extent and inevitability of such conflicts, and sharpens them at the expense of conflicts along the more traditional cleavages of class. Survey data regularly show that the public generational contract still enjoys high legitimacy among all ages and segments of the population. Among the young, this partly depends on whether they trust in the continued viability of this contract so that they themselves will also receive its benefits. Another reason is that pensions free the young from the obligation to support their parents, and even more important, that they can rely on their parents in times of need. We also have to examine the institutions, such as parties or unions (Kohli, Neckel, & Wolf, 1999), that mediate generational conflicts by favoring or disfavoring age integration in the political arena.

At this point, it is the gaps in our knowledge that come into focus. Although there is by now an extensive comparative literature on the welfare state in terms of old-age security and related programs, the institutions that shape the politics of aging societies—and by this, the way that generations are able to relate to each other—have mostly been neglected so far. The same is true for the articulation of the public with the private generational "contract." A second topic where we lack the necessary information concerns the relation between *intergenerational* and *intragenerational* equity. As to the former, the broad literature on generational accounting now provides a useful framework, even though the details of valuing costs and benefits remain highly contentious and in need of further analysis. As to the latter, many critical issues, such as the consequences of differential survival, still await closer scrutiny. A third topic where more research is needed is the structure of welfare state attitudes and the attitude-behavior link. Finally, it should be noted that most of the studies on economic well-being, as well as on attitudes, have been limited to cross-sectional data, or repeated cross sections at best. For a field in such rapid evolution, this is especially regrettable. Better monitoring and explanation of

changes will be possible only on the basis of individual-level longitudinal studies. It is to be hoped that new data sets now under construction will enable us to increasingly close these gaps.

## References

Ajzen, I., & Fishbein, M. (1980). *Understanding attitudes and predicting social behavior.* Englewood Cliffs, NJ: Prentice-Hall.

Andreß, H.-J., & Heien, T. (2001). Four worlds of welfare state attitudes? A comparison of Germany, Norway, and the United States. *European Sociological Review, 17,* 337–356.

Anttonen, A., Baldock, J., & Sipilä, J. (Eds.). (2003). *The young, the old and the state: Social care systems in five industrial nations.* Cheltenham: Edward Elgar.

Attias-Donfut, C., & Arber, S. (2000). Equity and solidarity across the generations. In S. Arber & C. Attias-Donfut (Eds.), *The myth of generational conflict: The family and state in ageing societies* (pp. 1–21). London: Routledge.

Becker, I., & Hauser, R. (2003). Zur Entwicklung von Armut und Reichtum in der Bundesrepublik Deutschland—eine Bestandsaufnahme. In C. Butterwegge & M. Klundt (Eds.), *Kinderarmut und Generationengerechtigkeit. Familien und Sozialpolitik im demografischen Wandel* (pp. 25–41). Opladen: Leske + Budrich.

Bengtson, V. L. (1993). Is the "contract across generations" changing? Effects of population aging on obligations and expectations across age groups. In V. L. Bengtson & W. A. Achenbaum (Eds.), *The changing contract across generations* (pp. 3–24). New York: Aldine de Gruyter.

Bernardi, B. (1985). *Age class systems.* Cambridge, UK: Cambridge University Press.

Binstock, R. H. (1983). The aged as scapegoat. *The Gerontologist, 23,* 136–143.

Binstock, R. H. (2000). Older people and voting participation: Past and future. *The Gerontologist, 40,* 18–31.

Binstock, R. H., & Quadagno, J. (2001). Aging and politics. In R. H. Binstock & L. K. George (Eds.), *Handbook of aging and the social sciences* (5th ed., pp. 333–351). San Diego: Academic Press.

Blekesaune, M., & Quadagno, J. (2003). Public attitudes toward welfare state policies: A comparative analysis of 24 nations. *European Sociological Review, 19*, 415–427.

Bonoli, G. (2004). *Generational conflicts over resource allocation: Evidence from referendum voting on social policy issues in Switzerland.* Paper presented at the Conference on Erosion oder Transformation des Sozialstaates?, Fribourg, Switzerland.

Callahan, D. (1987). *Setting limits: Medical goals in an aging society.* New York: Simon & Schuster.

Cohen, L. M. (Ed.). (1993). *Justice across generations. What does it mean?* Washington: American Association of Retired Persons.

Cook, F. L. (2002). Generational equity. In D. J. Ekerdt (Ed.), *Encyclopedia of aging* (Vol. 2, pp. 533–536). New York: Macmillan.

Daniels, N. (1988). *Am I my parents' keeper? An essay on justice between the old and the young.* Oxford: Oxford University Press.

Easterlin, R. A. (1987). The new age structure of poverty in America: Permanent or transient? *Population and Development Review, 13*, 195–208.

Elster, J. (1992). *Local justice: How institutions allocate scarce goods and necessary burdens.* Cambridge, UK: Cambridge University Press.

Esping-Andersen, G., Gallie, D., Hemerijck, A., & Myles, J. (2002). *Why we need a new welfare state.* Oxford: Oxford University Press.

Esping-Andersen, G., & Sarasa, S. (2002). The generational conflict reconsidered. *Journal of European Social Policy, 12*, 5–21.

European Commission (2004). *The future of pension systems (Special Eurobarometer 161/ Wave 56.1).* Retrieved January 7, 2005, from http://europa.eu.int/comm/publicopinion/archives/ebs/ebs_161 pensions.pdf.

Foner, N. (1984). *Ages in conflict : A cross-cultural perspective on inequality between old and young.* New York: Columbia University Press.

Forma, P., & Kangas, O. (1999). Need, citizenship or merit: Public opinion on pension policy in Australia, Finland and Poland. In S. Svallfors & P. Taylor-Gooby (Eds.), *The end of the welfare state? Responses to state retrenchment* (pp. 161–189). London: Routledge.

Förster, M., & Pearson, M. (2002). *Income distribution and poverty in the OECD area: Trends and driving forces* (OECD Economic Studies No. 34, 2002/I).

Goodin, R. E., Headey, B., Muffels, R., & Dirven, H.-J. (1999). *The real worlds of welfare capitalism.* Cambridge, UK: Cambridge University Press.

Hicks, P. (2001). *Public support for retirement income reform* (OECD Labour Market and Social Policy Occasional Papers No. 55).

Hudson, R. B. (1999). Conflict in today's aging politics: New population encounters old ideology. *Social Service Review, 73*, 358–379.

Igl, G. (2000). Zur Problematik der Altersgrenzen aus juristischer Perspektive. *Zeitschrift für Gerontologie und Geriatrie, 33,* Supplement 1, I/57-I/70.

Jesuit, D., & Smeeding, T. (2002). *Poverty and income distribution* (LIS Working Paper No. 293). Luxembourg: Luxembourg Income Study.

Johnson, D. S., & Smeeding, T. M. (1998). *Intergenerational equity in the United States: The changing well-being of the old and the young, 1960–1995.* Paper presented at the Twentieth Annual Research Conference of the Association for Policy Analysis and Management.

Kaufmann, F.-X. (2005). Gibt es einen Generationenvertrag? In F.-X. Kaufmann (Ed.), *Sozialpolitik und Sozialstaat: Soziologische Analysen* (2nd ed., pp. 161–182). Wiesbaden: VS.

Kingson, E. R., Hirshorn, B. A., & Cornman, J. M. (1986). *Ties that bind: The interdependence of generations.* Washington: Seven Locks Press.

Kluegel, J. R., Mason, D. S., & Wegener, B. (Eds.). (1995). *Social justice and political change: Public opinion in capitalist and post-communist states.* Berlin/New York: de Gruyter.

Kohl, J. (2003a). *Principles of distributive justice in pension policies. Cross-national variations in public opinion.* Paper presented at the Conference on New Challenges for Welfare State Research (International Sociological Association Research Committee 19), Toronto.

Kohl, J. (2003b). Citizens' opinions on the transition from work to retirement. Paper presented at the ISSA 4th International Research Conference on Social Security: Social Security in a Long Life Society, Antwerp.

Kohli, M. (1987). Retirement and the moral economy: An historical interpretation of the German case. *Journal of Aging Studies, 1*, 125–144.

Kohli, M. (1994). Work and retirement: A comparative perspective. In M. W. Riley, R. L. Kahn, & A. Foner (Eds.), *Age and structural lag: Society's failure to provide meaningful opportunities in work, family, and leisure* (pp. 80–106). New York: Wiley.

Kohli, M. (1996). *The problem of generations: Family, economy, politics. Collegium Budapest, Public Lecture Series No. 14.* Budapest: Collegium Budapest.

Kohli, M. (1999). Private and public transfers between generations: Linking the family and the state. *European Societies, 1*, 81–104.

Kohli, M. (2004). Generational changes and generational equity. In M. Johnson, V. L. Bengtson, P. Coleman, & T. Kirkwood (Eds.), *The Cambridge handbook of age and ageing* (in press). Cambridge, UK: Cambridge University Press.

Kohli, M., & Künemund, H. (2003). Intergenerational transfers in the family: What motivates giving? In V. L. Bengtson & A. Lowenstein (Eds.), *Global aging and challenges to families* (pp. 123–142). New York: Aldine de Gruyter.

Kohli, M., Neckel, S., & Wolf, J. (1999). Krieg der Generationen? Die politische Macht der Älteren. In A. Niederfranke, G. Naegele, & E. Frahm (Eds.), *Funkkolleg Altern, Bd. 2* (pp. 479–514). Opladen: Westdeutscher Verlag.

Kohli, M., & Szydlik, M. (Eds.). (2000). *Generationen in Familie und Gesellschaft.* Opladen: Leske-Budrich.

Kotlikoff, L. J. (1992). *Generational accounting: Knowing who pays, and when, for what we spend.* New York: Free Press.

Laslett, P., & Fishkin, J. S. (Eds.). (1992). *Justice between age groups and generations.* New Haven: Yale University Press.

Leisering, L. (2004). Paradigmen sozialer Gerechtigkeit. Normative Diskurse im Umbau des Sozialstaats. In S. Liebig, H. Lengfeld, & S. Mau (Eds.), *Verteilungsprobleme und Gerechtigkeit in modernen Gesellschaften* (pp. 29–68). Frankfurt/M: Campus.

Liebig, S., Lengfeld, H., & Mau, S. (2004). Einleitung: Gesellschaftliche Verteilungsprobleme und der Beitrag der soziologischen Gerechtigkeitsforschung. In S. Liebig, H. Lengfeld, & S. Mau (Eds.), *Verteilungs-* *probleme und Gerechtigkeit in modernen Gesellschaften* (pp. 7–26). Frankfurt/M: Campus.

Miller, D. (1992). Distributive justice: What the people think. *Ethics, 102*, 555–593.

Miller, D. (1999). *Principles of social justice.* Cambridge, MA: Harvard University Press.

Müller, H. K. (1990). Wenn 'Söhne' älter als 'Väter' sind. Dynamik ostafrikanischer Generations- und Altersklassen am Beispiel der Toposa und Turkana. In G. Elwert, M. Kohli, & H. K. Müller (Eds.), *Im Lauf der Zeit* (pp. 33–49). Saarbrücken: Breitenbach.

Musgrave, R. (1986). *Public finance in a democratic society* (Vol. 2). New York: New York University Press.

Myles, J. (2002). A new social contract for the elderly? In G. Esping-Andersen (Ed.), *Why we need a new welfare state* (pp. 130–172). Oxford: Oxford University Press.

Palme, J. (1990). *Pension rights in welfare capitalism. The development of old-age pensions in 18 OECD countries 1930 to 1985.* Stockholm: Swedish Institute for Social Research.

Pampel, F. C. (1994). Population aging, class context, and age inequality in public spending. *American Journal of Sociology, 100*, 153–195.

Pierson, P. (Ed.). (2001). *The new politics of the welfare state.* Oxford: Oxford University Press.

Preston, S. H. (1984). Children and the elderly: Divergent paths for America's dependents. *Demography, 21*, 435–457.

Quadagno, J. (1996). Social Security and the myth of the entitlement "crisis." *The Gerontologist, 36*, 391–399.

Reeher, G. (1996). *Narratives of justice: Legislators' beliefs about distributive fairness.* Ann Arbor, MI: University of Michigan Press.

Rothstein, B. (1998). *Just institutions matter: The moral and political logic of the universal welfare state.* Cambridge, UK: Cambridge University Press.

Schmidt, V. A. (2000). Values and discourse in the politics of adjustment. In F. W. Scharpf & V. A. Schmidt (Eds.), *Welfare and work in the open economy. Vol. 1: From vulnerability to competitiveness* (pp. 229–309). Oxford: Oxford University Press.

Schmidt, V. H. (1995). Soziologische Gerechtigkeitsanalyse als empirische Institutionenanalyse. In H.-P. Müller & B. Wegener (Eds.), *Soziale Ungleichheit und soziale*

*Gerechtigkeit* (pp. 173–194). Opladen: Leske + Budrich.

Schmidt, V. H. (2000). *Bedingte Gerechtigkeit: Soziologische Analysen und philosophische Theorien.* Frankfurt/M: Campus.

Sinn, H.-W., & Uebelmesser, S. (2002). Pensions and the path to gerontocracy in Germany. *European Journal of Political Economy, 19,* 153–158.

Smith, T. W. (2000). *Public support for governmental benefits for the elderly across countries and time.* Retrieved February 7, 2003 from http://www.oecd.org/dataoecd/52/61/2535827.pdf.

Svallfors, S. (1997). Worlds of welfare and attitudes to redistribution: A comparison of eight Western nations. *European Sociological Review, 13,* 283–304.

Svallfors, S. (2004). Class, attitudes and the welfare state: Sweden in comparative perspective. *Social Policy and Administration, 38,* 119–138.

Swift, A., Marshall, G., Burgoyne, C., & Routh, D. (1995). Distributive justice: Does it matter what the people think? In J. R. Kluegel, D. S. Mason, & B. Wegener (Eds.), *Social justice and political change: Public opinion in capitalist and post-communist states* (pp. 15–47). Berlin/New York: Walter de Gruyter.

Thomson, D. (1989). *Selfish generations: The ageing of the welfare state.* Wellington: Allen & Unwin.

United Nations Population Division. (2000). *Replacement migration: Is it a solution to declining and ageing populations?* New York: UN.

Walker, A., & Maltby, T. (1997). *Ageing Europe.* Buckingham: Open University Press.

Williamson, J. B., & Watts-Roy, D. M. (1999). Framing the generational equity debate. In J. B. Williamson, D. M. Watts-Roy, & E. R. Kingson (Eds.), *The generational equity debate* (pp. 3–37). New York: Columbia University Press.

Wohl, R. (1979). *The generation of 1914.* Cambridge, MA: Harvard University Press.

# Author Index

Page numbers in *italics* denote references for citations.

# Subject Index